CRC Handbook of Animal Diversity

Authors

Richard E. Blackwelder

George S. Garoian

Professors
Department of Zoology
Southern Illinois University
Carbondale, Illinois

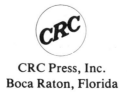

CRC Press, Inc.
Boca Raton, Florida

Library of Congress Cataloging-in-Publication Data

Blackwelder, Richard Eliot, 1909-
    CRC handbook of animal diversity.

    Bibliography: p.
    Includes index.
    1. Zoology--Variation.   I. Garoian, George S.
II.   Title.   III.   Title: Handbook of animal diversity.
QH408.B55   1986   591   85-21291
ISBN 0-8493-2992-2

Direct all inquiries to CRC Press, Inc., 2000 Corporate Blvd., N.W., Boca Raton, Florida, 33431.

International Standard Book Number 0-8493-2992-2

Library of Congress Card Number 85-21291
Printed in the United States

PREFACE

This book is a summary of the diversity between and within the classes of animals. It is intended for reference on all aspects of animals that can be studied comparatively, but such comparison requires that the occurrence of the feature in question be known for more than just one or two groups. It is in large part a book on invertebrate animals because the vertebrates form only a small part of the diversity of animals. This does not mean that vertebrates are excluded from consideration; in most respects they show an insignificant part of animal diversity as a whole, and they are here treated as 8 classes among the more than 100 classes of the Kingdom Animalia (about 5% of the species, but probably not over 1% of the diversity).

The basic purpose of this book is to bring together and display the extreme diversity found in animal structure and function. Because this diversity is present at all levels of structure and in all life cycle stages, the book would, if complete, cover all aspects of the existence of all animals.

Diversity is to us the most obvious feature of animal life, because the unity or uniformity that is said to exist is represented only by generalizations that hide the underlying diversity. All animals consist of protoplasm, but there are endless differences in the protoplasm of different animals. So far as known at present, all animals have genes to pass on their characteristics (although barely one thousandth part have actually been examined in this respect), but the known genetic mechanisms become more and more numerous as the geneticists study more and more animals.

There is a clear duality in the competition between unity and diversity. Louis Agassiz once wrote: "Since the ability of combining facts is a much rarer gift than that of discerning them, many students lost sight of the unity of structural design in the multiplicity of structural detail."

While acknowledging this, we must add that it is also easy to lose sight of the immense diversity of animals in the over-generalization of the extant similarities. As modern writers struggle with the voluminous data on even one aspect of animals, they feel forced to overlook some of the diversity and to simplify their generalizations of the rest. We sympathize with their problem but believe there can be no real justification for overemphasizing the existing unity while neglecting the ubiquitous diversity.

There is no possibility of bringing together all the known diversity; it is much too scattered and would prove to be far too abundant for even a series of volumes. It is thus our purpose to assemble the available knowledge of a variety of aspects of the diversity, especially in reproduction, development, structure and organ function, to classify these features and define the terms, to show the distribution of these features among the phyla and classes of animals, and to point out some of the implications of these distributions.

In preparing this book, the subject matter, as indicated by the part and chapter titles and as represented by the dichotomy of function vs. structure, has undergone frequent change — an actual evolution. Our prime consideration has been to find an arrangement that would permit display of the diversity with the fewest difficulties. For example, among the principal organ systems the reproductive system is usually listed. However, major aspects of animal reproduction have no controlling connection with any system of organs, therefore we deal with all reproduction in a separate section where organs are dealt with alongside the reproductive functions.

We believe that "an organism" is essentially a life history, including everything that the animal is and does during its life. With this approach, the present arrangement requires less cross-reference in the text than others tested. It is hoped that multiple tables of contents and a detailed index will enable the reader to find any subject needed.

To present the diversity in the best possible way would require us to analyze all the situations and activities and adopt definitions for the endless series of terms in use. These analyses and definitions would occupy more space than the diversity tabulations. We have tried to keep them to a minimum, but to justify our conclusions it has been necessary to introduce many definitions and choices between similar terms.

A few details of presentation require explanation. The subject arrangement is shown in detail in the Table of Chapters and in chapter tables of contents. It proceeds from reproduction through development to organ systems and all functions of the body and its parts. Some general aspects of behavior, coloniality, and death complete the sequence, which thus essentially proceeds from initiation of reproduction and origin of a new individual to its final disappearance as a separate living entity.

In lists of phyla and classes in the text, the names are often preceded by the letter s or m, as "s.Protozoa". This shows that some species in that group show the feature, but probably not all species. The m can be read as "many" or "most", again presumably not all species. If neither letter is used, it may be assumed that so far as we know all species show the feature, although it is to be expected that exceptions will occur. It is also likely that in some cases it is to be read merely as "occurs in Annelida".

In citing examples of animals showing a feature, the species is cited by name whenever known. If only the genus is cited, it should be read as "in appropriate individuals of at least one species in the genus". The same formula, of course, applies to citation of a class or phylum; it refers to some unidentified species in that group.

In a few cases where no species can be cited as example, a group below the class level is cited, but these are always placed in the class, thus: Insecta — Protura or Copepoda (Crustacea). Anyone unfamiliar with the classes of animals will find a complete list (as used herein) in Chapter 25.

Coverage: The parts of zoology dealt with in this book are shown in Table 1.

Acknowledgements: It is impossible, in a book that summarizes the entire Kingdom Animalia, to acknowledge the sources of all the information. We have been largely dependent on works of summary, such as those cited as references at the end of Chapter 1. We have occasionally cited as quotations the source of an unusual feature that seems to be strengthened by identification of the person reporting it. The author's name and date will serve to identify the work to most students, and the full citation will be in the references at the end of the chapter.

We acknowledge with thanks the authors of the several hundred books that have supplied the information tabulated here, but in many instances we have interpreted the data in fashion other than that of those authors.

Richard E. Blackwelder
George S. Garoian

Table 1

THE ASPECTS OF ZOOLOGY, ARRANGED AS 6 LEVELS OF INTEGRATION AGAINST 6 APPROACHES, TO SHOW THE SUBJECT COVERAGE OF THIS BOOK

Levels / Subject	Molecule	Cell	Tissue & Organ	Individual	Kind	Community
Nature	Chemistry	Cytology		Morphology	Comparative Zoology Classification	Ecology
Materials & Structure	Biochemistry	Cytology	Histology Organology	Anatomy	Protozoology Entomology Paleontology etc.	Ecology
Reactions	Biochemistry	Cell Physiology	Physiology Endocrinol.		Social Behavior Limnology	Ecology Parasitology
History			Physiology Behavior Parasitism	Reproduction Development Heredity Genetics	Evolution Paleontology Phylogeny	Ecology
Distribution	Biochemistry				Paleontology Zoogeography	Ecology
Interest to Man	Medical Research	Medical Research	Medicine	Public Health	Identification Limnology Bionomics	Conservation

Note: The shaded area includes the principal subjects in which comparative data have been collected.

THE AUTHORS

Richard E. Blackwelder was born in 1909 and received his Ph.D. from Stanford University in 1934. For 20 years he was associated with the Smithsonian Institution, as holder of the W. R. Bacon Travelling Scholarship and as Associate Curator of Insects. In 1956 he went to Southern Illinois University, broadening his interests to include all animals. He taught Zoology, Invertebrates, and Taxonomy, always emphasizing the extent of the diversity of animals. He retired from his Professorship in 1977. He was an officer of the Society of Systematic Zoology for 16 years from its founding and has published over 150 titles, including a dozen books.

Dr. George S. Garoian is a Professor of Zoology at Southern Illinois University at Carbondale. He received a B.A. in Zoology from Washington University in St. Louis (1949) and Ph.D. in Zoology from the University of Illinois, Urbana (1956). He has taught various general and advanced zoology courses at SIU-C since 1956, especially in the invertebrate offerings of the department, with advanced courses in Protozoology, Parasitology, Helminthology and two field courses, Natural History of the Invertebrates and Freshwater Invertebrates. In addition, he has participated in graduate research and teaching in the Department, having graduated 15 with Masters degrees and 5 with the Ph.D. degree.

Besides serving on many university and college committees, Dr. Garoian has been active in nine professional zoological and biological organizations, serving on the Executive Board and as President of the Association of Midwestern College Biology Teachers and as Executive Secretary/Treasurer for the Annual Midwestern Conference of Parasitologists. He has reviewed manuscripts for books and journal articles as well as published in protozoology, general biology, and science teaching. As the result of a National Science Foundation LOCI grant, he has produced a 5-unit cassette/slide self-instruction program on *Animal Diversity.*

TABLE OF CHAPTERS

PART I
Introduction...1
Chapter 1 Introduction to Diversity 3

PART II
The Origin of Individuals..13
Chapter 2 Animal Reproduction and Asexuality 17
Chapter 3 Bisexual Reproduction 45
Chapter 4 Parthenogenesis, Sequence, Sexuality 81

PART III
Development of Individuals..109
Chapter 5 Embryology...111
Chapter 6 Larva to Adult 143
Chapter 7 Life Cycles 159

PART IV
Adult Individuals 181
Chapter 8 Introduction to Structure and Function.....................185
Chapter 9 Morphology...193
Chapter 10 Cells 213
Chapter 11 Tissues 235
Chapter 12 Organs and Organ Systems......................................247
Chapter 13 Digestive System 265
Chapter 14 Circulatory Systems 293
Chapter 15 Respiration..307
Chapter 16 Excretion 327
Chapter 17 Nervous and Endocrine System 341
Chapter 18 Integuments..365
Chapter 19 Unique Organ Systems 385
Chapter 20 Miscellaneous Organ Functions................................397

PART V
Behavior 425
Chapter 21 Activities of Individuals...427
Chapter 22 Interactions of Animals 453

PART VI
Coloniality..483
Chapter 23 Colonies 485

PART VII
End of Existence 495
Chapter 24 Death..497

PART VIII
Classification 501
Chapter 25 Classification of Animals...503

Index..520

Part I
Introduction

"They are concerned with the diversities of the world instead of with its unities."

G. B. Shaw

Chapter 1

INTRODUCTION TO DIVERSITY

TABLE OF CONTENTS

I.   Diversity 4

II.   Problems of Viewpoint 4
      A.   Organismic Viewpoint 5
      B.   Human Orientation 5
      C.   Treatment of Adults Exclusively 6
      D.   Generalization 6

III. The Nature of Organisms 7
      A.   Protozoa as Animals 7
      B.   Cellularity 7
           1.   The Cell as a Unit 8
           2.   Cellularity of Protozoa 8
      C.   Individuality 9
      D.   Individuality vs. Coloniality 11
      E.   Polymorphism 12

General References 12

I. DIVERSITY

In modern biology books the word diversity is little used. It is well known that there are more than a million kinds of animals on earth and that they belong to at least several dozen groups that are often rather distinct from each other. But it is said that they all consist of cells made of similar protoplasm, originating in the same reproductive processes, developing by similar processes of differentiation and growth, and functioning by means of basically similar organs. This book may restore the balance to the word diversity, by its constant repetition, and it will show that the similarities as described above are either unwarranted generalizations or are meaningful only in some restricted sense while being surrounded by the almost endless diversity of animals.

The diversity is actually much greater than can be shown here. First, much diversity is lost to human knowledge through the extinction of types of animals evolved in earlier ages. These would be included if possible, but the only diversity that can be known for any of these groups now is that shown by the hard parts that were fossilized, and these give only indirect clues to bodily functions. There are more of these extinct groups than is usually recognized and together they hold almost all the keys to the course of evolution among animals as a whole. They are included whenever the available information warrants.

Second, biochemical diversity is limited by the nature of molecules and chemical bonds. The bonds are much more diverse than they were once thought to be. The molecules of living matter are limited by the apparently universal use of carbon in their basic structure and of water as the universal fundamental constituent of tissues and source of hydrogen and oxygen. The boiling and freezing points of water come close to setting limits to the existence of life, and actually do so for animals.

Third, there is a subtlety in the interaction of chemicals, genes, and internal and external environments that cannot be treated by comparative methods. The details of diversity seem endless, but the real extent of diversity in the mechanisms is either unknown or inexpressible.

Fourth, the interactions of animal organs, especially the nervous and endocrine system, are so complex in producing what is called animal behavior that the diversity is difficult to tabulate. Only a few aspects, such as parasitism, can be extensively dealt with here.

It is thus seen that *diversity is ubiquitous and greatly overshadows such unity (better called similarity) as does exist.* This diversity has largely been known for many decades, but it is so abundant and all pervasive, and often so deeply hidden in the literature of science, that general books give a seriously inadequate account of it. One could say that much of the diversity is forgotten by recent generations. It is hoped that these pages will restore the balance by tabulating the diversity that has been assembled and by providing a framework into which others can fit the no-doubt-large number of instances of which the authors are ignorant.

II. PROBLEMS OF VIEWPOINT

The reasons for the inadequate treatment of diversity in all textbooks are partly historical and partly curricular. These center around the fact that zoology courses often are forced to serve other goals than to make known the animal kingdom. They particularly serve the interests of men and women in medicine, nursing, public health, agriculture, and other "practical" fields. For these purposes, the interest is in *Homo sapiens,* but stand-ins are usually used in such activities.

These and other problems of viewpoint are dealt with under the following four headings.

A. Organismic Viewpoint

As biochemical knowledge and laboratory capabilities have increased in recent years, there has been a tendency to assume that only this "modern" experimental approach is fruitful in biology. It certainly has been fruitful, but it is a mistake to think that it is even now the only useful or the only interesting pursuit in biology. In this modern approach, it seems to be believed that time is better spent on the finer details revealed by new techniques and instruments. A student of invertebrates countered the argument thus: "The organismal viewpoint . . . maintains that biology should study entire living organisms, not merely the physics and chemistry of their isolated parts."

A person who examines the literature on the structure and physiology of animals in general will see at once that, although much is known, it is so widely scattered that it is unavailable to nonspecialists and so has never been treated comprehensively or comparatively. In this absence of ready knowledge of the comparative features of animals in general there has been a strong tendency to assume that in the "basic aspects" animals are all much alike. It is the authors' purpose to show the inadequacies of this assumption by displaying part of the existing diversity.

B. Human Orientation

Most of physiology and embryology, and much of the other branches of zoology, have been dominated by the study of the one species *Homo sapiens*. This was inevitable because of the immediate benefits to mankind, especially in regard to human health, and because man was the most interesting organism to many early workers. When other animals were studied, it was to compare with humans, again primarily for the increase of knowledge about the human organism.

By the time other animals came to be studied seriously, a large and detailed science of the biology of mankind had accumulated and, to record this, an extensive terminology. These terms were then applied to the lower animals, whether or not they were really appropriate. For instance, one may say that a jellyfish has eyes, even though there is little similarity between those simple light-sensitive organs and mammal eyes. One can speak of tracheae in both humans and insects, although there is no structural or developmental similarity and only a very general functional similarity.

The alternative would have been to have duplicate terms in vertebrates and invertebrates, and probably also between higher and lower invertebrates, which no doubt would have seemed a frightening prospect to zoology students of those days. Because this was usually not done, confusion has resulted, and gradually many different new terms had to be adopted for the fundamentally different situations that occur in the endless diversity in the animal kingdom.

Must one then conclude that this human-oriented terminology is unfortunate? In part yes, because, for example, it is unfortunate for any student to think that because "respiration", the sequence of biochemical reactions in the protoplasm, is basically the same in all animals, it follows that all animals "breathe". In the sense that this term is used in humans, insects might be said to breathe, with their very different tracheal breathing system, but a truly aquatic or parasitic animal certainly does not breathe. Thus, one must interpret such an expression each time from knowledge of the animal involved, because of recognition of the great differences that actually occur. However, generalizing is difficult; it is true that all animals require "food" and energy from the outside, but it is not true that all animals "feed" or "eat" in the vertebrate sense.

In studying any animal group outside of the vertebrates, and sometimes even among them, it is necessary to be alert to prevent being misled by a term that seems to say that this feature is similar to the one by that name in humans. Instead of trying to avoid such terms in this book, we try by tabulating the diversity to show that the general terms must be used with care and understanding. Where the structural differences are very great, it is probably better to use a different term, if one is available. For example, the kidneys in mollusks and humans are both excreting nitrogenous waste products, but they are not at all similar in structure, location, or embryonic origin. They are both "kidneys" only if that word is defined as equivalent to "excretory organ".

Thus, a major feature of this book is the attempt to bring terminologies into agreement with the true facts of structure and function in the diverse groups of animals. New terms are very seldom suggested, but distinctions between existing "synonyms" and careful definitions of terms are frequently used to make it possible to display the existing diversity.

C. Treatment of Adults Exclusively

There is a basic illogicality in nearly all treatments of animals, whether the subject is structure, function, or behavior, in that there is a tacit (and usually unrecognized) assumption that adult animals are alone involved. There is no way to justify this position, as the life of an individual extends from the moment it is isolated as an individual (zygote or fragment) until its death (or division).

Everything that occurs during the entire life is part of that animal. To cite only what occurs in the adult is utterly inadequate in a study of any organism, as we will try to make clear at many points in this book. We will cite structures, functions, and behaviors irrespective of the stage of the life history, which means citing these features in all stages in which they are known. Of course the subject of development itself covers all stages, and it could be treated as a time frame for discussing all the other features.

Inasmuch as animals are always in a state of change, even when they appear to be stable for a period, it is possible to define "an animal" as a life history. In speaking about one stage, one is in reality stopping the sequence, like stopping a movie projector on a single frame. The animal never stops in this continuous sequence of stages, although it appears to proceed now at a slower rate and now at a faster one. However, some so-called life cycles cover the lives of two or more individuals; in studying individuals it is necessary to watch out for interruption of the cycle by some hidden reproduction that brings an end to the individual long before the life cycle of the species is completed.

D. Generalization

Throughout this book there are references to or quotations of statements made in other books that seem to be inadequate for some reason. The most common reason is that the statement is a generalization that inadequately reflects the extent of the diversity of animals. Generalizing is not automatically bad, but in scientific writings it is dangerous; the pitfalls are many. For example, a physiologist recently wrote:

"I have deliberately restricted myself to such parts of the subject as are susceptible to broad generalization; but the broader the generalization the more exceptions it has to admit of. In disregarding such exceptions I realize that I have laid myself open to the charge of over-simplification . . . but the omissions have been deliberate. I cannot see much point in stating a generalization only to smother it with qualifications."

This is a very interesting comment, because the writer provides all the arguments necessary to refute his own contention. A generalization that *could* be smothered with exceptions is not worth stating. Where real exceptions occur, the generalization should acknowledge them as part of the facts being generalized. We agree that there is not much point in making such an unqualified generalization — in fact it is usually much better not to mislead the reader by making any statement that is just not true.

In this book also there are doubtless some generalizations. If these have known or even suspected exceptions, we have attempted to make that fact part of the generalization. Throughout this book an effort is made to emphasize exceptions, give examples rather than final, complete lists, and leave them all open to other interpretations, further expansion, and more detailed analysis. This, therefore, allows for addition of further exceptions not included in our lists and for the discoveries of the future.

III. THE NATURE OF ORGANISMS

Organisms exist in at least four levels of organization: single cells (including protozoans and zygotes of metazoans), colonies of single cells, multicellular individuals, and colonies of multicellular individuals. Most of these clearly consist of cells; in all four there is individuality of some sort, and all four of them may consist, within a single species, of several different kinds of individuals. These features all enter into the problem of the diversity of animals, greatly complicating it. The principal factors in this are discussed here. (Coloniality, polymorphism, and life cycles are discussed more extensively in other parts of this book.)

A. Protozoa as Animals

A user of this book will soon become aware that the diversity to be reported is greatly increased by the inclusion among animals of the large and diverse group of the Protozoa. These microscopic organisms are elsewhere often treated separately from animals, sometimes merely for convenience, but often because they are believed to be more closely allied to unicellular plants than to multicellular animals. All attempts to separate organisms into two or more clear-cut groups fail unless the ones usually called Protozoa are split up. Nevertheless, protozoans as a group show more similarity to animals than to plants, and nearly all zoological textbooks and treatises treat them as (or at least with) animals.

In spite of the relatively very small size of protozoans as compared to most metazoans, they show astonishing diversity. They may be photosynthetic, predaceous, or parasitic. They may reproduce sexually or only asexually, or both. They show more diversity in gametes than all metazoans together. They may be solitary or colonial, or even syncytial (as plasmodia). In most respects they are not sharply distinct from Metazoa, and we believe that it would falsify the nature of animals as well as the nature of protozoans to omit them from such distributional analyses as compose this book.

B. Cellularity

It is often stated (1) that all organisms consist of cells, (2) that Protozoa are not cellular, and (3) that cells are the fundamental units of life. None of these statements is quite correct, for Protozoa do show all the important features of metazoan cells in general, there are Protozoa (plasmodia) of some size without separate cells, and there are many parts in metazoan animals in which the cells are not separated by detectable membranes. Most normal cells do have nuclei and a surrounding membrane, and the fundamental unit of animals (and protozoans) would seem to be an *energid,* a tiny mass of protoplasm under the direction of a nucleus. Membranes are usual between cells; when they are absent the multinucleated mass is called a syncytium. The syncytium thus consists of energids, and no harm is done by referring to these as cells. These polyenergid masses, the syncytium and the plasmodium, are distinct in that the syncytium is part of an otherwise multicellular organism but the plasmodium is an independent amoeboid organism.

When such cells occur in masses in the organism, they form a syncytial tissue. Examples are

1. Epidermis (Coelenterata, Ctenophora, Temnocephaloidea, Acanthocephala, Rotifera, Gastrotricha, Kinorhyncha, Nematoda)

2. Parenchyma or mesenchyme (Turbellaria, Cestoda, Rhynchocoela)
3. Muscles (Acanthocephala, Vertebrata)
4. Coelomic peritoneum (Phoronida)
5. Calcigenous skeletal cells (Echinodermata)
6. Most body tissues (Rotifera, parasitic Copepoda, Acoela)
7. "Gut" epithelium (Hirudinea)
8. Retinal cells (Vertebrata)
9. Epithelium of rectal gills (Insecta)
10. Part of ovaries (Insecta)
11. Entire early embryos (Acanthocephala, Insecta)
12. Gemmules (s.Porifera)

1. The Cell as a Unit

Nearly every textbook of biology or zoology cites the cell as "the unit" of structure, function, development, and heredity. Justification or explanation for this statement is never given, and it is doubtful if it conveys any direct meaning to the reader.

Structure exists at numerous levels, from protoplasm to populations. In only one of the ten or so levels are cells the actual units or building blocks: they are the units of tissues or simple organs. Cells are not the units of structure of molecules, which are atoms or radicals; or of complex individuals, which are tissues or organs; or of colonies, which are individuals; or of populations, which are individuals or demes.

The unit of function in animals in general is the organ or organ system. The unit of behavior is the individual (or in some cases the colony or population). The unit of development is also the individual. The unit of heredity is the gene.

The cell is truly the unit of structure and behavior in individual protozoans. It is the unit of some functions, whereas for others the organelle is the unit.

This concept of the cell as the unit has been carried to ridiculous extremes. Besides the four items cited above (structure, function, development, and heredity), cells have been called the units of life, physiology, growth, reproduction, evolution, and irritability. Some of these can be meaningful in particular circumstances, but as generalizations they tell us nothing.

The diversity of cells is the subject of Chapter 10.

2. Cellularity of Protozoa

Great specialization of study on one group of organisms sometimes leads to viewpoints or theories that cannot be justified when one is considering all groups of organisms together. Although it is a universal generalization that all organisms are cellular, there is no longer agreement that protozoans are unicellular and metazoans multicellular. There is no rejection of the multicellularity of metazoans, though many of them start life as a single cell, but some protozoologists have recently argued that Protozoa are neither unicellular nor cellular; they prefer the terms acellular or noncellular.

The argument is that these organisms are whole individuals and are not merely divided into cells. It appears that some of the students feel that it is belittling to students of Protozoa to call their animals unicellular when they perform many of the basic functions of multicellular animals. To some zoologists (of Metazoa) this seems no more than quibbling, because both Protozoa and Metazoa may consist of single nucleated masses of protoplasm (energids) and both may consist of groups of such protoplasmic masses.

In this book the position is taken that although the individuality and completeness of protozoans must be recognized, we cannot refuse to recognize the structure of each as being one complete cell (or a colony of such cells). The words that are used to describe the singularity of one and the multiplicity of the other seem poor matters for dispute, but it will be noted that "unicellular" and "multicellular" are generally used in this book.

C. Individuality

In discussing many aspects of animals, it is necessary to refer to individuals. Individuality is familiar enough in vertebrates, but many difficulties arise when the vista is opened to include all animals.

First, every individual passes through some processes of development. If a grown man is an individual, was he also one as a child? As an unborn foetus? As a zygote?

Second, in colonial animals, does the bud become an individual only on detachment? Do colonies of attached zooecia consist of individuals? When a hydra produces a lateral bud, when does this bud become an individual?

Third, when a starfish tears itself in two, and each piece regenerates into a whole starfish, are there two new individuals, or one, or none?

Fourth, does it make a difference whether the new individual forms from original tissues or from newly formed tissues? The original tissues and organs may produce the two new individuals by fission, with little further growth, or single new cells from several tissues may assemble into the new fragment. Do both of these produce new individuals?

Fifth, is every living fragment a new individual when isolated? Are isolated gametes individuals because they are isolated and alive? How about the detached proglottids of tapeworms? Is a spermatophore an individual?

Sixth, does loss of normal structure followed by reformation produce a new individual or the same one? When a tardigrade dedifferentiates in a cyst to a formless mass and then grows and redifferentiates into an adult again, is it the same individual?

Such questions can be asked almost ad infinitum. They seem to raise difficult questions that would force one to make a complex definition of what is an individual. This would be necessary if one required a completely objective definition that left no doubts in any theoretical case, but there is no real need for such finality here. The factors that need to be covered in such a definition are these: (1) when, in development, a new individual comes into existence; (2) to what extent two individuals must be separate; (3) the extent of detachment of fragments; (4) the difficulty of distinguishing developmental processes from those that are reproductive.

A satisfactory definition should be made on the basis of the following choices:

1. A new individual arises (a) at the moment of fertilization, (b) at the moment of activation, in parthenogenesis, and (c) when the first inherent function begins in a part that will be isolated or autonomous.
2. They must be separated physically or functionally and perform at least some functions independently.
3. Detached fragments are new individuals only when they start some of the functions normal to that species *and* if they are fragments capable of complete regeneration.
4. The nature of processes can sometimes be distinguished only by their results. If they produce new individuals, they are reproductive, but they are usually at the same time developmental processes.

An individual is an organized mass of protoplasm in the form of (or capable of developing by itself into the form of) the usual members of that species and capable of performing the appropriate integrated activities necessary to its continued existence. The moment at which individuality is achieved varies from the instant of separation (in binary fission) to the instant of fertilization (in karyogamic species), and to the as-

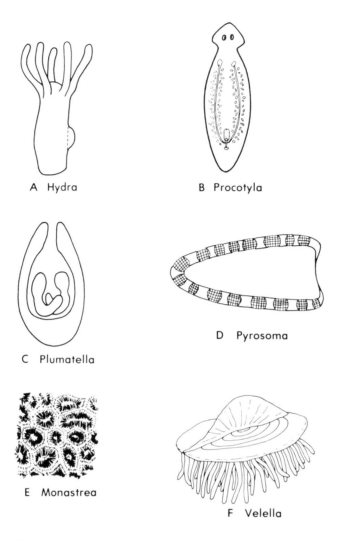

FIGURE 1.   Some forms of individuality in lower animals. A, Solitary polyp of coelenterate; B, hermaphroditic flatworm; C, dual embryo of a bryozoan; D, compound structure of a tunicate; E, encrusting colony of anthozoan; F, individualistic colony of siphonophore. (From Blackwelder, R. E. and Shepherd, B. A., *The Diversity of Animal Reproduction,* CRC Press, Boca Raton, Fla., 1981.)

sumption of the first inherent function (in a bud). The moment cannot be known in the case of parthenogenetic development of an ovum. In the case of twinning, the individual produced at the moment of fertilization will not be the same as the two or more individuals present after the next occurrence, its division into several. There are species in which embryos form inside unborn embryos, and tertiary embryos inside these. These are all individuals, because they are organized bodies in the normal form for that stage of that species (Figure 1).

Plasmodia, which are masses of protoplasm with nuclei but no cell separations, will be indeterminate as to individuality except for that of the mass itself. Similarly, the Porifera may be looked upon as colonies or as individuals. Many sorts of colonies have individuality, as in the protozoan *Volvox* and the coelenterate *Physalia,* and there seems to be no sharp division between reproduction by an individual and reproduction by a colony.

Even in the face of these situations no serious difficulty is found in treating as individuals all of the following:

1. Every fertilized zygote and the single animal which develops from it
2. Every unfertilized ovum which is activated rather than fertilized and is capable of development, and the single animal which develops from it
3. Every agamete capable of development and the single animal which develops from it
4. Every new cell formed by fission (binary or multiple) of a unicellular individual, whether or not separation is complete
5. Every new multicellular body formed by fragmentation, fission, or autotomy if capable of normal independent existence
6. Every new body formed by proliferation of new tissue at one place (budding or strobilation), if capable of normal existence whether separately or remaining attached
7. Every new body formed by cooperation of cells from various tissues, if capable of initiating normal independent existence (gemmules, statoblasts)
8. Individuals formed by division of a zygote or embryo to form several embryos capable of normal independent existence (twinning and polyembryony)

Living objects which would not be considered to be individuals would include spermatophores, ova which never develop, spermatozoa under any circumstance, tapeworm proglottids, autotomized appendages that do not themselves regenerate, and a reduction body which is merely the regressed body of one individual. It seems appropriate to sidestep the question of individuality or coloniality of sponges and plasmodia, as these are out of the range of either concept.

There are, however, real problems in the application of the concept of individuality to all animals. One normally thinks of male and female as separate individuals, but the sexes may be directly combined in a single individual (an hermaphrodite), which is a sort of dual individual.

Other sex combinations occur. A gynandromorph is an "individual" in which half of the body (one side) is male, in some features at least, and the other side is female. These can arise either through fusion of two fertilized eggs (each with sex genetically determined) or through loss of a sex chromosome in one blastomere at an early cleavage.

Even more rarely there are individuals with blends of the features of males and females. These are called intersexes.

D. Individuality vs. Coloniality

Levels of organization have so far been dealt with as if they were discrete, and as if their functions could be cited in similar discrete levels. These would be substantial misconceptions. Individual cells may be complete individuals or merely a small part of a multicellular individual. They may even be deprived of their cell limits and become blurred into a plasmodium or a syncytium. The multicellular individual very likely started life as a single cell, a zygote, and it may eventually lose its individuality in the formation of a colony. Some colonies start life by budding from one individual, either uni- or multicellular, but others start life as the individual does, by proliferation from a zygote.

Thus, all these levels become indistinct. Each merges with the others at some point, and it is not uncommon for there to be uncertainty at a given point as to which level is being observed.

Even if there is satisfaction with the definition of individual, one finds that individuals may be part of a larger mass, which is called a colony. This colony may be of nebulous size and shape, or it may have a fixed size and shape with all related colonies the same. In the former (indefinite shape) the individuals are usually distinct, and in general each performs all or most of the functions. In the latter (fixed shape) the individuals are less distinct and usually are clearly specialized in function.

Again the colony may be of even more definite size and shape, and the individuals may be highly specialized in function and in form. These colonies may have great individuality; they may function very much as an individual would, with its member individuals serving as organs.

Individuality can thus exist at the level of a cell, of a multicellular unit (the usual meaning of "individual"), or of a colony. There are even a few instances of behavior as an individual at the still higher organizational level of the population. The word individual thus serves at many levels, but this should produce little confusion.

In this book, colonies are treated in one of the last chapters, as they are in general a level of organization above the individual, which is the subject of most of the chapters. One must remember that this additional level of organization adds further to the already overwhelming diversity to be examined at the levels of cell, organ, and individual (or life history).

E. Polymorphism

Two other but related diversities of individuals must be recognized. First, in many species, in all parts of the animal kingdom, there are individuals of more than one form. This is polymorphism. Second, the sequence of forms that occur in a species is part of the life cycle of that species; as these sequences are themselves diverse, they add another level of diversity to life forms.

The diversities of polymorphism may be related to development, function, sex, environment, or to other factors that may not have been identified. They are discussed in Chapter 9, "Morphology".

The diversities of life history are closely involved with reproduction; they are discussed under "The Levels of Diversity" in Chapter 4, and under "Polymorphism" in Chapter 9.

GENERAL REFERENCES

Barnes, R. D., *Invertebrate Zoology*, 1st ed. (1963), 2nd ed. (1968), 3rd ed. (1974), W. B. Saunders, Philadelphia.

Beklemishev, W. N., *Principles of Comparative Anatomy of Invertebrates*, Vol. 1 and 2, University of Chicago Press, Chicago, 1969.

Encyclopaedia Britannica, 11th ed., Vol. 1 to 29 (same as 12th ed. 1921-1922), Encyclopaedia Britannica, New York, 1910-1911.

Florkin, M. and Scheer, B. T., Eds., *Chemical Zoology*, Vol. 1 to 3, Academic Press, New York, 1962-1969.

Gray, P., *The Encyclopedia of the Biological Sciences*, Reinhold, New York, 1967.

Gray, P., *The Dictionary of the Biological Sciences*, Reinhold, New York, 1967.

Hoar, W. S., *General and Comparative Physiology*, Prentice-Hall, Englewood Cliffs, N.J., 1966.

Hyman, L. H., *The Invertebrates*, Vol. 1 to 6, McGraw-Hill, New York, 1940-1967.

Kaestner, A., *Invertebrate Zoology*, Vol. 1 to 3, John Wiley & Sons, New York, 1967-1970.

Pennak, R. W., *Collegiate Dictionary of Zoology*, Ronald Press, New York, 1964.

Prosser, C. L., Ed., *Comparative Animal Physiology*, 1st ed. (1950) and 3rd ed. (1973), W. B. Saunders, Philadelphia.

Rogers, C. G., *Textbook of Comparative Physiology*, McGraw-Hill, New York, 1938.

Stern, C., *Principles of Human Genetics*, 3rd ed., W. H. Freeman, San Francisco, 1973.

Stern, C., Biology, in *An Orientation of Science*, Watkeys, C. W., Ed., McGraw-Hill, New York, 1938, chap. 7.

Wilson, J. A., *Principles of Animal Physiology*, Macmillan, New York, 1972.

Part II
The Origin of Individuals

DIVERSITY IN REPRODUCTION

A recent major biology textbook lists four major aspects of organic reproduction:

1.   It is basically a cellular process
2.   It nearly always involves sex
3.   It is production of like by like
4.   It is followed by an elaborate development

These are vertebrate-oriented ideas. In the animal kingdom as a whole they are scarcely half-truths:

1.   Cells are not directly involved in most asexual reproduction, which is very common
2.   Sex is involved only in sexual reproduction, which is widespread but frequently lacking
3.   Much reproduction does not produce likes but rather unlikes that may lead later on to like
4.   Many individuals reproduce and then disappear before there is any development (polyembryony); many others appear first as adults (division of an adult) and need to develop very little

The diversity of reproduction cannot be visualized by looking only at mammals, or by believing that functional sex is universal, or by believing that animals all develop in much the same way as vertebrates.

Chapter 2

ANIMAL REPRODUCTION AND ASEXUALITY

TABLE OF CONTENTS

I. Introduction..18
   A. Definitions..18
   B. Misconceptions..19
      1. Universality 19
      2. Simplicity of Reproduction...22
      3. Only Adults Reproduce 23
      4. Reproduction in Only One Body Form 23
      5. Reproduction Distinct from Development...............................23
      6. Bisexuality is All-Important..26
         a. Two Sexes, One, or None...26
         b. Bisexual Reproduction...27
         c. Sexual Reproduction...27
         d. Asexual Reproduction..27
         e. Gametes...27
         f. Conjugation..27
   C. Parameters 27
      1. Factors of Reproductive Diversity 28
      2. All New Individuals from Fragments 29
      3. One Process or Many 30
      4. Axioms Basic to this Discussion..30

II. Apomixis...31

III. Asexual Reproduction 32
   A. Definitions..32
   B. Clones 33
   C. Processes..34
      1. Agamogony and Sporogony...34
      2. Gemmulation 35
      3. Budding 36
      4. Fragmentation 38
         a. Fission 38
         b. Division 39
         c. Strobilation...41
         d. Epitoky..42
   D. Organs for Asexual Processes...43

References 44

I. INTRODUCTION

A. Definitions

The diversity of reproduction has been the subject of a monograph (Blackwelder and Shepherd, 1981) that treats the processes in detail, discusses the terms that have been used and the problems they introduce, and gives in detail the reproduction in each animal class and the distribution of the processes among the classes. Part of the material for the present chapter is adapted from that work. For the reasons behind the choices of terms herein, reference should be made to that monograph.

Principle of replacement: Because no animals are immortal, there must be continual replacement of lost individuals in each species to prevent its extinction. This replacement is by reproduction in any of its many forms.

The word reproduction has been used in many senses, for the replication of molecules in protoplasm, the duplication of structures in a cell, the multiplication of unicellular animals, the reproduction of multicellular animals, and the duplication of colonies. More appropriate terms than "reproduction" are available for some of these. The term is here restricted to the origin of new individuals from pre-existing ones, whether unicellular, multicellular, or an entire colony.

Reproduction in animals is extremely varied. It is difficult to do justice to this diversity in one section of a book. A complicated terminology often obscures similarities, but on the other hand loose usage of terms has confused some aspects. It is necessary to introduce definitions and a system to the terms before the occurrence of the individual processes can be presented.

Reproduction has been described as "the maintenance of a species from generation to generation", "the origination of new organisms from pre-existing ones", or "the capacity of living systems to give rise to new systems identical with themselves".

These quoted definitions are intentionally general. Their authors were trying to put the essence of a very diverse complex of processes, structures, and activities into simple language. None of these is wrong, but they are individually or all together inadequate to define, circumscribe, or explain reproduction. They gloss over the fact that there are problems in knowing what individuals are, what a generation is, what is and what is not "giving rise to new" ones.

These definitions do not give us any clue as to whether reproduction is the same in all animals. Although sexual reproduction is sometimes assumed to be universal and of prime importance, the very term implies that there are other forms of reproduction which are nonsexual, collectively known as asexual. Even when this distinction is made, it is usually forgotten that all reproduction involves fragmentation of some sort. The nature of the fragment is highly diverse, and sometimes two fragments fuse to form a new individual and sometimes not.

This puts a rather unusual slant on the customary distinction between sexual and asexual, because not all "sexual" processes involve fusion of two fragments (e.g., parthenogenesis) and there is fusion in some asexual processes (as in tunicate dual budding and in turbellarian composite eggs).

There is no clear way to isolate reproduction from other activities. Inasmuch as this book is concerned with diversity in all structures and processes, it is not necessary to make such a distinction. Some arbitrary decisions will therefore be made as to where a given process is to be discussed, or treatment of it will be placed in several parts of the book with reference to different aspects.

One of the difficulties is that some of the terms represent processes that can either be reproductive or not. Fusion of two individuals (in Protozoa) may produce one individual and thus actually decrease the total number in existence. Fragmentation may produce two or more pieces, of which only one can regenerate and live; this leaves the number of individuals unchanged. Division of tissue cells occurs universally in Metazoa without making new individuals. These are the processes called para-reproduction (meaning that they are "nearly" reproductive). They include conjugation and hologamy. They are some of the things that require us to make a more specific definition of the word reproduction.

Reproduction is multiplication of individuals, producing more members of the species but usually not immediate duplicates of the reproducing individual: the new individual will either grow into a duplicate (except for individual variation) or will itself produce either individuals that are near-duplicates or individuals that will produce such near-duplicates.

To understand this definition one must recall from the previous chapter the definition of the word individual: an organized entity capable of performing the appropriate integrated activities necessary to its continued existence. Under this definition a new individual is usually formed at the instant of activation of an ovum, or at the moment of functional separation of a fragment or bud. It can be seen from this that the new individual may be a zygote, a bud, or a piece that can regenerate to become like its parent. Thus, the new individual is usually not immediately a duplicate of its parent(s); it is a stage in the cycle of that species that will eventually produce such duplicates.

The processes of reproduction are so diverse that it is necessary to use a four-part grouping to distinguish their true natures. These four are Asexual Reproduction, Sexual Reproduction, Meiotic Parthenogenesis, and Ameiotic Parthenogenesis. They will be discussed in that order.

B. Misconceptions

There are several common misconceptions about reproduction; they seem to arise most frequently from a vertebrate orientation and a desire to keep things simple. Six of these misconceptions are discussed here.

1. Universality

Sexual reproduction is often thought of as universal. This is because some sexual process does occur in some form in most groups of animals. There are, however, many species of animals, in several groups, in which no sexual processes have ever been found. It is a further difficulty that there has been no way to say for sure what is sexual and what is not. Sexuality is a condition that may exist independently of any actual reproduction, and much so-called sexual reproduction does not clearly involve sexuality at all.

Many individuals take no part in bisexual reproduction, and it is entirely absent in widely scattered species (i.e., some Sarcodina, some Hydrozoa, some Rhynchocoela, some Polychaeta, and some Oligochaeta). It is entirely absent from all species in the Chrysomonadina (Protozoa), the Bdelloidea (Rotifera), and the Chaetonotoidea (Gastrotricha).

Even counting all kinds of reproduction, any individual may fail to reproduce or may even be incapable of reproduction; in fact there are thousands of species in which most individuals never reproduce in any way. Thus, at the individual level, reproduction is neither universal nor a necessity. It is at the level of species that it becomes essential. If biologists are right in believing that a given species can evolve only once, then it follows that no species can continue to exist without replacement of lost individuals.

In a recent biological encyclopedia, one contributor wrote: "Among the metazoa, asexual reproduction is significant only in the sponges, the simpler coelenterates such as hydra, and the flatworms and nemerteans." Such a gross misunderstanding of the extent and diversity of nonbisexual reproduction is unfortunate and highly misleading to any reader (see Table 2).

Table 2
OCCURRENCE OF ASEXUAL PROCESSES

	Budding	Architomy	Paratomy	Polyembryony	Strobilation	Gemmulation	Others
Protozoa	X	X	X	0	X	0	0
Porifera	X	0	X	0	0	X	Gemmules, sorites
Mesozoa	0	X	X	0	0	X	Pseudo-eggs, agamogony
Monoblastozoa	0	X	0	0	0	0	0
Coelenterata	X	X	X	X	X	X	Podocysts, sorites, pedal laceration, frustulation
Ctenophora	0	X	0	0	0	0	Pedal laceration
Gnathostomuloidea	0	X	0	0	0	0	0
Platyhelminthes	X	X	X	X°	X	X	Frustulation
Rhynchocoela	0	X	0	0	0	0	0
Acanthocephala	0	0	0	0	0	0	0
Rotifera	0	0	0	0	0	0	0
Gastrotricha	0	0	0	0	0	0	0
Kinorhyncha	0	0	0	0	0	0	0
Nematoda	0	0	0	0	0	0	0
Gordioidea	0	0	0	0	0	0	0
Priapuloidea	0	0	0	0	0	0	0
Calyssozoa	X	0	X	0	0	0	0
Bryozoa	X	X	X	X	X	X	Statoblasts, hibernacula
Phoronida	0	0	X	0	0	0	0
Brachiopoda	0	0	0	0	0	0	0
Mollusca	0	0	0	X	0	0	0
Sipunculoidea	0	0	0	0	0	0	0
Echiuroidea	0	0	0	0	0	0	0
Myzostomida	0	0	0	0	0	0	0
Annelida	X	X	X	X	X	0	Strobilation, epitoky
Dinophiloidea	0	0	0	0	0	0	0
Tardigrada	0	0	0	0	0	0	0
Pentastomoidea	0	0	0	0	0	0	0
Onychophora	0	0	0	0	0	0	0
Arthropoda	X	0	X	X	0	0	Stolonization

Chaetognatha	0	0	0	0	0	0	0
Pogonophora	0	0	0	0	0	0	0
Echinodermata	X	X	X	X	0	0	0
Enteropneusta	0	X	0	0	0	0	Stolonization
Pterobranchia	X	0	X	0	0	0	Strobilation
Tunicata	X	X	X	0	X	X	0
Cephalochordata	0	0	0	0	0	0	0
Vertebrata	0	0	0	X	0	0	0

a   Successional polyembryony.

2. Simplicity of Reproduction

Unity and diversity of animal structure and process are discussed throughout this book. When one comes to reproduction, the problems caused by this dual viewpoint are troublesome. There is temptation to simplify or generalize, partly because the diversity is so great.

Implications of bisexual reproduction in various aspects of biology (genetics, evolution, behavior) are so great and of such importance, that some biologists feel that any other form of reproduction is secondary or less fundamental or less worthy of study, and so they generalize that only sexual reproduction is important. In these fields, however, it is not sexuality itself that is important but outbreeding, the mixing of genetic materials from two unrelated individuals. Few biologists have taken note of Sonneborn's (1957) estimate that probably half of all animal individuals were the direct result of non-outbreeding reproductive processes. This large number cannot reasonably be labeled as exceptional.

The word reproduction is often used as if it were a single process, acting in a single organ system. In reality, it is always a complex of processes, often extending throughout the life of the individual. In general, it covers all the processes which lead to production of new individuals; in reproducing individuals this is substantially equivalent to its entire life, because there is little in that life that does not contribute to reproduction. Specifically, reproduction is the origination of new organisms from pre-existing ones. In fission it is direct and immediate, but bisexual reproduction involves operation of gonads and many associated organs. This results in two sets of gametogenesis, delivery of the spermatozoa to the ova, and fusion of the two.

When the term sexual reproduction is used to cover all reproduction by animals that produce gametes, there are a variety of unnoticed processes whose implications are omitted. These include several kinds of parthenogenesis, self-fertilization, pseudogamy or plasmogony, and autogamy. These are said to be sporadic in occurrence, but in some species in most groups of animals at least one of these reproductive processes is obligate. The species with no known true bisexual reproduction are more numerous than usually recognized. They occur in nearly all phyla of animals but are frequently overlooked.

Asexual reproduction can be very simple and direct. A bud grows or a fragmentation suddenly produces several individuals. Whether or not one can think of sexual reproduction as simple, it does involve a great many separate processes and often the entire life of the individual. When it is realized that reproduction in a species very often involved two or three distinct reproductive sequences (as described in a later section), then that reproduction can scarcely be thought of as simple. In many species of animals, reproductive processes are not only several and complex, but because of alternative pathways the reproduction can only be thought of as diverse.

There are a variety of reproductive methods. They range from simple binary fission to the quasi-sexual processes of parthenogenesis; the latter have evolved from the ordinary bisexual reproduction familiar in higher vertebrates. Although no simple scheme will cover all the diversity that occurs in reproductive processes, it appears that the various methods represent five basic ways in which new animal individuals arise:

1. Unicellular reproductive bodies
   a. Gametes
   b. Agametes (spores)
2. Division of the unicellular body into two or more substantial parts: fission of the cells
3. Multicellular individual, division of the body into two
   a. Fragmentation
   b. Polyembryony

4. Proliferation of tissue at one place
   a. Budding
   b. Strobilation
5. Multicellular reproductive bodies: gemmulation

These involve many subordinate processes, some of which are listed and described in later sections.

Most animals have only one choice of how they feed and digest, but many animals have a choice of the methods they can use to reproduce (see diagrams in Chapter 7).

3. Only Adults Reproduce

A third misconception is that reproduction is always performed by adults, adulthood being defined as sexual or reproductive maturity; however, any of a score of reproductive processes can occur in the larval stage, and most nonsexual processes can occur also in the embryo or even in the zygote. For example, reproduction by fragmentation can occur at the first stage of cleavage, where the two cells separate to start two new individuals. Budding can occur in an early embryo, immediately forming the individuals of a future colony. Several asexual processes may occur in a larval stage. When reproduction is defined most simply as the act of a living system giving rise to new living systems, it will be seen that this can occur at any stage in the life cycle (see Tables 3 and 4).

4. Reproduction in Only One Body Form

Whereas animals of all species exist as young and old, and many species exist as male and female, many species of coelenterates, bryozoans, annelids, social insects, etc., exist in several body forms. These forms may be very different, as seen in Figure 2. Here again, when reproduction is defined as the act of a living system giving rise to new systems identical with itself, it must not be forgotten that the "system" is an entire life cycle. It happens frequently that reproduction will produce offspring very different from the parent, because other reproductive processes intervene before an individual similar to the original parent appears. For example, in a colonial animal such as *Obelia,* the hydranth polyp can bud other hydranths like itself or it may bud a gonangium polyp which must bud medusae which must produce gametes to be fertilized before the sequence can produce a hydranth again.

It is also necessary to remember that even the simple reproductive processes do not *immediately* result in duplicates. They produce a fragment, bud, or zygote which is a new individual but must grow to maturity before it is a duplicate.

5. Reproduction Distinct from Development

In dealing with reproductive processes in any group of animals, it is essential to distinguish the reproductive processes from the developmental. Animals that reproduce bisexually have a series of processes whose sole or principal purpose is to lead to another generation of new individuals. The reproductive processes can be clearly distinguished from the later processes of development, by which the new individual (from the zygote stage) grows into an adult.

Roughly half of all animals reproduce in part by some asexual or at least nonbisexual process. In these, reproduction and development are not so clearly distinguished. For example, in the normal life cycle of the hydrozoan *Obelia,* a polyp will bud off tiny medusae which swim free of the parent. Each will then mature into a distinct individual. The budding is reproductive, but it is also part of the development of the new individual.

In many insects, an ovum is fertilized and begins to develop; this is bisexual repro-

Table 3
SOME OF THE DEVELOPMENTAL STAGES AT WHICH REPRODUCTIVE PROCESSES MAY OCCUR, WHICH THEN BECOME TERMINAL FOR THAT INDIVIDUAL

Stage	1st reproductive process	Last stage in development	2nd reproductive process	Stage produced	Example
1. Zygote	Bisex. repro.	Adult	Fragmentation	New adults	*Lineus,* Rhynchocoela
2. Zygote	Bisex. repro.	Larva	"Budding"	New larvae	Cestoda
3. Zygote	Bisex. repro.	Late embryo	Multiple bud	New embryos	Gymnolaemata
4. Zygote	Bisex. repro.	Early embryo	Polyembryony	New embryos	Parasitic Hymenoptera
5. Zygote	Bisex. repro.	Scyphistoma	Strobilation	Ephyrae	*Aurelia,* Scyphozoa
6. Zygote	Bisex. repro.	Larva	Strobilation	New larvae	Polyclinidae, Ascidiacea
7. Zygote	Bisex. repro.	Adult	Parthenogen.	Activated egg	Cladocera, Crustacea
8. "Zygote"	Hologamy	"Zygote"	Fission	"Young"	Lobosa, Sarcodina
9. "Zygote"	Sporogony	Oocyst	Mult. fission	Sporozoites	Myxosporidia, Sporozoa
10. "Zygotes"	Fission	"Zygote"	Autogamy	Changed adult	*Actinophrys,* Sarcodina
11. Activ. egg	Parthenogen.	Early embryo	Polyembryony	New embryos	Poss. in gall wasps, Insecta
12. Activ. egg	Parthenogen.	Larva	Fragmentation	New larvae	Poss. in Oligochaeta
13. Embryo	Mult. budding	Adult	Bisex. repro.	New zygote	Gymnolaemata
14. Embryo	Polyembryony	Adult	Fragmentation	New adults	Poss. in Oligochaeta
15. Larva	Budding	Larva	Bisex. repro.	Zygote	Cestoda
16. Larva	Fragmentation	Larva	Parthenogen.	Activated egg	Poss. in Oligochaeta
17. Larva	Strobilation	Larva	Bisex. repro.	Zygote	Polyclinidae, Ascidiacea
18. Adult	Fragmentation	Adult	Fragmentation	New adults	*Zeppelina,* Polychaeta
19. "Adult"	Fission	"Adult"	Conjugation	Exconjugants	*Paramecium,* Ciliata
20. "Adult"	Fission	"Adult"	Fission	New adults	Protozoa
21. Bud	Budding	Adult	Fragmentation	New adults	Hydrozoa
22. Bud	Budding	Adult	Frustulation	New larva	Hydrozoa
23. Bud	Budding	Bud	Fragmentation	New buds	*Distaplia,* Ascidiacea
24. Epitoke	Epitoky	Epitoke	Bisex. repro.	Zygotes	Polychaeta
25. Swarmers	Mult. fission	"Adults"	Bisex. repro.	Zygotes	Dinoflagellates, Flagellata

Notes: Read, for example, line 1 thus: a *zygote* produced by *bisexual reproduction* lives to the *adult* stage where *fragmentation* ends its existence and produces new *adults,* as in some Rhynchocoela. Again in line 5, a *zygote* develops to the *scyphistoma* stage where *strobilation* ends its existence and produces *ephyrae,* as in some Scyphozoa.

From Blackwelder, R. E. and Shepherd, B. A., *The Diversity of Animal Reproduction,* CRC Press, Boca Raton, Fla., 1981.

duction. Then the developing mass of cells come apart and each cell starts over and eventually forms a new individual. At least 1000 individuals may come from that 1 fertilized egg. This means that the sexual process that did occur is immediately masked by an asexual process, and the only sexually produced "individual" is the zygote. All the final individuals are the result of an asexual process called polyembryony. Although this latter process seems to be a feature in the development of any given offspring, it is in reality the beginning of many new life cycles.

In another case, in some Trematoda, an embryo develops from a zygote. Early in the larval development, some embryos are found inside the larva, and perhaps other embryos inside each of those. Exactly how they arise is unknown. They are sometimes implied to be successive generations, but it seems more likely that they are delayed fragments of the original embryo. This has been called successional polyembryony.

It is apparently because processes of this sort are often unrecognized or forgotten

Table 4

LIFE HISTORY STAGE AT WHICH REPRODUCTION OCCURS
IN SELECTED SPECIES

Starting stage	Initiating process	Next reproducing stage
Plasmodium vivax (Protozoa)		
Gametocytes (gametes)	Fertilization	Ookinete
Ookinete	Sporogony	Trophozoites
Schizont	Schizogony	Trophozoites or gametes
Obelia sp. (Hydrozoa)		
Medusa (gametes)	Fertilization	Hydranth
Hydranth	Budding	Hydranth
Hydranth	Budding	Gonangium
Gonangium	Budding	Medusa
Lineus sp. (Rhynchocoela)		
Adults (gametes)	Fertilization	Adult
Adult	Fragmentation	Adults
Asplanchna sp. (Rotifera)		
Adults (mictic ova + sperm)	Fertilization	Adult
Adult (mictic ova)	Activation	Adult
Adult (amictic ova)	Parthenogenesis	Adult
Bugula sp. (Bryozoa)		
Autozooid	Budding	(Avicularia, etc.)
Zooids (gametes)	Fertilization	Ancestrula
Ancestrula	Budding	Autozooid
Autozooid	Budding	Autozooid
Aphis sp. (Insecta: Homoptera)		
Adults (gametes)	Fertilization	Adult
Adult (ovum)	Activation	Adult
Ageniaspis fuscicollis (Insecta: Hymenoptera)		
Adults (gametes)	Fertilization	Adult (possible)
Adults (gametes)	Fertilization	Embryo
Embryo	Polyembryony	Adults
Dasypus novemcinctus (Mammalia)		
Adults (gametes)	Fertilization	Adult (possible)
Adults (gametes)	Fertilization	Zygote
Zygote	Polyembryony	Adults

that some writers can say that "asexual reproduction is not found in the Arthropoda . . . (it) is always sexual." In reality, parthenogenesis is fairly common, polyembryony occurs in several groups, and even budding occurs.

It is also stated that asexual processes are significant only in lower animals. While it is true that asexual processes are more common in some of the lower groups, especially the Coelenterata, they do not occur at all in others, such as the Gastrotricha, and they do occur in every large phylum, including the Vertebrata. There they probably occur in all classes, and certainly occur among mammals and even in humans (identical twinning is polyembryony).

Numerous problems of this sort arise, resulting in difficulty of defining "reproductive" and "developmental". There is no direct solution to the problem. It will suffice here to point out two things: (1) that reproductive processes include all those, and only those, that lead directly to additional individuals (either the original and one or more new ones, or only the two or more new ones); (2) that in developmental sequences there may occur processes which lead to new individuals, such as polyembryony or larval budding, and these are thus reproductive as well as developmental.

It must be recognized that reproduction always occurs during the course of development. It often occurs in the adult stage, but it may occur at any stage in develop-

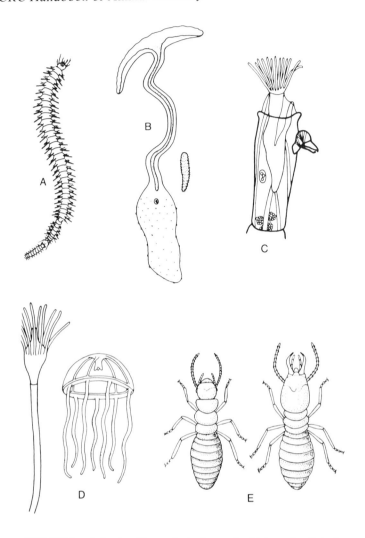

FIGURE 2.   Animals with two body forms. A, Atoke and epitoke in a polychaete; B, male and female of echiuroid; C, normal zooid and avicularium in a bryozoan; D, polyp and medusa in a hydrozoan; E, castes of termites.

ment, even in the zygote. It thus always occurs among developmental processes. The two sorts of processes can be distinguished only by their immediate results.

6. Bisexuality is All-Important

Another misconception appears when one finds in some book a great deal about sexual reproduction and its genetic consequences with only a brief reference to the existence of asexual reproduction. Here are some of the difficulties arising from this implication that sexual reproduction is dominant.

a. Two Sexes, One, or None

It seems easy to make a distinction among reproductive processes between those that are sexual and those that are asexual. Sexual reproduction is usually assumed to involve two sexes (bisexual) but there are many problems. There are several processes involving only one sex (unisexual and sometimes called asexual). Some other processes are not really sexual but still involve gamete-like bodies. Thus, the sexual/asexual division really does not work at all.

b. Bisexual Reproduction

This is supposed to involve production of spermatozoa and ova and their union to form a new diploid individual. The difficulties are (a) that this definition groups cross-fertilization between male and female individuals with self-fertilization of her-maphrodites; (b) that there are species that do not produce true gametes; (c) that the gametes may not be of two kinds (male and female) but rather be all alike (isogametes); (d) that the two gametes may not unite, or if they do, their nuclei may not fuse; and (e) that the new individual may be either haploid or diploid at the start.

c. Sexual Reproduction

This can be defined as any that utilizes gametes, or the definition can be based on the occurrence of meiosis, the process that reduces the number of chromosomes to the haploid number. Neither definition avoids all difficulties, but either may be used under some circumstances. It can also be defined as reproduction involving amphimixis, the mixing of chromosomes from two gametes. There are difficulties here also, as the gametes may come from the same individual (self-fertilization), members of a clone, or closely related individuals, such as siblings. In these, the reproduction will produce less genetic diversity than would be expected when "sexual reproduction" is specified, because this term generally presumes that there is cross-breeding (between unrelated individuals).

d. Asexual Reproduction

What is often dismissed as the exceptional asexual reproduction by budding and fragmentation turns out to be a score or more of quite distinct processes that do not involve sex. These processes are not at all exceptional, because they occur not only in some species in nearly every group of animals, but as the *only* reproductive method in certain groups and in occasional species in many other groups.

e. Gametes

Gametes can be either haploid or diploid, and they are sometimes indistinguishable from agametes (spores). These facts make gametes seem unsatisfactory as a defining feature of sexual reproduction. The alternative is the use of meiosis, the reduction of chromosome numbers, but this does not occur in *all* ova, and it can occur in processes that are not really reproductive, such as conjugation. Neither basis for definition is entirely satisfactory.

f. Conjugation

This is often cited as sexual and even as reproductive. In it the sexual process of meiosis does occur, and the two individuals fuse temporarily and are each changed in their genetic make-up by exchange of pronuclei. Because there is no increase in the number of individuals, there is no reproduction.

C. Parameters

In summary, to be sexual the reproduction must involve meiosis and to be bisexual it must involve the fusion of gametes (karyogamy); to be outbreeding the gametes must come from unrelated genomes. For reproduction to be asexual, there must be no gametes, no fusion, and no meiosis.

It is possible to combine these criteria into a definition, but there are no well-known terms for the resulting groups of processes. Sexual reproduction must utilize gametes

Table 5

OCCURRENCE OF REPRODUCTIVE PROCESSES

	Fission & division	Gemmulation	Agamogony	Gonochorism	Hermaphroditism	Parthenogenesis
Protozoa	X		X	X	X	X
Porifera	X	X		X	X	X
Mesozoa	X		X	X	X	?
Coelenterata	X			X	X	
Ctenophora	X				X	
Platyhelminthes	X			X	X	X
Rhynchocoela	X			X	X	?
Acanthocephala				X		?
Rotifera				X		X
Gastrotricha				X	X	?
Kinorhyncha				X		
Nematoda				X	X	X
Gordioidea				X		
Priapuloidea				X		
Calyssozoa	X			X	X	
Bryozoa	X	X		X	X	X
Phoronida	X			?	?	
Brachiopoda				X	X	?
Mollusca	X			X	X	X
Sipunculoidea				X	?	?
Echiuroidea				X		X
Myzostomida					X	
Annelida	X			X	X	X
Dinophiloidea				X		
Tardigrada				X		X
Pentastomoidea				X		
Onychophora				X		
Arthropoda	X			X	X	X
Chaetognatha					X	
Pogonophora					X	?
Echinodermata	X			X	X	X
Pterobranchia	X			X	X	?
Enteropneusta	X			X		
Tunicata	X			X	X	?
Cephalochordata				X	X	
Vertebrata	X			X	X	X

that have undergone meiosis and which will fuse in pairs. Meiotic parthenogenesis utilizes gametes that have undergone meiosis but do not require karyogamy (fusing of the male and female pronuclei). Ameiotic parthenogenesis utilizes gametes that have not undergone meiosis and do not require karyogamy. Asexual reproduction includes all that do not involve either gametes or meiosis.

The above definitions represent the scheme adopted in this book. However, it is not sufficient to use the term "sexual" in this restricted sense when it is so commonly used in a broader and generally much looser sense. To avoid this difficulty, we will use for the restricted sense of "sexual reproduction" the expression Basic Bisexual Reproduction (BBR), which is defined on the basis of unrelated gametes with meiosis and karyogamy (see Table 5).

1. Factors of Reproductive Diversity

Reproduction is extremely diverse among animals because of several factors:

1. There are more than two score of processes that may be employed
2. Most of these can occur at any stage in the life of the animal
3. Within a species there may be as many as four different reproductive pathways employed by different individuals
4. Some individuals exist from fertilization through adulthood to death, but others may cease to exist at much earlier stages because they undergo a type of reproduction that converts them into new individuals
5. Many individuals do not begin as a zygote but may start life as an apozygote, a multicelled embryo fragment, a bud, or a fragment of an adult
6. Sexual processes are not restricted to what is usually called sexual reproduction
7. In addition to individuals that can be recognized, there are composite structures consisting of parts of many individuals; there are pairs of individuals that exchange genomes; there are fused individuals that never separate; there are living masses formed by fusion of many individuals; there are colonies in which most individuals have disappeared in the production of the highly organized colony (an individual); any of these can reproduce themselves

2. All New Individuals from Fragments

The idea that reproduction is essentially a single process (sexual) was previously cited as a misconception. The methods were listed by which individuals may be formed. Another way to look at the formation of new individuals is to recognize that in reproduction they all arise from fragments separated from the parent or parents. These fragments may be cells, assembled bodies, half of the original individual, a portion broken off, or a bud; they may be referred to as reproductive bodies:

1. Gametes — haploid cells including all spermatozoa, most ova (sometimes improperly called spores)
2. Gametes — diploid cells (some parthenogenetic ova)
3. Agametes — diploid cells (most spores)
4. Blastomeres — from a cleaving zygote (polyembryony)
5. Multicellular bodies — such as gemmules (assembled bodies), where the cells come from various tissues
6. Body fragments — (by fission or division) either with advance preparation or duplication of organs (paratomy) or simple fragmentation followed by regeneration (architomy)
7. Buds — that develop into new individuals, either remaining attached or breaking away
8. Buds — that must fuse in pairs (pyloric buds)

As shown in (1) and (2) above, although gametes are usually assumed to be haploid, ova may be of two types genetically; they may be haploid or diploid, but this difference is usually not directly evident. Where there is to be karyogamy, the nucleus must be haploid. This fusion is loosely called amphimixis but most proceed through karyogamy to produce a new cell with a single nucleus which has a double chromosome complement. Where the ova are to develop parthenogenetically, there are three possibilities. First, many species produce diploid ova, simply omitting the reduction divisions; this is ameiosis, which is essentially asexual. Second, ova that are haploid but do not fuse in pairs may develop parthenogenetically; in this case the activated egg usually undergoes some process to double the chromosome number to restore diploidy. Third, in a few cases of haploid species there is diploidy only in the zygote, which then undergoes meiosis; thus the adult is haploid and produces haploid "gametes" without further meiosis. In both cases of haploid gametes, there has been meiosis, but the first is meiotic parthenogenesis and the second is bisexual.

Unfortunately for simple definitions and for the usual generalizations, there are a few animals in which the new individual is produced by the fusion of cells derived from more than two gametes. How the diploid chromosome number is achieved here does not seem to be known.

Multicellular reproductive bodies are occasionally formed in number by migration of cells from several tissues to form a body resistant to otherwise lethal environmental conditions. (These are not the same as reduction bodies, as that word is used in Tardigrada, formed one per individual, which later redifferentiates into a functioning individual again.) Different terms have been given in each group where they occur: gemmules, sorites, podocysts, statoblasts, resting buds, and hibernacula.

This view of reproduction by fragments throws a somewhat different light on the customary distinction between sexual and asexual. Some gametes do not require fertilization; some fragments called agametes and some buds, which are not supposed to fuse, actually do so. A large number of animals are produced by processes involving multicellular fragments, but this is not generally looked at from the viewpoint of these fragments.

It must be remembered that some fragments are merely broken-off pieces that never form new individuals, whereas others are formed bodies of definite size and shape. The latter are herein called *reproductive bodies*. These include: (1) gametes, which will fuse and are always haploid but may take several forms: anisogametes (spermatozoa and ova) and isogametes (which are indistinguishable from each other); (2) pseudova, which are diploid; (3) agametes or spores, which are diploid bodies that develop without fusion; and (4) gemmules, which are multicellular bodies made up of a variety of cells and usually liberated only at the death of the parent.

3. One Process or Many

The word ''process'' is extremely useful to describe the various methods by which animals accomplish each of their activities. It is at once seen, however, that the processes are at many levels, often with one process consisting of several others at a lower level. Thus, reproduction can be called the process which produces new individuals, but we know that reproduction can involve the process of fertilization, which itself can involve the process of gamogony, which itself involves the process of meiosis, which itself involves the process of fission, and so on. Thus, the word does not inform the reader of the level at which it is being used.

4. Axioms Basic to this Discussion

The diversity of reproduction tabulated in this study has forced a series of decisions and definitions that must be understood if the reader is to follow the conclusions. The following are nine axioms basic to the interpretation adopted:

1. New individuals may arise by: (a) reproduction, in which additional individuals are produced; (b) para-reproduction, in which one or two individuals are genetically changed without an increase in the number of individuals as in conjugation, thus producing new (i.e., changed) individuals.
2. Reproduction occurs only in an individual or from parts of two individuals.
3. Every reproduction produces a new individual. This can be by successive acts of reproduction by one individual or one pair, in each case of which a new individual is produced; or it can be by a succession of different processes, each of which produces a new individual, whether or not the original parent survives. There is thus only one reproductive process in the immediate background of each individual. These include: (a) the one that is produced by each bisexual process; (b) the one that is produced by each unisexual process; (c) the two that are produced by

binary fission or some form of fragmentation; (d) the many produced by multiple fission or fragmentation; or (e) the one produced by gemmulation.

An individual exists from the moment of fertilization (or activation) of an ovum or from the start of independent activity in a fragment or a bud.

In several asexual processes the parent ceases to exist, no matter how brief the time involved since its formation.

An individual may survive past a reproductive episode, but if its genome is changed it achieves a new individuality. Likewise if all its nuclear material is passed to new individuals (as in multiple fission) it ceases to exist.

There are species in which there occur a succession of reproductive processes, often alternating sexual and asexual, but no individual passes through two reproductive phases except in the sense of repeated episodes of the same process.

There are very many species in which there exist more than one pathway of reproduction; some individuals use one pathway (processes) and others another.

Although reproduction is not a necessity for any particular individual, and may not even be possible for it, some individuals in every species must reproduce, if the species is not to become extinct.

II. APOMIXIS

These three chapters on reproduction cover a great variety of processes. Some involve the mixing of genetic materials (usually called sexual, but should be called bisexual), some clearly involving no mixing (asexual), and some intermediate (parthenogenetic) in that they are usually implied to be one or the other but actually are inadequately distinguished on this feature. The latter (in parthenogenesis) also consists of two types clearly distinguishable genetically. To these must be added the processes here called para-reproductive (elsewhere called parasexual), which have features of sexuality but do not produce additional individuals.

A considerable terminology has grown up around these distinctions. Some of the terms are discussed in appropriate parts of these chapters, but ones such as apomixis find no place therein and so are dealt with here.

When there is mixing of chromosomes from two individuals by means of gametes and fertilization, the process is called *mixis* or *amphimixis* (Chapter 3). When there is no such mixing the process is labeled *apomixis* — the absence of mixis. It might seem that there would be no gametes in apomixis, but there may be gametes that do not fuse, resulting in apozygotes. Apomixis is all the means of reproduction that do not involve mixis (the mixing of different sets of chromosomes from two individuals). The terms relating to apomixis include these:

1. Amphimixis — union of gamete pronuclei to form a zygote with a fusion nucleus
2. Apozygote — a zygote that is formed without amphimixis
3. Automixis — includes autogamy and cytogamy, but only the latter is apomictic
4. Cytogamy — automixis which is essentially incomplete conjugation in which the exchange of pronuclei is inhibited and each "conjugant" undergoes autogamy
5. Endomixis — form of nuclear reorganization usually described as involving replacement of the original macronucleus with a new one formed by division of the micronucleus
6. Hemimixis (hemixis) — fragmentation or reorganization of the macronucleus without accompanying changes in the micronucleus or the cell as a whole
7. Mixis — the mixing of genetic material from two gametes; essentially the same as fertilization (karyogamy)
8. Nuclear reorganization — changes in the macronucleus at the time of cell division

Unfortunately, the distinction between apomixis and amphimixis is confused by the existence of clonal fertilization, fraternal fertilization, and other degrees of relationship between the two parents. These are not apomictic but are forms of inbreeding.

The term *agamic* has been used to describe reproduction from an unfertilized ovum (parthenogenesis); the word actually means "without gametes", which is both apomictic and asexual.

One additional apomictic term has been used. *Somatic fertilization* occurs when "spermatozoa enter somatic cells in the female reproductive tract and exert an influence on them" (Rothschild, 1956a). This is obviously not a reproductive process.

Thus, apomixis includes all asexual reproduction and all parthenogenesis, here treated in separate chapters. It thus occurs very widely in the animal kingdom, but it is completely lacking in the following groups, which are thus exclusively sexual in their reproduction: Temnocephaloidea, Cestodaria, Acanthocephala, Rotifera, Priapuloidea, Gordioidea, Echiuroidea, Myzostomida, Pentastomoidea, Onychophora, Merostomata, Pycnogonida, Diplopoda, Chilopoda, Crinoidea, Planctosphaeroidea, and Chondrichthyes.

III. ASEXUAL REPRODUCTION

A. Definitions

Asexual reproduction is any production of additional individuals without gametes. It is roughly equivalent to the expression vegetative reproduction, but includes more than a score of distinct processes that produce individuals without relation to sex. This includes all reproductive processes not involving sex (either two sexes or one). They may occur in animals which have sex, or in life cycles which include sexual reproduction, but they are independent of the sex or the existence of a second individual. The processes do not readily fall into groups, but they can be roughly categorized as fragmentation of the body (in the broad sense), budding, use of multicellular reproductive bodies, and use of spores or agametes. Some of these include several rather distinct methods.

One of the results of bisexual reproduction is the production of genetic diversity among the offspring of the pair of parents. This diversity is the result principally of meiosis and fertilization: (1) meiosis with its potential for random assortment and crossing-over that can diversify the gamete genomes, and (2) fertilization which mixes the genomes of the two gametes. Both of these sources of diversity are lacking in asexual reproduction, as there is no mixing (no fertilization) and no meiosis. The cells of the offspring arise mitotically from cells of the parent, automatically having the same genomes as the parent cells. Thus, all the asexual offspring of one individual have identical genotypes (barring mutations). These asexually produced and genetically identical offspring of a given animal are a clone.

A *clone* is a group of asexual offspring from one parent, all of which have the same genotype as that parent. Clones may vary in size from two individuals, as in identical twinning, to several thousands, as in some parasitic insects (Hymenoptera) (see also next section).

If asexual reproduction must produce clones, then one can see why parthenogenesis, as usually described, cannot be called asexual. In these cases there are gametes (at least ova) and the ova are produced by meiosis; therefore the offspring will be genetically diverse — they will not form a clone. As will be seen, there are many instances of parthenogenesis in which meiosis does not occur. The offspring thus are a clone, and the process is essentially asexual, even though the parent is obviously a female and the reproduction is initiated in an ovary.

Other terms that are essentially synonymous with asexual reproduction are *agamo-*

genesis (which might be mistaken for agamogony, reproduction by agametes), *hypo-genesis, monogony,* and *monogenesis.* None of these are well enough known to force adoption.

In a variety of animal species there is no reproduction except asexual. They include:

1. Flagellata — many species, such as *Trypanosoma*
2. Sarcodina — many amoebae
3. Turbellaria — said to be several species, including *Dugesia gonocephala*
4. Phylactolaemata — said to occur in some, where the sexual processes have degenerated
5. Polychaeta — at least in species of *Ctenodrilus* and of *Zeppelina*
6. Oligochaeta — in *Cognettia sphagnetorum* and some species of *Lumbriculus*

A much longer list emerges of those animals that have no form of asexual reproduction at all. First, there are nine phyla in which there is no known apomixis in any species. These are Kinorhyncha, Gordioidea, Priapuloidea, Echiuroidea, Myzostomida, Pentastomida, Onychophora, Chaetognatha, and Cephalochordata. These have neither asexual reproduction nor parthenogenesis and thus reproduce only bisexually.

In addition, there are ten phyla in which parthenogenesis does or may occur but no asexual reproduction is reported. These are Acanthocephala, Rotifera, Gastrotricha, Nematoda, Brachiopoda, Mollusca, Sipunculoidea, Tardigrada, Dinophiloidea, and Pogonophora.

This brings to 19 the phyla in which there is no directly asexual reproduction, but it must be added that polyembryony is believed to occur in the Mollusca and others, though apparently not directly reported. In addition to these, none is known in the class Hirudinea or Larvacea, or in the simple Ascidiacea.

B. Clones

When the offspring of a single individual all have identical genotypes, the group of the offspring are said to be a clone. It is thought at times that this statement so worded is redundant because such offspring would always have identical genotypes. There are complications, however.

In *Gray's Dictionary of the Biological Sciences* (1967) a clone is defined as "a group of organisms descended asexually from a single ancestor". This is the standard botanical usage, but it is also used by many zoologists. In *Pennak's Collegiate Dictionary of Zoology* (1964) a clone is defined as "All descendants derived from a single individual by asexual reproduction *or parthenogenesis;* members of a particular clone have the same genetic constitution" (italics added).

First, it can be noted that asexual offspring will have genotypes at first identical but later perhaps differing because of mutations; if these are in the germplasm, the next generation would be slightly different. This minute source of error can be neglected here.

Second, in the case of parthenogenesis, although the principal source of sibling diversity (mixis) is missing, the secondary source (meiosis and its crossing-over) may still be present (meiotic parthenogenesis; see Chapter 4). The diversity produced by this process may not be negligible.

Both of these situations must be recognized, but to use the same word for the group of siblings in both of them would seriously compromise the term. We therefore think it necessary to restrict the term clone to the asexual offspring (as in botany and many zoological books) and to use a new word for the pathenogenetic siblings. We have found the word *paraclonal* in our notes but cannot now tell whether it was our invention or came from some other work. From it would derive *paraclone.*

It must be pointed out that use of two terms will increase the explicitness of clone but does not completely solve the problem. Clones would be asexual, having identical genotypes; paraclones would be meiotically parthenogenetic, having the diversity of the mother's gene pool plus that of any crossing-over during meiosis. What then of those produced by ameiotic parthenogenesis? They would be intermediate, having the diversity of the mother's gene pool but none from crossing-over. Because the gene pool diversity is the greater, we class the two types of parthenogenesis together for this purpose, even though as a reproductive process we class ameiotic parthenogenesis as asexual (see Chapter 4).

C. Processes

The four basic types of asexual reproduction are (1) production of unicellular reproductive bodies (agametes and spores), (2) production of multicellular reproductive bodies such as gemmules, (3) budding, and (4) fission or fragmentation. Both budding and fragmentation, although usually described in adults, can occur as early as the embryo. Agametes can be produced either by adults or by other agametes. The several sorts of gemmules (see list below) have little in common in structure or tissue source.

Agamete and spore terms from various sources, include the following:

1. Amoeboid swarmers — produced by multiple fission (Sarcodina)
2. Ciliospores — produced by multiple fission (Ciliata: *Ichthyophthirius)*
3. Flagellated swarmers — produced by multiple fission (Flagellata)
4. Merozoites — produced by multiple fission of a sporont (merogony or schizogony) (Sporozoa)
5. Sporozoites — produced by multiple fission of a zygote (sporogony) (Sporozoa)
6. Spores — produced by multiple fission (Sporozoa: Myxosporidia)
7. Agametes — produced by fission of axial cells (Dicyemida)
8. Agametes — produced by fission of agametes (Dicyemida)
9. Axoblasts — in nematogen (Dicyemida)
10. Pseudo-eggs — from surface of infusorigen (Dicyemida)
11. Agametes — from a plasmodium (Orthonectida)
12. Ciliated swarmers — possibly produced by multiple fission (Monoblastozoa)
13. "Gymnospores" — from encysted gregarines (Sporozoa) (these are not spores but true gametes)

1. Agamogony and Sporogony

It is not entirely clear how many different things are represented by the terms spore and agamete (see list above). In various books it appears that certain protozoans reproduce by means of spores, whereas in other books certain protozoans and metazoans are said to produce agametes. It is sometimes claimed that agametes can be either diploid or haploid, with the latter requiring fusion (fertilization). In the latter case they could not be distinguished from isogametes, as both are produced by multiple fission.

It is clear also that spores are not all alike. Some spores are indistinguishable from agametes, being diploid and produced by multiple fission. Other spores start out with several nuclei and arise in groups as a pansporoblast.

From this emerges a picture of only two major types of diploid reproductive bodies. The first type are best called *agametes.* They are produced by multiple fission from either a zygote (sporogony) or a schizont (schizogony) (Telosporidia) or the internal cells or previous agametes of Mesozoa. (The latter is the only known case of multiplication of a reproductive body to form more of the same.)

The second type occur only in Myxosporidia and Microsporidia, where the term *spore* is still applied. The spore is never a simple nucleated cell but forms from a pansporoblast containing two or more multinucleate "spore cells" that will develop into mature spores that become infective to new hosts. Autogamy in the spore stage is usually the only form of sexuality. These spores are rather different from either spores in plants or agametes in either Telosporidia or Mesozoa.

Another term is employed in Protozoa for the process that produces nucleated "fragments" that eventually become gametes capable of sexual reproduction. This is *gamogony (gametogony)*.

A reproduction labeled "sporogony" has been described in the hydrozoan genus *Cunina*, in which only medusae occur. Undifferentiated sex cells (presumably still diploid) in either the male or the female develop into larvae by an unusual sequence. Each cell divides into two, with one becoming enveloped by the other. The outer cell is called a phorocyte, which nourishes the inner cell, which has been called a spore. The latter develops into a larva. There seems to be no way to distinguish this process from ameiotic parthenogenesis.

2. Gemmulation

In reproduction, gemmulation is the formation of a new individual by the enclosing of an accumulation of a variety of cells within a resistant capsule.

These *assembled bodies* are multicellular; they are occasionally formed in numbers by migration of cells from several tissues to form a body resistant to otherwise lethal conditions. They are so diverse that it seems necessary to retain the names given in each group, as follows:

1. Gemmules (Porifera)
2. Sorites (Porifera)
3. Podocysts (Scyphozoa)
4. Statoblasts (freshwater Bryozoa)
5. Hibernacula (Gymnolaemata)
6. Resting buds (Ascidiacea)

Gemmules are internal aggregations of several types of cells surrounded by a resistant covering. They may be released in large numbers from certain freshwater sponges. In marine sponges they then develop into larvae, and in freshwater sponges directly into adults. *Sorites* are aggregations similar to gemmules but without the protective covering. They develop into sponges, though the manner of liberation is not clear. *Statoblasts* in Bryozoa are masses of cells surrounded by chitinous protective bivalved shells; they are produced on the funiculus and consist of epidermal (ectodermal) and peritoneal (mesodermal) cells. *Resting buds* in Ascidiacea will develop only after a long interval; they seem to be formed from several tissues. In sponges, the so-called *reduction bodies* are groups of amoebocytes surrounded by epidermal cells in a degenerating individual that can develop into new sponges. It is not clear whether they are distinct from sorites. (Reduction bodies in bryozoans are more properly called statoblasts.) The unquestionable reduction bodies in Tardigrada are not productions but merely the regressed body of one individual. They are not reproductive, because they can only redevelop into the same individual again.

The above are all internally formed structures. There are also two types formed at the surface. *Podocysts* are chitinous cysts containing epidermal and mesenchyme cells in the pedal disk of certain scyphistoma larvae. They break away and develop into ciliated larvae. They appear to be multicellular reproductive bodies rather than fragments. *Hibernacula* are specially modified winter buds, multicellular reproductive bodies, in some Bryozoa. Each consists of a mass of undifferentiated cells surrounded by a thick sclerotized covering, which will later redifferentiate into a new individual.

3. Budding

Strictly speaking, budding is a form of fission or division in which the two fragments are of very unequal size. It is thus a form of paratomy, with advance preparation for the separation (growth of the bud itself). It is also a part of schizogenesis and scissiparity, both of which refer to reproduction by splitting.

Budding is formation of a new individual as an outgrowth from an existing individual. It has also been called *protogenesis.*

The new individual (the bud) grows from the surface, external or internal in either Protozoa or Metazoa, by proliferation of tissues at that spot. The terms exogenous and endogenous are also used, although the latter is rare. How there can be budding inside a protozoan which has no internal surface is illustrated in the small group Suctoria, where budding occurs in several unusual forms. Here the budding is the means for producing motile "swarmers", and it may be either exogenous or endogenous. The swarmers differ from the parent not only in size but in possession of cilia for swimming or creeping and also other organelles, and they undergo a metamorphosis into the stalked form.

In *Ephelota gemmipara,* the budding is exogenous and multiple, often producing four swarmers at once. Cilia develop for creeping but at metamorphosis are replaced by tentacles. In *Acineta,* only one swarmer is produced at a time, and this is endogenous. This is accomplished by unequal fission of the nucleus and the surrounding of it by an internal brood pouch that is connected to the outside by a pore; the pouch becomes the swarmer.

In the parasitic *Tachyblaston ephelotensis,* endogenous budding of the free-living but sessile stage produces several dactylozoites. These have no cilia but do have one tentacle. They penetrate the host (an individual of another suctorian, *Ephelota*), where they grow and produce the ciliated swarmers in rapid succession. The swarmers escape and then attach, usually to the stalk of another *Ephelota,* and metamorphose into the free-living stage. Thus, there is a real alternation of generations, as well as endogenous budding.

An example of endogenous budding in Metazoa will also illustrate a form of budding that involves fusion of two buds. In some Ascidiacea, two buds form internally, one from the oesophagus (endodermal and mesodermal tissues) and the other from the epicardial tubes (ectodermal tissues). The two fuse before liberation. This is called *pyloric* or *dual budding,* and in reality it is even more complex than described here because the epicardial bud is itself formed by the fusion of outgrowths from each of the tubes.

Organs in the bud do not always arise from the same tissues as in normal development. Buds may produce more of the same stage (adult from adult or embryo from embryo) or some other stage (in Suctoria, ciliated larvae from tentaculate, amoeboid, or biflagellate adult; in *Obelia,* medusa bud from gonangium polyps). The bud is at first dependent upon the parent, but it gradually assumes its normal functions. It may remain physically and physiologically connected, or it may break away to become completely independent. There is diversity in position, developmental timing, the form of the new individual, and the subsequent history of the bud.

Buds grow at specific sites in each species. These may be on the stalk (as in *Hydra*), on a tentacle (as in Anthozoa), on the mantle (as in Ascidiacea), from solenia (gastrodermal tubes between members of a colony) (as in Anthozoa), from a stolon (as in Bryozoa), from bladders (as in tapeworm larvae), from the radial canals of a medusa (as in Scyphozoa), or from various parts of a protozoan.

In some Tunicata, buds migrate over the surface to take up new positions on a special distant part of the body. The buds may divide into two or even more during this migration.

Budding is not limited to the adult stage. It may occur in any life stage, from the early embryo (as in most Bryozoa), to the larva (actinula of some Hydrozoa), and to the adult (as in *Hydra*). In the scyphozoan *Haliclystus,* "the planula is attached to a substratum by its anterior end, while at the posterior, free end of the planula, four planula-like larvae form by budding and later mature into adult organisms" and "in *Cassiopeia* the lower part of the scyphistoma gives rise by budding to a flagellated body which then develops into a planula" (Vorontsova and Liosner, 1960). Budding is also cited in some cases of polyembryony.

In many tunicates budding commences in the larval stage and continues in the adult stage. It produces colonies, compound "individuals", or separate zooids to start new colonies.

A peculiar double budding occurs in some Hydrozoa, where one part becomes another polyp and the other part becomes a medusa.

A sequence of budding called *multiple budding* occurs in both Protozoa and Metazoa. In the heliozoan *Acanthocystis,* fragments of the nucleus approach the surface and each forms a bud, which later separate. In the flagellate *Noctiluca miliaris,* such a nuclear fragment protrudes from the surface as a bud; inside the bud the nucleus divides to form further buds; in each of which there may form still more buds (up to 500). This process has been erroneously referred to as spore formation and the buds as zoospores.

In the phylactolaemate bryozoan *Plumatella fungosa,* ectoderm and mesoderm participate in forming a digitiform swelling (bud) on the polypide on which a daughter bud forms; the buds of a third generation also may appear while the daughter bud is still rudimentary. In some tunicates stolon buds, called pre-buds, may produce several generations of more specialized buds.

Budding occurs in all colonial animals: Protozoa, Porifera, Hydrozoa (polyp, medusa, actinula larva), Scyphozoa (planula and scyphistoma larva, strobilus), Anthozoa, Calyssozoa (adult, embryo), Phylactolaemata (embryo), Gymnolaemata (ancestrula, embryo, stolon), Pterobranchia (zooids), Ascidiacea (zooid, larva), and Thaliacea (stolon). Budding also occurs unexpectedly in some noncolonial animals, such as Cestoda (in all coenurus bladders and hydatid cysts and a few cysticerci), Polychaeta (adult), Oligochaeta (adult), and Crustacea (reported in Rhizocephala).

The word *stolonization* is not much used, but *stolon* has been used in a variety of animal groups for any lateral branch. Such branches are usually involved in the production of new individuals, but they may perform other functions. Some such stolons are hollow and connect the body cavities of individuals in a colony. Some apparently are solid. Initially, most of them are involved in producing new members of the colony by budding. They occur in Coelenterata, Calyssozoa, Bryozoa, Polychaeta, Crustacea (reported in Rhizocephala), Pterobranchia, and Tunicata.

In some books stolons are considered to be distinct individuals, highly modified, but there is usually no direct evidence that they are anything but extensions of polyps or zooids. They apparently can consist of one type of tissue or of several.

In Polychaeta, the tail region, which bears the reproductive organs, may become separated at sexual maturity and is then sometimes called a stolon. In other species, at the tail end clusters of reproductive structures may be formed (by budding), and these are also called stolons. This process is often part of the unique reproductive process called epitoky (described below). It is so different from stolon formation in Bryozoa, for example, that the word conveys little meaning when used in such a distinct sense.

In a few Polychaeta, stolonization into a chain has been called *gemmiparity.* This is strobilation because the terminal stolon is the oldest, and it is paratomy because most parts of the stolon are formed before separation.

4. Fragmentation

Many animals can break into two or more fragments that will become new individuals. The break may be at a special site, often with some new organs preformed, but it may be without preparation or not at a predetermined site. The term fragmentation is too general for some usages, but it can serve to cover all breaking of an animal into two or more. A variety of other terms are used to specify particular situations or methods of separation.

Both fission and division have been used for both single cell splitting and breaking of a multicellular body. It is here found reasonable to restrict fission to splitting of single cells (whether protozoan or metazoan).

Other terms that have been used in both Protozoa and Metazoa include *schizogenesis* and *tomiparity*, both as reproduction by splitting.

a. Fission

Cell division is, of course, one of the most universal processes in zoology. It can be binary, producing two cells, or multiple, producing many. There are three circumstances in which fission (or what is often called cell division) may be reproductive. These are (1) in many of the Protozoa, reproduction is by "cell division", fission of the whole individual into two (or more), in what is the most direct way to increase the number of individuals; (2) in Mesozoa, there may be fission of a unicellular agamete to produce more agametes; and (3) in many Metazoa, fission (cleavage) of a unicellular zygote to form two new separate cells that are both new individuals (polyembryony or twinning). In reproduction, fission is any division of a single cell (individual) that produces two or more new individuals. That single cell can be an organism (a protozoan), an agamete, or a zygote.

There are two principal forms of binary fission, depending upon the type of nuclear division, whether mitosis or meiosis. In reproduction the meiotic division is merely preparatory to production of gametes and the mitotic to that of two individuals or of agametes. Binary fission is also called *monotomy*. There are many variations of this process that is usually described as "simple division".

Protozoology books describe many varieties of mitotic binary fission. These differ in the formation of an equatorial plate in metaphase or its absence, presence or absence of a centriole, persistence of the nuclear membrane throughout mitosis, behavior of the centriole and the splitting of chromosomes, development of the centrosphere, behavior of the endosome, presence or absence of a spireme, whether the division is longitudinal or transverse, and so on. In all of these the division is roughly equal. Some of the same nuclear processes precede budding, which produces two cells of very different size. In Protozoa budding is thus usually a form of binary fission, whereas in Metazoa it is a form of paratomy.

Any cellular fission in which more than two nuclei are formed, followed by separation of the cytoplasm in fragments surrounding each nucleus, is *multiple fission*. New cell membranes then form, and more than two new individuals result. This may produce amoeboid young (Sarcodina), flagellated young (Sarcodina, Flagellata), spores (Sporozoa: Telosporidia), merozoites (Coccidia, Haemosporidia) and sporozoites (Sporozoa: Telosporidia), gametes (Sporozoa), and agametes (Sporozoa: Telosporidia, Mesozoa).

Other terms for multiple fission in Protozoa include:

1. Merogony — multiple fission of a schizont to produce merozoites; also called schizogony
2. Palintomy — "repeated division . . . leading to formation of spores"
3. Schizogony — multiple fission of a schizont, where the products develop into schizonts, not into agametes; also called merogony

4.   Syntomy — same as schizogony

When a multinucleate protozoan (such as an opalinid) divides into two or more parts without concomitant nuclear division and the nuclei become distributed among the daughter cells, the process is called *plasmotomy.* In Protozoa without a visible nucleus, such as *Protamoeba primitiva,* fission is by simple constriction termed *somatic fission.*

A peculiar form of multiple fission occurs under the misleading term "repeated budding" in a member of the Suctoria, *Tachyblaston ephelotensis,* in which "the mother cell is subdivided by repeated fission and no intervening growth into the so-called dactylozoites. These have only a single tentacle but no cilia" (Grell, 1973).

b. Division

In reproduction, division is the splitting of a multicellular individual into two multicellular fragments, regardless of their size. Comparing this definition with that just given for fission leaves the principal distinction as that between a cell and a multicellular body. The former is usually by mitotic division of a cell, whereas all such cell division occurs in the multicellular body only in building further tissues in preparation for the division.

Many invertebrate animals can reproduce by merely breaking into two or more pieces and then regenerating the missing parts of each. This can be a split down the middle, as in a sea anemone, a break across the body, as in several kinds of worms, or the breaking off of smaller fragments. The latter may be one arm of a starfish, a tiny piece of the base in a coelenterate polyp, or a shapeless strip from the side of a hydroid.

Division of a metazoan can usually be covered by the term fragmentation, and when reproductive it has been more technically called schizogenesis (reproduction by splitting). If the animal splits without preparation of new structures, the modern term is architomy, and included in this are pedal laceration, frustulation, and cases in Hydrozoa, Annelida, and Echinodermata in which there is a major body split without obvious preparation of the site. If the break is preceded by growth of new parts at the site of the break, the division is called paratomy; this obviously includes also the separation of a bud. There seems to be no real distinction between architomy and paratomy, although extreme cases of the two are quite different.

Division occurs in Dicyemida (as pseudo-eggs), in Monoblastozoa (adult), Hydrozoa (polyp, medusa), Anthozoa (polyp, planula larva), Ctenophora (suspected), Turbellaria (adult), Gymnolaemata (larva), Phoronida (adult), Polychaeta (adult, including epitoky), Oligochaeta (adult), Asteroidea (adult), and Ophiuroidea (adult).

Some form of division also occurs in Ctenophora, Gnathostomuloidea, Cestoda, and Phoronida. Pedal laceration occurs in Hydrozoa, Scyphozoa (scyphistoma larva), Anthozoa, and Ctenophora. Frustulation occurs in Hydrozoa. The divisions in Polychaeta take a variety of forms and sequences, sometimes being part of the process called epitoky; here the worm may transform to produce a separate gonad region and perhaps to divide into a nonreproductive "individual" and one that will take part in sexual reproduction.

Division can occur in any multicellular stage in the life cycle. When it occurs in the embryo, it is called polyembryony, producing identical twins (Mammalia), large clones in the parasitic Hymenoptera (Insecta), and genetically identical individuals in some species of Coelenterata, Bryozoa, Mollusca, Annelida, etc. At least these forms of division occur:

1.   Zygote or activated ovum — (polyembryony, which is fission because it is unicellular)
2.   Embryo — two-cell up to gastrulation (polyembryony)

3.   Larva — (paedogenesis, as fragmentation or strobilation)
4.   Adult — (fragmentation, including epitoky)
5.   Bud — (secondary budding)
6.   Colony — (including eudoxy; see Chapter 23)

Paratomy is separation of a multicellular body into two parts at a prepared region; to be reproductive this must be followed by regeneration into two individuals. The preparation consists of preformation of at least some of the structures of the future individuals, usually at a region prepared for separation.

The term *architomy* is for fragmentation with little or no prior formation of new organs. The term can be applied to protozoans or metazoans, but it is here restricted to the latter. It occurs in various life cycle stages and includes frustulation, pedal laceration, schizometamery, and all multiplicative autotomy.

In *frustulation,* an irregular piece of body exterior (apparently all epidermal) breaks off and forms either (1) a planula-like larva which will develop into a new polyp (in Coelenterata) or (2) a pseudo-egg which will develop into a new adult (in Dicyemida). (It is reported to occur also in Turbellaria.) In *pedal laceration* architomy approaches budding. As the polyp creeps slowly over a surface, small pieces of foot are left behind. These develop into new polyps (in Hydrozoa, scyphistoma larvae of Scyphozoa, Anthozoa, and the creeping forms of Ctenophora). In *schizometamery,* which is part of epitoky, separate individual segments out of the middle region of a worm *(Dodecaceria caulleryi),* regenerate both ends, multiply the segments, and then repeat the process, producing in all perhaps 50 individuals.

Architomy occurs in Orthonectida (plasmodium and larva), Hydrozoa (polyp), Scyphozoa (medusa or scyphistoma), Anthozoa (polyp, also in adult as pedal laceration), Tentaculata (pedal laceration), Turbellaria, Rhynchocoela, Polychaeta, Oligochaeta, Asteroidea, Holothurioidea, Enteropneusta (pedal laceration), Ascidiacea (buds, larva, zooid), Thaliacea (zooid).

Other terms referring to division of a multicellular body include these three ill-defined terms that are used in such general sense that they convey no more than the term division:

1.   Fissiparity — fragmentation with regeneration in such genera of Asteroidea as *Coscinasterias* and *Linckia,* and in *Sclerasterias* when they are quite young. In such Ophiuroidea as *Ophiactis* it seems not to be reproductive (only one piece regenerates)
2.   Schizogony — term applied to unequal division in some syllid Polychaeta; in Asteroidea, splitting through the disk
3.   Scissiparity — division that is reproductive if both parts regenerate; includes paratomy and architomy; cited for Anthozoa and Oligochaeta

It must be remembered that in Metazoa the division processes may not be reproductive. *Autotomy* is deliberate breaking off of an appendage or other structure, which will presumably then be regenerated. If the broken-off fragment itself regenerates into a new individual, there has been reproduction. This would have to be specified as "autotomy with regeneration of both parts", which occurs in fairly obvious form in Turbellaria, Rhynchocoela, Asteroidea, and Holothurioidea. It has also been termed *dichotomous autotomy.*

The group of processes encompassed by the term *polyembryony* amount to a form of fragmentation that can resemble budding or be merely separation of cells that have just been produced by cleavage; thus, division of the zygote or embryo into two or more (up to several thousand) can occur at any stage from the first cleavage up to the gastrula. In most animal groups there is inadequate information on how the embryo (or zygote) can divide into several or many. These divisions are all here treated as being the form of fragmentation called polyembryony. Some form of this occurs in Coelenterata, Trematoda, Cestoda, Gymnolaemata, Oligochaeta, Insecta, Mammalia, and very likely others. Something of this sort occurs in Sarcodina, where an hologamous "zygote" divides into several young. The same thing may occur in the unknown part of the cycle of Monoblastozoa. The process of embryonic multiplication in Insecta has been called gemmation, which appears to be an unnecessary synonym of polyembryony.

Identical *twinning* is polyembryony producing two or a few zygote fragments, each of which functions as a new zygote and develops into a complete individual. It occurs in Bryozoa, Insecta, all classes of Vertebrata, and is reported to be sporadic in all major phyla.

In several Trematoda, *successional polyembryony* produces a succession of groups of larvae not derived by metamorphosis or division of a previous stage, but by successive cleavages of the original zygote and its germinal daughter cells, which have been carried along in each larval stage.

c. Strobilation

Among animals, chains are produced by several processes. First, chains of individuals may be formed by the union of two or more, as in syzygy, but this is not reproduction. Chains may be formed by division of an existing body or by budding. The same processes, with rapid separation, can result in a series of separate individuals that are not connected after formation. The chains may consist of individuals, proglottids, or the annelid body regions called stolons.

Chains formed by division into two (repeatedly) are similar in formation, whether the successive parts are individuals, stolons, or proglottids. The term budding is sometimes applied to the formation of the new part, but the important feature is usually the growth of a septum between the old and the new parts. An incipient chain consisting of just two parts gives no visible clue to whether it is a strobilus or not. After the chain consists of three parts, it is possible to distinguish between ordinary chains and those in which the septum is always at the end next to the original individual. The latter is strobilation, which proceeds in such a way that parts are progressively younger from the extremity toward the base. In some chains there is development of new head and tail structures at each septum, as in Turbellaria; in others there are no new structures except the septum itself, as in tapeworms.

Chains that are not formed by strobilation may be found in Turbellaria, Polychaeta, Oligochaeta, and Thaliacea. The reproductive process in these is division, with actual separation indefinitely delayed.

In reproduction, strobilation is the formation of a chain of new individuals which are isolated by a series of septa at the base of the chain, so that the oldest of the new individuals is at the apex of the chain. In all known cases the new individuals eventually separate one at a time.

In its various forms, *strobilation* is successive partitioning of a body to produce either (1) a chain of proglottids or gonophores, to be liberated later, (2) a chain of individuals that remain attached for some time, or (3) a succession of individuals, each liberated before the next one is initiated. It is common to use the term budding in describing strobilation, but the new individual is not formed by mere proliferation, as in a normal bud, but by formation of a septum across the body, followed by growth of new organs in the smaller fragment, as in proglottid formation in tapeworms.

Strobilation produces chains in Flagellata (reproductive bodies from adults), Scyphozoa (ephyrae or scyphistomae from strobilae), Anthozoa (polyp from polyp), Ces-

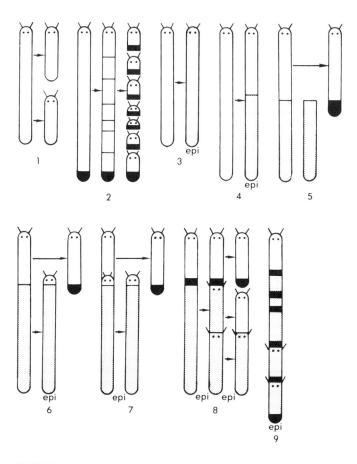

FIGURE 3.   Epitoky in the Polychaeta. The original worm is in white, the epitoke in stipple, and regenerating regions in black. (Adapted from Blackwelder, R. E., and Shepherd, B. A., The Diversity of Animal Reproduction, CRC Press, Boca Raton, Fla., 1981.)

toda (multiple gonophores, proglottids, from scolex), Polychaeta (adult or stolon from adult), and Ascidiacea (zooids from buds from zooids). Not all of these produce new individuals, but merely new compartments, so strobilation is not necessarily reproductive.

d. Epitoky

The term epitoky is used in quite different meanings for aspects of the life cycle of various polychaetes. In some textbooks and a few invertebrate compendia, it appears that these worms divide into a head end, which is called an atoke and is not reproductive, and a tail end, which contains gametes and is called an epitoke. The epitoke swims to the surface, spawns, and dies and thus has the nature of a gonophore, a detached fragment that contains the gonads.

In books that treat the subject of epitoky in more detail, it is clear that the word basically denotes the process of metamorphosis (with or without sexual or asexual reproduction or both), in which the rear (sexual) part of the worm changes in appearance, but may either detach or remain permanently attached. The diversity of expression of this process is much greater than any of the textbooks make clear (Figure 3).

The textbook usage would be the easiest to describe, but would leave a variety of borderline cases that would require other terms or specification. It is reluctantly concluded here that the second meaning (metamorphosis) is the correct one under the circumstances; it is adopted here with a diagram and a tabulation to show the range of the diversity.

Epitoky is the process or succession of processes in which one part of the worm body (usually the tail end) changes in structure and physiology in preparation for sexual reproduction. This part, the epitoke, may liberate its gametes after breaking away (as a detached gonophore), may remain attached and regress to the original condition after gamete liberation, or may regenerate the missing front end after breaking away and thus become a complete and new separate individual. It merges with ordinary sexual maturation at one point and with alternation of asexual and sexual generations at another and with strobilation at still another.

Epitoky may appear to be more of a developmental process than a reproductive one. It includes in its range not only sexual reproduction but fission, fragmentation, budding, and strobilation. It is at one point paratomous (the fission prepared in advance) and at the next architomous (the fission unheralded by new organs). The division may be single or multiple. The metamorphosed region may be broken off to spawn and die, or may remain attached and die with the head end (atoke) after spawning. It may also remain attached and later regress to the original form until the next breeding season. The isolated fragment may regenerate the missing head and thus become a separate individual for its brief life or it may remain a headless fragment. Stolons (the isolated parts in ordinary epitoky) may be formed in chains by "random" divisions or by strobilation, where all new sections develop at the base of the chain.

Even more unexpected is the form of epitoky called schizometamery. In *Dodecaceria caulleryi,* individual segments are separated out of the middle region of a worm, the tail pieces dying but the head end regenerating. The fragments then regenerate both ends, multiply the segments, and then repeat the process, producing in all at least 50 individuals.

In short, the possible ramifications of this process are numerous. It apparently occurs only in Polychaeta. Other terms associated with epitoky are *schizogamy,* which is the actual division into a sexual and an asexual individual, and *epigamy,* which is the metamorphosis that produces an epitoke without division.

D. Organs for Asexual Processes

All asexual reproduction in multicellular animals involves separation of part of the body, thereby forming a new individual without any fusions or gametogenesis. There are seldom any special organs involved, but the following situations occur:

Dichotomous autotomy. Breaking into two, where there is a region specially prepared to be the site of the break. This region can be thought of as an organ. For example, in annelids, there may be new tissues and structures forming in advance at the site of the break, in what is called paratomy. This tissue mass, preparing for the break, can be considered an organ, comparable to a meristem or abscission point in plants.

Budding. The bud is an organ of the parent until it separates or becomes self-sufficient. The buds may arise on a special structure called a blastostyle, but this term is also used for a sexual individual in some Siphonophora.

Strobilation. In Cestoda there is both a region of septum formation and the proglottid itself. The latter, especially, is an organ, because even when separated off it is incapable of living as a separate animal.

Polyembryony. There are here no special organs, as cells merely separate from neighboring cells.

Gemmules and statoblasts. Clearly multicellular organs until the moment of separation. They may be formed in specialized regions of the body which may then be looked upon as organs for their production.

Pedal disc. In the scyphistoma larvae of some Scyphozoa there are chitinous cysts (podocysts) that can produce larvae after release. They are surely organs of asexual reproduction also.

Germ balls. In Trematode larvae (sporocysts and rediae) these are surely embryonic organs, producing successive generations of embryos. The process is known as successional polyembryony, because at each step many new embryos are produced from the germ ball.

Organelles for protozoan processes. Because protozoans cannot have organs, by definition, only organelles could be cited here. In fact, in either sexual or asexual reproduction the only organelles primarily concerned are the spindle, chromosomes, etc., of the mitotic cycle. In a few colonial forms with polymorphic individuals, certain of these serve in the role of organs to conduct the reproductive processes.

REFERENCES

Barnes, R. D., *Invertebrate Zoology,* 2nd ed., W. B. Saunders, Philadelphia, 1968.

Blackwelder, R. E. and Shepherd, B. A., *The Diversity of Animal Reproduction,* CRC Press, Boca Raton, Fla., 1981.

Breder, C. M., Jr. and Rosen, D. E., *Modes of Reproduction in Fishes,* Natural History Press, Garden City, N.Y., 1966.

Campbell, R. D., Cnidaria, in *Reproduction of Marine Invertebrates,* Vol. 1, Giese, A. C. and Pearse, J. S., Eds., Academic Press, New York, 1974, chap. 3.

Davey, K. G., *Reproduction in the Insects,* Oliver & Boyd, Edinburgh, 1965.

Giese, A. C. and Pearse, J. S., Eds., *Reproduction of Marine Invertebrates,* Vol. 1 (1974), Vol. 2 (1975), Vol. 3 (1975), Vol. 4 (1977), Vol. 5 (1979).

Gray, P., *The Dictionary of the Biological Sciences,* Reinhold, New York, 1967.

Grell, K. G., *Protozoology,* Springer-Verlag, Berlin, 1973.

Hagan, H. R., *Embryology of the Viviparous Insects,* Ronald Press, New York, 1951.

Henley, C., Platyhelminthes (Turbellaria), in *Reproduction of Marine Invertebrates,* Vol. 1, Giese, A. C. and Pearse, J. S., Eds., Academic Press, New York, 1974, chap. 5.

Hyman, L. H., *The Invertebrates,* Vol. 1 (1940), Vol. 2 (1951a), Vol. 3 (1951b), Vol. 4 (1955), Vol. 5 (1959), Vol. 6 (1967), McGraw-Hill, New York.

Imms, A. D., *A General Textbook of Entomology,* 8th ed., Methuen, London, 1951.

Kudo, R. R., *Protozoology,* 5th ed., Charles C Thomas, Springfield, Ill., 1966.

Lasserre, P., Clitellata, in *Reproduction of Marine Invertebrates,* Vol. 3, Giese, A. C. and Pearse, J. B., Eds., Academic Press, New York, 1975.

Markewitch, A. P., *Parasitic Copepodes on the Fishes of the U.S.S.R.,* Indian National Scientific Documentation Centre, New Delhi, 1976.

Pennak, R. W., *Collegiate Dictionary of Zoology,* Ronald Press, New York, 1964.

Rothschild, (Lord), *Fertilization,* John Wiley & Sons, New York, 1956.

Sadleir, M. F. S., *The Reproduction of Vertebrates,* Academic Press, New York, 1973.

Sleigh, M. A., *The Biology of Protozoa,* American Elsevier, New York, 1973.

Sonneborn, T. M., Breeding systems, reproductive methods, and species problems in Protozoa, in *The Species Problem,* Mayr, E., Ed., American Association for the Advancement of Science, Washington, D.C., 1957.

Vorontsova, M. A. and Liosner, L. D., *Asexual Propagation and Regeneration,* Pergamon Press, London, 1960.

Waterman, T. H., Ed., *The Physiology of Crustacea,* Vol. 2, Academic Press, New York, 1961.

Wilson, E. B., *The Cell in Development and Heredity,* 3rd ed., Macmillan, New York, 1953.

Chapter 3

BISEXUAL REPRODUCTION

TABLE OF CONTENTS

I.   Bisexuality 46
     A.   Discussion 46
     B.   Bisexual Reproduction 48
     C.   Basic Bisexual Reproduction 48

II. Sexual Reproductive Processes 49
     A.   General Terms 49
     B.   Gametogenesis 49
          1.   Spermatogenesis 49
          2.   Oogenesis 49
     C.   Meiosis 51
     D.   Gamete Functions 52
          1.   Ova 52
          2.   Spermatozoa 52
     E.   Fertilization 53
          1.   Site of Fertilization 56
          2.   Insemination or Spermatozoon Transfer 56
          3.   Spermatozoon Migration 57
     F.   Syngamy 58
     G.   Karyogamy 59
     H.   Activation 59
          1.   Zygotes 59
          2.   Apozygotes 60
          3.   Blastomeres 60

III. The Reproductive System 60
     A.   Prologue 60
     B.   Reproductive Organs 61
     C.   Primary Organs 62
          1.   Gonads 62
               a.   Embryonic Source of Gonads 63
               b.   Position of Gonads in the Body 63
          2.   Gametes 64
               a.   Tissue Source of Gametes 65
               b.   Isogametes 65
               c.   Anisogametes 66
               d.   Spermatozoa 66
               e.   Polymorphism of Spermatozoa 67
               f.   Ova 68
               g.   Diversity of Ova 69
               h.   Polymorphism of Ova 69
               i.   Motility of Ova 70
               j.   Yolk 70
               k.   Egg Coverings 70
               l.   Ovum Types and Terms 72

         m.   Pseudova..72
         n.   Hologametes 72
    D.   Secondary Organs 72
         1.   Male Gonoducts...73
         2.   Female Gonoducts..73
         3.   Gonopores..74
         4.   Nutritional Organs 75
         5.   Storage Organs 75
         6.   Associated Glands 76

IV. Gonophores and Gametophores.......................................76
    A.   Comments 76
    B.   Gonophores 76
    C.   Spermatophores..77
    D.   Oophores 79
    E.   Zygotophores 79
    F.   Embryophores 79

References 79

I. BISEXUALITY

A. Discussion

Sexual reproduction is multiplication involving gametes that have undergone the reduction division of meiosis and which will fuse in pairs to form a zygote (a new individual).

Most zoologists would subscribe to this definition. However, most zoologists would probably not put great emphasis on the presence of meiosis or the eventual fusion. If the animals in question were obviously male and female (or even two cross-fertilizing hermaphrodites), and if they practiced some sexual behavior (especially copulation), the reproduction would unhesitatingly be called sexual.

There are difficulties and exceptions that make it necessary to take the definition seriously. Some apparently sexual animals in several phyla are of two sexes and do produce gametes with meiosis, but the gametes do not fuse: the spermatozoa disintegrate and the ova develop parthenogenetically. In an even larger number of phyla, there are apparently sexual animals whose "gametes" not only do not fuse but do not undergo meiosis. These ova also develop parthenogenetically, but they are more explicitly called pseudova.

It is obvious from this that the three criteria of sexuality in reproduction — gametes, meiosis, and fertilization — do not necessarily appear in all "sexual" reproductions. This means that in some animals reproduction may be more sexual than in others. It also means that the term "sexual reproduction" is not explicit; it must be used with great care or be replaced by some other term that is effectively definable. Synonyms include *amphigony* (any reproduction involving two individuals but usually taken as equal to bisexual reproduction) and *zoogamy*.

There is far more diversity in sexual reproduction than is ordinarily stated. Production of a zygote involves several structures and several processes; among these are gonads, gametogenesis, meiosis, gametes, and fertilization. Gonads are the body organs that produce the reproductive cells which, by mitosis and gametogenesis, produce the gametes. Meiosis is the process in gametogenesis which results in the gametes being haploid. Fertilization restores diploidy in the zygote by fusion of two haploid gametes. It is usually not mentioned that one or more of these structures or processes may be lacking in any given species.

The gonad, described in a later section, is the source of the gametes, but in several groups gametes may be produced in the lining of a cavity, where no gonad is distinguishable. This occurs in some Ctenophora, Brachiopoda, Sipunculoidea, Polychaeta, Hirudinea, and Tunicata. They may even be produced throughout the parenchyma, as in some Ctenophora and all Porifera.

The word gamete should be applied to haploid reproductive bodies produced in a gonad by gametogenesis. It is often forgotten that some apparent female "gametes" are actually diploid, not requiring fertilization. These are involved in parthenogenesis and should be termed pseudova. They differ from agametes in being produced in an ovary, but otherwise the two serve the same function and are essentially asexual (see a more complete definition in a later section on gametes; see also "Ameiotic Parthenogenesis" in Chapter 4).

Some ova, which are produced with meiosis and so are haploid, do not require fertilization, using one of several other processes to restore diploidy and activate development (see "Meiotic Parthenogenesis" in Chapter 4).

Fertilization can seldom be directly demonstrated, because insemination or even fusion of the gametes does not ensure that genes from both parents will be present in the offspring. The diversities here are also listed in Chapter 4 under "Parthenogenesis".

Even when the three stated conditions are met, "sexually" reproducing animals may not produce offspring that show the genetically expected results of gene recombination. This is because the life cycle includes also some nonbisexual process that interferes. These are discussed in Chapter 4 under "Sequence of Reproductive Cycles". The following problems occur, making it difficult to clearly delineate the process of sexual reproduction:

1. Parthenogenesis — which does not really belong here but is not always readily distinguishable: (a) there may be no males at all; (b) males may inseminate the females but the spermatozoa fail to unite with the ova; (c) males may inseminate and the gametes fuse, but the male pronucleus degenerates without karyogamy (pseudogamy); (d) males may inseminate and gametes fuse but the two pronuclei remain separate and presumably functional (gonomery)
2. Inbreeding — in which the fertilization is by related gametes such as those from sibling individuals
3. Clonal fertilization — which is by gametes from members of a single clone, so that they are essentially identical genetically
4. Self-fertilization — in the case of an hermaphrodite (this occurs in at least 21 classes in 12 phyla)
5. Asexual processes — following sexual reproduction will also upset the genetic picture, so the expected genetic results of sexual reproduction can occur only in a cycle where there are no asexual processes. An example: polyembryony in some parasitic wasps in which a zygote can give rise to as many as 1000 individuals by division of the early embryo into many parts, each of which becomes a new individual; obviously these 1000 individuals are genetically identical, i.e., they are a clone, and that particular part of the population will not show normal gene frequencies.

Several aspects of the reproduction that involves sex show unexpected diversity. They include sexuality (with sex distribution and sex determination), gonads, gametogenesis, meiosis, gametes, fertilization (more specifically karyogamy), activation, and the zygote. They are each discussed below.

B. Bisexual Reproduction

The expression "bisexual reproduction" is more explicit than sexual reproduction, because it refers to a process that can be clearly distinguished in most cases. Unfortunately, the cycles in many of these species also include other reproductive processes, ones that alter the genetic outcome of the cycle.

Thus, in discussing reproduction, it is not enough to define the processes and list their occurrences. It is necessary to realize that a given individual in a certain species resulting from a given reproduction may not develop to adulthood because it obliterates itself through another act of reproduction at some developmental stage. For example, the zygote may undergo polyembryony; whereupon it is transformed into two or more new individuals and thus itself ceases to exist. An individual, therefore, may exist as a zygote for only a brief span until another reproduction destroys it, or it may exist to the larval stage where fragmentation will destroy it, or it may exist to adulthood. There is great diversity among animals in this cycle-part which is the life span of a given individual (see later section "Sequences of Reproductive Cycles" in Chapter 4).

Bisexual reproduction occurs in all the species of animals except those entirely asexual listed in the previous chapter. There were 19 phyla which had no asexual reproduction, but 5 of those were known to reproduce parthenogenetically. Thus, 14 phyla are exclusively bisexual and at least 12 additional classes in other phyla, but the groups in which there is no bisexual reproduction in any species are the order Chrysomonadina in the Flagellata, the class Bdelloidea in the Rotifera, and the class Chaetonotoidea in the Gastrotricha. In addition, there are species without sexual reproduction in the Rhynchocoela *(Lineus sanguineus)*, the Polychaeta *(Zeppelina monostyla)*, and Oligochaeta (many of the family Naididae, and *Lumbriculus variegatus*).

Two other terms are synonymous with bisexual reproduction. These are *gamogenesis* and *zygogenesis*. In addition, *amphimixis, mixis,* and *amphigenesis* all refer to bisexual reproduction because they specify the union of ovum and spermatozoon.

C. Basic Bisexual Reproduction

It is necessary to pinpoint reproduction that will or can give the expected genetic ratios in the offspring and recognize the extent to which this is masked by the occurrence of other processes. There is no term that can effectively be used for this, and so the phrase Basic Bisexual Reproduction *(BBR)* is adopted here. This is reproduction in which gametes from two individuals unite in karyogamy to produce one new individual; without intervention of any other reproductive processes. Attempts to simplify this into a definition have led to this: production of a single offspring by immediate biparental karyogamy. In this definition, a single offspring must be specified to eliminate polyembryony; the immediacy is necessary to establish that there is no intervening other reproduction; biparental origin is necessary to specify (at least in part) that none of the forms of inbreeding occur; and karyogamy is necessary to show that true mixing of genomes occurs.

BBR is therefore not merely a process of reproduction but a reproductive cycle consisting of a single specified reproductive process, what might be called "pure" sexual reproduction. It can be looked on as an uncontaminated life cycle. The possible contaminants include polyembryony, additional reproductive processes (parthenogenesis or asexual), and substitution for outbreeding of either self-fertilization, activation by sperm without karyogamy (union of nuclei), clonal fertilization, or other inbreeding (the terms process, cycle, etc., are explained in the section "Levels of Diversity" in Chapter 4).

The term is thus used for bisexual reproduction unaltered in its genetic effects by any other reproduction in the cycle or by any "developmental" processes that are actually reproductive. There is no way to indicate where it occurs, except to say that it does *not* occur in any life cycle which includes *any* reproductive process listed in the chart as lacking karyogamy. It is thus much less universal than usually supposed; it can never be assumed unless the entire life cycle is known and no other reproductive processes occur.

BBR is what is usually understood by cross-fertilization, but as previously mentioned there must be additional stipulations both as to what is cross- and the absence of other processes in the cycle. Cross-fertilization is what is commonly meant by sexual or bi-sexual reproduction, and these terms are even less explicit.

II. SEXUAL REPRODUCTIVE PROCESSES

A. General Terms

Reproduction by means of gametes is *gamogony.* It thus includes all the amphimictic and parthenogenetic processes: heterogamy and isogamy, amphigony, exogamy, allo-gamy, dissogeny, endogamy, and automixis, as well as pseudogamy, plasmogony, and gonomery. The production of gametes in any individual is *gametogenesis,* including *spermatogenesis* and *oogenesis.*

The unicellular reproductive bodies produced by gametogenesis are gametes. Their production usually involves meiosis, which gives them just one genome. Thus, such gametes are haploid, but in some parthenogenesis the ova are mitotically produced and therefore diploid. In most animals the gametes are *anisogametes,* because they are ova and spermatozoa, sharply distinct in their structure and behavior. This condition is called either *anisogamy* or *heterogamy.* In a few Protozoa the gametes are indistin-guishable and are called *isogametes,* with the condition called *isogamy.* Anisogamy occurs in some Protozoa and in all gamete-producing Metazoa. In some Protozoa the entire organism acts as a gamete *(hologamete),* in a process called *hologamy*(Table 6).

B. Gametogenesis

All sexual reproduction in any sense is by means of gametes, whether two are used or only one, and whether they are isogametes, anisogametes (heterogametes), or holo-gametes. Formation of these gametes is gametogenesis; it is the first process in sexual reproduction.

Gametogenesis is not entirely uniform throughout the phyla of animals, especially if Protozoa are included. Gametes should be haploid, to prevent increasing the chromo-some number at each generation, but there is some diversity in how the reduction divisions (meiosis) occur, and there are diploid ova. In the case of hologametes in the Protozoa, something akin to meiosis must occur, either in each individual before union or in the "zygote" afterwards.

1. Spermatogenesis

This involves a series of cell divisions and cytological changes in the process of de-veloping functional spermatozoa. There is considerable diversity in the spermatozoa produced (as illustrated in Figure 4) but there is little diversity in the processes.

2. Oogenesis

This is somewhat more diverse than spermatogenesis. Primordial germ cells in the ovary divide by mitosis to form oogonia. Typically this is followed by meiosis in each oogonium. The homologous chromosomes become closely associated (synapsis) and are replicated, so that each chromosome consists of two chromatids and thus each

Table 6
THE REPRODUCTIVE AND GENETIC ASPECTS OF THE PROCESSES

	1 No. of individuals	2 Male and female	3a Gam-ogony	3b Gametes, etc.	4 No. of meioses	5 Kary-ogamy	6 Multi-plication
Bisexual	2	Yes	Yes	Aniso-	2	Yes	Yes
Outbreeding	2	Yes	Yes	Aniso-	2	Yes	Yes
Clonal fertilization	2	Yes	Yes	Aniso-	2	Yes	Yes
Self-fertilization	1	(Gonads)	Yes	Aniso-	2	Yes	Yes
Parthenogenesis I (pseudogamy)	(2)1[a]	(Yes)	Yes	Yes	(2)1[a]	No	Yes
Parthenogenesis II (meiotic)	1	No	Yes	Ovum	1	No	Yes
Parthenogenesis III (ameiotic)	1	No	Yes	Ovum	0	No	Yes
Parthenogenesis IV (polar body fertilization)	1	No	Yes	Ovum & polar body	1	Yes	Yes
Sporogony	1	No	No	Spores	0	0	Yes
Asexual (fission, budding)	1	No	No	None	0	0	Yes
Conjugation	2	?	No	Nuclei	2	Yes	No
Hologamy	2	?	No	Holo-	2	Yes	No
Automixis	1 or 2	No	No	Nuclei	1	Yes	No

[a] Two individuals but only one participates.

From Blackwelder, R. E. and Shepherd, B. A., *The Diversity of Animal Reproduction*, CRC Press, Boca Raton, Fla., 1981.

homologous pair forms a tetrad. The cell is then called a primary oocyte. Two maturation or meiotic divisions now occur, producing (1) one secondary oocyte and a polar body and (2) one ootid and another polar body. In the first of these divisions, the two chromosomes of each pair separate and pass to the daughter cells (secondary oocyte and polar body). In the second division, the two chromatids of the replicated chromosome separate as distinct chromosomes and pass to the two daughter cells (ootid and polar body). The ootid matures directly into an ovum, and the polar bodies ordinarily distintegrate (a subsequent anomaly in the functions of these polar bodies is described later under "Fertilization").

During the first maturation division, crossing-over may occur between the corresponding chromatids of the two chromosomes of the pair. This is the source of some of the diversity in the genetic make-up of those ova in which it occurs, but even more diversity comes from the random assortment of chromosomes in the first meiotic division.

Diversity in ovum production appears in several other ways. Some animals, such as mammals, produce one ovum at a time (they are said to be *uniparous*); others produce many ova at a time or continuously. Although ova are usually assumed to be immobile, in Porifera, Hydrozoa, Gastropoda, and Insecta there are species with eggs that show amoeboid movement. In some Coelenterata the egg is covered with microvilli or spines; in one species it is covered by a layer of nematocysts. In certain Copepoda (Crustacea), during maturation divisions, there may be elimination of chromatin. Differences in yolk content and polarity are discussed in a later section.

C. Meiosis

Meiosis is the process in gametogenesis by which diploid reproductive cells produce haploid gametes. To this basic definition must be added certain exceptional occurrences cited below.

In the usual case, animals that are produced asexually as a result of fertilization are diploid, because the haploid set of chromosomes contained in the spermatozoon and the haploid set in the ovum are combined at fertilization to form a diploid zygote, the new individual. In the process of gametogenesis, which is the formation of the gametes, meiosis is the mechanism by which the gamete receives its haploid set of chromosomes. This reduction of chromosome number from the spermatogonium or the oogonium to the gamete is *haplosis* — reduction from diploid to haploid.

In the process of meiosis there is not usually known to be much diversity. However, Protozoa occur in which there is only one division that reduces the number of gene sets; presumably there is no initial doubling, so haploidy is attained by a single division, which is reductional. In the nematode *Meloidogyne* there is also no doubling, so meiosis consists of a single division.

Although meiosis in both Protozoa and Metazoa is usually assumed to occur during gametogenesis (and is so defined above), there are some haploid Protozoa (Foraminifera) in which the haploid gametes are produced by simple mitosis. Fusion of the gametes produced diploid zygotes. (Here there is an alternation of generations of the type common in plants, where one "generation" is diploid and the other is haploid.) One of these produces a haploid generation by normal meiotic division; each of these haploid gamonts will eventually produce haploid isogametes by mitosis. The zygote resulting from fusion of the haploid isogametes will be a diploid agamont (trophozoite or schizont), which will eventually undergo the meioses and develop into haploid gamonts again.

In some Flagellata and the Sporozoa, the diploid zygote undergoes meiosis so that nearly all the cycle is haploid. In asexual species like those of *Trypanosoma,* there is neither meiosis nor fertilization at any time, and the cell may be considered to be either diploid or haploid, as there is no way to distinguish these processes when there is no meiosis.

In Metazoa it is usually true that meiosis occurs during gametogenesis (gametic meiosis). However, the existence of haploid ova in some parthenogenesis and diploid ova in others makes it likely that unusual meiotic sequences occur. Ameiotic parthenogenesis is known in Rotifera, Nematoda, Mollusca, Crustacea, and Insecta. Meiotic parthenogenesis occurs in Turbellaria, Oligochaeta, Crustacea, and Insecta. Both types probably also occur in other groups.

In some other Protozoa gametes may be replaced by hologametes. By meiosis, the entire gamont (parent cell) is converted into a haploid "gamete" *(hologamete)*. Fusion of two hologametes will restore the diploidy (see "Hologamy" under "Para-Reproductive Processes" in Chapter 4).

The results of gametogenesis are the gametes. They are usually thought of as haploid unicellular structures, two of which fuse to form a zygote — the start of a new individual.

Because gametes are in reality reproductive organs, their structural diversity is treated later in this chapter.

D. Gamete Functions

The primary function of gametes is to fuse in pairs to produce the zygotes that will each grow into a new adult individual. In reality, various gametes serve quite a variety of other functions.

1. Ova

The prime function of the ovum is to become activated into a zygote. The zygote is a new individual, and this must be diploid. There is a possibility that some ova are already diploid (pseudova), but usually the diploid number of chromosomes must be restored, by either of these occurrences: (1) fertilization (karyogamy) — actual union of spermatozoon and ovum pronuclei; (2) doubling its own chromosomes upon some internal stimulus. This stimulus appears to be "recognition" of subnormal chromatin content by the nucleus.

The functions of a given ovum might include one or more of the following:

1. Fuse with a spermatozoon to start a new diploid individual
2. Respond to activation stimulus and develop into a haploid individual
3. Respond to activation stimulus, duplicate its own chromosomes, and develop into a diploid individual
4. Change into a nurse cell for nourishing other ova
5. Carry one set of genes from one generation to the next
6. Carry food (yolk) for the future embryo
7. Provide cytoplasm for the zygote
8. Provide zygote envelopes

2. Spermatozoa

The spermatozoa of different animals are shown to differ in a variety of structural ways. It seems to be the case, however, that "many of these variations seem to be of little or no physiological significance; and beneath the structural diversity of spermatozoa exists a fundamental common plan of organization" (Wilson, 1953, p. 278). If so, this is an unusual example of lack of correlation between structure and function.

Although spermatozoa may occasionally take part in other processes, their unique function is simply stated: it is to activate the ovum and convert it into a zygote by contributing one set of chromosomes.

No spermatozoon, by itself, is known to grow into a new individual, although a spermatocyte that can do so is cited in an earlier section in the hydrozoan *Cunina*. Apparently none can differentiate into some other type of cell for any purpose whatever. However, spermatozoa may serve at least these (sometimes incidental) functions:

1. Fertilization (karyogamy) — complete fusion with an ovum
2. Activation — of some parthenogenetic ova
3. Nourishment — of female during production of eggs
4. Penetration — of barriers in the female, physical or chemical, so another spermatozoon can fertilize the ovum
5. Transportation — of one set of the genes from one generation to the next

E. Fertilization

Fertilization includes three events culminating in a zygote. These are syngamy (the penetration of an ovum by a spermatozoon), karyogamy (the fusion of the gamete pronuclei), and, at some point in this sequence, activation of the resulting zygote to develop. Real fertilization always accomplishes activation, but an ovum may be activated without fertilization.

The term *fertilization* is variously used for fusion of gametes, for such fusion followed by fusion of the pronuclei, or merely for insemination, or even for copulation. Because of this looseness in usage, the word is useless as a reproductive process unless it be made equivalent to the sum of syngamy-plus-karyogamy-plus-activation; these terms are preferred. The first and last of these required events can occur in situations where karyogamy does not occur. Physical fusion of the gametes may induce activation and development without karyogamy. Activation can be brought about by other factors without any spermatozoa being present. Therefore, in discussing these processes, it is always appropriate to use the most explicit term to convey the real nature of the process involved: syngamy for fusion of gametes or penetration of the ovum by the spermatozoon, karyogamy for nuclear fusion with mixing of the genomes, and activation for the initiation of development of the zygote.

The idea that fertilization is always the fusion of two gametes is firmly ingrained, yet it is not entirely accurate. Gametes are the haploid cells formed by meiosis from oocytes and spermatocytes, yet in Nematoda it is apparently common for the spermatozoon to fuse with an oocyte before it undergoes meiosis. This would be fusion of the cells, but it obviously would not mean karyogamy, which would be delayed.

As a reproductive process fertilization covers both the amphimictic karyogamy of BBR and that of self-fertilization and its relatives. In its broadest sense fertilization even includes activation and is then equivalent to amphimixis plus gametic apomixis.

In ova of parthenogenetic animals, where there will not be any spermatozoan chromosomes added by karyogamy, there still must be some stimulus to activate the "egg" to develop. Activation, therefore, is not dependent on fertilization, although it is often a direct result.

To speak of the beginning of life, in bisexual (dioecious) animals, as being at fertilization is never satisfactory for the animal kingdom as a whole because many eggs (from Protozoa to Vertebrata) develop without fusion of ovum and spermatozoon. The broader term is activation, to be discussed in a later paragraph.

Because the "nucleus" of the gamete is haploid, it is assumed to be of different significance from the nucleus of a diploid cell or a zygote. For this reason it is commonly designated by the term "pronucleus". The problem of diploid ova was apparently not considered when this term was adopted, and so even these are included under the term.

In the strict sense, fertilization is the complete series of events from the approach of the spermatozoon to the ovum to the formation of the fusion (zygote) nucleus and to activation of the fertilized egg to develop. This word has several meanings. In the most restricted sense, it is equivalent to *karyogamy* — the union of spermatozoan and ovum pronuclei. It is sometimes also used when there is no such union but the ovum is somehow stimulated to start development without any union with a spermatozoon. The latter is better called *activation.*

As mentioned above, the word fertilization is also used in a more general sense for physical contact of individuals. Correctly this is copulation, which normally leads to *insemination* — the introduction of spermatozoa into the body of the female. This is also called fecundation or impregnation.

In fertilization, the sources of the gametes (the gonads) can be diverse as regards their distribution among parent individuals. They are represented by the terms involving two individuals: cross-fertilization, fraternal fertilization, clonal fertilization; and the terms involving only one individual: self-fertilization, automixis, and polar-body fertilization.

When the two source gonads are in separate individuals, there are three possible situations: (1) reasonably unrelated individuals (cross-fertilization), (2) sibling individuals (fraternal fertilization), or (3) clonally related individuals — genetically identical (clonal fertilization); all of these are amphimictic but (2) and (3) produce increasingly less genetic diversity. Although it is implied here that the individuals are gonochorists, it is, of course, possible that they be hermaphrodites, but the fertilization is between individuals.

When the two source gonads are in the same individual, the syngamy is self-fertilization or autogamy or polar body fertilization, which are also amphimictic but produce less genetic diversity.

The possibilities of gamete source are these:

1.   From separate individuals (see gonochorism and dioecism, under "Sex in One Individual" in Chapter 4): (a) reasonably unrelated individuals (cross-fertilization), (b) sibling individuals (fraternal fertilization), (c) pairing with gamete from another member of one clone (clonal fertilization)
2.   From separate individuals (see hermaphroditism and monoecism in Chapter 4): (a) pairing with gamete from another individual (cross-fertilization between two hermaphrodites), (b) pairing with gamete from a sibling (fraternal fertilization), (c) pairing with gamete from another member of one clone (clonal fertilization)
3.   From a single individual: (a) pairing gametes from the one individual (self-fertilization), (b) union of an ovum with its own polar body. (Automixis in Protozoa would fit here except that it is not reproductive; see "Para-Reproductive Processes" in Chapter 4.)
4.   From individuals of different species; pairing with a gamete from an individual of another species: hybridization

The various types of fertilization are described here, followed by the definitive steps included in the sequence covered by that term.

Cross-fertilization is the situation in which the two gametes come from two individuals that are neither siblings nor members of a clone. It occurs in some species in many classes of animals, but is entirely absent in all species of the order Chrysomonadina of Protozoa, the class Bdelloidea of Rotifera, and the class Chaetonotoidea of Gastrotricha.

As so defined, cross-fertilization would be essentially the same as *outbreeding.* Opposed to this would be *inbreeding* (endogamy), which is the mating (with karyogamy) of individuals too closely related to be considered "unrelated". Siblings obviously qualify here, but there is no place to draw the line between this and cross-breeding or outbreeding.

A variation on cross-fertilization is gonomery (penetration without fusion), but because the chromosomes persist they apparently do eventually enter into development, making this merely a case of delayed or confused karyogamy.

Fraternal fertilization occurs when offspring (siblings) of one pair of cross-fertilizing parents produce the gametes which fuse. The resulting zygotes contain the combined genomes of the pair of related gametes, where there is potentially more genetic diversity than in the zygotes from clonal gametes but substantially less than in the case of cross-fertilization between unrelated parents.

Clonal fertilization occurs where asexually produced individuals (a clone) give rise to gametes that fuse. Whenever fertilization involves two individuals with basically identical genomes, such as two produced simultaneously by an asexual process from one parent (such as polyembryony), the fertilization is not "cross-" but similar to self-fertilization in effect. Clones occur in many classes, where they frequently go undetected, but clonal fertilization occurs principally in those colonial forms where gametes are produced and fertilized from within the clone (Hydrozoa, Anthozoa, Calyssozoa, Phylactolaemata, Gymnolaemata, Pterobranchia, Thaliacea), as well as in animals using polyembryony (especially some Insecta).

Self-fertilization occurs in hermaphrodites when an ovum is fertilized by a spermatozoon produced by the same individual. The gametes are thus from a common genome. It includes autogamy, paedogamy, and cytogamy. It is theoretically possible in most of the classes that include hermaphrodites, even where there is protandry or protogyny. It has been reported in these phyla: Coelenterata, Ctenophora, Platyhelminthes, Rhynchocoela, Nematoda, Bryozoa, Mollusca, Annelida, Arthropoda (Crustacea and Insecta), Chaetognatha, and Vertebrata (Osteichthyes).

It is generally assumed that self-fertilization must be disadvantageous and contrary to evolutionary expectation. It does not seem to be known whether there are any sexual species flourishing without any cross-fertilization, but the skepticism has been expressed as the Knight-Darwin Law, that nature abhors perpetual self-fertilization.

Usually not listed among these processes is the curious case in Crustacea and Asteroidea of polar body fertilization. In spermatogenesis, the two divisions of meiosis produce four haploid spermatozoa. In ovum formation, the two divisions of meiosis produce one ovum and two or three minute cells called polar bodies. These polar bodies are customarily described as nonfunctional, yet in some of these animals one of the polar bodies later fuses with the ovum, acting like a spermatozoon in providing the second (haploid) set of chromosomes and activating the ovum to develop. The resulting diploid cell is exactly comparable to a zygote, yet it does not quite fit the definition of a zygote formed by fusion of an ovum and a spermatozoon.

In Protozoa, because the "adult" (trophozoite or gamont) is unicellular, fertilization can involve either small gametes or the entire "adult" cell. The first is usually called *gamogony* and the second *hologamy,* but there is more diversity than this. A more elaborate scheme distinguishes three forms of fertilization, with one having five subforms: (1) fertilization (or reproduction) by fusion of gametes is *gametogamy,* which occurs in some Flagellata, some Sarcodina (s.Foraminifera), and some Sporozoa; (2) fertilization by fusion of gametes or nuclei derived from the same individual (gamont) is *autogamy,* which occurs in some Sarcodina (s.Heliozoa, s.Foraminifera); (3) fertilization by fusion of the gamonts themselves is *gamontogamy.* In the latter, both in some Foraminifera and some Sporozoa, the process is then followed by gamete formation and a cycle of gamogony. In some Flagellata, the gamontogamy is not followed by gamogony. In many Ciliata and most Suctoria the process is called *conjugation,* which may be *isogamonty* or *anisogamonty,* and the former may be in the form of *mating types* (because conjugation by itself never produces additional individuals, it is discussed under ''Para-Reproduction'' in Chapter 4).

An ovum may be penetrated by more than one spermatozoon, a condition called *polyspermy* (including *dispermy*). Presumably only one spermatozoon takes part in karyogamy, and the purpose of the multiple entry is not clear. It occurs commonly in Insecta and also in some Amphibia. The normal condition is then called *monospermy*.

1. Site of Fertilization

The formation of gametes in the gonads, usually in separate individuals of opposite sex, leaves the problem of bringing the ovum and the spermatozoon together for fertilization to occur. This may involve movement of the ovum to a new location, such as a brood pouch, and always involves movement of the spermatozoon to the ovum. The final location of the ovum determines the site at which fertilization will occur.

The ovum may remain inside the body of the mother *(internal fertilization)* or may pass outside before fertilization. On the outside it may enter a brood pouch or be liberated entirely. The brood pouch is thus an intermediate form in which a liberated ovum is still protected by the mother. Internal fertilization can be brought about by a variety of transmission processes (see list in next section).

Many aquatic animals release gametes into the surrounding water. This takes several forms. Both ova and spermatozoa may be released for chance contact in the water *(external fertilization)*. In some of the kinds in which the eggs are brooded somewhere outside of the reproductive organs of the female (in brood pouches or attached to appendages), fertilization can occur in these sites by the liberated spermatozoa.

In all cases where the spermatozoa are produced in a testis, they must be discharged along some pathway. These can be

1. Sperm ducts, as in mammals (vas deferens)
2. Common gonoducts, as in hermaphrodites of some Oligochaeta
3. From the coelom, via nephridia, as in most Annelida
4. Coelomoducts other than nephridia, as in some Oligochaeta
5. Through the alimentary canal and the mouth, as in Tardigrada and Echiuroidea
6. Rupture of the body wall, as in some Polychaeta
7. Directly through epidermis, as in some Coelenterata

2. Insemination or Spermatozoon Transfer

The methods used to transfer the spermatozoa to the female are unusually diverse, almost unbelievably so. They may not involve any purposeful activity on the part of either the male or the female animal. The principal methods of transfer are these:

Externally

1. By water currents and swimming, where both spermatozoa and ova are discharged into the surrounding water (Coelenterata, s.Ctenophora, s.Rhynchocoela, Priapuloidea, s.Phoronoida, s.Brachiopoda, s.Mollusca, Sipunculoidea, s.Echiuroidea, s.Annelida, s.Echinodermata, Enteropneusta, Pterobranchia, Cephalochordata, s.Vertebrata)

Internally, directly

2. By direct copulation of male and female (s.Gnathostomuloidea, s.Turbellaria, s.Trematoda, Cestoda, Acanthocephala, s.Rhynchocoela, s.Rotifera, s.Gastrotricha, Kinorhyncha, Nematoda, Gordioidea, s.Mollusca, s.Polychaeta, s.Oligochaeta, s.Hirudinea, m.Insecta, m.Vertebrata)

3. By mutual copulation of two hermaphrodites (s.Turbellaria, m.Trematoda, s.Cestoda, s.Oligochaeta)
4. By permanent copulation (s.larval Trematoda)
5. By hypodermic injection through body wall of the female (s.Gnathostomuloidea, s. Turbellaria, s.Rotifera, s.Hirudinea, Dinophiloidea, s.Crustacea)
6. By spermatozoon penetration, by "rotating and writhing" into the partner's body (s.Gnathostomuloidea)
7. By transfer within the body of an hermaphrodite (self-fertilization) (s. Trematoda, m.Cestoda, Phoronida, s.Insecta, s.Chaetognatha)
8. By permanent union of male and female, with sex pores in juxtaposition (s.Trematoda)

Internally, indirectly

9. By water currents to collar cells, which capture them and transfer them to an amoebocyte which carries them to the ova (Porifera)
10. By water currents into the digestive tract and then through the tissues to the ovary (s.Coelenterata, s.Ctenophora, Endoprocta, Bryozoa, s.Brachiopoda, s.Echinodermata)
11. By passage of a spermatophore (packet of spermatozoa); (a) via hectocotylized arm, also called a sematophore, into mouth of female (Cephalopoda), (b) via palpi of male (Arachnida: Phalangida), (c) as a capsule on stalk to be picked up by female (s.Arachnida), (d) as a capsule attached to female body wall (Myzostomida, Onychophora, s.Chaetognatha), (e) as a capsule attached to female gonopore (s.Crustacea), (f) by unspecified methods (s.Gnathostomuloidea, s.Trematoda, s.Rotifera, s.Gastrotricha, s.Gastropoda (slugs), s.Oligochaeta, Hirudinea, Myriapoda, s.Insecta, Pogonophora, s.Amphibia)
12. By artificial insemination of experimental or domesticated animals and humans
13. By parasite residence of a dwarf male in the vagina of the female (Nematoda: *Trichosomoides;* see Hyman, 1951b)
14. By parasitic residence of male inside female gonad (s.Echiuroidea)
15. By implantation of a testis into the female, permanently: organ transplant (s.Crustacea; see Yanagimachi, 1961).

3. Spermatozoon Migration

Where fertilization is internal, the manner in which spermatozoa reach the ova within the body of the female is also diverse. For example:

1. Immediate migration of spermatozoa through the female reproductive tract to the ovum (as in all copulating Vertebrata)
2. Storage of spermatozoa briefly in the female tract, for release as ova are individually laid (m.Insecta)
3. Long-term storage in special organs, until the female becomes reproductive, or until ova mature (which may be many months in some animals) (m.Insecta)
4. Migration of spermatozoa through the body cavity to the ovary, after hypodermic impregnation (Turbellaria, Rotifera)
5. Migration of waterborne spermatozoa from the digestive tract to the gonads (Coelenterata)
6. Transport of spermatozoa by amoebocytes, through the tissues to a sponge ovum (after capture of the spermatozoon in incurrent water by a choanocyte) (Porifera)
7. Movement of spermatozoa by swimming in the blood to the ovaries, from a random site on the body wall where a spermatophore was attached (Onychophora)

8. Conduction of each spermatozoon through the tissues to an ovum by a pair of special cells, the synergids (Chaetognatha)
9. Conduction of masses of spermatozoa through the tissues to the body cavity by syncytial carriers also called synergids (Myzostomida)
10. Conduction from a special "copulatory area" into which a spermatophore is "stabbed" by the male to the ova by a special vector tissue (Hirudinea)

F. Syngamy

Syngamy usually involves the physical penetration of the ovum by the spermatozoon (or at least its head) or the fusion of isogametes, but note that this does not have to include union of the pronuclei. This leads to a definition: *Syngamy* is fusion of two gametes (either anisogametes or isogametes or hologametes) without specification of what happens to the gamete pronuclei. It occurs in most species of most groups of animals, but as a terminal process not followed by fusion of the pronuclei, it is restricted to a few animals that reproduce parthenogenetically but only in the presence of spermatozoa.

Some writers assume that syngamy is the equivalent of fertilization, but, in the section on "Parthenogenesis" in Chapter 4, it will be seen that even when the spermatozoon enters the ovum, the pronuclei may not fuse, and therefore complete fertilization will not occur.

Syngamy, even when restricted to the mechanical penetration of the ovum by the spermatozoon, will also initiate certain processes in the egg. These will include the formation of a fertilization membrane (fertilization envelope). In certain forms of parthenogenesis the processes may also include activation of the ovum to develop.

There is some difficulty over the word "fusion" for the interaction of the gametes. In most animals the ovum is merely penetrated by the head of the spermatozoon, with the middle piece and tail remaining outside; the spermatozoon therefore enters the ovum only partially, rather than fusing with it. For example, in a sporozoan such as *Hyalosporina cambolopsisae,* only the nucleus of the microgamete enters the macrogamete.

The term syngamy can be misleading, because it does not include the cases in which the gametes may not completely merge. Actual complete fusion probably occurs only in the cases of isogametes and hologametes in Protozoa. Thus there are three activities to be specified in fertilization: (1) penetration or fusion of the gametes, (2) fusion of the pronuclei, and (3) activation of the ovum.

It should be clear that the climax of fertilization is not syngamy but karyogamy, which is the fusion of the two gamete *pronuclei* to form a *synkaryon* or *zygote nucleus.* Even this description is simplified and leaves less room for the diversity that actually does occur. Besides the various forms of parthenogenesis (development without karyogamy), there are several ways for diversity to enter the picture. Polyspermy, the entry of more than one spermatozoon, is said to be widespread, although only one pronucleus unites with the ovum pronucleus; the rest sooner or later disintegrate. Such double entry is abnormal and occasional in many Platyhelminthes, Nematoda, Mollusca, Echinodermata, and Mammalia. Double entry is normal in many Insecta and in some members of the other classes of Vertebrata.

The forms of activation without karyogamy are discussed under "Parthenogenesis" in Chapter 4.

One of the results of syngamy is the initiation of changes in the gamete nuclei that prepare them for fusion in the next phase. Although it is usually implied that nuclear fusion follows immediately after penetration by the spermatozoon, there is in reality great diversity over this length of time. The chromosomes of the spermatozoan nucleus may immediately join those from the ovum nucleus on a spindle in preparation for the first mitotic division of the zygote, or the spermatozoan chromosomes may have to await the maturation of the female pronucleus, a process that may take considerable time. The best known example of the latter occurs in the nematode *Ascaris*.

G. Karyogamy

Karyogamy is the fusion of a spermatozoon pronucleus with an ovum pronucleus (also applied to fusion of the nuclei of two isogametes or two hologametes). It is the process actually intended in most references to fertilization.

The definition of karyogamy cannot specify the source of the gamete pronuclei. Thus, karyogamy occurs in cross-fertilization, self-fertilization, autogamy, and hologamy, in all of which gamete pronuclei fuse.

Karyogamy can occur only by fusion of haploid pronuclei. It thus restores diploidy, which was lost in the formation of the gametes.

In all cases the result of karyogamy is a synkaryon, sometimes called *fusion nucleus*, which is the nucleus of the new zygote.

H. Activation

To speak of the beginning of life in bisexual (dioecious) animals as being at fertilization is not satisfactory when dealing with the full spectrum of animals, because many ova develop without fusion with any spermatozoon. The broader term is activation. The following forms occur (with the following being the essential steps):

1. Karyogamy, fusion of the two pronuclei; fertilization in the strict sense (most sexual animals)
2. Spermatozoon penetration without fusion of pronuclei; the entire spermatozoon may then be cast out; penetration provides the stimulus for development (s.Mesozoa, s.Turbellaria, s.Nematoda, s.Mollusca, s.Arthropoda, s.Vertebrata)
3. Spermatozoon presence, without penetration; accompanying substances probably provide the stimulus: (a) insemination by same species without spermatozoon entry (s.Turbellaria), (b) insemination by related species without spermatozoon entry (s.Amphibia)
4. Change of pH or other chemical change around the ovum, apparently includes most routine parthenogenesis: (a) mechanical change such as pricking the egg membranes with a needle; activation may be due to the same change as (4), reaching the ovum through the damaged membrane (s.Echinodermata, m.Vertebrata), (b) presence of males of the same species, without insemination, (c) presence of males of a related species without insemination (s.Reptilia)
5. Fertilization of an ovum by its own polar body (Crustacea, Asteroidea)

Only the first is fertilization, in the genetic/evolutionary sense. In the others there is no male complement of genes added to the ovum. Thus, normal genetic conclusions cannot be drawn about the offspring.

Activation is any process which starts an ovum developing into a new individual. It is part of fertilization, but can also be a separate process in parthenogenesis where there is no fertilization.

The processes that activate either an ovum or a pseudovum are diverse, as listed above. The principal one (with most ova) is karyogamy. In parthenogenesis, items (2) to (5) are methods of activation of the ovum without karyogamy.

1. Zygotes

The *zygote*, often referred to as the fertilized egg, is the end result of fertilization. It is at the same time a new individual and therefore not treated as an organ. It is unicellular and diploid. Although elsewhere there is definition of gametes as detached organs, the zygote or apozygote is a new individual, the start of a new life cycle. Like ova, zygotes are endlessly diverse in their genic endowment but present little visible differences. There are, however, several types of "zygotes", depending on how they are formed. These types and the methods by which they are formed include:

Zygotes

1.   Fusion of the pronuclei of two haploid anisogametes, as in most sexual animals
2.   Fusion of the pronuclei of two haploid isogametes, as in some Sporozoa
3.   Fusion of hologametes, as in some Protozoa (Sarcodina, Flagellata, and Sporozoa)

Apozygotes (see below)

4.   Activation of a haploid ovum with restoration of diploidy in the apozygote
5.   Activation of a diploid pseudovum (to form an apozygote)

Blastomeres (see below)

6.   Cleavage of a zygote into several or many blastomeres that separate to form what are in effect new zygotes

Each of these zygote-like structures is the first stage in the life of a new individual. The development of the individual is discussed in a later chapter.

2. Apozygotes
If a zygote is the result of fusion of two haploid gametes, then the cell formed without fusion by activation of a parthenogenetic ovum cannot be included under that term. The term apozygote is appropriate for this, as a new individual which was apomictic in origin.

3. Blastomeres
In polyembryony, the individual cells produced by the first few cleavages separate and each develops into a new individual. At that instant these blastomeres are thus the counterparts of zygotes, the diploid cell which is the beginning of a new individual.
An additional form of zygote occurs in Protozoa (Sporozoa) under the term *ookinete*. This is a zygote which has developed contractile fibrils to become motile for penetration of the intestinal wall of the host.

III. THE REPRODUCTIVE SYSTEM

A. Prologue
It is highly misleading to imply that sexually reproducing animals have "a reproductive system". In ordinary bisexual animals, individuals of dioecious species will normally have one reproductive "system", either male or female; in monoecious species, each normal individual will have two "systems", one for each sex. There is seldom any direct connection between the two, so they do not together form "a system". Furthermore, in many individual animals the "system" is multiple, consisting of a series of duplicate systems, even a series of systems for each sex.
In the vertebrates it is customary to list as part of the reproductive system not only the gonads and associated organs, but also the hormone system that is a major factor in the control of reproduction. This simply emphasizes that the organ systems of the

body cannot really be considered as isolated systems. In discussing the processes and behavior of reproduction in later sections, we will treat as part of the reproductive *system* only those structures directly, and usually exclusively, concerned with reproduction. Secondarily involved structures will be described principally under the heading of their primary function.

In animals which reproduce only asexually, there is no reproductive system, as there are no discernible permanent devices prepared to produce the new individuals. A possible exception to this is the stolon, whose sole function may be to bud new individuals, but the stolon is often looked upon as a specialized individual rather than an organ. Thus, this section refers principally to the organs of sexual reproduction — either bi- or unisexual.

The structures in the body that are directly involved in reproduction are numerous and of several sorts. The fact that most of them are associated with sexual reproduction, in the broad sense, tends to support the impression that all animals are sexual and that sexual reproduction is universal. These conclusions are not entirely correct, of course, but it is known that nearly all reproductive organs are concerned with bisexual or parthenogenetic reproduction. This results from the simple nature of most asexual reproduction. Of course, the organs of locomotion, coordination, nutrition, etc., also contribute to reproduction.

Diversity appears in these reproductive organs in at least the following ways:

1. Presence or absence of the organ
2. Tissue origin of the organs and of the gametes
3. Arrangement among the individuals: (a) dioecious, (b) monoecious, (c) protandrous, (d), protogynous, (e) simultaneous hermaphroditic
4. Location of the organs in the body: (a) pairing or suppression of one, (b) repetition in segmented body, (c) position among other organs
5. Ducts: (a) number and length, (b) point of discharge, (c) structure (histology), (d) multiple functions (nephridia, etc.)
6. Products: (a) gametes, (b) hormones, (c) accessory spermatozoa, (d) nurse cells, (e) spermatophores, (f) coverings (shells, etc.)
7. Secondary structures in association
8. Permanent or in temporary gonophores
9. Timing: (a) when they are formed, (b) when products are produced, (c) when they disappear as organs, (d) stimuli for these, (e) periodicity in function
10. Dissogony (with two periods of sexual reproduction)
11. Mechanisms to bring gametes together
12. Mechanisms to keep gametes apart

Most of these are discussed in later paragraphs, with examples of their distribution in the animal kingdom.

B. Reproductive Organs

The organs directly concerned with bisexual reproduction and with parthenogenesis are the same. They are the primary organs: gonads and gametes, the secondary organs (ducts, storage devices, and transfer organs), and the collateral structures such as glands, gonophores, and gametophores.

The organs include at least the following:

Primary organs

1. Gonads: (a) ovary, (b) "hermaphroditic gland" (Cestodaria, s.Gastropoda), (c)

testis or spermary or germarium, (d) ovotestis, (e) diffuse or temporary "gonads"
2.   Gametes: (a) ova, (b) spermatozoa, (c) isogametes, (d) hologametes

Secondary organs

3.   Ducts associated with reproduction
4.   Organs associated with the gonads
5.   Organs to serve the gametes: (a) for nutrition, (b) for protection, (c) for storage, (d) for transport (gonophores, etc.), (e) for oviposition
6.   Organs to serve the zygote: (a) for protection (including brooding), (b) for nutrition

This distinction between primary and secondary is not entirely clear-cut, but only gonads and gametes are described as primary organs below. Other structures are cited briefly as secondary (or collateral or associated) organs.

These terms have been somewhat confused in such groups as the insects by another pair of terms. *Primary sex characters* are those of the gonads *and* associated structures, including genitalia. *Secondary sex characters* are other features (of legs, body shape, color) that occur only on females or only on males. These are descriptive terms, not restricted to reproductive organs.

C. Primary Organs

The primary organs of reproduction are usually thought of as including only the gonads. To these can be added the gametes, as being detached unicellular organs; they are even more "primary" than the gonads, but they are usually treated merely as fragments or detached cells.

1. Gonads

In the vast majority of species, where gonads occur, they may be any of the following: testis (or spermary), ovary, ovotestis, or a diffuse area of an epithelium scarcely set off as an organ. In several phyla some species lack male gonads entirely (parthenogenetic) or both male and female gonads (asexual). At least the following occur:

1.   Testis or ovary in different individuals (dioecious)
2.   Testis and ovary in the same individual (monoecious)
3.   Ovotestis, called "hermaphrodite gland" (Rhynchocoela, Nematoda, Amphineura, Gastropoda, Bivalvia, Scaphopoda, Insecta, Asteroidea, Ophiuroidea, Echinoidea, Holothurioidea, Agnatha, Reptilia)
4.   No gonads (in those individuals that do not reproduce)
5.   Sex cells developing in body tissues not forming identifiable gonads (Polychaeta, Oligochaeta, Sipunculoidea, Echiuroidea, Phoronida, Crinoidea)
6.   A single propagatory cell, which at each division produces a cell that becomes an individual *and* a propagatory cell inside that new individual
7.   No gonads or sex cells at any time (all reproduction asexual)

The ovaries are unique in the Acanthocephala. There are one or two in early life, but during development they break up into *ovarian balls,* each consisting of a syncytium from which oogonia are formed. The ova are produced from these and are fertilized in the pseudocoel. Similarly, in females of the insectan group Strepsiptera, the gonads disintegrate and masses of eggs become scattered through the haemocoel; from here they pass out by way of special cuticular invaginations that form funnel-like oviducts.

Gonads are the real reproductive organs, often called the primary reproductive organs. They are usually cited as glandular, but any glandular function is secondary to the production of gametes by cell division.

The gonads in an individual may be arranged in a variety of combinations, including at least some species in each of the following groups:

1. No gonads (Protozoa, Porifera, Mesozoa)
2. Transient tissues (Porifera, Coelenterata, Turbellaria, Polychaeta, Oligochaeta, Sipunculoidea)
3. Single testis (male Tardigrada, Nematoda, Ascidiacea)
4. Single ovary (female Pentastomida, Nematoda, Temnocephaloidea, Tardigrada, Ascidiacea, Vertebrata)
5. Single ovotestis (Cestodaria, Nematoda, Insecta)
6. Paired testes (Nematoda, Insecta, Vertebrata)
7. Paired ovaries (Nematoda, Insecta, Vertebrata)
8. Two testes and one ovary (Trematoda, Acanthocephala)
9. Five testes (male Asteroidea)
10. Five ovaries (female Asteroidea)
11. Nine ovaries and one ovotestis (Asteroidea)
12. Several pairs of testes and several pairs of ovaries arranged in successive segments (Hirudinea)
13. Many pairs of testes (male Rhynchocoela, Hirudinea)
14. Many pairs of ovaries (female Rhynchocoela)
15. Many testes and one ovary (Cestoda)
16. Egg-masses scattered through the body space (Insecta: Strepsiptera) or as fragments adrift in the coelomic fluid (s.Polychaeta)

From this tabulation it should be clear why one cannot use the expression reproductive system. Only a few animals have a single unified system; the rest have two, many, or none. None of the asexual reproduction that occurs in virtually every phylum is performed by anything that can be called a system. In all but the simplest animals, wherever there is sexual reproduction there are organs of reproduction, but much reproduction is accomplished entirely without a definitive reproductive system, or even of special organs.

a. Embryonic Source of Gonads

The various sources of gametes are tabulated later under "Tissue Source of Gametes". Gametes are usually produced directly in the gonads, but occasionally they are not. Much information is lacking, but the known sources are

1. Egg-mother cell — an amoebocyte (Porifera)
2. Gastrodermis — endodermal (Coelenterata)
3. Mesoderm (mesenchyme) — (Turbellaria, Rhynchocoela, Nematoda, Bryozoa, Annelida, s.Arthropoda, Pogonophora, s.Asteroidea, Enteropneusta, m.Vertebrata, and probably most other animals)

b. Position of Gonads in the Body

The location of the gonads involves at least three factors: their embryonic origin, the cavity or tissue in which they are situated in the adult, and the number of gonads developed. The first and third of these have been dealt with above.

Ovaries and testes are generally located as follows:

1. None: (a) gametes form in mesenchyme tissues (Porifera, s.Turbellaria), (b) gametes form in peritoneum (Polychaeta, Bryozoa)
2. In epidermis (Hydrozoa)
3. In gastrodermis in general (Scyphozoa)
4. In gastrodermis of the septa and gastral filaments (Anthozoa)
5. In walls of digestive canals (Ctenophora)
6 In mesenchyme (m.Platyhelminthes, Rhynchocoela)
7. In pseudocoel (Rotifera, Gastrotricha, Kinorhyncha, Nematoda, Gordioidea, Calyssozoa, Acanthocephala)
8. In coelom, on peritoneum
9. In coelomic epithelium in the visceral mass, one or a pair (Mollusca, Pentastomida)
10. In haemocoel, one or a pair (Arthropoda)

2. Gametes

In keeping with our belief that an organ may be unicellular and that such detached objects as proglottids are organs, gametes are here classed as (detached) organs. (They are organized bodies performing a specific function, and they are *not* separate individuals.)

Gametes are produced by division of other cells, usually from gonadal tissue. The latter may be simply mesenchyme cells in the wall of the body cavity, or they are (in most animals) special cells in special organs called gonads. A gonad may produce spermatozoa (spermary, testis) or ova (ovary) or both (ovotestis, "gonad").

There are five types of "gametes": (1) isogametes, (2) spermatozoa, (3) ova that require fertilization, (4) ova that do not require fertilization, and (5) hologametes. They can be tabulated thus:

1. Isogametes, all alike in size and shape
   a. Haploid by meiosis (s.Sporozoa)
   b. Haploid without meiosis in gametogenesis, from haploid individuals in which zygotic meiosis always occurs (Sporozoa, s.Flagellata)
   c. Ploidy and meiosis unspecified (s.Flagellata, m.Sarcodina)
2. Spermatozoa or microgametes
   d. Haploid by meiosis of two divisions (most sexual animals)
   e. Haploid by meiosis of one division (Protozoa)
   f. Haploid without meiosis (zygotic meiosis in some Protozoa)
3. Ova or macrogametes
   g. Haploid by meiosis of two divisions and that will be fertilized (most sexual animals)
   h. Haploid by meiosis of two divisions but will not be fertilized: meiotic parthenogenesis (some species in most groups)
   i. Haploid with meiosis of one division (some Protozoa)
   j. Haploid without meiosis (zygotic meiosis in s.Protozoa)
   k. Pseudova, diploid "ova" in ameiotic parthenogenesis (in several groups)
4. Hologametes
   l. Whole protozoan individuals that fuse permanently (some Protozoa)

Not to be confused with gametes are two types of asexual reproductive bodies. Both spores (Protozoa) and agametes (Mesozoa) are diploid and do not fuse.

Gametes are produced by most species of animals, but there are still thousands in which they are not. The exceptions include:

1. Most members of the classes Flagellata and Suctoria, all of the class Ciliata, and some of the class Sarcodina, including most of the order Lobosa and all of the order Heliozoa
2. A few species of Hydrozoa
3. At least one species in Turbellaria *(Dugesia gonocephala)*
4. Some species of Bryozoa (Phylactolaemata)
5. One species of Polychaeta *(Ctenodrilus)*
6. Some members of two families of Oligochaeta

In most colonial groups and some others there are also many individuals that never produce gametes, because they reproduce asexually or not at all. These include:

1. Flagellata (many species)
2. Hydrozoa (hydranths)
3. Scyphozoa (strobila)
4. Anthozoa (siphonozooids)
5. Bryozoa (ancestrula, avicularia, vibracula, kenozooids, nannozooids)
6. Insecta (honeybee workers)
7. Pterobranchia (neuter zooids)
8. Tunicata (oozooids)

a. Tissue Source of Gametes

Gametes are produced only by division of pre-existing cells. These cells may occur in specialized organs, be scattered through certain tissues, or they may apparently arise as needed from certain tissues. Their embryonic origin is usually not clear and it is diverse among the phyla, but their functional location may be one of these:

1. In gonads: (a) ovaries (most classes of animals), (b) testes (spermaries) (most classes of animals), (c) ovotestes (in some species of Rhynchocoela, Nematoda, Calyssozoa, Mollusca, Annelida, Insecta, Echinodermata, Vertebrata: Cyclostomata)
2. In epithelial linings of body cavities: (a) gastrodermis (s.Hydrozoa), (b) epidermis (s.Hydrozoa), (c) peritoneum (Bryozoa)
3. In mesenchyme as free cells (s.Turbellaria: Acoela)
4. Interstitial cells (s.Hydrozoa)

Gametes thus may develop from any of the three germ layers (see epidermis and gastrodermis in Hydrozoa and mesenchyme in Turbellaria). They may be set aside very early in development, quite late, or may be produced from tissue cells as needed. From this it must be concluded that there is no sharp distinction between somatoplasm and germplasm in animals as a whole, as was once thought.

b. Isogametes

Isogametes are gametes that are structurally alike, but it seems clear that they are physiologically of two types and thus are different from anisogametes only in visible features. It is thus likely that one of each physiological type must be involved in fertilization. These gametes occur only in Protozoa (Flagellata, Sarcodina, and Sporozoa).

In the flagellate *Chlamydomonas perty,* there are many divisions resulting in many haploid isogametes, which fuse in pairs. In some other species the "isogametes" are diploid until after coming together, when they each extrude part of their chromatin. In still other species individuals are often haploid and produce isogametes without meiosis; after fusion the diploid zygote undergoes meiosis to become a new haploid individual.

The formation of the isogametes is apparently always by multiple fission, producing many gametes and resulting in destruction of the adult individual.

c. Anisogametes

This clumsy word refers to gametes that are not alike — spermatozoon and ovum. By analogy it must also include the ovum in parthenogenesis, because it is presumed that the second gamete, if it were present, would be a spermatozoon.

The anisogametes, which are the only form in many Protozoa and all Metazoa, are often assumed to be identical in all groups in consisting of relatively tiny spermatozoa that are motile by means of flagella and relatively huge yolky ova that are not motile, but with both forms showing considerable diversity. Obviously, no matter how much alike the spermatozoa of any two widely different kinds of animals are, in all visible ways, they must be strikingly different in their genes, which must produce all the different features of the two life cycles.

d. Spermatozoa

Spermatozoa are the male anisogametes. They are always smaller than ova of the same species and are also called microgametes. Spermatozoa are produced by individuals called males; thus they are also called male gametes.

In many animals, the spermatozoon is a motile, flagellated cell consisting of a head, a neck, a middle piece, and the flagellar tail. The head contains a nucleus and an acrosome or apical body, the neck (absent in many) contains centrioles and the beginning of the axial filament, the middle piece or connecting piece carries the axial filament with its mitochondrial sheath, the flagellum or tail consists of a pars principalis (which is the greater part of the flagellum through which the axial filament traverses), and an end piece which consists of the axial filament without covering envelopes.

The similarity of all spermatozoa has been exaggerated. Diversity appears in several ways. The sizes and shapes of the different parts present a considerable variety. Although the flagellated spermatozoa are most common, there are several diversities, as shown in Figure 4 and the list below.

A striking similarity among most spermatozoa is that the tail (flagellum) always consists of a shaft made up of a ring of nine pairs of tubular fibrils surrounding a central pair, which is the almost universal ultrastructure of all flagella and cilia in animals.

Spermatozoa may differ in gross form in these ways:

1. One flagellum (most groups except those cited below)
2. Two flagella (s.Sporozoa, s.Trematoda, s.Turbellaria, s.Polychaeta, s.Crustacea)
3. Many flagella (s.Trematoda, s.Gastropoda)
4. No flagellum: (a) amoeboid (Nematoda, s.Crustacea, Merostomata), (b) with stiff radiating processes (s.Crustacea), (c) with chitinous "explosive" capsule (s.Crustacea), (d) other forms (s.Turbellaria, s.Gnathostomuloidea, s.Archiannelida, s.Chilopoda, s.Arachnida, Acarina, s.Insecta)
5. Presence and form of the "middle piece"
6. Unusually large headed (s.Insecta)
7. Without nucleus (but with chromosomes) (s.Gastropoda, s.Insecta)
8. With less than normal number of chromosomes (s.Gastropoda)
9. Conjugate or double spermatozoa (s.Insecta)

Many other striking differences are found, from those that are extremely slender and elongate to those having short tails and bulbous heads. Some even show extending

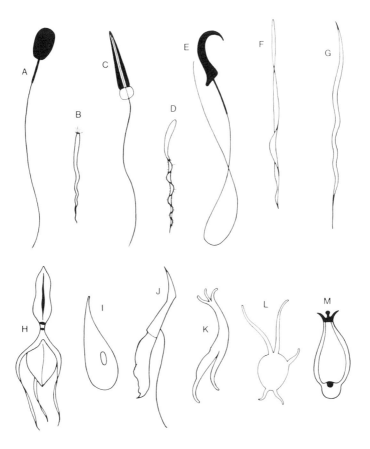

FIGURE 4. The diversity of spermatozoa. A,E, mammals; B,D,F,G, turbellarians; C, bivalve; H,J,K, crustaceans; I,M, nematodes.

hook-like acrosomes. Others appear to be double, with two heads or two tails. The middle piece may consist of a ring of spheroidal bodies, may be so short as to seem absent, or may be longer than the tail and appear spiralled. An oddity occurs in the form of an "explosive sperm" in some Crustacea: the "explosion" ejects a chitinous capsule, which presumably aids in penetration into the ovum.

Spermatozoa are apparently always produced in large numbers, but they may be "packaged" in various ways. In mammals, spermatozoa in the epididymis may be "in rouleaux", i.e., clumped in masses with all the tails protruding in one direction. In a few Gastropoda, Insecta, and Mammalia, spermatozoa may "conjugate", forming a temporary dual structure. In some Insecta, the spermatozoa are temporarily held in bundles by an elaborate corkscrew-shaped sheath. When packed in the spermatheca of some insects, the spermatozoa are aligned in one direction with their flagella beating synchronously. In many groups, spermatozoa are packed into spermatophores, for ease of transmission to the female.

e. Polymorphism of Spermatozoa

In many animals all the spermatozoa produced by the members of a species are indistinguishable externally or internally (except for the varying gene combinations). However, a variety of animals produce visibly different forms of spermatozoa as follows. In some there is sexual dimorphism, especially in the number of chromosomes. In Nematoda the spermatozoa may have either 5 or 6 chromosomes, being cited as male- and female-producing, respectively. Similar situations occur in some Insecta, Arachnida, Chilopoda, and Mammalia.

In some Nematoda, Rhynchocoela, Annelida, Insecta, Amphibia, Aves, and Mammalia there may be two classes of spermatozoa with respect to their head size or the size of their nuclei. This is termed *dimegaly* or *polymegaly*.

In some Gastropoda there may be oligopyrene (worm-shaped) and eupyrene (hair-shaped) spermatozoa. These are probably pathological rather than normal differences.

In some Monogononta (Rotifera), two kinds of spermatozoa are found: typical flagellated and atypical spermatozoa that are rod-shaped; these are believed to help penetrate the cuticle of the female during hypodermic impregnation.

Wilson (1953) reported: "A remarkable phenomenon is the regular occurrence in certain animals of "twin sperms" or "double sperms", consisting of two sperms closely united by their heads, leaving the tails more or less free . . . ." These are called conjugate spermatozoa. They occur in the beetle *Dytiscus* (Insecta) and in the mammal *Didelphys*.

f. Ova

An ovum is a female gamete; it is haploid and normally must be fertilized to start its further development. Where there are two sharply different gametes, the ovum is the one that is larger, it contains food reserves, is (usually) nonmotile, and is produced at the rate of one per mother cell. There are still several difficulties. When one thinks of the eggs of birds, turtles, praying mantises, and humans, one sees that there is diversity. The picture is somehow obscure, because the word egg has been used for several different things.

First, we must make a distinction between the ovum and an egg. An egg can be any of several things, but in the varying usages of different books the word is often used in place of ovum, especially by students of vertebrates. It is also applied to the hard shell of some eggs, being then roughly equivalent to eggshell. For example, in Acanthocephala, ova are produced in the pseudocoel and are released "when ripe", but at this time they already contain a mature acanthor larva. The change from ovum to egg came at fertilization but is often not recognizable.

Second, some reproductive bodies that appear to be ova are in fact diploid and cannot be fertilized. They otherwise differ from ova only in requiring activation by some means other than fertilization (see "Activation", above). They thus are parthenogenetic and are herein distinguished under the term pseudova.

The word egg is familiar for those animals in which the ovum is enclosed in a tough membrane or shell, and it is really this protective covering which is the "egg". In the case of the domestic chicken, the egg not only encloses the fertilized ovum but continues to enclose the embryo and baby chick that develops inside it.

It is clear that more careful use of terms is required if we are to communicate about these various structures. The following are the minimum terms necessary:

1. A haploid female gamete (an ovum)
2. A diploid female "gamete" (a pseudovum)
3. A fused spermatozoon and ovum (a zygote)
4. An activated pseudovum (an apozygote)
5. An encased ovum (an egg)
6. An encased zygote (a fertile egg)
7. An encased pseudovum (an egg)
8. An encased apozygote (an egg)
9. An encased embryo (an embryonated egg)
10. The investing capsule alone (an eggshell or tough egg membrane, regardless of how produced) (see next section)

The ovum is a cell with a membrane and a variety of internal organelles, but it seems never to be ciliated. It may have one or more coverings in the form of membranes or shells, some produced by the ovum itself. It is often furnished with a pore or micropile through the coverings, through which the spermatozoon may enter, although in other animals penetration at random position seems to occur before the extra coverings are formed.

As an object, there is often no way to distinguish an unfertilized from a fertilized ovum, and it would usually not be possible to distinguish a parthenogenetic ovum from one which will be or has been fertilized. In some animals a given ovum can develop with or without fertilization.

The extremely unequal divisions of meiosis result in the formation of a single ovum that contains all the yolk that otherwise would have been distributed among the four cells. This is one of the ways in which the developing zygote is provided with the necessary yolk food.

g. Diversity of Ova

Hidden above is the first diversity of ova, that some must eventually be placed in a protective capsule and others can remain comparatively naked. This is obviously related to where the eventual egg is to be, because, if the ovum or early embryo is "laid" (deposited on objects) or shed (liberated into water), it will need more protection than if it remains in the body of the mother. Thus, many developing ova are surrounded by protective coverings (see below).

Aside from the capsule there is little obvious diversity among ova. Nevertheless, ova are diverse in several ways:

1. Shape: spherical, oblong, or with their associated shells or other coverings forming a wide variety of shapes
2. Polarity: isotropy, without predetermined axis, and anisotropy, having a predetermined axis
3. Size
4. Surface texture and sculpturing
5. Association with nurse cells
6. Yolk content: quantity, quality, and location
7. Genome content
8. Ovum coverings
9. Ovum motility

h. Polymorphism of Ova

Ova may occur in a species in two or even three distinct forms, even produced by a single female at different times of the year. For example:

1. Winter and summer eggs — (s.Turbellaria, s.Rotifera, s.Crustacea)
2. Tachyblastic and opsiblastic eggs — in favorable and unfavorable environmental conditions (s.Gastrotricha)
3. Subitaneous and dormant eggs — both parthenogenetic (s.Gastrotricha)
4. Thin- and thick-shelled eggs — (s.Tardigrada)
5. Amictic (parthenogenetic) eggs, mictic but unfertilized eggs, and dormant (fertilized mictic) eggs — (s.Rotifera)

These sets of terms do not all represent different things. (1) to (4) are essentially the same, produced in response to environmental conditions. Number (5) is distinct and is at least partly independent of environment.

Such polymorphisms occur among the phyla thus:

1.   Turbellaria — winter and summer (subitaneous)
2.   Rotifera — mictic (winter, resting, fertilizable), amictic (summer, subitaneous, parthenogenetic), and dormant mictic (fertilizable to produce gametes)
3.   Gastrotricha — normal and dormant; tachyblastic and opsiblastic
4.   Dinophiloidea — larger (female-producing) and smaller (male-producing)
5.   Crustacea — summer (subitaneous) and winter
6.   Insecta — two forms, rarely, differing in chromosome number
7.   Aves — two forms differing in nuclear constitution

i. Motility of Ova

Ova are usually said to be immobile, in contradistinction to the motile spermatozoa. In at least four very distinct groups there are ova that show amoeboid movement at least during part of their life. These groups are the Porifera, Hydrozoa, pulmonate Gastropoda, and Insecta.

j. Yolk

Although there is much diversity in the amount and nature of yolk in animal ova (eggs), this feature is not clearly related to reproduction. Although development of the zygote is strikingly correlated with the amount and position of the yolk, the diversity of yolk itself is herein discussed principally in Chapter 13, under "Nutrients for Ovum and Zygote".

k. Egg Coverings

Ova are not merely masses of unprotected protoplasm. They are always surrounded by a plasma membrane and usually by other protective coverings. When fertilized (or activated) the ovum becomes a zygote (egg), which may have the same coverings as the ovum or additional ones. Some of these may persist to enclose the embryo.

Of these various coverings some are produced by the ovum itself, some by tissues of the ovary, and some by tissues of the genital ducts or organs attached thereto. There is not enough information about the sequence and origin of these investments to deal with them comparatively, but they include the following in various groups: vitelline membrane, jelly layer, chorion, shell, ootheca, cocoon, and zona pellucida.

Coverings produced by maternal tissues include at least the following:

1.   Cell membrane — of the ovum, formed during division from the cell membrane of the oogonium, often called vitelline membrane or plasma membrane (all groups)
2.   Shell — formed in the ootype (s.Turbellaria, Trematoda, Cestoda)
3.   Gelatinous envelope — secreted by epidermis of the mother (some Rhynchocoela)
4.   Mucinous or albuminous coats — (s.Mammalia)
5.   Protein membrane — outside of shell (Nematoda)
6.   Zona pellucida — (Mammalia)
7.   Chorion — chitinous or horny (Anthozoa, Gastrotricha, Amphineura, Cephalopoda, Tardigrada, Insecta)
8.   Ephippium — a pouch-like extra shell in winter eggs of Crustacea: Cladocera
9.   Cocoon — around some egg masses, as in Turbellaria, some Oligochaeta, and some Insecta
10.   Albumen layer — (Reptilia, Aves, s.Mammalia)
11.   Ootheca — (s.Mollusca, s.Insecta)
12.   Egg capsule — (s.Turbellaria, s.Trematoda, Rhynchocoela, s.Mollusca, Dinophiloidea, s.Pisces)

13. Layer of nematocysts — (s.Hydrozoa)
14. Jelly layers — (m.Amphibia)

Coverings produced by the ovum include at least these:

1. Fertilization membrane — (probably all animals)
2. Lipoid membrane — (Nematoda)
3. Shell — (Turbellaria)
4. Zona radiata — (Annelida, Vertebrata)
5. Jelly layer — (Mollusca, Vertebrata, etc.)

Apparently all ova have a cell membrane. When fertilized there is also a fertilization membrane. Further membranes or shells may be furnished by the maternal tissues, or membranes may be formed by the ovum, the fertilized egg, or by the embryo either inside or outside of previous ones. Some examples are cited.

Platyhelminthes. A shell is produced by the maternal tissues. "The turbellarian *Bothrioplana* is parthenogenetic . . . with one ovum from each ovary uniting and combining with cells of the vitellarium to form a cocoon" (Henley, 1974).

Rhynchocoela. Ova in viviparous and self-fertilized species may remain in the ovaries until hatching, covered by a cell membrane, a fertilization membrane, and the ovarian tissues. In other species the ova, with these same two cell membranes, are laid in gelatinous masses.

Acanthocephala. A membranous "shell" is produced by the ovum itself.

Rotifera. One or two membranes, which are probably the cell and fertilization membranes; these are inside an evident shell, formed by the egg. Outside the shell there may be an additional thin membrane or a gelatinous envelope.

Nematoda. The fertilization membrane thickens to form a shell. Inside of this shell, the egg produces a lipoid membrane, which is thin and delicate. The uterine wall may add a protein membrane outside of the shell.

Cephalopoda. The egg in its fertilization membrane is covered just before discharge by a paired membrane or capsule from the oviducal gland. A gelatinous outer covering may be added from a nidamental gland, which later may harden into a capsule.

Insecta. The ovum forms a cell membrane termed the vitelline membrane. Outside of this a shell (or chorion) is formed by the follicular epithelium of the mother. The chorion may consist of two layers, an exochorion and an endochorion. The chorion may be penetrated by one or more micropyles, or it may have an operculum for the eventual release of the larva.

Vertebrata. In addition to the plasma and fertilization membranes, an amnion, a chorion, and a yolk sac may be formed in differing sequences by the developing embryo. The allantois appears still later in development, formed from the archenteron and surrounding mesoderm.

It is usually not possible to tell visually whether a given egg capsule contains an ovum, a pseudovum, a zygote, an apozygote, an embryo, or even a larva ready to hatch. It may also contain yolk cells, spicules, nematocysts, or nutritive substances other than yolk. It may also contain more than one zygote, as in several Turbellaria, where they are called composite eggs.

Many animals produce more than one kind of "egg". Presumably these differences must have existed also in the ova before fertilization. Various terms, such as mictic/amictic and winter/summer have been applied. Because these features are usually treated as part of development, and because the terms are usually not applied to ova as such, this subject will be treated in the chapters on development.

l. Ovum Types and Terms

Many terms are applied to ova (and eggs) to distinguish various features. Some of these have already been cited (see also the yolk terms listed in Chapter 13):

1. Amictic ovum — one that will not be fertilized
2. Cleidoic egg — one that is enclosed in a moisture-proof enclosure (Aves)
3. Dormant ovum — usually thick-shelled and destined to remain for some time before developing (s.Coelenterata, s.Turbellaria)
4. Ephippial egg — the winter egg of Cladocera (Crustacea)
5. Isotropic ovum — one without a predetermined axis
6. Mictic ovum — one that may be fertilized; mictic egg, one that has been fertilized
7. Opsiblastic egg — one thick-shelled for weather resistance; winter or resting egg (Gastrotricha)
8. Resting egg — one that is thick-shelled and fertilized, that hatches after dormancy (s.Rotifera, s.Crustacea)
9. Subitaneous egg — one thin-shelled and destined to hatch promptly (s.Turbellaria)
10. Summer egg — parthenogenetic; see subitaneous egg (s.Rotifera, s.Turbellaria, s.Crustacea)
11. Tachyblastic egg — one that hatches rapidly (Gastrotricha)
12. Winter egg — resting egg, dormant egg (s.Rotifera, s.Crustacea)

m. Pseudova

There are two types of reproductive bodies comparable to ova that are formed in an ovary but do not require fertilization. They are of two sorts: (1) haploid ova — produced by oogenesis with meiosis, but which nevertheless can develop without fertilization; they restore diploidy in some other manner; and (2) diploid "ova" — (pseudova) produced without meiosis; they can be activated by some method other than fertilization.

Both of these are the "ova" of parthenogenesis, the first meiotic and the second ameiotic. For the first, there is no special term, especially as many haploid ova can develop either with or without fertilization. Thus, all haploid female gametes are covered by the term ova. For the second, where there will be no mixis, the term pseudova is appropriate. Both of these develop into zygotes, but because of the lack of mixis the term apozygote is used with pseudova.

n. Hologametes

In some Protozoa (Flagellata, Sarcodina), whole individuals may fuse into one in the manner of gametes. This is different from conjugation, because the fusion is complete and permanent. The process of hologamy is sometimes listed as reproductive, but as it produces no additional individuals it scarcely fits our definition. However, it does produce a new (i.e., changed) individual and therefore is one of those sexual processes that are here called para-reproductive.

It is clear that some processes such as meiosis have served to make these fusing individuals haploid; it is reported that they are usually not exactly the same size, one being smaller than the other.

In the flagellate *Copromonas subtilis,* there is a complete nuclear and cytoplasmic fusion of the two hologametes. However, the individuals had each previously cast off a portion of its nuclear material, presumably thus becoming haploid. After fusion, the zygote contains a diploid synkaryon.

D. Secondary Organs

Secondary organs are those that directly assist the gonads in the formation and delivery of gametes, and they may also continue to function in relation to the developing zygote and embryo. They are so numerous and so diverse that they are difficult to classify. Among them are ducts and pores and nutritional systems; transfer organs to place the spermatozoa into the female; storage devices for spermatozoa, yolk, seminal fluid, or shell material; glands to produce these materials and others; and packaging devices such as spermatophores.

The secondary organs may serve the gonads as ducts, glands, and storage devices, they may serve the gametes as nutritive mechanisms and packaging devices, or they may serve to facilitate delivery of the gametes to the fertilization site. They are here briefly cited according to their function.

1. Male Gonoducts

Some testes open directly to the outside without any duct, but in most animals the spermatozoa are carried to the discharge point by ducts of considerable length. In vertebrates these are called *vas efferens* and *vas deferens*. In invertebrates they are usually called *sperm ducts* (other ducts may also be involved in spermatozoan movement; see below). These ducts are single, paired or multiple to correspond with the number of testes present.

Sperm ducts occur in most male animals, with some parts given special terms. There is one duct from each testis, often uniting to a single common duct, but there are five in most Echinodermata. There may be as many as four segmental pairs, each with duct, in Oligochaeta. These ducts may open independently to the outside (in many groups) or they may open into the pericardium (Mollusca), into the intestine (s.Nematoda), or directly through the remnants of the stomodaeum (Echiuroidea).

The duct may be very short or absent (s.Pisces), with the spermatozoa discharged into the body cavity, from which they escape via the nephridia (Priapuloidea, Phoronida, Xenoturbellida, and Cyclostomata). They are called vasa deferentia in such groups as Cestoda, Nematoda, Hirudinea, Insecta, and Chaetognatha, but such terms have only very general meanings. In these Chaetognatha this duct consists of just two cells, which become hollow to form a short tube.

In Ctenophora, the sperm ducts lead to a pore in the epidermis; there may be one such duct or as many as 600 in one individual.

In *Petrobius* (Insecta: Thysanura) "each vas deferens is double throughout the greater part of its course, the two canals thus formed being united by a series of fine transverse connecting tubes" (Imms, 1930). No special function is known for this ladder-like duct.

2. Female Gonoducts

The products of the ovary normally leave by a duct system usually called *oviduct*. In some animals this system consists of distinct parts, such as an oviduct nearest the ovary, a *uterus* where ova are often stored, and a *vagina* which is often more properly part of the sperm-receiving system. The ovary may have no duct at all, discharging into the body cavity directly, as in some Rotifera, Polychaeta, and all Amphibia, or to the outside as in Hydrozoa.

Ovaries may not discharge their ova, holding them until fertilized and then allowing the zygotes to escape (or even brooding them).

When oviducts are present, there will be one for each ovary. They may unite to form a single uterus, or the entire system may be paired or multiple so that there are two or more uteri.

Oviducts also occur in most groups. They lead from the ovary to an external gonopore in many, but may open into the pericardium (as in Mollusca) or into a uterus (Trematoda, Cestoda, Gastrotricha, Nematoda, s.Mollusca, Pentastomida, Vertebrata), or into a vagina (Hirudinea, Chaetognatha). They may open into the body cavity, with the ova then escaping via nephridia (Priapuloidea, Phoronida, Brachiopoda, and Sipunculoidea). They may be absent in Porifera, Xenoturbellida, and Cyclostomata. There may be one for each ovary (up to 5 as in Echinodermata) or a common duct.

In general, distal parts of the duct may be modified for various purposes and then be called uterus or vagina. And they may open by an exterior gonopore or into the digestive tract as the cloaca. In Bryozoa there may be an intertentacular organ, a temporary oviduct formed from the dorsal tentacles.

In both Priapuloidea and many Vertebrata both the male and the female ducts are referred to merely as urinogenital ducts. In some Gastropoda the combined male and female duct is called an hermaphrodite duct, which opens into the mantle cavity.

Oviducts are sometimes formed by nephridia. One or more pairs may be modified to serve this function, or the structure may be a nephromixium and serve both excretory and oviducal functions, as in some Echiuroidea and some Polychaeta.

In Chaetognatha, "the oviduct is composed of a cuboidal to cylindrical epithelium. Inside the oviduct there is another tube with syncytial wall that extends posteriorly into . . . the seminal receptacle" (Hyman, 1959). Neither tube connects to the ovary, but spermatozoa pass up the inner tube and fertilize the ovum, which then passes down the outer tube to an undiscovered exit.

A most unusual organ called a uterine bell operates with the oviduct in Acanthocephala. "Eggs" coming down the duct are sorted (by size) into mature and immature ones. The mature ones pass to the vagina and outside; "immature eggs are rejected and returned via an aperture in the ventral bell to the dorsal pseudocoele" (Smyth, 1976).

3. Gonopores

Although gonoducts do not always open to the exterior of the body (e.g., into the cloaca), they generally do so, and the word gonopore is here restricted to such external openings.

The almost endless diversity in the number of gonads per individual, partially tabulated above, is to some extent reflected in the number of gonoducts and thus of gonopores. There may be one per gonad, which means from one duct or one pair to pairs in each segment and to many temporary pores formed when each gonad is mature. There may even be pores for each sex in one individual. Two or more gonads may have ducts merging into a common duct, so that the single or few pairs of pores may serve many gonads. In hermaphrodites the paired male and female organs may open through a single common pore. In addition to the usual female genital opening, a few Crustacea (parasitic Copepoda) have a special opening for copulation; it admits spermatozoa into the spermatheca (see Markewitch, 1976).

There is much diversity, even within some groups as to how the eggs reach the outside, but the following are among the groups in which there are no external female genital pores, in which other exits are utilized:

1.   Osculum (Porifera)
2.   Epidermis rupture (s.Coelenterata)
3.   Proctostome (s.Coelenterata, s.Ctenophora, and apparently the Xenoturbellida)
4.   Body wall rupture (s.Turbellaria, presumed also in Cestoda: Aporidea)
5.   Mouth (s.Turbellaria)
6.   Nephridia (females of Priapuloidea, Phoronida)
7.   Antrum (genital atrium) (Temnocephaloidea)
8.   Cloaca (s.Rotifera, s.Tardigrada, Myzostomida, Aves)

4. Nutritional Organs

Nutrition of the ovum is outlined in Chapter 13 on the digestive system. It is generally accomplished through the inclusion in the ovum of yolk (deutoplasm). The organs that provide the nutritives are of two main types as in these examples, but terms are used loosely:

Yolk cells or glands

1. Vitelline cells — (s.Turbellaria, s.Insecta)
2. Nurse cells — (Porifera, Coelenterata, Ctenophora, Platyhelminthes, Rotifera, Mollusca, Annelida, Arthropoda, Echinodermata, Tunicata, Cephalochordata, Vertebrata)
3. Rhorocyte — (Scyphozoa)
4. Yolk glands — (Trematoda)
5. Vitellarium — (s.Turbellaria, Rotifera)
6. Germovitellarium — (s.Turbellaria, s.Rotifera)

Placentas

7. Uterine secretions through a placenta in the uterine wall (s.Onychophora)
8. Uterine blood vessels in a placenta (m.Mammalia)
9. Periblast implantation (m.Vertebrata)
10. Diffusion placenta (Tunicata)
11. Brood pouch (s.Protozoa: Suctoria)
12. Marsupium (s.female Crustacea)
13. "Placenta" (s.Porifera)

Excess gametes phagocytized

14. Ova (or oocytes) (s.Platyhelminthes)
15. Spermatozoa (may be phagocytized but do not supply yolk)

The embryos of many animals can feed at an early stage. In Porifera some blastulae can engulf surrounding cells. In many Platyhelminthes yolk may be supplied from the vitelline glands as the ovum is fertilized and enclosed in a shell by the ootype. In Hydrozoa the yolk may be obtained by ingestion of neighboring cells. In animals with a placenta nutrients are obtained from the mother.

5. Storage Organs

Storage devices for spermatozoa are diverse. They include the following examples:

In the male before transfer

1. In a seminal vesicle (Nemertodermatida, Trematoda, Rhynchocoela, Nematoda, Cephalopoda, s.Annelida, Insecta)
2. In coelomic sperm sacs (Oligochaeta, Pogonophora)
3. In a coiled epididymis (Hirudinea, Mammalia)
4. In a spermiducal vesicle (s.Turbellaria)

In the female after transfer

5. In bursa copulatrix, receptaculum seminis, seminal receptacle, or spermatheca (most groups in which insemination of the female occurs)

6.   In ovisac (s.Oligochaeta)
7.   In ovarian epithelium in such Pisces as *Heterandra formosa,* where immobilized
       spermatozoa may remain alive for months.

Organs (5) to (7) do not seem to form an homologous group, but their nature is
seldom made clear. Different authors use different terms in a given group, and there
seem to be no reasonably distinctive definitions. They are all simply organs of the
female which usually or sometimes are involved in storage of spermatozoa.

In some animals it is known that spermatozoa have a short life, so storage time is
short. In others, they may be stored in the female for use in successive cycles of ovum
production, thus retaining their potency for as much as 6 years. In still other groups
the spermatozoa may survive for several months in the male system, but even these
may die quickly after transfer into the female if they do not soon fertilize an ovum.

Ova are seldom directly stored, but in free-living marine Nematoda the Demanian
system has been thought by some to store ova, but there is also doubt. In Polychaeta
there may be a "coelomic storage organ". In Oligochaeta there may be an ovisac for
temporary storage of ova. No doubt marine animals that spawn large quantities of ova
at one time also store the ova briefly in the oviduct or uterus. The materials used in the
formation of the "egg" are usually stored in the lumen of the gland that produces
them.

6. Associated Glands

The glands associated with sexual reproduction produce yolk and other materials to
be incorporated into the egg, fluids to carry the spermatozoa or to nourish them when
stored, substances to form eggshells or cases, adhesives, lubricants, and chemical messengers (both hormones and pheromones). The following are examples:

Shell glands. In a wide variety of animals whose eggs leave the body of the mother
before fertilization or immediately therafter, one of the coverings is hardened enough
to be called a shell. It is produced in the oviduct, uterus, or ootype with materials from
a shell gland. A supplementary egg covering may be secreted in some Insecta by an
accessory gland called a corysterium.

The Mehlis' gland in Trematoda apparently secretes lubricants into the oviduct.

In Mammalia, there are two sets of glands that contribute to the seminal fluid; these
are the single prostate gland and a pair of small Cowper's glands. The seminal fluid
provides a medium for the swimming spermatozoa and materials for their metabolism.
The term prostate gland is used for glands in several aberrant groups of flatworms
(Nemertodermatida, Temnocephalida) and in Monogononta (Rotifera).

Glands may secrete the cover of a spermatophore or any of the various egg cases,
such as oothecae or cocoons.

IV. GONOPHORES AND GAMETOPHORES

A. Comments

The gametes may be enclosed in either of two ways: (1) by isolation of a body section
to carry the gonads, a gonophore, or (2) by enclosure of one or more gamete in a
separate carrier, a gametophore. It is well known that spermatozoa are sometimes
transferred from the male to the female in a container called a spermatophore. It is
much less common for eggs to be packaged in an oophore. Because the same coverings
are often involved, it can also be cited that there are zygotophores and even embryophores.

B. Gonophores

Structures are formed in a few animals in which the entire sexual reproductive apparatus is situated. This is a special portion of the body that becomes detached. These fragments that contain the gonads are alive and continue to perform appropriate functions (gametogenesis, metabolism, locomotion). They are not here considered to be separate individuals but merely detached organs. They include proglottids and epitokes.

The usual place for gonads is in the body cavity of the individual. There are exceptions of a curious type. Somtimes part of the body, including part of the internal organs, is separated off as a partitioned unit or as a completely isolated fragment. In tapeworms, each proglottid in the chain contains a complete set of sexual organs capable of reproducing the species. It is usually hermaphroditic, so that it is truly complete and may even be capable of self-fertilization. Each proglottid is a gonophore, a structure formed to carry the gonads.

In polychaete worms, some marine individuals have the gonads in the rear part of the body. This *epitoke* then breaks off, swims away, liberates its gametes, and dies. It also is a gonophore. This process is called *epitoky*.

In many hydroid Coelenterata, there are structures producing gametes; these are sometimes called gonophores. They may be reduced to evaginations of the surface called sporosacs. In *Dicoryne,* the ciliated sporosacs may become free and swim about.

C. Spermatophores

Several types of spermatozoan packages occur and operate in several manners.

Rotifera. In the Seisonidea, the flagellated spermatozoa may adhere in bundles, which have been called spermatophores.

Turbellaria. In some the spermatozoa are bundled into spermatophores before they are placed in the copulatory pouch of the partner.

Gastropoda. In some slugs part of the vas deferens secretes a spermatophore, which may be of very complex shape, or the spermatozoa may be enclosed within a mass of jelly.

Cephalopoda. Spermatozoa are enclosed in an elaborate spermatophore while in the seminal vesicle. The structure has several membranes, almost a shell, and includes a device for ejecting spermatozoa. A special reservoir, *Needham's sac,* near the mantle cavity, stores spermatophores. Each male has a specially modified arm, designed to transfer the spermatophore to the mantle cavity of the female. This arm or its specialization is called a *hectocotylus.* (This phenomenon is *hectocotyly,* and the animal which possesses the arm is said to be hectocotylized.) The arm may include a cavity for storage of spermatozoa. There is physical contact between male and female, during which the hectocotylus places spermatophores in the mantle cavity of the female near the openings of the oviducts. The hectocotylus may be broken off and left in the cavity. Each spermatophore releases the spermatozoa over a period of time; these then fertilize the ova as they emerge from the oviduct. In some octopuses there is a seminal receptacle near the mouth, into which the spermatophores are placed.

Myzostomida. Two hermaphroditic individuals each attach a spermatophore to the integument of the other. The spermatophores contain cysts filled with spermatozoa and also other cysts containing cells that are probably modified spermatozoa. These cysts fuse to form a syncytium that penetrates the body wall and forms masses which migrate to the coelom by amoeboid movement. The spermatozoa are liberated into the coelom, where they fertilize the ova. The penetration is apparently not hypodermic injection but a penetration by the syncytium between the epidermal cells in the manner of amoebocytes.

Polychaeta. In some of the Protodrilidae spermatophores are attached to the ''dorsal organs'' of the female, which are seminal receptacles.

Oligochaeta. ''In tubificids spermatozoa agglutinate in the atrium and form elongated spermatophores which are stored after copulation in the spermathecae'' (Lasserre, 1975).

Hirudinea. A common atrium just behind the male gonopore may form a spermatophore of hardened protein. The latter consists of two bundles of spermatozoa, one from each ejaculatory duct. The spermatophore is inserted through the body wall (at the clitellum) and discharges its spermatozoa into the coelom. This is thus a combination of spermatophore transfer with hypodermic injection. A further peculiarity is that the injection is made at a predetermined site or copulatory area, beneath which lies a special conducting tissue that connects with the ovisacs.

Onychophora. In the united sperm duct, the spermatozoa are enclosed in spermatophores with a chitinous envelope. The spermatophore is attached at random upon the female, sometimes many on one individual. The underlying cuticle is dissolved from beneath by amoebocytes, and the spermatozoa thus make their way into the haemocoel.

Arachnida. A spermatophore may be attached to the ground, often on a stalk, and discharged into the female genital pore by a trigger (as in scorpions and pseudoscorpions). It may be placed in the female pore by the male, using his chelicerae (Solifugae, s.Acarina), pedipalps (Pedipalpida), or legs (Ricinulei). In some, what is called a spermatophore may be merely a special reservoir on the pedipalp, from which the spermatozoa are placed in the female gonopore (s.Araneida).

Crustacea. ''In (some Copepods), internal fertilization is brought about by a remarkable device. When sexually mature, the male produces from a gland a plastic-like substance with which it forms a kind of ''bottle'', the spermatophore, with an exceedingly long tubular neck; it passes its sperm into this and then swims off to attach it to an opening on the first abdominal segment of a female. . . . The sperms now pass from the spermatophore into the female . . . '' (Hardy, 1956).

Chilopoda. A spermatophore on a stalk is taken in by the female gonopore.

Symphyla. The male places a spermatophore on a stalk on the ground. The female takes this into her mouth, where the spermatozoa fertilize her eggs as she is transferring them from her gonopore and attaching them to substratum with her mouth.

Pauropoda. A spermatophore is formed and deposited on the ground, where it may be found by the female.

Insecta. Usually a spermatophore is deposited directly in the female duct, but rarely it may be left on the ground to be taken up by the female. In some insects the heads of the spermatozoa form a single cyst and are held together by a hyaline cap, which may persist through transfer. In others they are held together by an elaborate corkscrew-shaped sheath which persists until just before the ova are fertilized.

Chaetognatha. A spermatophore is formed in the seminal vesicle, from which it escapes upon rupture of the vesicle. It is placed on the ''female'' (mutually by hermaphrodites), after which it breaks open and liberates the spermatozoa on the surface. The spermatozoa then migrate backward to the two openings into seminal receptacles of the female system.

Amphibia. In a few salamanders a gelatinous spermatophore is deposited on the bottom, to be picked up later by the cloaca of the female.

Thus, a spermatophore is a device for delivering spermatozoa to the female. The manner of delivery is diverse. The organ producing the spermatophore is not always the same. The site of fertilization may be in the ovary, in the ducts, in the body cavity, or outside at the opening of the oviduct (or even in the mouth of the female).

The spermatophore itself, in the dozen classes where it may occur, may be (1) a complicated organ with locomotory and penetrative powers, (2) a stalked or attached capsule that waits to be picked up by the female, (3) a simple sac, handled by appendages, or (4) merely a cavity in an appendage, in which loose spermatozoa are carried for transfer.

D. Oophores

These are not common, because the ova are not usually liberated from the body. They occur (1) when several cells, usually nutritive, are enclosed with the ovum in a membrane or shell, (2) when several zygotes are enclosed in a capsule, or (3) when separate eggs are united into an enclosed egg mass. The last occurs in Polychaeta and Amphibia, and in Pisces (where the masses are called egg rafts). (The term is seldom used but some of the investments cited under "Egg Coverings" earlier would qualify.)

In Coelenterata, the egg of *Bougainvillea multitentaculata* is surrounded by a layer of cells, consisting of thousands of nematocysts. These cells are contributed by the parent, and they remain through cleavage.

Egg masses of various sorts are produced in many arthropods, including Crustacea and Insecta. They may consist merely of eggs adhering or cemented together, or they may be oophores because the clusters of eggs are surrounded by a complex gelatinous, silky, or papery covering. In Rhynchocoela such masses have been called composite eggs, but that term is better reserved for the truly composite single eggs of some Turbellaria (see Chapter 5).

E. Zygotophores

The proglottids of tapeworms contain the ova before and during fertilization (see "Gonophores", above). In some orders (such as Pseudophyllidea) either zygotes or developing eggs leave the proglottid via the uterine pore continuously. In other orders (such as Cyclophyllidea) the zygotes are not liberated until destruction of the proglottid outside of the host.

F. Embryophores

Less obvious in this connection are the protective devices provided for the developing embryos:

1. Eggshells or membranes may still serve
2. Special embryonic membranes may be formed: (a) by tissues of the mother, (b) by cells of the blastoderm of the developing embryo itself
3. (See also section on "Exploitation" in Chapter 22)

REFERENCES

Baccetti, B., Ed., *Comparative Spermatology Symposium*, Academia Nazionale dei Lincei, Roma, Academic Press, New York, 1969.

Barnes, R. D., *Invertebrate Zoology*, 2nd ed., W. B. Saunders, Philadelphia, 1968.

Blackwelder, R. E. and Shepherd, B. A., *The Diversity of Animal Reproduction*, CRC Press, Boca Raton, Fla., 1981.

Breder, C. M., Jr. and Rosen, D. E., *Modes of Reproduction in Fishes*, Natural History Press, Garden City, N.Y., 1966.

Campbell, R. D., Cnidaria, in *Reproduction of Marine Invertebrates*, Vol. 1, Giese, A. C. and Pearse, J. S., Eds., Academic Press, New York, 1974, chap. 3.

Davey, K. G., *Reproduction in the Insects*, Oliver & Boyd, Edinburgh, 1965.

Giese, A. C. and Pearse, J. S., Eds., *Reproduction of Marine Invertebrates*, Vol. 1 (1974), Vol. 2 (1975), Vol. 3 (1975), Vol. 4 (1977), Vol. 5 (1979).

Hagan, H. R., *Embryology of the Viviparous Insects*, Ronald Press, New York, 1951.

Hardy, A. C., *The Open Sea*, Collins, London, 1956.

Henley, C., Platyhelminthes (Turbellaria), in *Reproduction of Marine Invertebrates*, Vol. 1, Giese, A. C. and Pearse, J. S., Eds., Academic Press, New York, 1974, chap. 5.

Hyman, L. H., *The Invertebrates,* Vol. 1 (1940), Vol. 2 (1951a), Vol. 3 (1951b), Vol. 4 (1955), Vol. 5 (1959), Vol. 6 (1967), McGraw-Hill, New York.

Imms, A. D., *A General Textbook of Entomology,* 2nd ed., E. P. Dutton, New York, 1930.

Imms, A. D., *A General Textbook of Entomology,* 8th ed., Methuen, London, 1951.

Kudo, R. R., *Protozoology,* 5th ed., Charles C Thomas, Springfield, Ill., 1966.

Lasserre, P., Clitellata, in *Reproduction of Marine Invertebrates,* Vol. 3, Giese, A. C. and Pearse, J. B., Eds., Academic Press, New York, 1975.

Markewitch, A. P., *Parasitic Copepodes on the Fishes of the U.S.S.R.,* Indian National Scientific Documentation Centre, New Delhi, 1976.

Rothschild, (Lord), Unorthodox methods of sperm transfer, *Sci. Am.,* 195(5), 1956b.

Sadleir, M. F. S., *The Reproduction of Vertebrates,* Academic Press, New York, 1973.

Sleigh, M. A., *The Biology of Protozoa,* American Elsevier, New York, 1973.

Smyth, J. D., *Introduction to Animal Parasitology,* 2nd ed., John Wiley & Sons, New York, 1976.

Sonneborn, T. M., Breeding systems, reproductive methods, and species problems in Protozoa, in *The Species Problem,* Mayr, E., Ed., American Association for the Advancement of Science, Washington, D.C., 1957.

Waterman, T. H., Ed., *The Physiology of Crustacea,* Vol. 2, Academic Press, New York, 1961.

Wilson, E. B., *The Cell in Development and Heredity,* 3rd ed., Macmillan, New York, 1953.

Yanagimachi, R., The life cycle of *Peltogasterella, Crustaceana,* 2, 183, 1961.

Chapter 4

PARTHENOGENESIS, SEQUENCES, SEXUALITY

TABLE OF CONTENTS

I. Parthenogenesis 82
    A. Introduction...82
    B. Meiotic Parthenogenesis 83
    C. Ameiotic Parthenogenesis 84
    D. Activation 84
    E. Pseudova..84
    F. Apozygote 84

II. Sequences of Reproductive Cycles..85
    A. Discussion 85
    B. Single-Segment Sequences 87
    C. Multiple-Segment Sequences 89
    D. The Levels of Diversity...93
        1. Reproduction During Developmental Stages.......................94
        2. Multiple Pathways of Reproduction 95

III. Sexuality 96
    A. Definitions...96
    B. Sex within a Given Species..98
        1. Males 98
        2. Females..98
        3. Hermaphrodites 99
        4. Neuters 99
        5. Mating Types 99
    C. Sex in One Individual...99
    D. Sex Distribution and Change...100
        1. Sex Reversal...102
        2. Gonad Transplant 102
    E. Sex Determination 102
    F. Fusion 103

IV. Miscellaneous Concepts 104
    A. Introduction...104
    B. Para-Reproductive Processes 104
    C. Paedogenesis..107
    D. Germ Cell Line 107

References 108

I. PARTHENOGENESIS

A. Introduction

Parthenogenesis is activation and development of either haploid ova or diploid pseudova without karyogamy (fertilization). It involves only one or two of the three features of sexual reproduction; i.e., although gametes are formed (sometimes only "ova"), meiosis may or may not occur, and there is no fusion of pronuclei of gametes. Thus although males may not exist, they *may* be present, insemination *may* occur, and there *may* be syngamy (penetration of the ovum by the spermatozoon), but there will be no complement of male chromosomes in the offspring, because there is no fusion of two pronuclei (no karyogamy).

The key to a clear understanding of parthenogenesis is the fact that karyogamy (fusion of the paternal and maternal pronuclei) does not occur, not that males are absent. There are several forms of parthenogenetic reproduction that require males to be present to stimulate activation of the haploid ovum.

The difficulties of bringing about the meeting of the ovum with a spermatozoon and successfully consummating karyogamy are very great in many animals. This may have led to widespread occurrence of an abbreviation of the process, in which some of the steps are omitted. When an ovum is fertilized (completed karyogamy), it is thereby stimulated to embryonic development. Ova that are not fertilized may die, but in some animals they may be stimulated in some other way to start development. At some point in this development, if the diploid number of chromosomes is to be restored, there must be some process that is the counterpart of karyogamy in this respect.

The process that stimulates the development of the ovum is activation. Fertilization usually provides this activation, but other means of activation include chemical and mechanical stimulation. Such activation other than by fertilization occurs in all forms of parthenogenesis. After such parthenogenetic activation, the ovum becomes an apozygote.

Parthenogenesis appears in at least the following situations:

1. Ameiotic parthenogenesis — the ovum is diploid (s.Turbellaria, s.Rotifera, s.Nematoda, s.Mollusca, s.Crustacea, s.Insecta, s.Reptilia)
2. Meiotic parthenogenesis — the ovum is haploid; activation occurs without influence of males (s.Protozoa, s.Turbellaria, s.Rotifera, s.Gastropoda, s.Annelida, s.Insecta)
3. The ovum is haploid — activation occurs with influence of males: (a) insemination by males of same species, without spermatozoon entry (s.Mesozoa, s.Turbellaria, s.Nematoda, s.Pisces); (b) without insemination but with males of a related species present (s.Pisces, s.Amphibia); (c) insemination by males of another species must occur, but there is no syngamy (s.Pisces, s.Amphibia, s.Reptilia); (d) spermatozoon penetration with nuclei remaining separate (i.e., without karyogamy): (i) gonomery (s.Turbellaria, s.Gastropoda, s.Crustacea, s.Pisces, s.Amphibia); (ii) pseudogamy (s.Protozoa, s.Turbellaria, s.Nematoda, s.Oligochaeta); (iii) with male pronucleus cast off by the activated egg (s.Mesozoa)

In addition to phyla and classes cited in the tabulation, some form of parthenogenesis also occurs in some species of each of the following: Protozoa (Flagellata and Sporozoa), Gastrotricha, Bryozoa, Gastropoda, Sipunculoidea, Echiuroidea, Tardigrada, Oligochaeta, Dinophiloidea, Arachnida (Acarina), Symphyla, Echinodermata, Pterobranchia, and Reptilia.

Various forms of parthenogenesis have received these special names; some occurrences are found in these groups:

1. *Arrhenotoky* or *androgenesis* or *arrhenogeny* — in which only males are produced (Insecta, Amphibia)
2. *Thelytoky* or *gynogenesis* — in which only females are produced (Gastrotricha, Nematoda, Insecta, Amphibia)
3. *Deuterotoky* or *amphitoky* or *anthogenesis* — in which both males and females are produced (Insecta)
4. *Pseudogamy* — in which the spermatozoon activates the egg, usually without entering it (Protozoa, Turbellaria, Nematoda, Oligochaeta)
5. *Plasmogony* or *plasmogamy* — in which the spermatozoon enters the ovum but the nuclei remain separate (Protozoa: Sarcodina; Nematoda)
6   *Gonomery* — in which there is nuclear fusion but the chromosomes remain in separate groups (Turbellaria, Gastropoda, Crustacea, Chrondrichthyes, Osteichthyes, Amphibia)
7. *Progenesis* — which is parthenogenesis in the metacercaria stage of some Trematoda
8. *Polar body fertilization* — in which the second polar body fuses with the ovum and the nuclei fuse; the term *automictic parthenogenesis* has been used (Insecta)

There have been two sets of descriptive terms used to indicate genetic aspects of the ovum:

1. Zygoid parthenogenesis — development of an unfertilized ovum that is diploid, either by remaining diploid (ameiotic parthenogenesis) or by restoring its diploidy during development
2. Hemizygoid parthenogenesis — development from haploid ova
3. Ameiotic parthenogenesis — development from an ovum which is diploid because it undergoes no meiotic division (see under "Asexual Reproduction" below)
4. Meiotic parthenogenesis — development from an ovum which has become haploid by a normal process of meiotic reduction divisions

The occurrence of parthenogenesis in any given species is either obligatory (a necessary part of the life cycle) or facultative (may occur or not, depending on circumstances). They occur in some species of the following groups:

1. Facultative parthenogenesis — (Turbellaria, Nematoda, Gymnolaemata, Gastropoda, Sipunculoidea, Dinophiloidea, Oligochaeta, Arachnida, Crustacea, Insecta, Ophiuroidea, Echinoidea, Pterobranchia, Osteichthyes, Amphibia, Reptilia)
2. Obligate parthenogenesis — (Bdelloidea, Monogononta, Chaetonotoidea, Heterotardigrada, Symphyla, Insecta)

Among these latter groups, in three there is no reproduction other than parthenogenesis, neither bisexual nor asexual. These are in the Rotifera (Bdelloidea and Monogonta) and in the Gastrotricha (Chaetonotoidea). One species in the Oligochaeta *(Cognettia glandulosa)* reproduces both asexually and parthenogenetically.

B. Meiotic Parthenogenesis

Parthenogenesis in which the ovum is haploid because of meiosis.

The result of meiosis is that the ovum is haploid, having only one set of chromosomes. Although a few exceptional animals can develop into haploid adults, in most the diploid condition is restored by one of a variety of methods. In most animals these methods are little understood.

Meiotic parthenogenesis occurs in some species in the Protozoa, Turbellaria, Nematoda, Annelida, Arthropoda, and Vertebrata, and probably elsewhere. In the Reptilia, "the parthenogenetic egg is surprisingly not haploid but diploid, as the haploid cell nuclei formed in a second cell division fuse together instead of passing into daughter cells" (Sadleir, 1973).

In *pseudogamy*, a spermatozoon activates the ovum, and its nucleus may enter the ovum. If so, it degenerates without fusing with the ovum nucleus. Thus a synkaryon is not formed, even though there is fertilization in every other sense. This is known to occur in some Protozoa, some Turbellaria, some Nematoda, and a few Oligochaeta.

C. Ameiotic Parthenogenesis

Parthenogenesis in which the "ovum" is a diploid pseudovum.

This form of parthenogenesis is said to be more widespread than the meiotic form, but it is not clear whether males are always absent. It is ameiotic because there are no reduction divisions in this oogenesis but merely a single mitosis. Thus, the ovum is diploid (zygoid) and the reproduction is asexual because there is neither mixis nor meiosis. Apparently the pseudova are produced without meiosis, and there is a possibility that meiosis does occur, but is unrecognized because there is later some process that restores diploidy.

This process occurs in some species in the Protozoa, Rotifera, Nematoda, Mollusca, Crustacea, Insecta, and probably others.

D. Activation

Activation was cited earlier as part of the process of fertilization. In parthenogenesis the karyogamy part of fertilization is lacking, so activation becomes a distinct process with some diversity. The nature of the stimulus that produces this activation is usually not known. It may be any of these:

1. Contact or penetration by a spermatozoon which takes no part in development
2. Presence of spermatozoa of another species
3. Presence of a male of another species, without insemination
4. Internal reactions, perhaps due to the presence of only half the normal amount of chromatin
5. Experimentally, by pricking the ovum membrane
6. Experimentally, by changing the pH or other condition of the surrounding water

It can be seen that most of these are chemical influences.

E. Pseudova

Gametes are defined above as haploid because they are produced by meiosis. How then can one refer to female gametes that are diploid? These unusual but not rare "ova" are so little talked about that there is no common word to distinguish them from haploid ova. A word useful for this type of gametes is *pseudovum* — a diploid "ovum", formed without meiosis, which can be activated by some process other than karyogamy. When a pseudovum is activated, it becomes an apozygote.

F. Apozygote

In defining a zygote as a new individual which is the product of the fusion of two gametes, we exclude the comparable new individual formed in parthenogenesis by the activation of an "ovum" without fertilization. These are nearly always diploid, either because the "gamete" (pseudovum) was diploid or because the haploid ovum doubled its chromosomes in some manner. (Exceptions to this are the males in a few arthropod species, which remain haploid throughout their life.) These new diploid individuals, formed without fertilization, are called *apozygotes;* their development is exactly comparable to that of zygotes. (The term parthenospore has also been used in Protozoa.) Because the two chromosome sets of each are both of maternal origin, it is different from a zygote, in which there is one maternal and one paternal set.

Some apozygotes arise from unfertilized haploid ova that made themselves diploid, as in some Turbellaria, some Annelida, Arthropoda, and Pisces. Other apozygotes arise from unfertilized diploid pseudova, as in some species of Rotifera, Nematoda, Mollusca, Crustacea, and Insecta.

The problem of the restoration of diploidy in parthenogenesis by haploid ova, where the parent is diploid, is a fascinating one for which the only answers are hints. Of the protozoan *Actinophrys,* Grell (1973) writes, "It is likely that the chromosome number...is regulated to diploidy." In Insecta, it is reported (Davey, 1965) that diploidy is restored "by fusion of two nuclei", which may be the ovum nucleus and that of the second polar body or else two cleavage nuclei. In Reptilia, it is reported by Sadleir (1973) that a similar fusion with the polar body nucleus occurs. There are also hints that in facultative parthenogenesis the ovum may somehow recognize its chromatin deficiency and mitotically double its chromosomes to give itself the second set.

II. SEQUENCES OF REPRODUCTIVE CYCLES

A. Discussion

The actual reproduction of all animals consists of processes leading directly to new individuals. These processes are diverse, as cited in the preceding sections under "Asexual Reproduction", "Sexual Reproduction", and "Parthenogenesis". They sometimes occur singly so that reproduction in a given species may consist of just one such process, repeated in each generation, or it may instead consist of more than one process, each of which results in a new individual (or individuals) and which may occur in sequence in the reproductive cycle of the species or in its multiple (parallel) pathways. Each of the individuals will undergo appropriate development, and the species reproduction will be the sum of all the processes producing new individuals among all its members.

Several words basic to this subject require explanation or definition. They do not form a single system but are different ways of looking at reproduction in relation to the life cycle. *Process* in this connection is the one event that produces a new individual, not necessarily a new adult or a similar form. Many, probably most, species employ more than one reproductive process. Reproduction in many animals is a *sequence* of processes and the sequences are even more diverse than the processes. A sequence is the pathway by which one individual produces a duplicate of itself; this is often indirect, after a series of processes. All of the sequences in a species constitute its composite *cycle;* thus, many life cycles involve two or more alternative sequences, two or more parallel pathways to reach the final goal of a similar individual.

In each pathway, the sequence of reproductive processes is a series of steps, always diverse. Each step is here called a *segment,* a step in the reproductive cycle involving one occurrence of one of the processes. If a pair reproducing bisexually, or an individual reproducing either parthenogenetically or asexually, survives the process and repeats it several times, each repetition is an *episode.* Successive episodes produce the successive new individuals by repetition of a given process (see Figure 5).

There is some ambiguity in the word cycle, as it seems to require completion of a circle back to a second individual of the same sort. In some species one individual completes this cycle, but in other species it takes a sequence of unlike individuals to complete it. We thus refer to the reproductive cycle of a species as consisting of all the reproductions that can occur in the entire life cycle of all individuals. The life cycle is

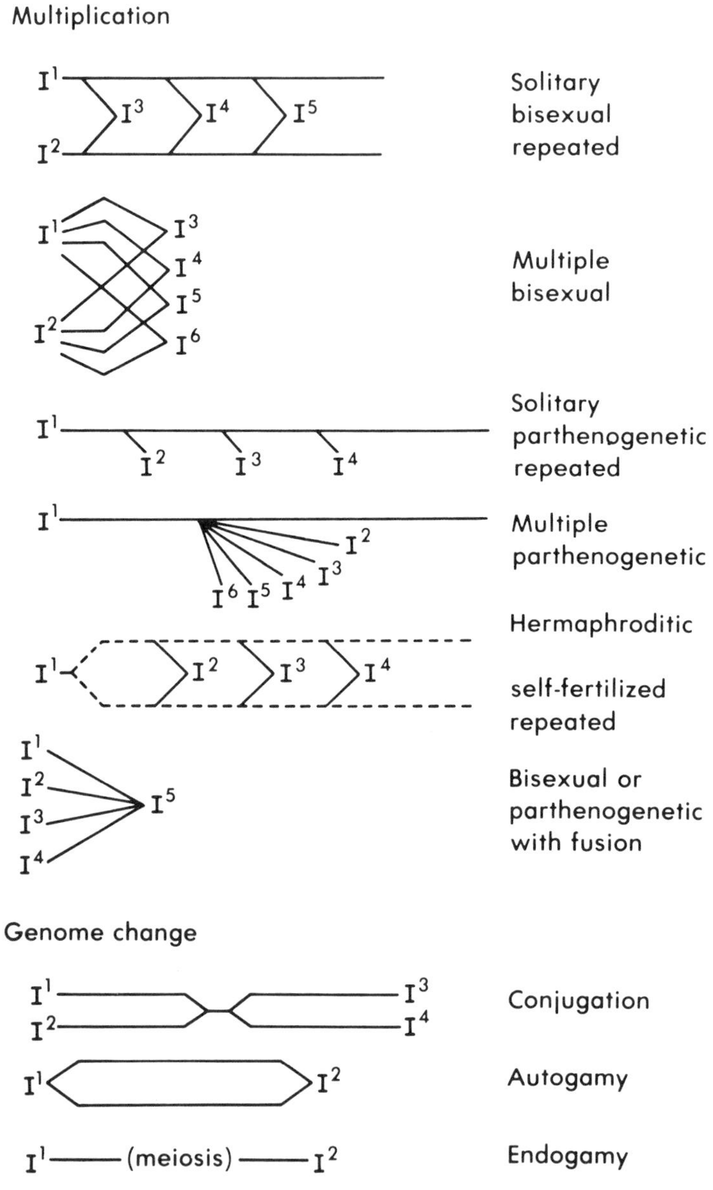

Multiplication

FIGURE 5. Diagrams of reproductive episodes. I^1, I^2, I^3, etc., are succes-sive individuals. (From Blackwelder, R. E. and Shepherd, B. A., *The Diver-sity of Animal Reproduction,* CRC Press, Boca Raton, Fla., 1981.)

dealt with in Chapter 7. In discussion below, the word cycle is usually replaced with the word sequence.

Our previous definition of an individual (in Chapter 1) shows that it is that part of the reproductive cycle of the species from the moment of one reproduction to the moment at which that new individual dies or is replaced through fragmentation by several new ones or loses its identity by fusion with another. In each process the indi-vidual is just one segment in one of the sequences found in the reproduction of that species. (See Table 7.)

Table 7

THE VARYING SPAN OF INDIVIDUALS BETWEEN REPRODUCTIVE OCCURRENCES

First individual	End of life stage	Because of this process	Producing next new individual	Example (occurs in)
1. Zygote	Early embryo	Polyembryony	New embryos	Armadillo
2. Zygote	Late embryo	Multiple budding	New embryos	Phylactolaemata
3. Zygote	Larva	Fragmentation	Larvae	Scyphozoa
4. Zygote	Adult	Any asex. repro.	Fragments	Polychaeta
5. Activated ovum	Early embryo	Polyembryony	New embryos	Insecta
6. Activated ovum	Larva	Fragmentation	Fragments	Gymnolaemata
7. Embryo	Embryo	Fragmentation	Fragments	Insecta
8. Larva	Larva	Fragmentation	Larvae	Ascidiacea
9. Adult	Adult	Fragmentation	Fragments	Rhynchocoela
10. Adult	Adult	Conjugation	Exconjugants	Ciliata
11. Adult	Adult	Autogamy	Differ. adult	Protozoa
12. Adult	Adult	Fission	Adults	Sarcodina
13. Bud	Adult	Any asex. repro.	Fragments	Anthozoa
14. Fragment	Adult	Any asex. repro.	Fragments	Polychaeta
15. Adult	(Irrelevant)	Gamet. & fertil.	Zygote	Humans

Note: Read line 1 (for example) thus — a new *zygote* ends its life at the *early embryo* stage because of *polyembryony* which produces *new embryos,* as occurs in the armadillo. Again in line 9, an *adult* ends its life at the *adult* stage because of *fragmentation* which produces *fragments* that regenerate into adults, as occurs in some Rhynchocoela.

From Blackwelder, R. E. and Shepherd, B. A., *Diversity of Animal Reproduction,* CRC Press, Boca Raton, Fla., 1981.

There are thus three levels of complexity. First is the individual and the process by which it was produced; these are the processes discussed earlier in this chapter. Second, it is common for the life of the species to involve a sequence of reproductions (see *Obelia* below), involving individuals of several types (and often produced by different processes), before an individual comparable to the initial one is produced. Third, many species can reproduce by any of several sequences, as shown in Figure 6.

In *Obelia,* the budding of a hydranth (feeding polyp) is followed by the budding of a gonangium (reproductive polyp) which is followed by the budding of a medusa, before the sexual part of the cycle (from the gonads of the medusae) produces the initial polyp type again. The hydranths, the gonangia, and the medusae are separate and different individuals in the reproductive cycle of the species.

B. Single-Segment Sequences

These are the simple cycles that are often assumed to be universal or nearly so. They will produce populations of predictable genetic make-up. There are three basic ones and several varieties:

1. Basic Bisexual Reproduction (BBR) $\quad\quad\quad$ S — S — S — S
2. Parthenogenesis $\quad\quad\quad$ P — P — P — P
3. Asexual reproduction $\quad\quad\quad$ A — A — A — A

Each formula represents four generations, passing from left to right. Each letter represents a new individual produced by a process denoted by that letter (S = bisexual, P = parthenogenetic, A = asexual). Between (1) and (2) there are actually two other

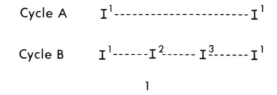

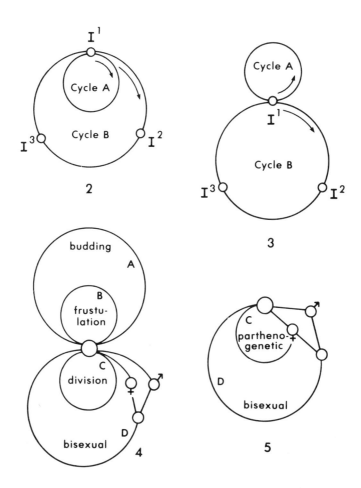

FIGURE 6.   Diagrams of reproductive sequences. 1, Simple life histories; 2 and 3, a species with two alternative pathways; 4, a species with four alternative pathways; 5, a species wtih two alternative pathways, of which one is parthenogenetic. (From Blackwelder, R. E. and Shepherd, B. A., *The Diversity of Animal Reproduction*, CRC Press, Boca Raton, Fla., 1981.

varieties: clonal fertilization (CF — CF — CF — CF) and the obligate self-fertilization of hermaphrodites (SF — SF — SF — SF); these produce greatly reduced genetic diversity among the gametes and thus in the offspring. The clonal fertilization is actually a form of BBR, but the self-fertilization is akin to parthenogenesis.

Furthermore, the parthenogenesis can be of either of two sorts (meiotic or ameiotic, with differences in the genetic ratios among the resulting offspring), and the asexual reproduction can be of any of at least four processes (budding, stolonization, agamogony, or fragmentation). It must be recognized that to be a single-segment sequence there must be no other reproduction in that species.

A further diversity occurs in the sex arrangement of the individuals in species in which BBR occurs. The species may be dioecious or monoecious. The hermaphrodites would then necessarily be obligately cross fertilizing, if the reproduction is to be considered to be BBR.

Among the diagrams of Figure 6, there could be normal bisexual reproduction, parthenogenesis, or any of a variety of asexual processes. The most common process is the bisexual, and it is the authors' major intent here to isolate this from all other reproductive processes. For this purpose it is not enough to examine the process that is obvious; it is necessary to determine whether there is in the sequence, or among the alternative sequences, any other process which will upset the expected genetic ratios of the population. The sexual reproduction which will produce the predicted gene ratios is herein called *BBR*. This has been defined earlier as production of a single offspring by immediate biparental karyogamy. Any deviation from this or addition to it may alter the gene ratios to a greater or lesser extent.

To determine whether a reproductive sequence qualifies as BBR, three things are necessary: (1) there must be only the one reproductive sequence employed by that species, rather than several alternate sequences; (2) there must be only one reproductive process in that one sequence; and (3) that reproductive process must be a fusion of gametes with karyogamy.

Thus, this is contrasting BBR (as a single sequence of just one particular process — karyogamy) with *all other reproduction* (whether nonkaryogamic, or involving mixtures of processes or sequences of processes or mixtures of sequences).

Lest it appear that reproductive sequences are all very much alike, it must be noted that there are more than 200 different sequences, and these can be reduced to about 50 basic types. The one most often assumed by biologists, BBR, is by no means universal, and one must not take for granted its occurrence in any animal species (see Table 8).

C. Multiple-Segment Sequences

In addition to the single-segment sequences, shown here again as (1), there are three sorts of sequences involving more than one reproductive process; (2) they may be obligate sequences, where two or more processes alternate in some fixed series; (3) they may be obligate and fixed as to the sequence but variable as to the number of episodes of each process in the sequence; or (4) they may involve a fixed basic sequence with the possibility of occasional interruptions by some other process. These four types of sequences are

1. A fixed sequence of one process .... S-S-S-S
2. A fixed sequence of two processes .... S-A-S-A
   Two segments repeated; A stands for an asexually reproducing individual (s.Hydrozoa)
3. A variable sequence of two processes... S-P-P-P_n-S
   Five or more segments and individuals; P stands for a parthenogenetically reproducing individual; P_n stands for an indefinite number of repetitions (Insects: aphids)
4. Occasional alternatives of processes ....

$$
\begin{array}{c}
\text{S--S--S--S} \\
\quad\quad | \\
\quad\quad \text{A--S} \\
\text{A--S} \\
\quad | \\
\quad \text{A}
\end{array}
$$

Eight or nine segments; can be drawn either way, to show emphasis on sexual or asexual; any individual could reproduce by either method (Hydrozoa: *Hydra*)

Table 8
OCCURRENCE OF VARIOUS TYPES OF SEGMENTS IN THE PHYLA AND MAJOR CLASSES

	Dioecious cross-fert.	Hermaphrod. cross-fert.	Hermaphrod.	Self-fertil.	Clonal fert.	Fraternal fertiliz.	Parthe-nogen.	Agamo-gony	Adult division	Larval division	Embryonic division	Polyembryony	Para-reprod. and others
Protozoa	X					X		X	X	X		X	X
Mesozoa	?		X			X		X	X			Succ.	X
Monoblastozoa	X					?			X				
Coelenterata													
Hydrozoa	X		X	X	X	X	?		X	X	X	X	
Scyphozoa	?		X	?		X			X	X			
Anthozoa	X		X	?	X	X			X	X			
Ctenophora			X	?		X			X				
Platyhelminthes													
Turbellaria	X		X	X		X	X		X				
Trematoda	X		X	X		X						Succ.	
Cestoda	X		X	X	X	X	X			X		X	X
Cestodaria		X		?		X							
Rhynchocoela	X	X		?		?	?		X				
Acanthocephala	X					?	?						
Rotifera	X					X	X						
Gastrotricha	X		X	X		X	X						
Kinorhyncha	X					X							
Priapulida	X					X							
Nematoda	X		X	X		X	X						
Gordioidea	X					X							
Calyssozoa			X	?	X	X			X		X		
Bryozoa	X		X	X	X	X	X		X		X	X	
Brachiopoda	X		X	?		X	?					?	
Phoronida	X		X	?		X			X				

Mollusca
  Amphineura
  Solenogastres
  Gastropoda
  Bivalvia
  Scaphopoda
  Cephalopoda
Sipunculoidea
Echiuroidea
Tardigrada
Annelida
  Polychaeta
  Oligochaeta
  Hirudinea
  Archiannelida
Dinophiloidea
Myzostomida
Pentastomida
Onychophora
Arthropoda
  Merostomata
  Pycnogonida
  Arachnida
  Crustacea
  Pauropoda
  Symphyla
  Diplopoda
  Chilopoda
  Insecta
Chaetognatha
Pogonophora
Echinodermata
  Crinoidea
  Asteroidea
  Ophiuroidea
  Echinoidea
  Holothurioidea

Table 8 (continued)
OCCURRENCE OF VARIOUS TYPES OF SEGMENTS IN THE PHYLA AND MAJOR CLASSES

	Dioecious cross-fert.	Hermaphrod. cross-fert.	Hermaphrod.	Self-fertil.	Clonal fert.	Fraternal fertiliz.	Parthe-nogen.	Agamo-gony	Adult division	Larval division	Embryonic division	Polyembryony	Para-reprod. and others
Pterobranchia	X		X	?		X	X		X				
Enteropneusta	X					X			X				
Tunicata													
Larvacea	X		X	?		X	?						
Ascidiacea	X		X	?		X			X	X			
Thaliacea		X		?	X	X			X	X			
Cephalochordata	X		X			X							
Vertebrata	X		X	X		X	X					X	

From Blackwelder, R. E. and Shepherd, B. A., *Diversity of Animal Reproduction*, CRC Press, Boca Raton, Fla., 1981.

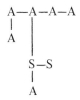

In this scheme reproduction in humans would usually be assumed to qualify as a fixed sequence of one process (exclusively sexual) as in (1), but identical twins are two new individuals produced asexually by the early embryo, so that the zygote-individual is very short-lived and is replaced by the two new ones. Humans thus fall into (4), where the cycle would be diagrammed thus:

$$
\begin{array}{c}
\text{S–S–S—S} \\
\mid \\
\text{A–S}
\end{array}
$$

Any sexually produced individual (zygote) could theoretically by this asexual process produce new individuals which would later become sexual reproducers again.

In the fixed sequences, besides the one shown, there may be S — P — S — P and P — A — P — A. In the variable sequences, P_n signifiees an indefinite number of parthenogenetic generations. Besides the one shown, these can involve P and A or S and A.

The occasional alternations are numerous and diverse. In a sexual series an individual may also reproduce by self-fertilization, or by clonal or fraternal fertilization. It may occasionally reproduce by asexual reproduction (as shown in (4) or by parthenogenesis). There may be individuals which can reproduce either bisexually or parthenogenetically or asexually, or all three. There may be a sequence of two different As, as in a hydroid which reproduces sexually (S) as well as by budding (A) and occasionally by pedal laceration (A′).

$$
\begin{array}{c}
\text{S—S—S — S} \\
\mid \qquad \mid \\
\quad\ \text{A′–S} \\
\mid \\
\text{A—A—S} \\
\mid \\
\text{A′–S} \\
\mid \\
\text{A′}
\end{array}
$$

The diagrams of Figure 6 show that many species can complete this reproductive sequence, from I¹ around to I¹ again, by more than one route. These are shown as the A and B pathways in the diagrams, and there may be four or more in some species. We call these alternative sequences because they are facultative; they do not occur in a fixed sequence. Depending on how they are drawn, the diagrams will be parallel (linear), concentric, or tangential.

D. The Levels of Diversity

Reproductive processes are diverse in so many ways, as already seen, that they are difficult to classify or to arrange. When these processes are combined into sequences involving several different processes, the complexity is greatly increased.

Life cycles are usually thought of in connection with development of an individual, but because many life cycles include a succession of different individuals produced by several reproductive processes, it is also possible to think of the reproductive cycle of a species. Most ways of diagramming this become very complex because of the great diversity. The diagrams above show only the simpler forms of cycles that occur in animals.

Furthermore, it is usual but not universal for any particular type of reproductive process to be repeated several times by that individual (or pair). Thus, there may be successive episodes of sexual reproduction in a pair of adults, repeated strobilation (as in Coelenterata), or there may be repeated budding by an adult. These repeated episodes each produce new individuals.

Diversity has so far been suggested at these four levels:

1. The segment occupied by one individual from one reproduction to the next. In Figure 6, the individual segments are (in A) I^1 to I^1, in which they are the same as reproductive sequences (one segment each); and (in B) I^1 to I^2, I^2 to I^3, and I^3 to I^1, in which there are three individual segments in the one reproductive sequence (Table 8).
2. Single reproductive sequence of a species. Two or more individual segments forming a single sequence from I^1 to I^1 in all 6 cycles, but in the B cycles there are several steps involved in each reproductive sequence.
3. Sum of the reproductive sequences of a species. Each species has at least one pathway, but many have alternative pathways, as shown in each pair of diagrams; cycles A and B together in each case. (Diagrams could be drawn for other species that would show more than two alternating cycles.)
4. Episodes are the repetitions of a single-process sequence by one individual (parthenogenetic or asexual) or two (bisexual), as in all animals that live long enough to take part in two or more breedings (see Figure 5).

Two additional diversities appear over this entire tabulation; first because of the fact that very many species reproduce during other developmental stages than just the adult, often in several of them, and second because many reproduce by several parallel pathways.

1. Reproduction During Developmental Stages

Nearly all of the individual processes listed above may occur at other stages than just the adult; for example, budding and fragmentation may occur in the embryo, or gametogenesis may occur in a larva.

In the cited developmental stages below, there may be reproduction of some type as indicated. Some of these are widespread among the phyla, but some are rare; the occurrence of the latter is shown:

1. Zygote — separation at first fission, which is polyembryony
2. Germ ball — in embryo, successive fragmentation to form successive generations of larvae, each carrying its germ ball fragment (Trematoda)
3. Embryo — from first cleavage to gastrula, budding, or fragmentation, which is polyembryony and colony budding
4. Larva — fragmentation, budding, or strobilation, and sexual reproduction that may be either fertilization or parthenogenesis
5. Adult — fragmentation, budding, fertilization, or parthenogenesis
6. Bud — budding (Thaliacea)
7. Stolon — budding, strobilation (Tunicata)

8. Agamete — fission (Dicyemida)
9. Colony — fragmentation or budding or fertilization

The reproductive processes of the embryos and larvae, as above, are often followed by a sexual process in the adult, producing a sequence of reproductive processes in what seems to be a single life cycle; for example, a larva (L^1) may reproduce by budding (L^2), and each budded L^2 larva goes on to become adult to reproduce again — sexually, but the first larva (L^1) and the L^2 adult are different individuals. Actual examples of these short-lived individuals are shown in Table 4, line 4 of *Obelia* and lines 2 and 3 of *Bugula*.

2. Multiple Pathways of Reproduction

As described above, there may be two individuals within a species which reproduce by different methods. One may use budding, whereas the other may use karyogamy. There may even be as many as four different reproductive sorts of individuals in a given species. Thus, each one of these species can reproduce by several pathways, sequences of processes, or alternative reproductive sequences.

These individuals frequently succeed each other in either fixed or variable sequences, producing what is often called *metagenesis,* or alternation of generations. The alternations may involve bisexuality, parthenogenesis, and asexual reproduction, each in several forms, and at least 50 basic alternation sequences that occur have been tabulated.

In addition to the words defined above, there are several terms in the literature referring to sequences of reproductive processes or features of them:

1. Alternation of generations — used in several senses in animals, for sequences of processes or polymorphs, generally quite different from the meaning in plants of sporophyte vs. gametophyte
2. Digenetic — having an alternation of sexual and asexual processes (m.Trematoda)
3. Heterogamy — same as Heterogony (in this usage)
4. Heterogenesis — same as Metagenesis
5. Heterogony — the alternation of parthenogenetic with syngamic processes (s.Insecta, s.Rotifera)
6. Hypogenetic — same as Monogenetic
7. Metagenesis — alternation of generations in animals, usually alternation of sexual and asexual individuals
8. Monogenetic — not showing metagenesis

Some sort of reproductive alternation occurs in most classes in animals. Four types can be listed, with examples, although many variations of them occur:

1. Sexual/asexual — (s.Protozoa, m.Coelenterata, m.Platyhelminthes, s.Rhynchocoela, s.Annelida, s.Insecta, s.Tunicata)
2. Sexual/parthenogenetic — (s.Rotifera, s.Crustacea, s.Insecta)
3. Parthenogenetic/asexual — (Dicyemida, Calyssozoa, Gymnolaemata)
4. Cross-fertilization/self-fertilizing — (s.Nematoda, s.Insecta)

A quite different sort of alternation occurs in the Ctenophora under the term *dissogeny.* Here the larvae become sexually mature, produce ova and spermatozoa, and presumably there are fertilizations and offspring. However, most authors leave some doubt of this, and Hyman (1940) remarks "whether the larva actually produces normal offspring does not seem to be known.'' The gonads degenerate before the adult stage, they are formed anew, and the definitive adult bisexual reproduction occurs.

Because many generalizations have been made about the processes that occur in a class or phylum, it is appropriate to take note also of the diversity that can occur in such a group. These range from a single sequence consisting of a single (bisexual) process, as in all species in such small groups as Kinorhyncha and Onychophora, to the ten or more possible sequences found among the species in the Hydrozoa and the Trematoda (see Figures 8 to 15 in Chapter 7).

III. SEXUALITY

A. Definitions

Sexuality is the phenomenon of members of a species existing in two forms, generally identified as male and female, that contribute hereditary factors to the next generation. It is the state of organisms that exhibit sex. *Sexuality is thus the condition in a species that consists of individuals showing the differences called sex.*

Sex is the sum of the differences in structure, process, and behavior that leads to production of gametes. Among these processes only meiosis is essential. If a series of processes includes meiosis, it is sexual; if it does not, it is not sexual. However, it must be remembered that meiosis is not always reproductive (does not always lead to multiplication). It may change the nucleus of a protozoan, for example, without producing any additional individuals, in such processes as conjugation, automixis, and nuclear reorganization.

It is not correct of say, however, that "sex" is the existence of male and female, or that every sexual species must consist of two sexual types of individuals. The basic meaning of the word must be modified to accommodate the various situations that have evolved from whatever was the primitive sexual system.

These include: (1) normal gonochorism, in which male and female organs are in separate individuals; (2) various combinations of sexual features in one individual (hermaphroditism, gynandromorphy, intersexuality); (3) parthenogenesis, with various devices for restoring the chromosomes to diploidy without fertilization; (4) isogamety, implying that the two parents were identical (no different sexes); (5) sex reversal; (6) conjugation; and (7) nuclear reorganization processes.

Not all species of organisms show sex; a few reproduce entirely without sexuality. They include some Protozoa, Rhynchocoela, and Annelida. In many groups, there are species that consist of but one sex, always female — these are parthenogenetic. In many groups there are at least a few individuals that show no evidence of sex — these are neuters, and they reproduce only asexually or not at all. They occur in Protozoa, Coelenterata, Rhynchocoela, Bryozoa, Annelida, Insecta, Pterobranchia, and elsewhere (see Table 9).

One must here forget the current everyday careless use of the word sex to refer to mammalian behavior leading to copulation. Biologically, sex is a condition among the individuals of a species; it often has nothing to do with behavior or delivery of gametes.

Sex is thus fundamentally dual, but in many species one of the sexes is absent or some other complication occurs. Thus, sexuality is shown by the males, females, and hermaphrodites in bisexual species as well as by the females in unisexual species.

Our recognition of maleness and femaleness may be based on differences in (1) sex chromosomes, (2) appearance of gametes (cytological), (3) anatomical and/or morphological characteristics of the animal as a whole or of specific visible structures (sexual dimorphism), and (4) behavioral or subtle physiological differences. There is diversity in all of these. In (1), sex chromosomes do not always occur and they do not determine sex in most animals even though they influence the determination within limits. In (2),

Table 9
OCCURRENCE OF SEXUAL REPRODUCTION AND SEXUALITY

	BBR	No bisexual	Dioecious	Hermaphroditic	Parthenogenetic	Alternations	♂	♀	⚥	♀	Insemination methods
Protozoa	X	X	X		X	S/A	X	X		X	Water, autogamy
Porifera	X		X	X	X	S/A	X	X	X		Water — inside
Mesozoa			X	X	?	S/A	X	X	X		
Coelenterata	X	X	X	X		S/A	X	X	X	X	Water — in & out
Ctenophora	X			X		S/A	X	X	X		Water — in & out
Gnathostomuloidea	X			X	?						Copulation
Platyhelminthes	X	X	X	X	X	S/A	X	X	X		Copulation, mutual copul., self-fert., hypodermic injection
Rhynchocoela	X	X	X	X	?	S/A	X	X	X		Water — outside, copulation
Acanthocephala	X		X		?		X	X			Copulation
Rotifera	X	X	X		X	S/P	X	X			Copulation, hypodermic injection
Gastrotricha	X	X	X	X	?		X	X	X		Water — outside
Kinorhyncha	X		X				X	X			Copulation
Nematoda	X		X	X	X	S/P	X	X	X		Copulation, self-fert.
Gordioidea	X		X				X	X			Copulation
Priapuloidea	X		X								Water — outside
Calyssozoa		X	X	X		S/A	X	X	X		Water — inside
Bryozoa		X	X	X		S/A, P/A	X	X	X	X	Water — inside, self-fert.
Phoronida	X		X	X		S/A	X	X	X		Water — outside, self-fert.
Brachiopoda	X		X	X	?		♂ X	X	X		Water — outside
Mollusca	X		X	X	X	S/A	X	X	X		Water — inside, self-fert., spermatophore, copul.
Sipunculoidea	X		X	X	X		X	X	X		Water — outside
Echiuroidea	X		X				X	X			Parasitic male, water — outside
Myzostomida	X			X					X		Spermatophore
Annelida	X	X	X	X	X	S/A, P/A	X	X	X	X	Water — outside, spermatophore, copul. & mutual copul., hypod. inj.
Dinophiloidea	X		X				X	X			Hypodermic injection
Tardigrada	X		X		X		X	X			Shed skin
Pentastomoidea	X		X				X	X			
Onychophora	X	X	X				X	X			Spermatophore
Arthropoda	X		X	X	X	S/A, S/P	X	X	X	X	Water — outside, spermatophore, copul. & mutual copul., hypod. injection
Chaetognatha	X			X					X		Self-fert., spermatophore
Pogonophora	X		X		?		X	X			In tube
Echinodermata	X	X	X	X	X	S/A	X	X	X		Water — out & in
Enteropneusta	X		X			S/A	X	X			Water — outside
Pterobranchia		X	X	X	?	S/A	X	X	X		Water — inside
Tunicata	X		X	X	?	S/A	X	X	X		Water — out & in
Cephalochordata	X		X	X			X	X	X		Water — outside
Vertebrata	X		X	X	X	S/A	X	X	X		Water — outside, copul.

Note: A, asexual; P, parthenogenetic; S, bisexual.

gametes are generally a large sperical ovum and a tiny motile spermatozoon (anisogametes — "not-identical gametes"), but in some Protozoa they may be isogametes (visually indistinguishable), or even hologametes (where the whole protozoans fuse in pairs).

There is endless variety in (3), from animals with very obvious "sex differences", as in many birds, to animals in which the sex can be determined only by microscopic examination of the gametes produced. In (4) there is also a range from those species in which most activities of the males and females are very different to those in which the sexes can scarcely be distinguished by their activities.

An additional diversity can occur that is directly related to sex. In both Rotifera and Insecta, there are species in which two kinds of females may be found. In Rotifera they are called mictic and amictic in reference to the type of ova they produce. In termites they are the queens and the workers. This condition is called *heterogyny.*

B. Sex within a Given Species

Sex can appear in a variety of combinations in the different individuals of one species:

1. Males and females, with testes and ovaries, respectively (gonochorists)
2. Hermaphrodites, with both testis and ovary
3. Males, females, and hermaphrodites
4. Males and hermaphrodites
5. Females only (parthenogenesis)
6. Males only (this cannot occur except if the individuals are reproductively neuter, reproducing asexually; there are a few species known only from males, but females will presumably be found)
7. Mating types

It should be noted that in (1) and (3) there may also be neuter (nonsexual) individuals. Furthermore, there are species in which only neuters are known, all reproduction being asexual. In (1) and perhaps others there may also occur gynandromorphs or intersexes.

1. Males

Males are the individuals that normally produce spermatozoa. They thus occur in all species reproducing bisexually, but they also occur in some parthenogenetic species. Some species have males, females, and hermaphrodites.

In several groups, the males are so unexpectedly small compared with the females that they are called *complementary males* or *dwarf males.* In the Rotifera these are apparently actually degenerate, occur rarely, and are often nonfunctional. In Nematoda, in some species of *Rhabditis* and *Diplogaster* the normal males produce spermatozoa but do not copulate and all reproduction is parthenogenetic. In *Dinophilus,* the males have been described as very similar to those of the Rotifera.

In some of the Echiuroidea, the males are very much smaller than the female and lack many organs. They live parasitically in the intestine or nephridia of the female. In the Myzostomida most individuals are hermaphrodites, but there may be also dwarf or complementary males. These are similar to the dwarf males found in some Crustacea (Copepoda, Isopoda, Cirripedia). Such accessory males are also reported in Insecta, but details are not available.

2. Females

This word is sometimes defined as that form of a dioecious species which produces ova, but of course all parthenogenetic females also produce ova, whether males are present or not. Females are the essential sex in all gametic reproduction. The presence of two kinds of females in Rotifera and termites was cited above.

3. Hermaphrodites

These are individuals with the organs of both sexes. They may produce ova and spermatozoa simultaneously, but more often produce first one and then the other: in *protandry,* spermatozoa first, in *protogyny,* ova first.

4. Neuters

There are also individuals in many groups that do not have the organs and features of either sex. They are without sexual function, and if they reproduce it is asexually. Examples are the avicularia in the Bryozoa, along with many types of individuals in polymorphic colonies where sexual reproduction is reserved to certain specialized individuals.

Animals may lose their sexual function through accident or senescence. They do not thereby become neuters in this sense. Such "neutering" may be by damage in fighting, surgical procedure, or parasitic castration.

There may be present in certain Crustacea both males and hermaphrodites in one species. This condition is described as *androdioecious.* (This appears to be an error for andromonoecious, since hermaphroditism is not related to dioecism but to monoecism.)

5. Mating Types

In many ciliate protozoans there may be in a given species two or more classes of individuals, distinguished in subtle physiological ways similar to sexual differentiation. In the process of conjugation members of any one class do not conjugate together, but individuals from two different classes may do so. This is suggestive of cross-fertilization. The classes are termed *mating types,* and there may be more than two types in some species. These mating types are not really features of sexual reproduction.

C. Sex in One Individual

Gonochorism is the existence of separate males and females. It is widespread but probably no more common than hermaphroditism.

Hermaphroditism is the occurrence of the primary organs of both sexes in one individual. From different points of view these hermaphroditic features may be classified in several ways.

1. By sequence in the life cycle
   a. Being male and female simultaneously but with separate ducts and no self-fertilization
   b. Being male and female simultaneously in one gonad or with common duct and therefore self-fertilization possible
   c. Being male first and then female (protandry)
   d. Being female first and then male (protogyny)
2. By type of organs
   a. Male and female organs separated in the body
   b. Organs combined in an ovotestis with tissues separate
   c. Organs combined with the male and female tissues indistinguishable
3. By type of individual
   a. Always hermaphroditic
   b. Gonochorists mixed with the hermaphrodites

4. By frequency of occurence
   a. Sporadic
   b. Cyclic
   c. Frequent
   d. Obligate

In Protozoa the terms *monoecy* and *dioecy* are sometimes used for hermaphroditism and gonochorism, respectively. The botanical terms *monoecism* and *dioecism* are also used in animals. These processes are widespread, sometimes even both occurring in closely related and otherwise similar species. "Both monoecy and dioecy are found within small taxonomic groups" (Grell, 1973) in Protozoa. "Both monoecious and dioecious forms are richly interspersed throughout the various groups of Cnidaria" (Campbell, 1974).

In some species in many groups there are also a few exceptional individuals that are the result of abnormal mixing of sex features. These are *gynandromorphs* (usually one side male and the other side female) or *intersexes* (where the features of the two sexes are mixed or merged). These are most obvious in such insects as butterflies, where the sexuality is expressed in the pattern and color. Intersexes are also reported in Echiuroidea and Vertebrata.

Gynoecy or *gynoecism* is the condition in which only females are known for the species. This means no males and no hermaphrodites. Neuters are usually neglected in such distinctions. There are gynoecious species in at least these groups: Rotifera, Gastrotricha, Nematoda, Gastropoda, Sipunculoidea, Crustacea, and Insecta.

Androecism is the condition in which only males are known. This is really possible, of course, only in asexually reproducing animals. Only one exception is known, in the Pterobranchia, where *Cephalodiscus sibogae* is known only from a colony with male and neuter individuals. It is presumed that females do exist, but in such a budding animal there is a possibility that all sexual reproduction has been lost.

A curious form of hermaphroditism occurs in certain Hypermastigida (Flagellata) where "sexual reproduction is initiated by a mitosis which...leads to the formation of a male and a female gamete..." (Grell, 1973). Presumably these are not hologametes, although the parent cell disappears.

D. Sex Distribution and Change

In the ordinary vertebrate heritage, sex is distributed among individuals in the familiar form of males and females. In every species some are one and the rest are the other. Occasionally one hears of an individual that changed from one to the other, and even of individuals that seem to be mixtures of a sort. Then one learns of earthworms that each have both sexes, and the simple vertebrate understanding of bodily sex becomes blurred. When all animals are examined, a variety of sex conditions are found.

A species is said to be *dioecious* if it consists of separate individuals that are either male or female. This condition is *dioecism,* commonly referred to as "having the sexes separate", i.e., in separate individuals. The species is said to be *monoecious* if all individuals contain the organs of both sexes, in which case the condition is *monoecism.* (These terms are more common in botany; they are sometimes mixed up with the next set, which properly apply to individuals rather than to species.)

Dioecism obtains in most species in all classes having any sexual processes, but not in the universally hermaphroditic Gastrotricha, Gnathostomuloidea, Phylactolaemata, most Oligochaeta, and Hirudinea. These include the individuals that would be called "unisexual", although they would usually reproduce bisexually.

Monoecism obtains in all hermaphrodites (listed below).

An individual is said to be *gonochoristic* if it has the organs of only one sex, and this is *gonochorism*. An individual is *hermaphroditic* if it contains both types of gonads, either at the same time or at different times, and this condition is *hermaphroditism*. Such hermaphroditic individuals therefore have the ability to produce both spermatozoa and ova, either simultaneously or in sequence. If in sequence, they may first be male and then female *(protandry)*, or first female and then male *(protogyny)*. There are a few species in which three types of individuals occur: males, females, and hermaphrodites, or males, females, and neuters (with no sex), but there seems to be no term to indicate these unusual sexual arrangements.

Gonochorism occurs in all dioecious species; i.e., in all except those that are completely parthenogenetic or those that are entirely hermaphroditic.

Hermaphroditism is widespread. It occurs in each of the classes of these 17 phyla: Porifera, Coelenterata, Ctenophora, Platyhelminthes, Rhynchocoela, Nematoda, Gordioidea, Calyssozoa, Bryozoa, Phoronida, Sipunculoidea, Myzostomida, Annelida, Chaetognatha, Pterobranchia, Tunicata, and Cephalochordata (possibly). It also occurs in these classes in 8 other phyla: Orthonectida, Macrodasyoidea, Articulata, Solenogastres, Amphineura, Gastropoda, Bivalvia, Cephalopoda, Crustacea, Insecta, Asteroidea, Ophiuroidea, Echinoidea, Holothurioidea, Agnatha, Osteichthyes, Reptilia, and Mammalia.

It thus appears in all phyla *except* these 11 small ones: Acanthocephala, Rotifera, Kinorhyncha, Priapuloidea, Echiuroidea, Dinophiloidea, Tardigrada, Pentastomida, Onychophora, Pogonophora, and Enteropneusta.

The term *syngony* has been used in Nematoda, where it is synonymous with hermaphroditism. It is not uncommon among terrestrial species, where it is usually protandric.

There are at least eight different arrangements of sex organs in animals. Sex can occur in two sexes, one sex (female or neuter), or in various combinations of sequences of the three "sexes". There seems to be no term to indicate these unusual sexual arrangements.

As indicated above, within a given individual, the sex may change during its life from male to female or vice versa. We are not here dealing with the manipulations of sex in humans by hormonal or surgical procedures but with processes in those animals in which the individuals normally pass through phases of producing first one type of gamete and later the other type. These are also included in the term hermaphrodite, along with those that have both sexes simultaneously. The possible sequences in an individual are these, showing the terms that are sometimes used:

1. Sexes permanently in separate individuals (gonochorism)
2. Occasional pathological sex reversal in an individual (no special term)
3. Normal reversal of sex in the life cycle
   a. Single change of sex (dichogamy): male first (protandry) or female first (protogyny)
   b. Alternating sex changes (multiple dichogamy)
4. Permanent union of sexes in one individual (hermaphroditism)
   a. Producing spermatozoa and ova simultaneously (synchronogamy): in separate gonads with separate ducts and therefore with no internal self-fertilization or in a single gonad (ovotestis) and therefore with internal self-fertilization possible or in two gonads that have a common duct and therefore with internal self-fertilization possible
   b. Gametes maturing at different times (dichogamy, as above): male first (protandry) or female first (protogyny)
   c. Abnormally half male and half female (gynandromorphism)
   d. Abnormal mixture of sexual features (intersexuality)

5. Transplantation of a testis into a young female, which thereafter functions as a self-fertilizing hermaphrodite (gonad transplant; see below)

It is sometimes assumed that there is no self-fertilization within an hermaphrodite. If that is in fact impossible, the condition is called *dichogamy*. This includes the two forms of protandry and protogyny described below. However, self-fertilization is at least possible in many groups. It has been reported in some species of Porifera, Coelenterata, Ctenophora, Platyhelminthes, Rhynchocoela, Nematoda, Bryozoa, Mollusca, Annelida, Arthropoda (Crustacea, Insecta), Chaetognatha, Echinodermata, and Vertebrata (Osteichthyes).

Hermaphroditism may involve two types of gametes produced simultaneously. When this occurs it is called *synchronogamy*, but this is not as common as to have the individual produce first one form of gamete and then the other, in succession. If spermatozoa are produced first, the sequence is called protandry. This occurs in some species of Anthozoa, Gnathostomuloidea, Rhynchocoela, Gastrotricha, Nematoda, Gymnolaemata, Phoronida, Solenogastres, Gastropoda, Bivalvia, Myzostomida, Annelida, Chaetognatha, Asteroidea, and Ophiuroidea. Protandrous (protandric) animals may produce the gametes from separate testis and ovary or from a single gonad which is first a functioning testis and then an ovary.

If ova are produced first, either in a separate ovary or first in sequence from a single gonad, the sequence is called protogyny. This occurs in some species of Anthozoa, Gastrotricha, Calyssozoa, Gymnolaemata, Bivalvia, and Osteichthyes.

Synchronogamy occurs in all hermaphrodites where there is no change. Dichogamy occurs in all those listed under protandry and protogyny. Gynandromorphism occurs in Insecta. Intersexuality occurs in Echiuroidea, Insecta, and Vertebrata.

1. Sex Reversal

The existence of protandry and protogyny indicates that the sex of an individual changes as its life proceeds. In fact, there may be several changes, back and forth. In some cases one gonad serves in both stages, and sometimes the gonad degenerates and is replaced for the next stage. Sometimes, as in some Insecta, the sex changes because of the presence of a parasite. Sex reversal obviously occurs in all the groups listed above under Protandry and Protogyny.

2. Gonad Transplant

This is an artificial sort of change, from female to hermaphrodite. It occurs in one species of Crustacea, where, at an early age, the male injects (by hypodermic injection) a few de-differentiated cells into the female body cavity; these then develop into a gamete-producing testis which makes the female ostensibly hermaphroditic; the zygotes are apparently produced by "self-fertilization", but genetically they are the result of normal cross-fertilization. This could be called pseudohermaphroditism, in which the ova are actually cross-fertilized (see Markewitch, 1976).

E. Sex Determination

At one time it was believed that the sex of the individual is determined at the time of fertilization by the type of sex chromosomes contributed by gametes. In some animals it was the presence of a Y-chromosome (the female being XX, the male XY); or in other species the XY being female and the XX male); and in still others there may be other chromosomal mechanisms (such as XO-XX). It is now realized that *all* animals with sex, so far as known, are potentially bisexual and may differentiate as either male or female regardless of their genetic or chromosomal sex. This is because any genetic determination can be overridden or superseded by other factors. Therefore, while it was true that the genetic sex of an individual is determined at fertilization, that individual may develop as either male or female.

Among the factors that may override the genetic factors are the following: (1) unusual temperatures, (2) presence of certain hormones or pheromones, (3) nutritional differences, (4) crowding, (5) sexual dimorphism of the spermatozoa, (6) fertilization of the ovum, and (7) influence from the other sex.

The actual methods of sex determination so far known are these:

1. The XX-XY chromosomes, as in humans
2. The XX-XO chromosomes, as in some Insecta
3. The fertilized/unfertilized method in the rotifers and in the honeybee
4. Action of a single gene as in some fishes
5—7. At least three other systems in Phasmida (Insecta)
8. By the action of a series of multiple homozygotic and heterozygotic alleles situated at corresponding locations (Insecta)
9. An accidental environmental determination, as in *Bonellia* (Echiuroidea) and some Crustacea
10. Automatic determination by simultaneous production of one gamete of each type, as a single differential cellular or nuclear division (Protozoa: Flagellata)

Terms involved in sex determination include the following:

1. Androgenesis — determination of maleness (s.Amphibia)
2. Chromosomal determination — by the presence of an extra chromosome (XO) or by one pair of chromosomes being unlike (XY)
3. Digamety — some spermatozoa have chromosomes for male-determining, others for female-determining
4. Genetic sex determination — that in which sex depends on genes
5. Genotypic sex determination — same as genetic
6. Gynogenesis — determination of femaleness (s.Amphibia)
7   Haplodiploidy — in which unfertilized (haploid) eggs produce males (arrhenotoky) and fertilized (diploid) eggs produce females (thelytoky)
8. Heterokinesis — the movement of the sex chromosome to one pole of the spindle
9. Modificatory sex determination — same as phenotypic
10. Phenotypic sex determination — not due to genetic factors but to some outside influence

F. Fusion

The usual bisexual reproduction culminates in fusion of the gamete pronuclei. It is sometimes implied that the word fusion can be restricted to this karyogamy. There are, however, several other instances of fusion in reproduction and elsewhere; they need to be kept distinct, as they do not all involve gametes. In the broadest sense, the following permanent fusions occur:

1. Two isogametes (s.Sarcodina, s.Flagellata, s.Sporozoa)
2. A spermatozoon and an ovum (as in all bisexual reproduction)
3. A spermatozoon and a somatic cell, "somatic fertilization (as in laboratory experiments with mammals)
4. An ovum and a nurse cell (s.Porifera, s. Mollusca, and probably others)
5. An ovum and one of its polar bodies (s.Crustacea, s.Asteroidea)
6. The blastomeres from several cleaving zygotes (s.Turbellaria)
7. Two buds, in pyloric budding (s.Ascidiacea)

8. Two whole individuals, hologamy (s.Flagellata, s.Sarcodina)
9. Two "adults", syzygy (Sporozoa: Gregarinida)
10. Two diporpa larvae (s.Trematoda)
11. Two ova, to produce one embryo (Hydrozoa: *Sagartia*)
12. Larvae or postlarvae of some sponges, to form "heterogenomic specimens"
13. Oocytes with epidermal or gastrodermal cells, apparently for nourishment (s.Hydrozoa)
14. Fertilized eggs fuse after being spawned, developing as a single large embryo (s.Anthozoa)
15. Two whole metazoans, fusing to form one (s.Anthozoa)
16. Two colonies, fusing to form one (s.Anthozoa)
17. Many amoeboid larvae (myxamoebae) to form a plasmodium (Sarcodina: Myce-tozoa)

The strange union of individuals in some gregarine Sporozoa is known as syzygy. Here the sporozoite larvae develop into gamonts, which tend to adhere in chains of two or more. The adherence to two gregarines seems to be a forerunner of gamogony, because it later develops that the anterior member is female, the posterior male. This is a case of the permanent union of individual animals. Other types of this same process occur in this same group, when two larvae encyst together, each becoming a gameto-cyte. Each gametocyte produces many gametes by multiple fission, whereupon each of the gametes from one gametocyte unites with one from the other, forming many zygotes.

IV. MISCELLANEOUS CONCEPTS

A. Introduction

There are a few features of reproduction at large that have not found a place in the foregoing accounts of processes, organs, and sequences. They are the para-reproductive processes, paedogenesis, and germ cell line.

B. Para-Reproductive Processes

When the word "reproduction" is hurriedly used in referring to animals that are normally sexual, it may include not only all varieties of sexual reproduction but also some similar processes that do not actually form new individuals and also some behavior that is associated with reproduction. The latter are here termed pre-reproductive; they do not formally enter into this book, as comparative treatment of them is difficult. They can be considered to include such things as transfer of spermatozoa, which is discussed in the previous chapter.

The processes that seem to be sexual but do not produce additional individuals have been called parasexual but are here termed *para-reproductive:* they are on the periphery of reproduction. These processes are restricted to the unicellular Protozoa. Although there may seem to be some form of sexuality involved, these processes are not in themselves multiplicative. They therefore cannot be included in reproduction as defined above. They do, however, produce changes in genetic make-up of the individuals involved, and they probably always include something akin to meiosis. They are sometimes followed by asexual reproduction (see Table 10).

These processes have been cited under various names, but we recognize the following: conjugation, hologamy, automixis, and nuclear reorganization.

When two individuals fuse permanently, with mixing of genetic materials, the process is called *hologamy,* the entire (protozoan) animal acting as a gamete. Temporary fusion is termed *conjugation,* but whereas there is normally transfer of nuclei and

Table 10

MULTIPLICATION AND GENOME CHANGES IN
REPRODUCTIVE AND RELATED PROCESSES

	Multiplication	Genome change
Bisexual reproduction	Yes	Yes
Pseudogamy	Yes	Yes
Parthenogenesis (meiotic)	Yes	Yes
Parthenogenesis (ameiotic)	Yes	No
Sporogony	Yes	No
Nongametic reproduction (asexual)	Yes	No
Conjugation	No	Yes
Hologamy	No	Yes
Automixis	No	Yes
Nuclear reorganization	No	Yes

From Blackwelder, R. E. and Shepherd, B. A., *The Diversity of Animal Reproduction.* CRC Press, Boca Raton, Fla., 1981.

karyogamy, there are species in which conjugation involves no exchange; this is *cytogamy.* There are Protozoa that undergo changes in the nuclei without gamogony, which are called *automixis* or *nuclear reorganization.*

In the similarity of these processes to fertilization, these processes differ as follows. Conjugation is comparable to cross-fertilization of two hermaphrodites, hologamy is comparable to ordinary cross-fertilization, autogamy is comparable to self-fertilization, and cytogamy is comparable to two individuals practicing autogamy individually.

Because all of these processes involve meiosis, they alter the genetic make-up of each of the individuals, and thereby increase the genetic diversity of the eventual progeny.

In many of these animals the processes of conjugation and hologamy are similar. In both of these processes diversity has recently been indicated by use of the terms isogamonty and anisogamonty. However, the important fact distinguishing these two processes is not the identity of form (iso-) or nonidentity (aniso-), but whether the fusing is temporary (conjugation), resulting in two changed individuals, or permanent (hologamy), resulting in one new individual from the fusion of two.

The temporary union of two ciliate protozoans of the same species with exchange of nuclear material is conjugation. It involves a series of events, including the following: (1) the two cells (conjugants) first join by their anterior ends, lying side by side along their oral surfaces, with membrane fusion and cytoplasmic bridges; (2) in each cell the micronucleus enlarges and its chromosomes become arranged into homologous pairs; (3) reduction of chromosome number is achieved by meiosis; (4) of the four haploid daughter nuclei, three are resorbed into the cytoplasm; (5) the remaining nucleus divides once more into two pronuclei, called stationary pronucleus and migratory pronucleus; (6) the migratory pronucleus of each cell passes into the other conjugant; (7) the stationary pronucleus and the new migratory pronucleus now fuse to form a fusion nucleus sometimes called a synkaryon; (8) the cells separate, being now referred to as exconjugants; (9) the fusion nucleus in each divides into two daughter nuclei, one becoming a new micronucleus and the other developing into a new macronucleus. The old macronucleus has disintegrated during the preceding steps. There is considerable diversity in these processes, including multiple conjugation, and the sequence may include also autogamy or cytogamy.

Although conjugation occurs only in the Ciliata (and the Suctoria), there are several diversities in its features. When the two individuals come together, it is normal for the micronuclei to be exchanged, but this may not happen, and the two nuclei that fuse may be derived from the same individual (autogamy). The conjugants themselves may be of three types: (1) similar to the original vegetative cells (hologamy or isogamonty), (2) much smaller and motile (merogony), or (3) the two widely different, especially in size (heterogamy or anisogamonty).

The two partners may be similar or different in size (1 and 3 above) and are then called isogamous or anisogamous, respectively. The "conjugation" may be total (karyogamy plus cytogamy, which is equivalent to hologamy) or partial (karyogamy alone, which is true conjugation). The conjugants may be of different ancestry (exogamy) or of the same ancestry (endogamy). The conjugation may be multiple, involving more than two individuals; in *Paramecium bursaria* there may be three, all undergoing nuclear changes but only the anterior two exchanging pronuclei.

The restoration of the normal nuclear constitution following conjugation is by a variety of mitoses and fusions of the synkaryon or fusion nucleus (details are to be found in Sleigh, 1973).

Fusion of sister nuclei from a previous division is *automixis*. If the sister nuclei are still in one cell, it is *autogamy* (but other usages of this term also occur). If they are now in separate cells, it is called *paedogamy* (but see also another usage of this word in the next section). In both forms of automixis the two "gamete nuclei" that eventually fuse are formed within a single cell by meiotic division; thus only one initial individual is involved, in what is similar to self-fertilization. It occurs in Sarcodina, Ciliata, and Sporozoa.

The process of *cytogamy* is a mixture of the features of conjugation and autogamy, in which two individuals unite temporarily without exchanging pronuclei. The two "conjugants" come together, but instead of exchanging migratory nuclei, the two pronuclei in each cell unite in autogamy. Some species use both autogamy and cytogamy, but not conjugation. Cytogamy occurs only in the Ciliata.

The process called *nuclear reorganization* is not clearly different from the preceding ones. In these the macronucleus may break up and re-fuse *(hemimixis)* or both macro- and micronucleus may be reformed from derivatives of the original micronucleus in the cytoplasm of the cell *(endomixis)*.

In Protozoa, *hologamy* is the permanent fusion of two whole individuals acting as gametes, with fusion of their pronuclei. Approximately the same steps occur as in conjugation, but there are basic differences. The two individuals are always of slightly different size (aniso-), and only one of them survives. When the two cells come together, their nuclei have undergone changes that leave in each cell a single pronucleus. (In the flagellate *Notila proteus,* these changes consist of a single meiotic division.) The smaller cell is then absorbed by the larger, and the two pronuclei fuse to form a synkaryon. The result is one individual with a nucleus changed by both meiosis and karyogamy, and a nearly doubled size.

In discussing the para-reproductive processes, it is desirable to eliminate clearly some processes that are not even pre-reproductive. Fusion in pairs is also cited under "Fertilization" as including some pairing that does not lead directly to reproduction. These include syzygy in gregarine Protozoa, fusion of larvae in Porifera, fusion of larvae or adults of flatworms, fusion of buds of some Tunicata, somatic fertilization (fusion of spermatozoa with somatic cells), composite zygotes of some Cestoda and Insecta, and fusion of cells in various tissues, including oocytes in Hydrozoa and Dinophiloidea. None of these are relevant to this discussion of reproduction.

One other form of nonkaryogamic union of single cells occurs in the Mycetozoa, which are sometimes considered to be sarcodine Protozoa. The individuals fuse without fusion of nuclei, producing a multinucleate plasmodium. This is called *plastogamy,* but it is scarcely reproductive.

C. Paedogenesis

Paedogenesis is reproduction by nonadult individuals, which occurs in several groups. Some writers restrict it to sexual reproduction, some to asexual. In the broad view of animal processes, there seems to be no advantage to either such restriction. There is reproduction in all stages of life, as shown in the list under "Levels of Reproductive Diversity" (above) and in the list below arranged by process:

1. Larval bisexual reproduction (Ctenophora)
2. Embryonic budding (Calyssozoa, Ascidiacea)
3. Larval budding (Hydrozoa, Scyphozoa, Cestoda, Ascidiacea)
4. Larval cyst budding (Cestoda)
5. Embryonic division (Insecta, Mammalia)
6. Zygote fission (Insecta)
7. Larval fragmentation (Orthonectida, Scyphozoa, Cestoda, Ascidiacea)
8. Larval frustulation (Hydrozoa)
9. Larval germ ball fragmentation (Trematoda as successional polyembryony)
10. Larval parthenogenesis (Insecta, Trematoda as progenesis)
11. Pupal parthenogenesis (Insecta)
12. Larval pedal laceration (Scyphozoa)
13. Polyembryony (Coelenterata, Trematoda, Cestoda, Gymnolaemata, Oligochaeta, Insecta, Asteroidea, Chondrichthyes, Amphibia, Reptilia, Aves, Mammalia)
14. Larval stolon formation (Scyphozoa)
15. Larval strobilation (Scyphozoa)

Production of gametes by a larval individual has been called *paedogamy*. This occurs only in Ctenophora and Trematoda. The term *neoteny* is sometimes used in place of paedogenesis, but it is better reserved for the evolutionary concept of a species which becomes sexually mature as larvae and then loses the adult stage altogether. This occurs in Amphibia (salamanders of the family Ambystomidae) and in Insecta (certain castes of termites).

In some Trematoda a metacercaria larva may attain sexual maturity and produce ova, parthenogenetically, that will develop into infective larvae.

D. Germ Cell Line

An important consideration in gametogenesis is the ancestry of the cells. It is often stated that the gametes are derived from a cell traceable through cleavage and therefore forming a continuity of the germplasm through all generations. There is no formal way in which this can have meaning in all animal groups alike, but since all cells arise from pre-existing cells there always is a continuity of some sort. It is not true that the germ cell line is distinguishable in all stages of all animals.

In fragmenting worms, for example, the gonads and gametes in some of the fragments arise by fresh differentiation of some somatic cells that happen to be in that fragment. A hydroid polyp that develops from a tiny fragment of the base, probably all ectodermal, can develop normal gonads and gametes.

On the other hand, there are rotifers in which the gametes are derived from a germ cell line distinguishable and isolated at the 10-cell stage of cleavage.

Every gamete, like nearly every other cell, is formed by division of a pre-existing cell, and thus every gamete can be traced back to the preceding generation. There is no real continuity of the germplasm in the sense that germplasm is discrete from somatoplasm through the life of the individual. There is an approach to this in some animals, but in many the germplasm is formed from somatoplasm.

It has long been believed that the idea of continuity of the germplasm from generation to generation meant that there is a rigid separation of somatoplasm (body) and germplasm (sex cells). Inasmuch as germ cells, like all other body cells, arise by many divisions from the original zygote, there *is* continuity. However, there is no clear separation of the germ line during development in most animals. Some of the reported sources of germ cells are

1.   Ectoderm (some Hydrozoa)
2.   Gastrodermis (s.Hydrozoa, Scyphozoa, Anthozoa, Ctenophora)
3.   Interstitial cells (some Hydrozoa)
4.   Mesoderm, epithelium (s.Gastropoda, s.Echinodermata, Mammalia: *Homo sapiens*)
5.   Peritoneal cells (Phoronida, Bryozoa, Brachiopoda, Polychaeta, s.Echinodermata)
6.   Primordial germ cells, from first cleavage (s.Trematoda, s.Rotifera, Nematoda)
7.   Mesenchyme, any amoebocyte (Porifera, Turbellaria, Cestoda, Rhynchocoela, Gordioidea)

REFERENCES

Barnes, R. D., *Invertebrate Zoology,* 2nd ed., W. B. Saunders, Philadelphia, 1968.
Blackwelder, R. E. and Shepherd, B. A., *The Diversity of Animal Reproduction,* CRC Press, Boca Raton, Fla., 1981.
Campbell, R. D., Cnidaria, in *Reproduction of Marine Invertebrates,* Vol. 1, Giese, A. C. and Pearse, J. S., Eds., Academic Press, New York, 1974, chap. 3.
Davey, K. G., *Reproduction in the Insects,* Oliver & Boyd, Edinburgh, 1965.
Giese, A. C. and Pearse, J. S., Eds., *Reproduction of Marine Invertebrates,* Vol. 1 (1974); Vol. 2 (1975), Vol. 3 (1975), Vol. 4 (1977), Vol. 5 (1979).
Grell, K. G., *Protozoology,* Springer-Verlag, Berlin, 1973.
Hagan, H. R., *Embryology of the Viviparous Insects,* Ronald Press, New York, 1951.
Henley, C. Platyhelminthes (Turbellaria), in *Reproduction of Marine Invertebrates,* Vol. 1., Giese, A. C. and Pearse, J. S., Eds., Academic Press, New York, 1974, chap. 5.
Hyman, L. H., *The Invertebrates,* Vol. 1 (1940), Vol. 2 (1951a), Vol. 3 (1951b), Vol. 4 (1955), Vol. 5 (1959), Vol. 6 (1967), McGraw-Hill, New York.
Imms, A. D., *A General Textbook of Entomology,* 8th ed., Methuen, London, 1951.
Kudo, R. R., *Protozoology,* 5th ed., Charles C Thomas, Springfield, Ill., 1966.
Lasserre, P., Clitellata, in *Reproduction of Marine Invertebrates,* Vol. 3, Giese, A. C. and Pearse, J. B., Eds., Academic Press, New York, 1975.
Markewitch, A. P., *Parasitic Copepodes on the Fishes of the U.S.S.R.,* Indian National Scientific Documentation Centre, New Delhi, 1976.
Sadleir, M. F. S., *The Reproduction of Vertebrates,* Academic Press, New York, 1973.
Sleigh, M. A., *The Biology of Protozoa,* American Elsevier, New York, 1973.
Smyth, J. D., *Introduction to Animal Parasitology,* 2nd ed., John Wiley & Sons, New York, 1976.
Waterman, T. H., Ed., *The Physiology of Crustacea,* Vol. 2, Academic Press, New York, 1961.
Yanagimachi, R., The life cycle of *Peltogasterella, Crustaceana,* 2, 183, 1961.

Part III
Development of Individuals

"The process whereby a single cell may multiply and differentiate, becoming a flower, a man, or a butterfly, depending upon its antecedents, is one calling for regulatory devices of incomprehensible complexity."

Williams and Beerstecker, 1948

"Discussions of development often stop with the completely matured adult. But development in its full biological sense does not cease then. The adult organism is not a static entity; it continues to change, and hence to develop, until death brings the developmental process to an end."

Keeton, 1972

"So life becomes a ceaseless striving for a peaceful heterogeneous equilibrium, the attainment of which would result only in death."

Holmes, 1948

Chapter 5

EMBRYOLOGY

TABLE OF CONTENTS

I.   Orientation 112
     A.   Introduction 112
     B.   Developmental Stages 112
     C.   Unity in Early Development 113
     D.   Diversity in Development 113
     E.   Cycles of Development 114
     F.   Problems of Sponge Embryology 116
         1.   Tissues and Organs 116
         2.   Inversion 117
     G.   Zygotes and Apozygotes 118
         1.   Location of Zygote 120
         2.   Special Terms 121
         3.   Fate of the Zygote 121
         4.   Composite Eggs 121

II.   Cleavage 122
     A.   Commentary 122
     B.   Cleavage Terms 123
     C.   Cleavage Patterns 124
     D.   Blastoderm Formation 125

III.   Embryogenesis 126
     A.   Blastula 126
     B.   Gastrula 126
         1.   Germ Layers and Gastrulation 127
         2.   Blastopore 129
         3.   Fate of the Blastopore 129
         4.   Mesoderm Formation 132
     C.   Morphogenesis 134

IV.   Embryo 135
     A.   Commentary 135
     B.   Cavities of the Embryo 136
     C.   Determination 138
     D.   Site of Embryonic Development 139
     E.   Emergence 140

References 141

I. ORIENTATION

A. Introduction

In its broadest sense, which is the only one that can be defined realistically, development includes all processes and activities from inception to death. These extend from fertilization (or activation) through embryonic and juvenile stages to adult and include morphogenesis, growth, and senescence. It also includes the sequence of changes from the moment of separation (in budding or fragmentation) until death.

Some aspects of this life-long sequence of processes are specified by special words: cleavage, embryogeny, birth or hatching, larval development, metamorphosis, growth, maturing, senescence, and death.

It is impossible to separate reproduction from development or either of these from physiology. Reproduction is here defined as including all processes that result in multiplication of individuals. Weiss (1939) distinguished physiology from development thus: "If an effect passes without leaving a trace, it is physiological; if it leaves a permanent residue in the organism, it is developmental . . . No vital processes are in themselves either specifically developmental or specifically physiological. Developmental and functional processes are essentially of the same making."

In Chapter 8 an attempt is made to justify the statement that structure and function are really inseparable; one can discuss things from either view, but each inevitably involves the other.

It must be emphasized, however, (1) that the division between "development of individuals (Part III) and features of adult individuals (Part IV) is arbitrary — development really includes the entire life cycle, and (2) life cycles may vary extremely from what we normally think of in mammals or any other strictly bisexual animals. Thus, whereas this section deals with the structures and processes of animal life histories up to the adult stage, emphasis should be on change, for change of process leads to change of form which leads again to change of process. Change may be sequential or cyclic, but in general it is a combination of both in bewildering profusion.

It must also be remembered that life cycles frequently do not lead in a straight line from egg to adult. Many animals make sharp deviations in producing highly specialized larvae that show few features of the eventual adult; in insects with a pupal stage there may be no continuity between larval organ systems and those of the adult.

In fact, it has been said (Rudnick, 1961) that "The general principles underlying the relation of embryonic to adult function have yet to be enunciated."

This does not mean that development within a given species is disorganized or variable; it is highly controlled. As Gerard (1949) put it: "The (rare) monsters . . . serve to emphasize the amazing accuracy of the normal process of development."

B. Developmental Stages

Development overall can be divided into several components, usually sequential. These include the processes of activation or onset, differentiation, organization, growth, senescence, and death. Dedifferentiation, resorption (so-called negative growth), and even reorganization may also be interspersed.

From a slightly different approach the sequence can be viewed as stages: zygote, cleavage, blastula, gastrula, embryo, larva, adult. In many cases a period of quiescence or dormancy is inserted at some point.

The structural forms assumed by animals during their development are almost unlimited. They include: (1) zygote, (or apozygote), (2) embryo, (3) foetus, (4) larva, which may be anything from an early embryo to any of scores of independently living forms, (5) pupa, (6) juvenile, and (7) adult. In addition there may be several larval stages in sequence, and still further in asexual animals development may start from (8) buds, (9) gemmules (including sorites and statoblasts); or (10) fragments (including frustules, epitokes, or eudoxids — fragments of colonies).

Most life cycles include several of these. The average number in a life cycle must be about six. This means that the 1 million species of animals now known present themselves in at least 6 million forms. Every one of these forms undergoes its own development.

C. Unity in Early Development

It has been written that there is a high degree of unity in the early development of all multicellular animals, and that there is great similarity in gametogenesis (including maturation), fertilization, cleavage, and gastrulation. In reality, there is substantial diversity in all of these. For example, gametogenesis may be meiotic or ameiotic, resulting in either haploid or diploid gametes. What is called fertilization may be either karyogamic or mere activation. Cleavage is diverse in many ways and in asexual cycles is completely absent. Gastrulation is performed in at least 10 different ways.

A more realistic statement is " . . . the various animal groups by no means behave identically in their development."

D. Diversity in Development

The development of animals from the beginning of their separate existence until their death is generally assumed to always include an embryogeny — a period in which cleavage forms a blastula, followed by gastrulation and embryo formation. This is, of course, a gross misconception.

Among the asexual processes cited in Chapter 2, there are seven in which the individuals produced develop entirely without cleavage, gastrulation, or embryo formation. These seven processes are agamogony, gemmulation, fragmentation, budding, strobilation, pedal laceration, and frustulation. A very large number of kinds of animals representing roughly half the phyla reproduce in this manner, usually not merely as an exceptional occurrence. Even among animals that develop from a zygote, the stages of blastula and gastrula may be completely bypassed. In the forms with superficial or discoidal cleavage, the embryo is formed directly on the surface of the egg by delamination and differentiation, with many of the usual processes and stages omitted. The latter include at least 80% of the animal kingdom.

The diversities in developmental processes of the asexually produced individuals are not always different from those of zygote individuals because in polyembryony the separated blastomeres cleave in a manner identical to the zygotes. These blastomeres then pass through the stages of embryo and larva. In some individuals, the asexual reproduction will bypass all the usual developmental stages and produce a new adult directly.

Among those animals that do arise from a zygote or apozygote, there is much diversity at several points. Only a suggestion of the diversity in certain parts of development can be given in this book, which tabulates some of the diversity in the following features (some subjects treated in other chapters are so indicated).

1. Activation methods ("Parthenogenesis", Chapter 4)
2. Adult features and processes ("Adult Individuals", Part IV)
3. Anabiosis ("Dormancy", Chapter 7)
4. Archenteron fate ("Larval Tissues", Chapter 11)
5. Asexual origin ("Cycles of Development", Chapter 5)
6. Basic life cycles ("Life Cycles", Chapter 7)
7. Blastopore fate ("Gastrula", Chapter 5)
8. Blastula structure (Chapter 5)

9. Body cavity formation ("Embryogenesis", Chapter 5)
10. Body cavity types ("Body Spaces", Chapter 20)
11. Cleavage (Chapter 5)
12. Cleavage patterns (Chapter 5)
13. Dormancy (Chapter 7)
14. Embryo reproduction ("Asexual Reproduction", Chapter 2)
15. Eutely, cell constancy (Chapter 7)
16. Gastrulation methods ("Gastrula", Chapter 5)
17. Germ layer formation ("Gastrula", Chapter 5)
18. Growth (Chapter 7)
19. Larval organs (with "Adult Individuals", Part IV)
20. Larval types ("Larva", Chapter 6)
21. Maternal care ("Exploitation", Chapter 22)
22. Metamorphosis (Chapter 6)
23. Polymorphism (Chapter 9)
24. Regeneration (Chapter 7)
25. Reproductive cycles ("Sequences", Chapter 4)
26. Retrogression ("Dormancy", Chapter 7)
27. Zygote (Chapter 5)

E. Cycles of Development

Before starting with the diversity of the zygote stage, it is well to note how diverse is the sequence of stages through which different animals pass and how many animals arise and live without ever passing through a real development at all.

In many animals the *life history* of an individual is not the same as the *life cycle* of the species. For example, in *Obelia* the zygote gives rise to polyp (hydranth) and this development is the life history of that individual. The polyp is an adult. The polyp then buds other polyps, which have more abbreviated life histories. One of these may bud a different polyp (gonangium), also with a simple life history. The gonangium may then bud off medusae, also adult. The medusa is the sexual stage, with its own life history. The zygotes it produces may start the original life cycle again. From the first zygote to the next takes at least four steps, each involving its own life history. All together the zygote to hydranth plus the hydranth to gonangium, plus the gonangium to medusa plus the medusa to hydranth — four life histories — form the life cycle of the species. All four life histories are necessary to this particular cycle.

In a few books it is implied that the processes usually called reproduction are part of development. We prefer the viewpoint that development starts at the formation of a new individual and extends to the point at which it ceases to exist separately (because of death, subdivision into two or more, or union with others to form one). Reproduction often occurs during this life and is part of it. However, the production that produced that individual in the first place is not part of its life but an activity of the one or two individuals that produced it.

A new individual is not started until fertilization, activation, or asexual reproduction has occurred. Therefore, reproduction is herein treated more as an activity of individuals than as a developmental or systemic process, except that sexual maturation is a milestone in the development of some animals.

A major part of this chapter and all of most of the comparable ones in other books is devoted to the development of animals from fertilization to death. This is evidently looked upon as the "normal" cycle. There are, however, a wide variety of animals that do not pass through this standard sequence.

On the assumption, which seems inescapable, that a new individual can be formed by any of a variety of processes, the life cycles of animals may vary *in extremis*. With an example of each, these include:

1. Zygote — embryo — juvenile — adult — Death (Vertebrata)
2. Zygote — embryo — larva — adult — Death (Polychaeta)
3. Zygote — embryo — adult — Division (Anthozoa)
4. Apozygote — embryo — larva — adult — Death (Turbellaria)
5. Zygote — adult — Fusion (Flagellata: Phytomonadina)
6. Apozygote — adult — Fusion (possible in Protozoa: no example known)
7. Zygote — embryo — Division (polyembryony) (parasitic Insecta)
8. Apozygote — embryo — Division (polyembryony or embryo budding) (likely in Oligochaeta; no example known)
9. Bud (from adult) — adult — Death (Bryozoa)
10. Bud (from larva) — adult — Death (Hydrozoa)
11. Bud (from adult) — larva — adult — Death (Hydrozoa)
12. Bud (from adult) — Fusion (Ascidiacea)
13. Bud (from larva) — larva — adult — Death (Hydrozoa)
14. Fragment (of embryo) — embryo — larva — pupa — adult — Death (parasitic Hymenoptera)
15. Fragment (of embryo) — embryo — juvenile — adult — Death (Oligochaeta)
16. Fragment (of adult) — adult — Death (Hydrozoa)
17. Fragment (of adult) — adult — Division (Oligochaeta)
18. Gemmule — adult — Death (Porifera)
19. Fused eggs — larva — adult — Death (Turbellaria)
20. Fused larvae — adult — Death (Trematoda)
21. Fused adults — adult — Fission (Ciliata)
22. Adult — Fusion (Flagellata)
23. Adult — Fission (Sarcodina)

It must be noted that further variations in these cycles occur, such as occurrence of several larval forms in sequence (*hypermetamorphosis*), addition of a resting stage (such as a pupa) at some point, and regressions followed by regenerations.

In the examples given, as in (1) Vertebrata, the end of life of the adult is always metabolic death, but in other animals (such as some of the Anthozoa) the end of life would be at a division that produced two new ones. Thus, in the list the word "Death" may include both forms of "life ending".

Only (1) and (2) above fit the common conception of a developmental cycle. Although these two no doubt cover the cycle of most familar animals, a large majority of all individuals of all species together exist only in one of the beheaded or bobtailed cycles of (5) through (23). A developmental cycle will start when a new individual is formed, and this cycle may *start* in any of these stages:

1. Zygote
2. Apozygote (activated ovum)
3. Fragment (at any age: embryo, larva, adult)
4. Bud (at any age: embryo, larva, adult)
5. Gemmule or other assembled body
6. Fused individuals (at any age: zygotes, embryos, larvae, adults)

Looking at this another way, a cycle may *end* at:

1. Natural death (at any age)
2. Accidental or violent death (at any age)
3. Division of the individual (at any age)
4. Fusion with another individual (at any age)

F. Problems of Sponge Embryology

Two features of sponges are frequently cited as requiring the isolation of this group from other metazoan animals. These are the claims that they do not have tissues or organs and that their embryology is unique. There is considerable room for question of the validity of each of these claims.

1. Tissues and Organs

The peculiarities of early embryology of sponges have sometimes been stated to be so great that any cell layers or tissues formed cannot be correlated in manner of origin with layers of other animals. These cells are described as not forming anything that can be called germ layers or tissues. The justification for this statement is seldom given, but it consists in part in the looseness of the layers, often with the cells not in contact with one another, even in the epidermis. (The fact that the exterior cells are unhesitatingly called an epidermis scarcely emphasizes any great peculiarity.)

Presumably because of this looseness of cell layers, it was concluded by Hyman (1940) that the Porifera are at "the cellular grade of construction as distinct from the rest of the Metazoa which are at "the tissue grade of construction". (The peculiar Mesozoa were conveniently separated out first, so they did not appear in either grade.) The claimed difference between the two grades is that in the "tissue grade" there are clear-cut tissues with two or more types of cells formed into organs (which must consist of two or more kinds of cells or tissues), whereas in the "cellular grade" there are no tissues and no organs.

Although the sponges are described as consisting of a loose aggregation of cells hardly formed into tissues, they actually consist essentially of epithelia and mesenchyme with some differentiation into epithelial, muscle, amoeboid, and possibly glandular cells.

A person who recognizes that there are many complete unicellular organs among higher animals (receptors, glands, gametes) will recognize organs in sponges, including phagocytic collar cells, gametes, and gemmules. In the structure of a sponge, a very satisfactory epidermis exists, along with a feeding layer of the collar cells (choanocytes) interspersed with pore cells. There is also a mesenchyme of a proteinaceous matrix with several types of amoeboid cells. The ova may be surrounded by a mass of nurse cells, which may be interpreted to form a simple ovary, where the ovum awaits the approach of spermatozoa carried by amoebocytes.

Sponges are no doubt very simple animals, but there seems to be no way to deny that they consist of several simple tissues and organs. There has to be some coordination of activity in an animal that produces many identical spicules and transports spermatozoa to the ovum from a distance. Even though the cell layers do not always correspond in origin to those usually ascribed to other animals (some of which also do not correspond to each other!), there *are* layers and there are three of them. The obvious looseness of the construction of these tissues is no greater than in some tissues elsewhere; they merely are *all* of this loose nature.

To return to the sidetracked Mesozoa, some zoologists believe them to be degenerate flatworms. If so, they must be basically triploblastic. However, they actually consist of two layers, a syncytial outer layer of epidermis and an inner mass consisting of one or a few reproductive cells. Again the embryology is such that these "layers" cannot be correlated with germ layers of higher animals. There *are*, however, at least two layers, with functional similarity to epidermis and mesenchyme. It does not seem adequate to label these animals as merely cellular. These and the sponges consist of layers of cells (simple tissues), perhaps of different embryological nature from those of other animals (or those of each other).

In the animals that have unquestioned tissues of the type familiar in higher animals, and produced by similar processes, two are said to be diploblastic and all other triplo-blastic. Hyman (1940) accepts Coelenterata and Ctenophora as diploblastic with epidermis and gastrodermis. Earlier in the same volume, she unaccountably states that "Porifera, Cnidaria, and Ctenophora are not really diploblastic . . . " In a later volume (IV, 1959) she reviews newer information and concludes that the latter comments, on the earlier page in her book, are correct and "that in fact all Metazoa except hydrozoan polyps are triploblastic". The hydrozoan polyps simply have a mesogloea without many cells or the usual collagen fibers, but it still seems reasonable to call it a tissue layer because it serves the same function as a cellular mesogloea in other coelenterates.

Thus the distinction so clearly shown by Hyman in the titles of her chapters and part of the text, between cellular grade and tissue grade, turned out to be unacceptable even to her.

2. Inversion

Nearly all recent textbooks of zoology state that development in sponges is very different from that of other animals and puzzling in these differences. It appears that these textbook opinions are largely derived from Hyman (1940), who is the most frequently quoted modern author on invertebrates other than annulates. She states that "The embryonic history of sponges is peculiar and cannot be homologized with that of other metazoans."

Nearly all writers describe one process as the main peculiarity of sponges and the source of most of the difficulty. This is inversion, which carries apparent endoderm cells to the outside to become epidermis.

In trying to find adequate descriptions for the processes and the basic facts necessary to explain them, the present study has uncovered only greater confusion. It is unquestionable that inversion is not a widespread phenomenon among sponges and actually occurs only in the class Calcarea. It seems to be unchallengable that it is not universal even in Calcarea, but occurs in only a few species. It is true that in some sponges inversion is an identifiable process and that it is unusual among animals. It is also true that a few other features of sponge development are unusual, including the temporary mouth, the relocation of entire tissues by cell migration, and gastrulation by cavitation.

Beyond this there is a mass of contradictory opinion, evident cases of misleading use of terms, and misquotation of earlier works. The following facts and conclusions do not settle this problem, but they do seem to reduce its proportions and remove some of the confusion.

First, there is no point to citing situations that occur unless the species is identified, because different species within one genus may be very different in development. There are clear descriptions of the development of about 1 dozen named species. Three of these are Calcarea, 7 are Demospongea, and 2 are Hyalospongea (Hexactinellida). One of the Calcarea *(Leucosolenia variabilis)* is described as having inversion (Kume & Dan, 1968), but the species *Leucosolenia blanca* is described in four books as NOT showing inversion. Only two other species are specifically cited as showing inversion; they are both Calcarea but they are identified only to genus (by Hyman, 1940): *Sycon* and *Grantia* spp. *Sycon raphanus* is described in at least three books as NOT showing inversion, however. The name *Grantia* is commonly applied to species of *Sycon*. None of the other species described in any class show inversion.

Second, in most textbook descriptions of inversion, in unnamed species, a temporary mouth is described that ingests neighboring cells. Then by inversion the interior cells pass out through "the mouth". In most detailed descriptions, the temporary mouth closes promptly, and the interior cells migrate individually to the surface.

Third, most examples of sponge peculiarity are based on the fact that the early cleavages produce some large and some small cells. It is claimed that in Metazoa the small blastomeres become the ectoderm and the large ones the endoderm, whereas it is just the reverse in sponges. This is said to make the resulting "germ layers" so different in nature that they cannot be homologized with those of higher animals. Metazoa are not all alike in this regard, and it is not necessary to see radical divergences in this feature.

Fourth, the peculiarities in further development are exaggerated. For example, Meglitsch (1972) stated that "From this point on, however, the sponge embryo does everything wrong". However, in earlier works (Tuzet, 1963, quoting Jaegersten in 1955 and 1959) it is clearly recognized "that the developmental features of sponges do not separate them from other metazoa". Tuzet added, "Nothing is opposed, it seems to me, to the derivation of the Hydrozoa from the sponges", and she quoted Jaegersten again to that same end.

Fifth, several authors have discussed sponge species that would be of interest here. Their own primary interest appears to have been in the effects of oviparity and viviparity to such an extent that they omitted essential developmental features from their descriptions. (Whether the so-called viviparity of some sponges is similar to the nourishment-providing viviparity of higher animals is questionable, as pointed out by Harrison and Cowden in 1976.)

There is much further confusion over the use of terms, such as inversion itself which seems to be used for two quite different processes by some textbook writers, and in describing morphogenetic cell movements by terms usually used for major features such as gastrulation. We conclude that only two features of sponge embryology need be specially recognized: inversion (which occurs in only a few species of Calcarea) and gastrulation by cavitation, which is the appearance of a cavity within a solid blastula. Hyman did not list cavitation in 1940 (pp. 260 to 262) among her eight methods, presumably because she thought that in sponges it should not be called gastrulation at all.

The usual textbook summaries of peculiarities in sponge development are thus without direct foundation. Some of the peculiarities are unique among animals, but none are outside of the range of diversity in animals at large. That there should be peculiarities in the development of animals that can regenerate (reconstitute) themselves from a pile of separated cells, as some sponges do in nature, should not surprise one at all, but there seems to be no compelling reason to believe that sponges are substantially different from all other animals in the features of early development as so far understood.

Inversions in some other groups are reported to be similar to that described for these few sponges. One such is cited for the colonial flagellate *Volvox*, where the cleavage of the zygote (or apozygote) inside the parent results in a sphere of cells with flagella on the inside. These flagella are described as reaching the outside by a rupture and inversion of the sphere of daughter cells. An unusual hydrozoan named *Polypodium hydriforme* is also involved in an inversion. During the early stages of development, this small polyp parasitizes the eggs of a sturgeon. It is turned inside out, with the endoderm layer toward the yolk of the host egg. It develops a stolon on which form a score or so of buds, all with endoderm outside. Finally, the stolon bursts, and the polyps turn their ectoderm outward and leave the host for a free life outside. The parasite is said to resemble an inverted intestine, as it feeds through its "outer" (endoderm) layer (after Dogiel, 1966).

G. Zygotes and Apozygotes

When animals arise from a single cell formed by fusion of two gametes (either spermatozoon and ovum or two isogametes or two hologametes), the new cell is termed a *zygote*. In the numerous animals that arise from an ovum that is not fertilized but merely activated (induced to start development) by other means than fertilization, the term zygote is not really appropriate. No commonly used term is available for this situation, but apozygote is both apt and useful. Fertilization will be used herein only when there is fusion of a spermatozoon pronucleus with that of the ovum (karyogamy) and activation when an ovum starts to develop without such complete fertilization. Karyogamy produces a zygote; activation alone results in an *apozygote*. In much of the following diversity, when the term zygote is used, it should be understood that apozygotes are included, as their development is usually indistinguishable from that of zygotes.

There is diversity among these zygotic structures, which are classed both as whole animals and as new individuals at the start of their life cycles. As always, there is diversity in their genetic make-up, as well as in size, shape, polarity, coverings, etc. In their genetic make-up, zygotes may be

1.   Diploid — the result of: (a) cross-fertilization between unrelated parents, (b) cross-fertilization between members of a clone, (c) self-fertilization, (d) production without meiosis or fertilization from a diploid ovum
2.   Haploid — the result of development of an unfertilized ovum (no karyogamy)
3.   Diploid/haploid — (a) fusion of egg and spermatozoon, and of their pronuclei, but with the two chromosome sets remaining separate in the nucleus (gonomery); the fusion nucleus has two sets of chromosomes but only one functions at this time

The range of size in eggs is tremendous, but comparable figures for the extremes are difficult to find. Near one extreme is the ostrich, with an egg 155 × 130 mm, with a volume of 1.25 ℓ or ¹/₃ gal. Near the other extreme would be the eggs of parasitic insects, that are small enough to be laid inside the eggs of other insects. These are probably as small as 0.05 mm in diameter, with a volume roughly 0.0001 mm³. The size of zygotes is in part related to the amount of enclosed yolk.

Even greater size was attained in the extinct elephant bird of Madagascar, *Aepyornis titan*, in which the egg had a volume of approximately 2 gal and a weight of 18 lb. It had the volume of 6 ostrich eggs combined, or of 12 dozen chicken eggs!

It must be emphasized that these bird eggs are extremely rich in yolk, the volume corresponding roughly to the size of the adult. In many other groups eggs tend to be fairly uniform in size among the species, a fact exemplified in the eggs of some Nematoda. In this phylum individuals of all species — very large as in *Ascaris* or very small as in *Meloidogyne* — have eggs of much the same size, usually in the range of 50 to 90 μm in length and half that in width. Another diversity appears here within some species, as in *Ascaris lumbricoides* itself, the eggs range from 52- to 84-μm long.

Zygote shape is often dependent on the membranes or shell of the ovum inside which the zygote develops. The shape is fairly close to a sphere in most eggs that develop by ordinary cleavage. It is often elongate in eggs that will develop by meroblastic cleavage (as in many Insecta).

Polarity of the zygote is likely to be the same as that of the ovum, defined by shape, position of the nucleus, a micropyle, the point of sperm entry, etc., but it may be recognizable only after the first or the first two cleavages.

Yolk in the zygote is always the yolk that was contained in the ovum (and any nurse cells that fuse with it). The terms for the quantity and distribution of this yolk are defined in the section on nutrients for ovum and zygote in Chapter 13. Yolk may be divided among the blastomeres during cleavage or may remain outside of all the daughter cells (see Section II. A. Cleavage).

Zygote coverings are in part the same envelopes as those of the ovum, because the egg always develops from the ovum after activation of some sort. Of these coverings, the original cell membrane is expanded to surround the individual daughter cell (blastomere), but it does not cover the embryo as a whole. The fertilization membrane simply disappears with the onset of cleavage. These and additional coverings of the ovum are listed under Ova in Chapter 3.

Other zygote coverings may be present, often produced by a variety of maternal tissues, especially in cases of maternal care (examples follow).

Rhynchocoela. Ova in viviparous and self-fertilizing species may remain in the ovaries until hatching, covered by a cell membrane, fertilization membrane, and the ovarian tissues. In other species the ova, with these same two cell membranes, are laid in gelatinous masses.

Acanthocephala. There is a shell formed by the syncytial 32-cell stage.

Rotifera. One or two membranes occur, which are probably derivatives of the cell and fertilization membranes of the ovum; these are inside the shell, which is also formed by the egg. Outside the shell there may be an additional thin membrane or a gelatinous envelope.

Nematoda. The fertilization membrane thickens to form a shell. Inside of this shell, the egg produces a lipoid membrane, which is thin and delicate. The uterine wall may add a protein membrane outside of the shell.

Cephalopoda. The egg in its fertilization membrane is covered just before discharge by a paired membrane or capsule from the oviducal gland. A gelatinous outer covering may be added from a nidamental gland, which later may harden into a capsule.

Insecta. The ovum forms a cell membrane termed the vitelline membrane. Outside of this a shell or chorion is formed by the follicular epithelium of the mother. The chorion may consist of two layers, an exochorion and an endochorion. The chorion may be penetrated by one or more micropyles, or it may have an operculum for the eventual release of the larva.

Vertebrata. The plasma and fertilization membranes cover the zygote, but become indistinguishable as the embryo is formed. In some vertebrates a shell is formed around the zygote and its membranes. Extra-embryonic membranes are later formed by the embryo, and some of them enclose it.

It is usually not possible to tell visually whether a given egg capsule contains an ovum, a pseudovum, a zygote, an apozygote, an embryo, or even a larva ready to hatch. It may also contain yolk cells, spicules, nematocysts, or nutritive substances other than yolk. It may also contain more than one zygote, as in several Turbellaria (composite eggs).

1. Location of Zygote

A zygote may start its development inside the mother, attached to various external objects, floating free in the sea, or elsewhere. Zygotes may be found:

1. In tissues of the mother's host (Mesozoa, s.Trematoda)
2. In the plankton of the sea (Porifera, Coelenterata, Brachiopoda, s.Mollusca, Sipunculoidea, Echiuroidea, s.Asteroidea, s.Echinoidea, s.Holothurioidea, Enteropneusta, Tunicata, Cephalochordata, Agnatha, Pisces)
3. In the plankton of freshwater (s.Coelenterata)
4. In a brood chamber of a parent (Calyssozoa, Bryozoa, Brachiopoda, s.Mollusca, s.Ophiuroidea, s.Echinoidea, s.Holothurioidea, s.Pterobranchia, Tunicata)
5. In exterior cavities, where brooding is incidental to other functions, such as respiratory currents in a mantle cavity (Mollusca, s.Crustacea: Cirripedia)
6. In body wall of the parent (s.Coelenterata)
7. In a cocoon (Oligochaeta, Hirudinea, s.Arachnida)
8. In maternal uterus, with placenta (Onychophora, Mammalia)
9. Attached to outside of female or male (Pycnogonida, s.Arachnida, Crustacea, s.Amphibia)

10. In the maternal genital system (s.Arachnida, s.Insecta, Pogonophora, s.Ophiuroidea, s.Holothurioidea, s.Tunicata)
11. In the ground (s.Arachnida, Reptilia, s.Mammalia)
12. Attached to land objects (s.Insecta)
13. In a structure guarded by parents (Aves, Mammalia)

2. Special Terms

Some special terms are sometimes applied to certain zygotes. For example:

1. Apozygote — one formed without karyogamy
2. Fertilized egg — one containing a synkaryon
3. Homozygote, heterozygote, allozygote, and others that indicate the genetic make-up of the zygote
4. Hypnozygote — a dormant zygote
5. Oocyst — an encysted zygote, as in Sporozoa
6. Ookinete — a motile zygote of such protozoan parasites as *Plasmodium* (malarial pathogen)
7. Sporont — a zygote destined to undergo sporogony, in Sporozoa

3. Fate of the Zygote

A zygote usually exists only for a short period of time. The karyogamy that created it is promptly followed by cleavage; however, there is diversity in what happens to the developing zygote. For example:

1. It may develop into an embryo, as in most life histories of familiar animals
2. It may divide into two or more (sometimes more than a thousand) daughter cells, each of which will then develop into an embryo (twinning or polyembryony)
3. It may unite with other zygotes to form a single embryo (composite eggs, see below)
4. It may fail to develop

A few zygotes (always called eggs in this connection) are capable of surviving for considerable periods. These are usually called dormant, resting, or winter eggs. After the dormant period, the development is in the same manner as other zygotes. (Many eggs of parasites are normally capable of surviving for extended periods.)

4. Composite Eggs

In the Tricladida (Turbellaria) it is usual to find, within one eggshell (capsule), a large number of yolk cells — sometimes as many as several thousand — surrounding a few zygotes (possibly as many as 40). The cleavage of these zygotes is extremely peculiar, in that the blastomeres become isolated from each other and distribute themselves among the yolk cells. The latter proceed to fuse together, forming a syncytium, while some of the blastomeres transform into wandering amoeboid cells and, separating from the other blastomere masses, migrate to the vicinity of the yolk syncytium. There they form a thin membrane, which acts as a boundary between the ordinary yolk cell masses outside and the yolk syncytium inside. At the same time another group of wandering cells assembles at one point on this membrane; eventually a cavity appears in this cell mass and the whole thing takes the shape of a small sac. Next, a mouth opens to the outside of the membrane and an embryonic pharynx is formed, at the inner end of which is a sac that functions as a temporary intestine. This mouth sucks in the yolk from the outside, swells enormously, and its wall pushes away the blastomeres and yolk which lie outside of it, gradually approaching the outer membrane, and together with it, forms the embryonic wall. Inside this the blastomeres, suspended in yolk, proliferate actively, and the resulting cells eventually gather at the ventral side where they form a germinal cord (destined to become the endoderm of the adult). The embryonic pharynx and the outer membranes degenerate, while the germinal cord forms the adult intestine. Other organs begin to develop from other masses of the enclosed cells (blastomeres). (After Kume and Dan, 1968).

A similar development is shown by eggs of some species in two other orders of Turbellaria, which form a capsule with many yolk cells but only one egg. It seems inescapable that in the case described above, the cells of the adult will come from a number of different zygotes and will therefore not have identical genotypes.

II. CLEAVAGE

A. Commentary

In all eggs, so far as known, fertilization is followed, sometimes after a dormant period, by a period in which the zygote and its nucleus undergo a rapid series of mitotic divisions. These early divisions together are what is called *cleavage.* The first division (also called first cleavage) is thus the usual first obvious process of the new individual. (The exceptions, where other processes come first, include: [1] chromosome doubling in the case of haploid parthenogenesis; [2] fusion with yolk cells; and [3] reorganization of the egg contents.)

The first physiological purpose fulfilled by cleavage is the restoration of the balance between the size of the nucleus and the amount of cytoplasm in the cell. Egg cells are generally very large as cells go, because of the included yolk. The second purpose fulfilled is to start the building of the multicellular individual by increasing the number of cells.

The zygote itself, but not its shell or coverings, ceases to exist at the first nuclear division; it has now become the simplest possible embryo. Cleavage and embryogeny are, of course, not really distinct but a continuous sequence of cell multiplication and differentiation, with continuous change. It is convenient, however, to have words for the stages as well as for the processes. When the zygote cleaves, it is converted into a mass of daughter cells. These cells are blastomeres. When there are only a few of them, they usually form a solid mass, often called a *morula.* Further multiplication forms either a layer of cells around a central cavity (derived from intercellular spaces) or a solid sphere of many cells. Each of the latter is called a *blastula,* the last stage before clear differentiation begins.

The word morula is sometimes defined as equivalent to a stereogastrula, but it should be restricted to the earlier stage before any blastula, hollow or solid, is formed. The word is best known in the embryology of placental mammals, for it is at this early stage that the "embryo" is implanted in the wall of the uterus of the mother.

When the cleaving mass or morula, followed by the blastula and gastrula, begins to differentiate into identifiable structures (embryonic organs), the mass is called an *embryo.* These processes are the first steps in *embryogenesis.*

In the earliest development, there is great diversity in the time at which the fate of the blastomeres is fixed, in the amount of yolk they contain, in whether the cleavage planes pass completely through the zygote or blastomeres or merely penetrate them, and in the structure of the blastula which results from cleavage.

Cleavage of the zygote (or apozygote) is usually represented as the division of the cell into two by a plane which divides it into more or less equal parts. This complete cleavage of the zygote into two is called holoblastic. Successive cleavages in this manner would produce a spherical mass of cells with little visible differentiation. More rarely the mass may depart at times from the sphere, as in the Nematoda where the four-celled stage may be T-shaped, or in Porifera where the early embryo is a plate of cells in one plane.

The actual cleavage may result in cells varying from equal to very unequal size. The cleavage planes usually each pass through the egg at an angle (to one of the egg axes) that is fixed for that species, but the angle varies in different groups. The successive cleavages are then at a fixed angle to each other, giving a recognizable pattern to the mass of cells. This division of the cell can be a critical phase in the life of the animal, because it may reveal the polarity of the egg and may make the initial division of it into a symmetrical body. In a few animals the first cleavage plane appears to be in a random position, with the polarity or symmetry established later by other mechanisms.

Zygotes in several groups, actually a majority of all animals because insects are included, do not cleave in this fashion. In some, the nucleus divides and the separation plane of the cytoplasm does not pass clear through the zygote but merely passes a short way into the cell from the surface, partially separating the two nuclei as if by a curtain. This is called meroblastic, partial, or incomplete cleavage. In others, the nuclear divisions take place deep in the egg center, with the many daughter nuclei later migrating to the surface, where separating membranes gradually develop. These meroblastic forms of cleavage are much more complex than the holoblastic forms listed above. They may be influenced by egg shape, egg polarity, and amount and distribution of yolk. They result in more complex processes of embryogeny.

There are several animals in which the first division of the zygotes does not result in blastomeres that form the earliest embryo. For example, in the medusa *Cunina proboscidea*, "the eggs on fertilization divide into two cells, only one of which gives rise to the embryo. The other grows, pushes out pseudopodia, at first engulfs the embryo and later carries it on its surface . . . This cell, the phorocyte, nourishes the embryo and transports it (to the outside)" (Dogiel, 1966).

B. Cleavage Terms

Many terms have been used to describe the position and penetration of the first cleavage, or the effect of that cleavage on the fate of the blastomeres produced. For example:

1. Bilateral — early cleavage resulting in blastomeres arranged to produce a bilaterally symmetrical embryo
2. Biradial — cleavage producing an eight-cell plate, two cells from front to rear, and four cells wide (only in Ctenophora)
3. Complete cleavage — see Holoblastic
4. Determinate — cleavage in which the future of the blastomeres is already determined
5. Discoidal — meroblastic cleavage in which the blastomeres at the animal pole form the entire embryo on the surface of the egg
6. Equatorial — through the equator; cleavage dividing the egg into one blastomere at the animal pole and one at the vegetal pole
7. Holoblastic — cleavage in which the developing zygote is completely divided into blastomeres
8. Incomplete cleavage — see Meroblastic
9. Indeterminate — cleavage in which the fate of the blastomeres is not yet determined: they retain some ability to differentiate into several types
10. Meridional — through the longitudinal axis
11. Meroblastic — cleavage in which the developing zygote is not completely divided; the nucleus divides and the cell membranes eventually form between them; the daughter cells being incompletely separated (includes superficial, discoidal, and peripheral)

12. Peripheral — meroblastic cleavage resulting in a blastula by division of the central nucleus and migration of the daughter nuclei to the periphery, where separating membranes are then formed
13. Superficial — meroblastic cleavage starting at the surface at one pole and progressing around the egg
14. Radial — holoblastic cleavage in which the tiers of blastomeres form on top of each other parallel to the polar axis
15. Spiral, holoblastic cleavage in which the blastomeres lie at an angle to the polar axis and thus tend to form a spiral

C. Cleavage Patterns

There are two ways to classify cleavages — by the completeness of the cleavage planes (whether the zygote is divided into two blastomeres or merely its nucleus is divided) or by the arrangement of the blastomeres with respect to each other. Both of these follow:

Holoblastic cleavage through the longitudinal axis (meridional)

1. Between the right and left halves of the future embryo (Ctenophora, Bryozoa, Chaetognatha, Rhynchocoela, Enteropneusta, Tunicata, s.Vertebrata)
2. Between the front and back halves of the future embryo (Gastropoda, Pelecypoda, Araneida, Polychaeta, s.Vertebrata)
3. Not related to the future embryonic sides (Turbellaria, Acanthocephala, s.Mollusca, s.Annelida)

Holoblastic cleavage at right angles to the longitudinal axis

4. Equatorial (Nematoda, Merostomata, s.Acarina)
5. Above the equator (Oligochaeta, Hirudinea)
6. Below the equator (Trematoda)

Holoblastic cleavage at an angle unrelated to the future axis of the larva or the adult

7. (Dicyemida, Hydrozoa, s.Insecta, Crinoidea, Echinoidea, Pogonophora)

Meroblastic cleavage, incomplete cleavage

8. (s.Anthozoa, Cephalopoda, m.Arthropoda, s.Crinoidea, s.Thaliacea).

Three terms appear in the descriptions of meroblastic cleavage. Although they have inherent meanings that can be identified, they are applied confusingly in the literature. They all require division of the zygote nucleus to form daughter nuclei around the egg. These terms are discoidal, superficial, and peripheral, all referring to cleavage. Arthropoda are cited in all three. Cephalopoda are listed in the first and second. Frogs are listed as discoidal but are elsewhere usually described as holoblastic.

In some Arthropoda the nucleus divides in the center of the egg and the daughter nuclei migrate out in all directions to form a blastoderm. In others the central nucleus itself migrates to the periphery before it divides. In still others the nucleus is peripheral and divides there to form blastoderm and blastodisc (embryo). It does not seem possible to attach to these the terms given above.

Nearly all books on invertebrate embryology classify the forms of cleavage on a geometric system. They are said to be

1. Radial (Bryozoa, Chaetognatha, Echinodermata)

2. Biradial (Ctenophora)
3. Spiral (s.Hydrozoa, s.Turbellaria, Rhynchocoela, Acanthocephala, s.Rotifera, s.Gastrotricha, Calyssozoa, s.Brachiopoda, Amphineura, Gastropoda, Scaphopoda, Bivalvia, Sipunculoidea, Echiuroidea, Annelida)
4. Bilateral (Gordioidea, Nematoda, s.Enteropneusta, Cephalochordata, Vertebrata)

This classification is thought to show agreement with major groupings of animals. Unfortunately, there are many exceptions. For example:

1. Although Hydrozoa are listed as spiral, they are normally radial
2. Turbellaria are listed as having spiral cleavage, but some do not and may be highly irregular
3. Although Acanthocephala are usually listed by spiral, they are elsewhere said to follow a bilateral pattern
4. Rotifera are said to be spiral but some are not, or they may start out as spiral and then continue as bilateral
5. Gastrotricha belong to the group that is spiral but are said to be otherwise
6. Although most Aschelminthes are cited as spiral, both Gordioidea and Nematoda are bilateral and others are also not clearly spiral
7. Although Bryozoa are radial, the two other phyla of the Lophophorata are spiral (or other)
8. Phoronida are not listed, but they may be radial or spiral or irregular
9. Some Brachiopoda are not spiral but bilateral
10. Although most Mollusca are spiral, the Cephalopoda are not
11. Although Enteropneusta are listed as bilateral, they are mostly radial
12. Although most Vertebrata are bilateral, some are said to be otherwise

About one third of the classes of animals are so poorly known that we have little information on their cleavage. Even if the exceptions in each class can be satisfactorily explained as specializations, it is hard to explain away the fact that lophophorates may be either radial or spiral, item (7) above, Aschelminthes may be either spiral or bilateral, item (6), and the Cephalopoda and all the Arthropoda cannot be placed in the system at all because of the peculiarities of their meroblastic cleavage.

D. Blastoderm Formation

Cleavage of the zygote produces blastomeres (cells) which at first form a solid mass of cells which may later develop a cavity. In all such cases the cells are considered to form a blastoderm, even if it is not an actual layer. This typical arrangement of cells is called a blastula.

There often is no complete cleavage — merely division of the zygote nucleus into many nuclei, with cell separation following much later. If the nuclear divisions are at the surface, a blastoderm is formed by these spreading and multiplying "cells", which gradually enclose the original zygote. If the nuclei are deep in the yolk, the blastoderm will be formed by their migration to the surface and development of cell membranes between them. The latter (one cell or more thick) is the first real germ layer. It is converted into two layers, ectoderm and endoderm, by the next process which is gastrulation.

Thus *blastoderm* is formed in these ways:

1. Cleavage of zygote into a solid mass of cells

2. Cleavage of zygote into cells around a cavity
3. Multiplication of nuclei at the surface, eventually with cell separations
4. Migration of nuclei from interior of zygote, again with cell separations appearing later

III. EMBRYOGENESIS

A. Blastula

The cleavages that form the blastoderm will result in a blastula. Although usually described as hollow, the blastula in many animals is a solid mass of cells. The number of cells may vary from a few dozen to a few hundred, but there is as yet no clear indication of structural differentiation of tissues or organs. Several types of blastulae occur:

From holoblastic cleavage

1. Coeloblastula — a hollow sphere with blastocoel cavity (Demospongia, s.Coelenterata, Rhynchocoela, Gastrotricha, Nematoda, Gordioidea, Bryozoa, Brachiopoda, Phoronida, s.Mollusca, Echiuroidea, s.Annelida, s.Arthropoda, Chaetognatha, Echinodermata, s.Pterobranchia, Enteropneusta, Cephalochordata, Vertebrata)
2. Stereoblastula — a solid sphere with no cavity (Mesozoa, s.Coelenterata, Ctenophora, Acanthocephala, Rotifera, s.Mollusca, s.Annelida, s.Arthropoda, Pogonophora, s.Pterobranchia)

From meroblastic cleavage

3. Discoblastula or periblastula — a layer 1-cell thick enclosing the central yolk, with a disk of cells on one side to become the embryo (Porifera, Cephalopoda, Hirudinea, s.Arachnida, s.Crustacea, s.Insecta)

Some of these blastulae (e.g., some Coelenterata) need to change very little to become embryos or even larvae, as the planula larva is little more than an elongate blastula. The difference between hollow and solid blastulae is shown to be of no phylogenetic significance by the fact that in groups such as the Coelenterata the blastula may be either.

Two other blastula terms occur in works on the Porifera. These are stomoblastula and amphiblastula. In the account of Hyman (1940), the former is a ball of eight macromeres and many micromeres, the latter being flagellated, in which a temporary mouth may form among the macromeres to ingest adjacent material. This stomoblastula is then said to undergo a process of inversion, turning inside out by way of the mouth "so that the flagellar ends of the flagellated micromeres are brought to the outside" forming an amphiblastula. After this a gastrulation occurs. No drawings of a stomoblastula have been found, and it is not clear how flagellated blastomeres can have the flagella inside a ball that is solid. (See the account of sponge embryology earlier in this chapter.)

B. Gastrula

The blastula develops into the next stage, the gastrula, but the transformation is not uniform among the groups of animals or even within most groups. The gastrula is sometimes defined as the stage starting with the inpushing and overgrowth of blastoderm at the animal pole, with the pocket so formed enlarging into an archenteron, which nearly or entirely obliterates the blastocoel. From this it is evident that the word will not fit well for animals with a stereoblastula (i.e., with no blastocoel).

In most animal groups an archenteron develops, and it is thus clear that there must be alternative ways of forming a gastrula. For this reason a better definition of *gastrula* is that it is that stage in embryogeny in which there is an archenteron but no nervous system. This leaves room for there to be more than one method of forming the archenteron.

The gastrula is thus the stage formed by the establishment of the archenteron, usually the first organ of the developing embryo, and the stage in which the three germ layers become clearly established. At the same time there is development of a definitive body cavity, either from the blastocoel or independent of it. These steps will be briefly examined for diversity.

Special terms have sometimes been used to specify gastrulae of supposedly different sorts. These include the following:

1. Archigastrula — one produced by embOly; thus, the same as "gastrula" as usually used without qualification
2. Coelogastrula — one derived from a coeloblastula
3. Discogastrula — one produced by cell or nuclear movements after meroblastic cleavage
4. Paragastrula — one formed by invagination of the amphiblastula, in Porifera
5. Parenchymula — a form of stereogastrula, in Porifera
6. Stereogastrula — a solid gastrula, sometimes being a planula larva

1. Germ Layers and Gastrulation

The actual first "germ layer" is the blastoderm, already described as surrounding the blastula. The term *germ layer* is, however, usually restricted to the three layers formed from the blastoderm. It is customary to assume that these layers, ecto-, endo-, and mesoderm (or at least the first two), are formed by one of the processes included under the term *gastrulation*. These are again assumed to be formed by invagination of cells (presumably at the vegetal pole) to form endoderm — the archenteron or primitive digestive tract. By thus setting off some blastomeres to be endoderm, the rest simply become ectoderm. (Mesoderm may appear at approximately the same time or in a later stage, as discussed in a later section.)

In many animals, these germ layers are formed by less abrupt processes that do not involve invagination. They result in an embryo without passing through the obvious stage called the gastrula. In such books as Hyman (1940) eight methods of gastrulation are thus listed, but only two of these actually produce a gastrula. It seems to be necessary to recognize that germ layer formation by gastrulation is significantly different from that by cell rearrangement. We emphasize this by separating them below.

Endoderm by gastrulation. There are two methods of converting a blastula into a gastrula, an early embryo with an archenteron. They are

1. By invagination or *embOly* — accompanied by cell division; the new pouch is the archenteron with a cavity, and the opening into it is the blastopore (Porifera, Scyphozoa, Anthozoa, Turbellaria, Gordioidea, Brachiopoda, Gastropoda, Cephalopoda, Polychaeta, Crustacea, Chaetognatha, Enteropneusta, solitary Ascidiacea, s.Vertebrata)
2. By epiboly — the smaller cells at the animal pole grow down over the vegetal pole cells and enclose them, leaving the large cells as endoderm to form an archenteron and a sort of blastopore (Porifera, Turbellaria, Nematoda, Gastropoda, Polychaeta, Onychophora, Ascidiacea)

Endoderm by rearrangement. In animals where gastrulation does not occur, the germ layers of the embryo are formed by other sorts of cell movements and differentiation. These have been called "gastrulation by involution" or "gastrulation by ingression". In the present framework they should be cited as methods of germ layer formation rather than of gastrulation. With some modifications and additions, the list given by Hyman (1940) includes these (numbered consecutively with the previous list because they are all methods of germ layer formation in the broad sense):

3.   By *involution* — the cells at the edge of the disk in a discoblastula migrate under the surface cells, between them and the underlying yolk, forming a second layer (Cephalopoda)
4.   By *delamination* — the inner halves of the cells of the coeloblastula are cut off by cleavages parallel to the surface and become the endoderm (s.Hydrozoa, s.Anthozoa, Pogonophora)
5.   By *separation* — the inner cells of a solid stereoblastula become the endoderm. This has been called secondary delamination (s.Hydrozoa, s.Anthozoa, Pogonophora)
6.   By *polar ingression* — cells from the vegetal pole region of a coeloblastula migrate into the interior as endoderm (s.Hydrozoa)
7.   By *general ingression* — cells from many points on a coeloblastula migrate inward to form the endoderm (?Porifera, s.Hydrozoa, s.Anthozoa, Phylactolaemata)
8.   By *proliferation* — of cells from the tips of the ectodermal stomodaeum and proctodaeum in a late embryo to form an endodermal mid-gut connecting the two (Insecta)
9.   By *cavitation* — appearance of a cavity in a solid blastula (s.Porifera, s.Platyhelminthes)

In addition to these nine methods, which account for the development of most animals, there are several groups in which there are complications or combinations of these. First, some form gastrulae by combinations of two or more methods: (A) emboly with epiboly and sometimes cell movement (Ctenophora, Nematoda, Sipunculoidea, s.Vertebrata, (B) emboly with ingression (Crustacea), and (C) epiboly with cell rearrangement and cavitation (Trematoda, Cestoda).

Second, there is one group in which the processes and sequence are so different as to require special description. In Acanthocephala, after the 34-cell stage of cleavage, cell walls disappear and some of the nuclei migrate to the center of the syncytium, where they form the gonads and the ligament sacs; no archenteron or clear endoderm is formed, then or ever.

It can be seen from the above list that these processes are not distributed systematically through the animal kingdom. In the following groups more than one method occurs, either in different species or as combinations of methods:

Porifera (emboly, epiboly, cavitation)
Coelenterata (emboly, delamination, differentiation, ingression, and combinations)
Platyhelminthes (emboly, epiboly, cavitation, and combinations)
Aschelminthes (emboly, epiboly, and combinations)
Brachiopoda (emboly, delamination)
Mollusca (emboly, epiboly, involution)
Annelida (emboly, epiboly)
Arthropoda (emboly and combinations)
Tunicata (emboly, epiboly)
Vertebrata (emboly, epiboly)

2. Blastopore

In most embryologically well-known groups there is at least some form of invagination (emboly) or some form of blastopore. This usually is the spot at which the single layer of blastomeres pushes inward to form the archenteron. This is a tubular pouch, often like the finger of a glove, which at its formation becomes an endoderm and is destined to form at least part of the digestive tract of later stages.

The site of this invagination and the nature of the structures formed from it are thought to be evidence of phylogenetic relationship and so are used in classifying major groups, using the terms *protostome* (mouth first) and *deuterostome* (mouth later). In its simplest form, there seems to be good basis for this, but difficulties are more numerous than usually admitted. Not only does the blastopore become the mouth in some and the anus in others, a fact which has never been explained, but in still others it may form both or neither. Similar invaginations occur in many animals, forming quite different structures, such as the proboscis cavity in Rhynchocoela, a mouth after the anus in many, a hydropore in Holothurioidea, and an adhesive sac in Gymnolaemata.

Many efforts have been made to tabulate these diversities for use in classification, but the excessive range of timings and details of these events has made any simple distinctions impossible. Some such differences are correlated with and may be due to the various amounts of yolk in the eggs of different species in a group.

Blastopores are rare in the Arthropoda. It is said that they form the mouth, but description or justification of this has not been found.

3. Fate of the Blastopore (Table 11)

Gastrulation by emboly or epiboly leaves a central cavity (archenteron) in the gastrula and thus a blastopore opening into it. This pore has a very different fate in different groups. For example:

1. It may become the future mouth and thus the front end of the archenteron.
2. It may become the future anus, and thus the hind end of the archenteron.
3. It may elongate and form both
4. It may close permanently and both mouth and anus form anew.
5. An invagination (or two) occurs but no true mouth or anus are ever formed (Porifera)

In an early chapter of Volume I of *The Invertebrates* (1940), Hyman gives a diagram of the animal phyla to show which are deuterostomatous and which are protostomatous. Although the diagram is designed to show Hyman's ideas of phylogeny of the animal groups, it is clearly annotated to show the fate of the blastopore. First, the Protozoa, Porifera, Mesozoa, Coelentarata, and Ctenophora are removed, although in the latter two at least some are protostomatous.

Hyman divides the Bilateria (all the Metazoa except the Coelenterata and Ctenophora) into two: the Protostomia and the Deuterostomia. As Protostomia she lists Platyhelminthes, Rhynchocoela, Aschelminthes, Mollusca, Echiuroidea, Annelida, and Arthropoda. As Deuterostomia Hyman lists Chaetognatha, Echinodermata, Hemichordata, and Chordata. These two groupings are founded also on other features, such as whether the cleavage is determinate and the manner of formation of the coelom. In this way these three features are shown to support this division of the Bilateria into the two groups.

In the groups that Hyman lists, the following exceptions seem to occur:

Supposed to form a MOUTH (protostomatous)

1. Platyhelminthes — in some the blastopore closes and forms neither mouth nor anus; in others no blastopore ever forms

Table 11
FATE OF THE BLASTOPORE

	Blastopore forms					Never forms
	Proctostome	Mouth	Anus	Both	Neither	
Porifera					X	
Mesozoa						X
Coelenterata	X					X
Ctenophora						X
Gnathostomuloidea						X
Platyhelminthes						
Turbellaria				X		
Trematoda						X
Cestoda						X
Cestodaria						X
Rhynchocoela					X	
Acanthocephala						X
Rotifera						X
Nematoda					X	
Calyssozoa					X	
Bryozoa						
Gymnolaemata					X	X
Phylactolaemata						X
Phoronida		?		?		
Brachiopoda						
Articulata					X	
Inarticulata					X	
Mollusca						
Solenogastres		X				
Amphineura		X				
Gastropoda		X[a]	X[a]			
Bivalvia		X				
Scaphopoda		X				
Cephalopoda						X
Sipunculoidea					X	X
Annelida						
Archiannelida				X		
Polychaeta		X				
Oligochaeta		X				
Hirudinea		X				
Onychophora		X				X
Arthropoda						
Merostomata						X
Pycnogonida						
Arachnida						
Crustacea			X		X	X
Myriapoda						X
Insecta		X[b]	X			
Chaetognatha					X	
Pogonophora						X
Echinodermata						
Crinoidea					X	
Asteroidea			X			
Ophiuroidea			X			
Echinoidea			X			
Holothurioidea			X			
Pterobranchia			X			
Enteropneusta			X			

Table 11 (continued)
FATE OF THE BLASTOPORE

	Blastopore forms					Never forms
	Proctostome	Mouth	Anus	Both	Neither	
Tunicata						
Ascidiacea			X			
Thaliacea					X	
Cephalochordata					X	
Vertebrata			X			

^a Either mouth or anus.
^b Mouth before anus.

2. Rhynchocoela — in some it forms the anus; in others it closes and both form later
3. Aschelminthes — in some it forms the anus; in some the mouth; in some it closes; and in some it never occurs
4. Mollusca — in some it becomes the anus; in some the mouth
5. Annelida — in some it forms the mouth; in some it elongates into a slit and forms both

Supposed to form an ANUS (deuterostomatous)

6. Hemichordata — in some it forms the anus; in some it closes and forms neither
7. Chordata — in Ascidiacea it forms the anus; it Thaliacea it closes and forms neither; in Cephalochordata none ever forms; in Vertebrata it forms the anus

In later volumes Hyman adds other phyla to these lists. By her own descriptions elsewhere there are discrepancies as follows:

Supposed to form a MOUTH

8. Acanthocephala — none ever forms
9. Calyssozoa — it forms neither
10. Bryozoa — it is variously described as never forming or as closing without forming either
11. Phoronida — it is variously described as elongating to form both or as forming the mouth
12. Brachiopoda — it closes and forms neither
13. Sipunculoidea — it closes and forms neither
14. Onychophora — it is said to form both in one genus and neither in another

Supposed to form an ANUS

15. Pogonophora — none is formed

In the groups that Hyman leaves out as Radiata, a blastopore may be formed, with these results:

1. Hydrozoa — none is formed

2. Scyphozoa — it becomes the proctostome
3. Anthozoa — it becomes the proctostome
4. Ctenophora — none is formed

It appears that these exceptions have not been taken into account adequately. They throw doubt on the use of the fate of the blastopore in either phylogeny or classification (see Table 11).

It should be pointed out that similar invaginations are reported in several animals, producing a variety of organs. In addition to the mouth, anus, and proctostome, these may form various structures or cavities:

1. Adhesive sac — in Gymnolaemata
2. Hydropore — in Holothuriodea
3. Rhynchocoel — the proboscis cavity of Rhynchocoela
4. Bursae — in Ophiuroidea
5. Imaginal discs — in holometabolous Insecta
6. Neural tube — in Vertebrata

In the embryology of vertebrates, much attention is given to what is called the *dorsal lip of the blastopore*. This is presumptive notochord cells and seems to act as an important organizer or center of influence on the differentiating cells. There is no such organizing center apparent in invertebrates, although doubtless there are influences of this sort at work in embryogeny of all animals.

4. Mesoderm Formation

Either before, during, or after gastrulation, or extending over a considerable period, the third germ layer of cells, the mesoderm, is formed by multiplication and migration of cells from one or more of the earlier layers. It is of less definite structure and more varied in origin than the ectoderm or the endoderm. In the source of its cells and the manner of becoming a layer, there are the following situations:

From proliferating nuclei

1. Formed directly from the nuclei wandering out from the center of the egg, of which others give rise to the ectoderm simultaneously (s.Arthropoda)

From the blastoderm

2. Inwandering of cells from the blastoderm, usually not much before the latter becomes ectoderm (s.Platyhelminthes, s.Aschelminthes, Bryozoa, Phoronida, Mollusca, s.Annelida, s.Arthropoda)
3. From two teloblasts, separated from blastoderm at the time the endoderm first appears (Polychaeta, Hirudinea)

From the ectoderm

4. Inwandering of cells after the surface blastoderm has differentiated into the ectoderm (s.Rhynchocoela, Bryozoa)

From the endoderm

5. Wandering of single cells out from the endoderm (archenteron) (Phoronida)
6. A sheet of mesoderm cells produced along the archenteron on each side near the blastopore, later splitting into two layers (groups with schizocoely)

7. Pouches of endoderm cells produced from the walls of the archenteron and becoming detached as mesoderm (groups with enterocoely)

From both ectoderm and endoderm

8. Wandering of cells from both layers simultaneously to form a mass in the space between them (s.Rhynchocoela, s.Bivalvia, s.Arthropoda, Ascidiacea)

The tissues resulting from 1 to 4 are usually loosely called ectomesoderm, in spite of the differences.

Some books imply that ectomesoderm and endomesoderm are distinct and cannot even be homologous. For example, Hyman (1940) describes ectomesoderm as "always mesenchymal, never epithelial". Loose connective tissue may be distinct from epithelium, but we find no statement that they can be distinguished by anything but their origin. In fact, it is said that they all originate from epithelium and may promptly differentiate into other types of cells. "It (the mesoderm) may begin as mesenchyme or mesothelium, and each may later assume the other tissue form." In many animals the adult mesoderm is said to be a mixture of the two types.

It is difficult to see any fundamental difference between these methods of mesoderm formation. In all cases the mesoderm arises from cells that are or have recently come from blastoderm. There do not seem to be consistent cytological differences between these two types, which are distinguished at best at this early stage by position and sometimes extent.

These formation methods can also be arranged in relation to the type of blastula, thus:

a. Formation of ectoderm and endoderm

In the case of a stereoblastula

1. Epiboly
2. Differentiation (secondary delamination)

In the case of a coeloblastula

3. Emboly
4. Epiboly
5. Delamination (primary)
6. Ingression: (a) polar, (b) general

In the case of a discoblastula

7. Involution

In the case of a periblastula

8. Proliferation from stomodaeum and proctodaeum

b. Formation of mesoderm

From blastoderm

1. Inwandering
2. Teloblasts

From endoderm

3.   Isolation of endoderm cells: (a) singly wandering out, (b) sheets (schizocoely), (c) pouches (enterocoely)

From ectoderm

4.   Cell wandering

From both endoderm and ectoderm

5.   Cell wandering

Although, as pointed out above, adults do not have ecto-, endo-, or mesoderm, but only tissues derived from these embryonic germ layers, these words are used in the list below for convenience in showing the tissue origin.

There is more diversity, however, than is shown by recognition of three basic germ layers. The following are the varieties recognized in this study, with examples:

1.   A single layer functionally corresponding to a combined ecto-endoderm (Monoblastozoa)
2.   Two layers, functionally corresponding to epidermis and mesenchyme (Mesozoa)
3.   Two layers, in stomoblastula and amphiblastula, with future choanocytes and pinacoderm (future epidermis) sometimes reversing position (Porifera)
4.   Two layers, ectoderm and endoderm (some planula larvae, s.Hydrozoa)
5.   Two layers, ectoderm and mesoderm (Cestoda, s.Bryozoa, Acanthocephala, Pogonophora)
6.   Three layers, ecto-, endo-, and mesoderm (presumably all other groups)

C. Morphogenesis

The completion of cleavage and gastrulation is the beginning of a period of differentiation of cells and the establishment of a particular form typical of that species. This latter is morphogenesis. Several terms are applied to these changes, but they seem to confuse rather than help in our comparative study. For example:

1.   Embryogenesis — the conversion of the zygote into an embryo
2.   Embryogeny — same as embryogenesis
3.   Histogenesis — the differentiation of tissues
4.   Morphogenetic movements — movement (translocation) of cells and layers or masses of cells, to mold the developing embryo
5.   Organogeny — the production of the embryonic organs, usually starting with the archenteron
6.   Topogenesis — the same as morphogenesis but sometimes restricted to development of form in gastrulation

Movement of cells, tissues, and organs without apparent propulsion is more common than usually admitted. These movements start in the early embryo, at the time of gastrulation and may continue at times clear into the adult, where organs such as gonophores (in Hydrozoa) and buds (in Tunicata) may move some distance along the surface, and thereby attain a new and specifically required location. The embryonic movements may include the movement of entire areas of cells, as in the invagination of embolic gastrulation and the convergence of notochordal tissue behind the lip of the blastopore. Other embryonic movements may involve isolated cells rather than tissues, for example, the movement of the two teloblasts into the blastocoel.

It is an interesting fact that morphogenesis at the embryo level is independent of conducted impulses in a nervous system, for no such system has yet been formed. The likelihood of complicity of chemical influences, on the other hand, is high.

Morphogenetic processes are not restricted to embryogenesis but also occur in later development. Some of the processes that participate in the morphogenesis of invertebrates have received special names, viz:

1. Anabiosis — arrested development, as in Rotifera and Tardigrada
2. Blastokinesis — the double inversions of the embryo within embryonic envelopes, in some Insecta
3. Evagination — of scolex from a cysticercus, in Cestoda
4. Inversion — in embryo of some Porifera
5. Metamorphosis — in many groups but especially in Insecta
6. Regeneration — as in adult Asteroidea
7. Resorption — as of the tail in larvae of Tunicata
8. Rotation (also called torsion) — of larvae in Echinodermata
9. Torsion — in larval Gastropoda

IV. EMBRYO

A. Commentary

Logically considered, an embryo is formed when the zygote first cleaves into a two-celled stage. In many books, however, an embryo is not presumed to appear until completion of gastrulation. Embryogenesis thus usually includes a period of cleavage, followed by formation of germ layers, leading to the definitive embryo that has distinct organs. This view gives a reasonable accounting of the occurrences when complete cleavage occurs.

In meroblastic cleavage, on the other hand, the sequence of stages or processes is much obscured, although the terms blastula and gastrula are often used. Starting with a zygote, there is multiplication of nuclei and later completion of cell separations. It gradually becomes evident that there has been change and growth at one point of the surface, and finally it can be said that an embryo has formed there. The definitive point is sometimes the enclosure of the embryo by the embryonic membranes, which are themselves part of the developing egg. One of the most striking early differentiations of organs occurs in Insecta, where the embryo, developing on the surface of the egg as a discoblastula, may very early show clearly the buds of developing limbs, even before the digestive tract appears. Because there is no archenteron formed in meroblastic animals such as Insecta, the digestive tract is formed in three parts; two invaginations of ectoderm (also called stomodaeum and proctodaeum) form the anterior and posterior parts (foregut and hindgut), whereas the mid-gut is formed by proliferation of (endoderm) cells from the tip of both.

One of the earliest formed lasting ''organs'' is the germ ball in Trematoda. It divides to form the germ balls of the next generation of ''embryos'' that form very early. The neural plate, the dorsal lip of the blastopore, the notochord, and the somites in vertebrates may be considered to be early organs, long before the liver or brain or gill arches appear. In many coelomate animals the coelomic sacs develop early and serve several purposes; they are a sort of organ.

Another early structure is the neural groove of vertebrates, which, especially in Amphibia, heralds the stage called the *neurula* — the beginning of the nervous system.

Although most embryology is discussed around holoblastic cleavage, the vast majority of animals have meroblastic cleavage. It is therefore appropriate to define the *embryo* as the developing phase when either (1) the gastrula produces clear organs or (2) the meroblastic egg shows a localized organization distinct from the embryonic membranes.

There are special terms applied to the embryos of certain animals (in the most general sense):

1. Blastocyst — same as blastodermic vesicle
2. Blastodermic vesicle — an embryonic stage, especially in Mammalia, consisting of an outer trophoblast and an inner cell mass with a blastocoel
3. Blastodisc — the area on the surface of a discoblastula which is becoming the embryo
4. Blastula — the mass of cells (blastomeres) produced by cleavage of the zygote, with or without a blastocoel
5. Composite egg (late in their development) — "embryos" formed by fusion of blastomeres from several zygotes
6. Foetus — a well-developed mammalian embryo, in humans from the 4th month
7. Gastrula — an initially diploblastic stage resulting from formation of an archenteron, later becoming triploblastic
8. Germ band — early area of the blastoderm of Insecta which thickens and grows into an embryo
9. Morula — the mass of cells formed by the cleaving zygote
10. Neurula — the stage in the vertebrate embryo during which the neural plate is invaginated to form the neural tube
11. Thecated embryo — one which secretes a capsule around itself, as in some Hydrozoa

The end of the embryo stage is also equivocal. In viviparous animals, it is usually assumed that the embryo becomes a juvenile (or larva) at birth. In oviparous animals the hatching of the egg is usually the end of the life of the embryo, but there are animals in which a clear-cut larva exists inside the egg — even passing all of that stage there. There are animals in which the "larva" is no more than an early embryo, as in the planula of Coelenterata.

This same problem of timing is evident in the terms usually used for the layers of cells in embryos and adults. It is an arbitrary decision ot use the term germ layer for the embryonic layers and the term tissue for all later ones.

B. Cavities of the Embryo

In descriptions of embryos and their early development, there is frequent reference to cavities in the interior. A cavity is, of course, not an empty space, but is simply an enclosed region full of fluid and not occupied by organs. There are four general sorts of cavities in embryos:

Water channels. The water channels of sponges begin to form in the later embryo but are primarily cavities of the adult. They are discussed in Chapter 19 under "Spongiocoel as a System".

Intercellular spaces of blastula. In most animals the first cavity to appear is the blastocoel, the space between the first four cells, enlarged as they cleave into many. In many animals this blastocoel is obliterated by development of archenteron, mesoderm, and organs in later development, but in Aschelminthes and Arthropoda it persists into the adult and becomes the pseudocoel or haemocoel, respectively. In the many animals in which superficial or peripheral cleavage occurs, the space finally surrounded by the layer of cells is filled with yolk. It is not especially identified, but is the only "cavity" in the early embryo of these forms. A pseudocoel is formed in Rotifera, Gastrotricha, Kinorhyncha, Nematoda, Gordioidea, and Calyssozoa. It was at one time cited in Acanthocephala because the cavity lacks the inner lining, but it is described as forming by a split in the mesoderm. It has recently been reported that in Chaetognatha the "coelom" is structurally like a pseudocoel even though it appears to arise by enterocoely.

Archenteron. The archenteron is potentially a cavity, but generally has no lumen until it is transformed into a digestive tract, either for the larva or for the adult.

Coelomic spaces. The coelomic spaces are ones developed in the mesoderm. They form in several different ways and are sometimes forerunners of the adult body cavity (see below).

Two other terms are employed for cavities. These are *stomodaeum* and *proctodaeum,* commonly used for the fore and hind invaginations that form the ends of the embryonic digestive tract. The former gives rise to the mouth cavity and the latter to the anal cavity and related parts of the tract.

A confusing situation arises with the terms stomodaeum and proctodaeum. In animals other than Arthropoda, gastrulation forms an invagination, called the archenteron, which is the beginning of endoderm. This may be at the site of the future mouth (protostomatous) or of the future anus (deuterostomatous). In either case, a second invagination produces the other opening. These openings are universally called stomodaeum and proctodaeum. In the Insecta neither invagination, if any occurs, will form endoderm, but the animals are said to be protostomatous.

The embryonic origin and development of the mesoderm is closely involved with spaces that develop inside the embryo, some of which persist into the adult. Body cavities are identified by terms defined with reasonable clarity and distinctiveness, viz: *pseudocoel,* a cavity situated between the mesoderm and the digestive tract and derived from the blastocoel; *coelom,* a cavity in the mesoderm, surrounded on all sides by mesothelium, and unrelated to earlier cavities. Nevertheless, this feature has proven to be more disturbing than helpful in classification because of the exceptions that occur, very similar to the ones listed for the fate of the blastopore. For example, one phylum (Priapuloidea) that is placed with the pseudocoelomates has an unquestioned coelom. The second largest phylum of animals (Mollusca) is placed with the coelomates yet seems to be without any such cavity in identifiable form. The largest phylum (Arthropoda), with its meroblastic cleavage, produces all of the mesoderm by quite different processes, but the coelomic cavities still appear as spaces inside the mesoderm bands. (Thereafter, in this phylum, the coeloms are much reduced, and as body cavities, are replaced by the haemocoel.)

Among the animals that develop a coelom, there is considerable diversity in the method of formation and in the eventual distribution of parts of the cavity. There are two principal ways in which coelom may develop. They differ principally in the timing of events, as in each case they form in mesoderm that is recently formed from the archenteron (endoderm) or the blastoderm (teloblasts). The first method is *schizocoely,* in which a mass of mesoderm accumulates by cell migration between the ectoderm and the endoderm. The mass splits into layers that separate and come to line the body wall on the one hand and surround the digestive tract on the other. The space between is coelom, called a *schizocoel;* it is lined all around with peritoneum.

The second method is *enterocoely,* in which pouches appear from the archenteron and pinch off as hollow masses of cells, now called mesoderm. The space is coelom, and it is called an *enterocoel.* It is also completely lined with peritoneum. The paired cavities usually coalesce dorsally and ventrally; the longitudinal rows of pouches may become united or may be compartmentalized in separate regions of the body.

The distribution of the two among the phyla and classes should warn us that the two methods do not represent fundamentally different processes:

1.   Enterocoelous — Brachiopoda: Articulata, Tardigrada, Pentastomoidea, Chaetognatha, Pogonophora, m.Echinodermata, Enteropneusta, Tunicata, Cephalochordata
2.   Schizocoelous — Brachiopoda: Inarticulate, Sipunculoidea, Echiuroidea, Annelida, Arthropoda, s.Echinodermata, Vertebrata

These 13 phyla are less than one half of the number that should be listed. The reason is that there is uncertainty in the other phyla, or no information at all. These situations are as follows:

1.   Doubtful status but *not enterocoelous* — Priapuloidea (usually included with the pseudocoelomates), Bryozoa, Phoronida, probably Pterobranchia in which mesoderm pouches have not been seen
2.   Status in doubt — Mollusca where the very existence of a coelum is questioned or schizocoely of a much modified sort is described, Myzostomida, Dinophiloidea, Onychophora

Beyond this, in the eight groups listed as forming the coelom by enterocoely (pouches from the archenteron) the pouches are described in varying numbers of pairs. At least the following occur:

1.   1 pair of enterocoelic pouches — Brachiopoda: Inarticulata, Chaetognatha, Echinodermata, Tunicata
2.   1 pair plus one terminal pouch — Pogonophora, Cephalochordata
3.   2 pairs plus one terminal pouch — Enteropneusta
4.   4 pairs — Pentastomida
5.   5 pairs — Tardigrada

There is also diversity in the division of anterior pouches into two laterally, in the division of paired pouches into segmental cavities, and in the definiteness of the peritoneal lining. Coelom formation is obviously not a notably good character for use in classification.

C. Determination

An important concept in development is the fixation of the fate of the cells in the embryo — the channeling of their future development to produce some specific organ or part of the animal in later stages. These are differences in how and when this fixation occurs in various animals, but no data are available to produce any general tabulation of the processes.

There is difficulty about how the term *determination* is to be used. In the first place, it can refer to the means by which one discovers what the fate of a cell is to be, or it can refer to the actual channeling of the cell and its progeny into some particular fate. There is such great difference in the applicability of this term that we conclude it should never be used without specification of the parameters. To say that an animal produces determinate eggs raises the questions of when each type of offspring cell is determined, how complete the determination is (absolute or normal with possibility of being overridden by other factors), and whether the concept applies to the cell and all of its descendants or to only one line of them, etc.

A few examples to show the diversity is all that can be offered here on this important but esoteric subject.

In studies of the occurrence of determination, the standard subject was historically the egg of some amphibian. In these, and apparently other, vertebrates the early cleavage divisions of the embryo do not impart specific qualities to the daughter cells. This is *indeterminate cleavage*. It is demonstrated by dissecting out one cell from a cleaving mass of 16 and finding that it develops into a normal individual. In these animals the first restriction of potency seems to come at gastrulation, where some cells are determined to be fated to become endoderm and its derivative organs. This occurs in vertebrates and is sometimes stated as a law covering all animals (see the next example).

In the Ctenophora, if the two blastomeres produced at the first cleavage are mechanically separated, they will each develop into a sort of half-larva. This means that each blastomere is already determined to produce one of the halves of the future animal. This doubtless means that the zygote itself was in some way organized into two regions.

An unusual cleavage occurs in Nematoda, where the first cleavage plane is equatorial, dividing the zygote into an "anterior" and a "posterior" cell. Some of the progeny of the posterior cell will become organs that are never formed by any offspring of the anterior cell, so there has been some restriction on the fate of each. This cleavage is called *determinate*.

In the parasitic Hymenoptera (Insecta), on the other hand, after a few cleavages of the zygote, the cells separate into small masses which will then act like embryos. In other species the first cleavage will produce two cells which may separate and form two embryos.

It is reported that some Bryozoa and Annelida can produce many embryos by the breakdown of one as advanced as the gastrula stage. In these, determination must not be effected until this relatively late stage.

In many animals the first indication of restriction of the fate of any cell is the unequal cleavages that produce some large and some small cells. This gives a polarity, which leads to invagination of one of the groups at gastrulation. This latter process also is part of determination, as the invaginated portion produces the digestive tract. In some animals gastrulation is preceded by isolation of two cells which tend to remain near the blastopore; these are called *teloblasts* and where they occur they form the mesoderm. It is often found, however, that these early "determinations" are only tentative, and later influences can upset them and lead to unexpected formations.

Furthermore, all through life there are a series of determinations of the future of specific tissues. For example, the embryo in some Crustacea contains cells capable of producing an eye. In the adult, if the eye is extirpated, there are not cells left that are still able to produce an eye, so the regeneration cannot produce an eye but will produce some other structure. This means that all the cells in the adult which are available to the eye site have already been determined to become something other than an eye.

These differences are covered by such a term as *potency*, the ability of a tissue or a cell to deviate from its normal fate and differentiate into something normally unexpected.

Determination may last only to some intermediate stage. For example, Bryozoa have a "peculiar embryology in which all parts of the larva except ectoderm degenerate and all definitive structures arise from the ectoderm" (Hyman, 1959).

In Trematoda, the successive larval stages are not developments one from the tissues of the previous one. Each stage is produced anew from a germ ball carried through the sequence. The adult organs bear no relation to any larval or even embryonic structures, except that they arise from parts of the same mass of germplasm.

In Insecta with a complete metamorphosis, no adult tissues except possibly the body wall are derived from larval structures, all arising anew during pupation.

D. Site of Embryonic Development

At some point the egg membranes or shell surrounding the embryo will rupture to release the new individual into the outside world. This individual may be an early embryo, a blastula, or a late embryo, or it may be a postembryonic stage — a larva or juvenile. This simply means that the time of appearance of the new individual is adjusted to the nature of the independent life it must now start leading. The basic differences in this timing are the amount of maternal care and the environment in which the early eggs will be placed. These features combine to produce the following situations:

1. "Eggs" shed into surrounding water before fertilization, for chance meeting with spermatozoa (s.Coelenterata)
2. "Eggs" laid early but placed in a brood pouch to await approach of spermatozoa (the ovicell in s.Bryozoa)
3. Eggs laid on a substrate immediately after fertilization (m.Insecta)
4. Eggs fertilized and laid early but placed in a brood pouch for development (s.Amphibia)
5. Eggs retained in the mother's reproductive tract until a larva is formed inside: (a) the egg laid just before rupture, oviparity (s.Insecta), (b) the egg ruptured just before being laid, so there appears to be "live birth", ovoviviparity (s.Insecta)
6. There never is a real "egg", but the developing embryo is retained inside the mother until it can survive (viviparity): (a) embryo survives to late embryo, which then still requires protection in a pouch of the mother (Mammalia: Marsupialia), (b) embryo survives to juvenile stage that can then survive with parental care and feeding (s.Mammalia), (c) embryo survives virtually to adult stage, ready to feed and care for itself (m.Reptilia)

It should be noted that although oviparity is cited in (5a), to contrast with ovoviviparity in (5b), the term oviparity also covers the occurrences in (1) through (4).

E. Emergence

If the beginning of the embryo is difficult to pinpoint, the end of its span is usually clear, because it usually occurs at a point of drastic change in its surroundings. The earliest embryo is always enclosed in protective membranes and often in some sort of a shell. One of the greatest diversities in timing is the stage at which the "animal" inside breaks out and first meets directly the world in which it will live. The words that are used for this emergence do not cover all the situations that occur. For example:

1. Birth — emergence of the young (larva or foetus) from the reproductive tract of the mother
2. Eclosion — hatching from the egg; sometimes used also for breaking out of the pupa or puparium
3. Emergence — general term for either birth or eclosion
4. Exovation — same as eclosion from the egg
5. Hatching — layman's term for eclosion
6. Parturition — strictly the separation of the embryonic and maternal placentas, but more often used as synonymous with birth (complete separation from the mother)

The hatching of the egg may occur when the embryo is scarcely more than a blastula, or the embryo may develop into a distinct larva or even into a virtual adult before hatching. The stage of eclosion or birth is shown by various terms:

1. Oviparity — the laying of eggs (all egg-laying animals are oviparous)
2. Ovoviviparity — retention of embryonated eggs, inside the mother, until hatch-

ing, so that "living young" are born (s.Trematoda, s.Amphineura, s.Insecta, s.Pisces, and s.Reptilia are ovoviviparous)

3. Viviparity — bearing living young, usually a juvenile (s.Bdelloidea, s.Nematoda, s.Insecta, s.Ophiuroidea, and m.Mammalia are viviparous)
4. Larviparity — ovoviviparity that produces a larva (s.Insecta)
5. Pupiparity — ovoviviparity that produces a pupa (s.Insecta)

In some animals emergence from the egg is not in itself the effective moment of facing the outside world; various forms of parental care may intervene. These terms describe the stage of release and the presence of direct maternal care (for further details see Chapter 22):

1. Brooding — in an exterior pouch, in some cases with nourishment provided
2. Placentation — attachment to a special internal surface of the mother, through which nourishment passes

All of these terms fit into a system that emphasizes the role of the mother:

Retention inside the mother

1. Of embryonated eggs that will hatch before birth; ovoviviparity
2. Of embryo or larva or foetus; viviparity

Release from the reproductive tract of the mother

3. To the outside, laying of eggs, oviparity
4. Into brood pouch; brooding after "laying"

REFERENCES

Balfour, F. M., *A Treatise on Comparative Embryology,* (2 volumes), Macmillan, London, 1885.

Counce, S. J. and Waddington, C. H., Eds., *Developmental Systems: Insecta,* (2 volumes), Academic Press, London, 1972.

Frost, S. W., *Insect Life and Insect Natural History,* Dover, New York, 1959.

Gerard, R. W., *Unresting Cells,* Harper & Row, New York, 1949.

Gray, P., Ed., *The Encyclopedia of the Biological Sciences,* Reinhold, New York, 1961.

Hagan, H. R., *Embryology of the Viviparous Insects,* Ronald Press, New York, 1951.

Harrison, F. W. and Cowden, R. R., *Aspects of Sponge Biology,* Academic Press, New York, 1976.

Holmes, S. J., *Organic Form and Related Biological Problems,* University of California Press, Berkeley, 1948.

Hyman, L. H., *The Invertebrates,* McGraw-Hill, New York, Vol. 1 (1940, Vol. 2 (1951a), Vol. 3 (1951b), Vol. 4 (1955), Vol. 5 (1959), Vol. 6 (1967).

Imms, A. D., *A General Textbook of Entomology,* 8th ed., Methuen, London, 1951.

Jaegersten, G., On the early phylogeny of the metazoa; the Bilaterogastraea theory, in *Zool. Bidrag fran Uppsala,* 30, 321, 1955.

Jaegersten, G., Further remarks on the early phylogeny of the Metazoa, *Zool. Bidrag fran Uppsala,* 33, 79, 1959.

Kaestner, A., *Invertebrate Zoology,* Interscience, New York, Vol. 1 (1967), Vol. 2 (1968), Vol. 3 (1970).

Keeton, M. T., *Biology Science,* 2nd ed., W. W. Norton, New York, 1972.

Kume, M. and Dan, K., *Invertebrate Embryology,* NOLIT, Belgrade, 1968.

Marshall, A. J., *Parker & Haswell, A Text-Book of Zoology,* Vol. 2, 7th ed., Macmillan, London, 1964.

Meglitsch, P. A., *Invertebrate Zoology,* 2nd ed., Oxford University Press, New York, 1972.

Raven, C. P., *An Outline of Developmental Physiology,* Pergamon Press, London, 1959.

Rudnick, T., *Synthesis of Molecular and Cellular Structure,* Ronald Press, New York, 1961.

Tuzet, O., The Phylogeny of Sponges . . . , in *The Lower Metazoa,* Dougherty, E. C., Ed., University of California Press, Berkeley, 1963, chap. 10.

Waddington, C. H., *Principles of Embryology,* Macmillan, New York, 1956.

Weiss, P., *Principles of Development,* Henry Holt, New York, 1939.

Williams, R. J. and Beerstecher, E., Jr., *An Introduction to Biochemistry,* Van Nostrand, New York, 1948.

Chapter 6

LARVA TO ADULT

TABLE OF CONTENTS

I.   Direct and Indirect Development 144

II.   Larva 144
    A.   Orientation 144
    B.   Types of Larvae... 145
    C.   Function of the Larva 147
    D.   Fate of the Larva 148

III. Metamorphosis... 148
    A.   Discussion 148
    B.   Metamorphosis Terms... 150
    C.   Sequences Within Metamorphosis 151
    D.   Terms for Postembryonic Stages... 154
    E.   Hypermetamorphosis 155
    F.   Unusual Processes of Change.. 155
        1.   Torsion.. 155
        2.   Epitoky.. 155
        3.   Pupation 155
        4.   Anamorphosis 156
        5.   Strobilation.. 156
        6.   Retrogression 156
        7.   Inversion 157

IV. Neoteny and Paedogenesis.. 157

References 157

I. DIRECT AND INDIRECT DEVELOPMENT

The development of an embryo into an adult animal is either direct (with little change and that quickly accomplished) or indirect (involving much greater change usually over a much greater time).

Direct development usually occurs in one of the three following circumstances:

1. All development to the juvenile stage passed inside the mother (viviparity)
2. All development to the juvenile stage passed inside the egg, after early laying (oviparity)
3. All development to the juvenile stage passed inside the egg which is retained until late inside the mother (ovoviviparity)

Indirect development is that which produces substantial change (metamorphosis). A new body form is in some way necessary to the changing life of the individual. This new body form is represented by the term *larva*, used in its most general sense — any body form assumed in development between the embryo and the adult. There is great diversity in this larval form and the stage it occupies.

The concept "larva" does not, however, occur in direct development. It is found only where there is clear change, beyond a slow gradual development. Thus, "larva" is always accompanied by *metamorphosis*, a word with several meanings.

It must be remembered, however, that many, perhaps most, animals depart from the egg-embryo-adult or the egg-embryo-larva-adult sequences by the presence of processes or occurrences such as these (which are not entirely distinct):

1. Asexual reproduction — (a) in place of sexual reproduction, (b) in alternation with it, or (c) as optional paths alongside the sexual
2. Retrogressive reproduction — where fragmentation of an adult produces a larva, or where fragmentation of an embryo produces new individuals of one or a few cells by polyembryony
3. Dormancy — of some sort (see Chapter 7)
4. Anabiosis — especially de-differentiation or reduction

The first two of these were discussed in Chapter 2. The last two will be discussed in Chapter 7.

It must also not be assumed that what occurs in one species will occur in others of that group. For example, in Echinodermata there is assumed always to be a distinct larval form, but Ubaghs (1969) cites one (unidentified) species in which the larval form is entirely suppressed, so that development is direct.

II. LARVA

A. Orientation

The word larva is difficult to define in a really general sense, even though in any group the larvae can be readily identified. The factors usually included in a definition are (1) that it is postembryonic, (2) that it differs markedly from the parent in form, (3) that it attains adult form by a sharp change (metamorphosis), (4) that it lives independently, (5) that it is active, (6) that it feeds, and (7) that it occurs before the stage of reproductive maturity (adult).

Only one of these stipulations is universal: the difference in form from the adult, which is universal simply because it is agreed not to cite as larvae any stages that are *not* different. (It is customary to use the term *juveniles* for such "immature" forms as are basically similar to the adult (see below).

Of the other six factors cited, all are open to exception. For example, there are larvae which are in reality mere gastrulae or even blastulae. There are larvae which never metamorphose into adult form, either because they are neotenic (precociously able to reproduce and therefore never become adult) or because they change into other forms of larvae (hypermetamorphosis). There are many larvae which are not independent; they live in brood chambers, may be nourished by the parent, etc. There are larvae that do not "feed", because the zygote included enough yolk to last for development to the adult stage or because they live as parasites.

Although most larvae are active to some extent, their translocation movement may be passive and other movement slight; it is true that they are seldom actually attached. There are many larvae that are capable of reproduction by one or more of a variety of asexual methods, and in the Ctenophora they can reproduce bisexually.

Most animals (except the neotenic forms) do have a stage that can be recognized as adult, even without clear-cut definition, and the larval stage, if it occurs, is between the early embryo and the adult.

Larvae, however, do not necessarily arise from embryos. They may be budded from another larva or from an adult. They may be formed by the fusion of two embryos (diporpa). They may actually be multiple, being already larval colonies (as in Bryozoa). They may be parasitic when the adult is free-living (Gordioidea), or free-living when the adult is parasitic (parasitic copepods).

It must be noted that the word "larvae" has rather different connotations in different groups. In sessile animals it is the motile dispersal stage. In insects it is the feeding stage, which is usually less motile than the adult (which usually eats little or nothing). In many parasites it serves to transfer the organism to a new host. In many animals it is the principal reproductive state, because its asexual reproduction produces far more new individuals than the sexual reproduction of the adult. The larva may be little more than a flattened blastula (planula larva) or scarcely different from the adult (nymphs). Thus, many generalizations about "larvae" are of limited application and must be accepted in the framework of the development of that particular group of animals.

B. Types of Larvae

There is great difficulty in classifying the diverse larvae found in the animal kingdom. The number of distinct types is larger than usually implied, and grouping on the basis of gross form produces almost as many larval types as there are groups of animals.

A simple grouping on the basis of general ecological and behavioral nature of the larvae seems to be the best for our purposes:

Aquatic larvae

1. Planktonic (swarmers in Protozoa, trochophore, bipinnaria)
2. Benthonic (amoeboid in Protozoa, ciliated planula, unciliated planuloid)

Terrestrial larvae

3. In soil
4. On surfaces

Symbiotic larvae

5. Ectoparasites
6. Endoparasites
7. Commensals

Inasmuch as the vast majority of phyla are aquatic, at least in part, and most of them marine, the greater part of the named kinds of larvae are marine and especially planktonic. Nevertheless, even greater diversity of form occurs among the terrestrial species (in part because food must be actively sought) and among the parasitic species (where there may be severe requirements for acquiring a host).

It would be impracticable to give a complete list of the names for larval stages in all animals. The following list is intended to give those that are normally associated with specific types found in one or more groups of invertebrates or aquatic vertebrates:

1.   Acanthella — second larva of Acanthocephala
2.   Acanthor — first larva of Acanthocephala
3.   Acanthosoma — larva of some marine Crustacea (Decapoda)
4.   Actinotrocha — larva of Phoronida
5.   Actinula — larval polyp of Hydrozoa
6.   Alima — first larva of s.Crustacea (Stomatopoda)
7.   Ammocoetes — larva of the lamprey
8.   Amoebula — swarmer of Protozoa
9.   Amphiblastula — first larva of Porifera
10. Amphigastrula — second larva of Porifera
11. Appendicularia — tadpole larva of Ascidiacea
12. Atrocha — larva of Polychaeta
13. Auricularia — larva of Holothurioidea
14. Bipinnaria — first larva of Asteroidea
15. Brachiolaria — second larva of Asteroidea
16. Caddis — larva of s.Insecta (Trichoptera)
17. Caterpillar — larva of s.Insecta (Lepidoptera, etc.)
18. Cephalotrocha — larva of Turbellaria
19. Cercaria — fourth larva (rarely third) of Trematoda
20. Coenurus — "larva" of s.Cestoda
21. Coracidium — first larva of s.Cestoda
22. Cydippid — late larva of s.Ctenophora
23. Cyphonautes — larva of s.Bryozoa
24. Cypris — second larva of s.Crustacea (Cirripedia)
25. Cysticercoid — solid-bodied larva of s.Cestoda
26. Cysticercus — bladder-worm of s.Cestoda
27. Desor's larva — of Rhynchocoela
28. Dipleurula — bilateral larva of Echinodermata
29. Doliolaria — first larva of Crinoidea and second larva of Holothurioidea
30. Echinopluteus — larva of Echinoidea
31. Echinospira — a shelled veliger of s.Gastropoda
32. Ephyra — larval medusa of Scyphozoa
33. Erichthus — larva of s.Crustacea (Stomatopoda)
34. Fucilia — last larva of s.Crustacea (Euphausiacea)
35. Glochidium — larva of s.freshwater Mollusca (Bivalvia)
36. Gotte's larva — of s.Turbellaria
37. Grub — legless larva of s.Insecta
38. Hexacanth — first larva of m.Cestoda (same as oncosphere)
39. Infusorigen — larva of s.Mesozoa
40. Kentrogen — larva of s.Crustacea (Cirripedia)
41. Leptocephalus — larva of some eels
42. Lycophore — larva of Cestodaria
43. Maggot — legless larva of s.Insecta (Diptera)

44. Megalops — larva of s.Crustacea (Decapoda)
45. Merozoite — swarmer of s.Protozoa (Sporozoa)
46. Metacercaria — fifth larva of m.Trematoda
47. Metanauplius — later larva in s.Crustacea
48. Metazooea — intermediate larva of s.Crustacea (Decapoda)
49. Miracidium — first larva of Trematoda
50. Mitraria — early trochopore of s.Polychaeta
51. Mueller's larva — of s.Turbellaria
52. Mysis — later larva of s.Crustacea
53. Nauplius — first larva of m.Crustacea
54. Nectochaeta — larva of s.Polychaeta
55. Oligopod — larva of s.Insecta
56. Oncomiracidium — first larva of s.Trematoda
57. Oncosphere — first larva of m.Cestoda (same as hexacanth)
58. Ophiopluteus — larva of Ophiuroidea
59. Parenchymula — larva of s.Porifera
60. Pentacrinoid — second larva of Crinoidea
61. Phyllosoma — larva of s.Crustacea
62. Pilidium — trochophore larva of s.Rhynchocoela
63. Pladinium — early larva of s.hypermetamorphic Insecta (Hymenoptera)
64. Planula — early larva of m.Coelenterata
65. Planuloid — asexually produced larva in s.Coelenterata (Hydrozoa)
66. Plerocercoid — late larva of s.Cestoda
67. Pluteus — larva of Ophiuroidea and Echinoidea
68. Polypod — early larva of s.Insecta
69. Polytrochula — trochophore larva of s.Polychaeta
70. Procercoid — early larva of s.Cestoda
71. Protaspis — first larval stage of s.Trilobita
72. Protoconch — larva of s.Gastropoda
73. Protozooea — early larva of s.Crustacea
74. Protrochula — larva of s.Turbellaria
75. Pseudozooea — larva of s.Crustacea (Stomatopoda)
76. Redia — third larva of m.Trematoda
77. Schizopod — mysis larva of s.Crustacea (Decapoda)
78. Scyphistoma — sessile larva of Scyphozoa
79. Sporocyst — second larva in Trematoda
80. Sporozoite - swarmer of s.Sporozoa
81. Tadpole — larva of s.Amphibia
82. Tadpole larva — of s.Tunicata
83. Tenuis larva — second larva of some eels
84. Tetrathyridium — larva of s.Cestoda
85. Tornaria — larva of Enteropneusta
86. Triungulin — first larva of hypermetamorphic Insecta (Strepsiptera and Meloidae)
87. Trochophore — larva of s.marine Turbellaria, Rhynchocoela, Bryozoa, Phoronida, Brachiopoda, Mollusca, Sipunculoidea, Annelida
88. Veliger — later larva of marine Gastropoda, Scaphopoda, Bivalvia
89. Vexillifer — first larva of some eels
90. Zooea — early larva of s.Crustacea (Decapoda)

C. Function of the Larva

Like most other things in biology, there is no answer to the question, "Why are there larvae?'' It is possible, however, to see some important functions served by larvae, and it is sometimes obvious that when these particular functions are not needed, the stage is reduced or omitted. From this one may be forgiven for concluding that larvae were evolved to serve these functions in the life cycle.

First one must realize that many kinds of animals are as immobile as plants. Most of these, Coelenterata (polyps), Calyssozoa, Bryozoa, Brachiopoda, some Echinodermata and Tunicata, have active larval stages, and an obvious function that these can serve is dispersal, inasmuch as the adult cannot move about much. All of these are marine or at least aquatic. Dispersal not only serves to enlarge the area occupied by the species but at the same time may prevent competition between the larva and the adult, for both space to occupy and food.

In terrestrial forms, such as insects, it is common for the adult to be short-lived and not to feed at all. In these the major function of the larva is to feed — accumulating enough reserves in the body to produce the adult, to keep it alive at least until reproduction, and to stock its egg with yolk.

In parasitic animals, the larva may be adapted for penetration of the host (or its organs) or to accomplish the transfer from one host to another.

It has also been cited as a function of the larva that it can reproduce asexually. Inasmuch as asexual reproduction can occur in any stage of the life cycle, it is not a special function of the larva. It is true that a few larvae, such as scyphistomae of Scyphozoa, may duplicate themselves in addition to the more normal production of the adult.

D. Fate of the Larva

By definition, the larva is an intermediate stage in the life cycle and ends its existence by changing into an adult. There are, however, many exceptions (See items 2 and 3 in the list below and the section on ''Neoteny and Paedogenesis'' at the end of this chapter). The events that end the life span of a larva include:

Metamorphosis of the larva

1. Into an adult (Polychaeta, Echinodermata, s.Insecta)
2. Into a pupa (m.Insecta)
3. Into another larval stage, *hypermetamorphosis* (m.Insecta and others listed below)

Death of the larva

4. After producing other larvae via its germ ball, in successional polyembryony (Trematoda)
5. After sexual reproduction, in *neoteny* (s.Amphibia)
6. As food for predators

Metamorphosis and hypermetamorphosis are discussed in the next section of this chapter. Successional polyembryony is described under ''Asexual Reproduction'' in Chapter 2.

III. METAMORPHOSIS

A. Discussion

The subject of development from the larva to the adult has proven to be an especially difficult one to present, partly because there is so much diversity — diversity both

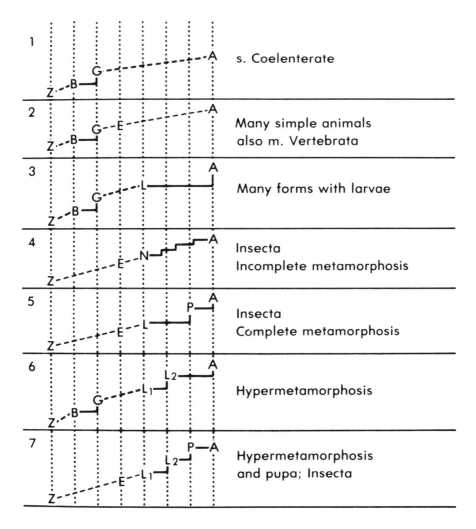

FIGURE 7.   Life cycles and metamorphoses. Dashes = gradual change; line with angles = abrupt change. Z, zygote; B, blastula; G, gastrula; E, embryo; L, larva; N, nymph; P, pupa; A, adult.

among the groups of animals and in the way terms have come to be used in different fields. An effort to treat this part of development in a uniform manner for all groups runs into unusual difficulties.

If "larva" is defined as the life-cycle stage that changes (metamorphoses) into an adult, it should be simple to define metamorphosis: it is the process of change that produces an adult from a larva. This is deceptively simple, beset with numerous difficulties (see Figure 7).

The word metamorphosis means the process of changing form (note that "form" is equivalent to "shape" and does not refer directly to structure; see Chapter 9). Note that this definition contains no reference to larvae, and when the word is applied to animals in general, there are seen in most kinds to be several episodes of change, some slight and some drastic. In some animals the initial stage, the zygote, changes form very little when it undergoes cleavage, merely changing from a smooth sphere to a spherical mass of blastomeres. In others the cleavages may produce a form that is very different from a sphere, so that it is clear that there has been a change in form. (Note that some textbooks neglect to mention such an early stage if it is passed within an egg shell, where it is not obvious.) When the spherical blastula becomes a gastrula, a variety of internal changes may occur, but often they produce little clear change in overall form. When the embryo gives rise to a larva, there is usually a rather drastic change in form. If this occurs inside the egg, i.e., before hatching, the change will not be apparent until later.

The larva may eventually change into an adult, a change often very obvious. It may also involve an intermediate resting stage of a still different form, so that there are actually two changes of form to produce an adult from a larva. There may also have been a succession of two or more different larvae, with clearly visible change between them.

There are thus many changes in some life histories and almost always several, but in actual use the word metamorphosis is always applied to the change of form from a larva to an adult, whether or not there are additional stages between them. To be more specific, metamorphosis is the change or series of changes from the first postembryonic stage (larva) to the sexually mature adult.

Difficulties arise when one encounters the myriad situations that are found among the phyla. Here one finds "larvae" that do not become adult but become other larvae, larvae that die without becoming anything else (carriers of the germ balls), larvae that need to change little to become adult, larvae that are in fact "adult" already because they are neotenic.

There are thus problems caused by (1) the varying number of changes in the cycles of different species, (2) the diversity of postembryonic stages, and (3) the varying use of even such common words as "larva" and "metamorphosis".

B. Metamorphosis Terms

In order to tabulate the diversity in metamorphosis among animals, it is necessary to define at least roughly the various terms that have been employed:

1. Abrupt metamorphosis — (see "Complete Metamorphosis")
2. Ametabolous — developing without metamorphosis
3. Complete metamorphosis — development from a larval stage to the adult by way of a pupal stage
4. Gradual metamorphosis — (see "Incomplete Metamorphosis")
5. Hemimetabolous — developing from a nymph or a naiad (immature terrestrial or aquatic forms) without abrupt metamorphosis
6. Holometabolous — developing from larva to adult through a distinct pupal stage (complete metamorphosis)
7. Homoeosis — same as Metamorphosis
8. Incomplete metamorphosis — change from larva or nymph to adult by a series of small changes
9. Metabolous — pertaining to metamorphosis
10. Metamorphosis — properly used for abrupt change of form between successive stages in a life cycle; frequently used to cover all the changes between the initial larva and the adult
11. Paurometabolous — developing from a nymph to adult with appearance of wings as the only metamorphosis

All of the above expressions except the first two are used principally for Insecta, where they are universal and are standardized. It is, of course, potentially confusing to speak of "incomplete metamorphosis" when the word metamorphosis itself is used to imply complete change.

C. Sequences within Metamorphosis

The various developmental sequences, from the viewpoint of metamorphosis, can be indicated in simplified form by three general terms:

1. Direct Development — without abrupt changes from immature stages to adult
2. Indirect development — with one or more abrupt changes
3. Hypermetamorphosis — a form of indirect development in which two or more larval stages occur in succession

There terms are not sufficiently explicit or uniform throughout the animal kingdom to be used to compare the development in different groups. It is thus necessary to be more direct in stating the nature of the development.

The occurrence of larval forms and metamorphoses in the life cycles of the classes of animals is outlined here.

PORIFERA. Calcarea. Amphiblastula "larva" undergoes gastrulation, so it is not really a larva; later a parenchymula larva is formed. It attaches and grows into adult via a simple metamorphosis.

Hexactinellida. No real larva and no metamorphosis.

Demospongia. A coeloblastula "larva" undergoes gastrulation, so it is not really a larva; it attaches and develops without metamorphosis.

MESOZOA. There is no stage recognized as a larva and thus no metamorphosis.

MONOBLASTOZOA. In the partially unknown cycle there may be amoeboid "swarmers", which would be larvae; if so a simple metamorphosis would no doubt occur.

COELENTERATA. Hydrozoa. (1) No larva and no metamorphosis. (2) Planula larva and a simple metamorphosis. (3) A blastula "larva" that gastrulates to form a planula larva which undergoes a simple metamorphosis. (4) The planula may develop into an actinula which metamorphoses (hypermetamorphosis). (5) Planula larva develops directly to colony without metamorphosis.

Scyphozoa. (1) Planula larva with simple metamorphosis to polyp. (2) A planula becomes a scyphistoma which produces ephyrae by strobilation; these ephyrae are larvae but develop into medusae without metamorphosis; the succession of these larvae do constitute a hypermetamorphosis.

Anthozoa. (1) No larva and no metamorphosis (Epiactis orikufera). (2) Planula larva with simple metamorphosis.

CTENOPHORA. (1) Cydippid larva with simple metamorphosis (Cydippida). (2) Cydippid larva with strong metamorphosis (Lobata, Cestida). (3) Planula larva and metamorphosis (Gastrodes).

GNATHOSTOMULOIDEA. No larva and no metamorphosis.

PLATYHELMINTHES. Nemertodermatida. Development not reported but assumed to be as in Acoela in Turbellaria.

Xenoturbellida. Development not reported.

Turbellaria. (1) Mueller's larva and metamorphosis to adult. (2) Gotte's larva and metamorphosis to adult. (3) A stereogastrula that never changes greatly (s.Acoela). (4) Embryo to juvenile to adult, without metamorphosis (Tricladida).

Temnocephaloidea. Development not reported.

Trematoda. (1) A "larva" with a simple metamorphosis to adult. (2) A "larva" changes into a diporpa larva which unites with another, both gradually metamorphosing into an adult, still attached (Diplozoon). (3) Miracidium develops into a sporocyst which produces rediae which produce cercariae and develop into encysted metacercariae. These gradually develop into adults. (4) Miracidium to redia to cercaria and on to adult. (5) Miracidium to sporocyst to cercaria, etc. (6) Miracidium to sporocyst I to sporocyst II to cercaria, etc. (In these last four types, the successive intermediate larvae are produced in a unique way, one inside the other; see "Successional Polyembryony".)

Cestoda. (1) From a motile coracidium an oncosphere emerges and develops into a procercoid which develops into a plerocercoid and then into an adult (as in Pseudophyllidea). (2) Oncosphere to cysticercoid to adult (s.Taenioidea). (3) Oncosphere to cysticercus or bladder worm to adult (s.Taenioidea). (4) Oncosphere to tetrathyridium to adult *(Mesocestoides)*. (5) Oncosphere to hydatid cyst to adult *(Echinococcus)*.

Cestodaria. (1) A lycophore or decacanth larva develops into a procercoid and then to adult *(Amphilina foliacea)*. (2) Lycophore metamorphoses into adult *(Gyrocotyle)*.

RHYNCHOCOELA. (1) Gastrula gradually to adult; no metamorphosis *(Cephalothrix)*. (2) Pilidium larva metamorphoses into a juvenile *(Cerebratulus)*. (3) Desor's larva metamorphoses into a juvenile *(Lineus)*.

ACANTHOCEPHALA. Acanthor larva in a shell emerges and becomes an acanthella to metamorphose into a juvenile.

ROTIFERA. Eggs hatch as juveniles; no metamorphosis.

GASTROTRICHA. Eggs hatch as juveniles; no metamorphosis.

KINORHYNCHA. (1) A larva which molts with anamorphosis but gradual metamorphosis. (2) A "larva" which is actually a juvenile; no metamorphosis.

NEMATODA. (1) Hatched as a juvenile which molts but undergoes no metamorphosis (free-living forms). (2) Hatched as "larvae" (including microfilariae) which grow by a series of molts.

GORDIOIDEA. Larva, sometimes called echinoderid larva, develops into juvenile without metamorphosis.

PRIAPULOIDEA. Larva that is essentially a juvenile; no metamorphosis.

CALYSSOZOA. (1) Larva, by some said to be a modified trochophore, with metamorphosis to adult *(Pedicellina)*. (2) Larva similar to that of a rotifer, with metamorphosis to adult *(Loxosoma)*.

BRYOZOA. Gymnolaemata. (1) Cyphonautes larva metamorphoses into an adult *(Electra pilosa)*. (2) Unnamed larva metamorphoses to adult (*Bugula*, etc.); this adult may be the ancestrula of a colony.

Phylactolaemata. "Larva" is actually a juvenile colony *(Plumatella)*.

PHORONIDA. A "larva" which is scarcely more than a gastrula is later called an actinotroch; metamorphoses to adult after very extensive development.

BRACHIOPODA. Inarticulata. A bivalved "larva" which is usually a juvenile; without metamorphosis *(Lingula)*.

Articulata. "Larva" without shell but with metamorphosis *(Terebratulina)*.

MOLLUSCA. Monoplacophora. Development unknown.

Amphineura. Trochophore larva metamorphoses into adult.

Solenogastres. (1) A "larva" which metamorphoses *(Nematomenia banyulensis)*. (2) No larva and no metamorphosis, in brooding species.

Gastropoda. (1) Trochophore to veliger, which metamorphoses to adult *(Haliotis)*. (2) Veliger, first visible stage, metamorphoses *(Melampus)*. (3) Echinospira larva, a veliger with two shells, which metamorphoses *(Capulus hungaricus)*. (4) Trochophore and veliger pass inside egg membranes, hatch as juvenile (most Pulmonata).

Bivalvia. (1) Trochophore to veliger to metamorphosis (most forms). (2) No larva or metamorphosis (Sphaeriidae), although trochophore and veliger may be detected briefly. (3) Glochidium layer with metamorphosis (Unionidae).

Scaphopoda. Trochophore to veliger with gradual metamorphosis to adult.

Cephalopoda. No metamorphosis from the juvenile, although this is sometimes called a larval stage.

SIPUNCULOIDEA. Trochophore to juvenile via metamorphosis *(Golfingia)*.

ECHIUROIDEA. Trochophore to adult via metamorphosis.

TARDIGRADA. No larva, no metamorphosis.

MYZOSTOMIDA. Larva to adult via metamorphosis.

ANNELIDA. Polychaeta. (1) Trochophore to adult by an extended metamorphosis (most species). (2) Larval stage passed in egg, in whole or in part, so no obvious metamorphosis *(Clymenella)*. (3) Other larvae in these sequences include: metatrochophore, nectochaeta, polytrocha, and aulophora. (Details not available.)

Archiannelida. Trochophore larva to adult via metamorphosis.

Oligochaeta. No larva and no metamorphosis.

Hirudinea. No larva and no metamorphosis.

DINOPHILOIDEA. Not a real trochophore (details not available.)

ONYCHOPHORA. No larva and no metamorphosis.

ARTHROPODA. Trilobita. In this extinct group, larval stages have been identified among fossils. Protaspis larva to meraspis larva to holaspis larva but no further metamorphosis *(Olenus)*.

Merostomata. A "trilobite" larva molts repeatedly to become adult without metamorphosis.

Pycnogonida. A protonymphon "larva" undergoes a slight metamorphosis.

Arachnida. (1) All early development is before emergence, so no metamorphosis (viviparous species). (2) Several "larval" stages are described, more often called nymphs; no clear metamorphosis (Acarina).

Crustacea. (1) Nauplius larva produces a zooea larva which gradually becomes a postlarva or juvenile, with anamorphosis but no metamorphosis. (2) Juvenile which molts but no metamorphosis (freshwater crayfish, Amphipoda). (3) Nauplius to several copepodid stages but no clear metamorphosis (Copepoda). (4) Postlarva or manca stage but no metamorphosis (Isopoda). (5) Either slightly metamorphic or metamorphic with stages such as nauplius-protozooea-mysis-zooea, or protozooea-zooea-postlarva, or phyllosoma-zooea, or mysis-postlarva, or zooea-megalops (m.Decapoda). (6) Many other named larval forms.

Chilopoda. No named larva, no metamorphosis, but with or without anamorphosis.

Diplopoda. No named larva; no metamorphosis, but with anamorphosis.

Symphyla. No named larva, no metamorphosis, but with anamorphosis.

Pauropoda. No named larva, no metamorphosis, but with anamorphosis.

Insecta. (1) No larva or metamorphosis (Apterygota). (2) Nymph but no metamorphosis (terrestrial Hemimetabola). (3) Naiad but no metamorphosis (aquatic Hemimetabola). (4) Larva (caterpillar, grub, maggot) to pupa to adult, a "complete" metamorphosis (Holometabola). (5) Larva to different larva to pupa to adult; typical hypermetamorphosis (s.parasitic Hymenoptera). (6) Triungulin to unnamed larva to larva to pupa to adult (Coleoptera: *Epicauta*). (7) Stylopid (triungulin) larva to maggot, through molts to pupa to adult (Strepsiptera). (8) Numerous variations of these.

CHAETOGNATHA. No metamorphosis, although the juvenile is usually called a larva.

POGONOPHORA. There is said to be a larva but metamorphosis is not reported.

ECHINODERMATA. Crinoidea. Doliolaria larva to pentacrinoid larva to adult, but without clear metamorphosis.

Asteroidea. (1) "Larva" to bipinnaria larva to brachiolaria larva, which metamorphoses to adult. (2) "Larva" to bipinnaria, which metamorphoses. (3) "Larva" metamorphoses directly.

Ophiuroidea. (1) "Larva" to ophiopluteus, with metamorphosis. (2) Embryo to juvenile in bursal sac, no metamorphosis *(Amphipholis squamata)*.

Echinoidea. (1) Echinopluteus larva metamorphoses into adult. (2) No free larva but metamorphosis occurs *(Heliocidaris)*.

Holothurioidea. Auricularia larva to doliolaria larva to juvenile, without further metamorphosis.

ENTEROPNEUSTA. (1) A "larva" but no metamorphosis *(Saccoglossus horsti)*. (2) "Larva" to tornaria larva, with regressive metamorphosis *(Balanoglossus clavigerus)*.

PTEROBRANCHIA. (1) "Larva" to tornaria larva, but no real metamorphosis *(Cephalodiscus)*. (2) Juveniles occur but the complete cycle is unknown *(Atubaria)*. (3) Apparently no larva and no metamorphosis *(Rhapdopleura)*.

TUNICATA. Ascidiacea. Appendicularia or tadpole larva with regressive metamorphosis.

Thaliacea. (1) No larva and no clear metamorphosis *(Pyrosoma)*. (2) A "larva" that metamorphoses into adult (Doliolida).

Larvacea. A tailed larva which is neotenic; without metamorphosis.

CEPHALOCHORDATA. "Larva" but no real metamorphosis.

VERTEBRATA. Agnatha. (1) Ammocoete larva with metamorphosis *(Petromyzon)*. (2) No larva and no metamorphosis *(Myxine)*.

Chondrichthyes. No larva and no metamorphosis.

Osteichthyes. (1) Leptocephalus larva ("glass-fish") to adult with metamorphosis (some eels). (2) Vexillifer larva to tenuis larva to juvenile to adult *(Carapus acus)*. (3) A neotenic larva is cited, with no metamorphosis *(Clariallabes petriola)*. (4) A larva "practically adult" in form *(Protopterus)*. (5) No larva and no metamorphosis.

Amphibia. (1) Hatch as tadpoles, with metamorphosis to adult. (2) Neoteny may occur. (3) Aquatic larva to terrestrial larva (eft) to adult with metamorphosis *(Notophthalmus viridescens)*.

Reptilia. No larva and no metamorphosis.

Aves. No larva and no metamorphosis; juveniles are called nestlings.

Mammalia. No larva and no metamorphosis but usually a juvenile.

D. Terms for Postembryonic Stages

The preceding list shows that there is diversity in usage of such words as larva and juvenile. In some cases a questionable status is indicated by quotation marks, however, there are definitions that serve to standardize these, and they also serve to emphasize the intermediate cases.

The terms "instar" and "stadium", used for insects between successive molts, are cited in the next chapter under "Molting."

Larva. A postembryonic stage, living free of the parent, and attaining adult form by a metamorphosis (see also discussion in the previous section on "Larva").

Naiad. An aquatic nymph stage of an insect.

Nymph. In an earlier section, the two major forms of postembryonic development in arthropods are described as complete and incomplete metamorphosis. In terrestrial Arthropoda that undergo incomplete (or gradual) metamorphosis, it is customary to designate the successive stages as nymphs, as they are not truly larvae. These occur in Insecta, and something similar in Arachnida (Acarina), where the stages have received separate names.

Pupa. In Insecta with complete or abrupt metamorphosis, the change from larva to adult also involves a resting stage or pupa. The pupa is outwardly inactive, but extensive anatomical change and physiological activity take place inside it. The living animal is enclosed in a chrysalis, a puparium, or a cocoon. The latter term is also used for an egg case in some Annelida and in some Arachnida.

Juvenile. A larval stage occurs in the life cycle of nearly all marine animals and also in most arthropods, thus in something like 90% of animal species. In the other 10% there is in place of a larva a juvenile that more or less closely resembles the adult, except that the reproductive system is immature. They do not undergo metamorphosis. These include free-living Nematoda, Oligochaeta, Onychophora, Diplopoda, Chilopoda, most Arachnida, Thaliacea, and most Vertebrata.

Adult. In development (the life cycle), the final form attained; usually the sexually reproductive stage. Also called imago (pl. imagines) in Insecta.

E. Hypermetamorphosis

It will be noted that in the preceding list hypermetamorphosis is frequently cited, even though this term is not commonly used in some of the groups. The term is usually applied only to a few special insects whose development is unusually complicated. In these the definition is that development passes through two or more markedly different larval forms. By this definition the phenomenon must be recognized in at least these groups:

1. Scyphozoa — (planula, scyphistoma, strobila, ephyra)
2. Trematoda — (miracidium, sporocyst, redia, cercaria, metacercaria)
3. Cestoda — (oncosphere, cysticercus, and others)
4. Cestodaria — (lycophore, procercoid)
5. Some Gastropoda — (trochophore, veliger)
6. Crustacea — (nauplius, cypris, and others)
7. Some Insecta — (larval stages not formally named; in Meloidae, Strepsiptera, Mantispidae, some endoparasitic Hymenoptera, etc.)
8. Crinoidea — (doliolaria, pentacrinoid)
9. Asteroidea — (bipinnaria, brachiolaria)
10. Some Holothurioidea — (auricularia, pentactula)
11. Some Crinoidea — (doliolaria, pentacrinoid)
12. Some Osteichthyes — (leptocephalus, tenuis)

F. Unusual Processes of Change

Various other processes of change occur and have been given distinctive names in various groups. These include torsion, epitoky, pupation, strobilation, retrogressive metamorphosis, and inversion. Some of these occur too early in the development to be treated as metamorphosis.

1. Torsion

A 180° rotation of the visceral mass of gastropods with respect to the head and foot is torsion; not related to spiralling of the shell; sometimes reversed later; gastropods are distinguished as untorted, torted, or detorted.

2. Epitoky

The development of a special body region for carrying the gonads is termed epitoky, with often complete separation of this region as a detached gonophore (epitoke); in Polychaeta only (see Chapter 2).

3. Pupation

The word pupation is used only with reference to some Insecta. In these the larva changes into a resting stage, usually in a case derived from the larval exoskeleton, inside of which nearly all body organs disintegrate and are rebuilt. In general, the rebuilding is directed by a series of imaginal discs on the inside of the body wall.

The imaginal discs or histoblasts are a fascinating factor in the story of the development of a fly or butterfly from a caterpillar. They are first clearly seen in the pupa or puparium, but it is known that they form in the early larva and even in the embryo. They form in many parts of the body, but those that produce the new integument are probably the most obvious; these arise from the larval epidermis (called hypodermis by entomologists). From these are gradually formed a new integument inside the larval one. Organs and appendages are produced by special discs, the latter everting to the outside. The larval organs disintegrate and are replaced by those growing form the discs.

Some features of pupation are duplicated in a little-known process in some Rhynchocoela, where a remarkable and unique metamorphosis occurs. There seems to be no special term for this process, in which a pilidium larva *produces* an adult but does not develop into one. (This is also reminiscent of the process of successional polyembryony, except that it is not multiple.) Inside the larva "metamorphosis is initiated by invaginations of the ectoderm at several places (imaginal discs) . . . , these invaginations become connected to each other, secondarily forming a new body wall surrounding the gut, and the process is completed when cilia appear on this body wall . . . " The adult is thus free in the interior of the larva, which continues to swim about. Finally, the adult bursts out and the pilidium remnant dies (Kume and Dan, 1965).

4. Anamorphosis

Although zoological dictionaries omit this term or refer to it in another sense, it is regularly used to refer to the process by which additional body segments are added at times of molting.

In Annelida, there seems to be some question whether there is regular molting such as is seen in the Arthropoda, but it is clear that segments are added to some worms during their life. These apparently are not added at the time of any molting. A different process is described by Beklemishev (1969), as follows:

"Most arthropods emerge from the egg with the full number of segments characteristic of their species, as is also the case with many annelids (e.g., Lumbricidae and all leeches). A number of arthropods, however, emerge from the egg as larvae having an incomplete number of segments and developing later by successive formation of new segments from a growth zone, like most annelids. In arthropods this method of development is called *anamorphosis* . . . Full anamorphosis is characteristic of trilobites, Pantopoda (Pycnogonida), and very many crustaceans; limited anamorphosis, of some crustaceans, e.g., *Leptodora* (Cladocera) and the family Sergestidae (Decapoda) . . . , Eurypterida, Diplopoda, Pauropoda, Symphyla, some Chilopoda, and all Protura . . . "

The opposite of anamorphic development is called *epimorphic*, "having their segmentation essentially complete on emerging" as adult.

5. Strobilation

The term strobilation covers two rather different situations which arise in a similar manner. First, it has been described in Chapter 2 as an asexual reproductive process, where it produces new complete individuals. Second, in the Cestoda, strobilation produces a chain of segment-like structures called proglottids, which are simply multiple gonophores. These are detachable organs, or packets of organs, that can complete their function before they die. The worm with the strobilus is very different in appearance from the pre-adult that precedes it; thus a type of metamorphosis has occurred.

6. Retrogression

In several animals a change of form occurs that involves loss or modification of important features and so is a form of metamorphosis. For example, in ascidian Tunicata, the retrograde metamorphosis involves elimination of the tail and destruction of most of its tissues. The body form changes from a swimming tadpole larva to a sessile pitcher stage.

7. Inversion

In development, inversion is the abrupt turning inside out of a sponge stomoblastula, bringing what seemed to be endoderm cells to the outside, where they may later be drawn inside again by gastrulation (see Chapter 5).

IV. NEOTENY AND PAEDOGENESIS

Larvae are usually defined on the basis of not having the distinctive feature of adults, which is the ability to reproduce sexually. Larvae do, however, usually have a distinct form and way of life that can readily be recognized. When such an apparent "larva" is seen to reproduce sexually, the situation arouses special interest.

In one such case, in the Ctenophora, it was found that not only does the larva reproduce sexually but it then changes into an adult where it reproduces sexually for a second time. The term *paedogenesis* refers to this reproduction by a larva (although it is sometimes also used to cover asexual reproduction in a larva).

In certain Amphibia, on the other hand, an obvious larva will become sexually mature and reproduce. This process is sometimes called paedogenesis, which it is, but it is also frequently called "neoteny", reproduction by an unmetamorphosed larva which will never complete its cycle into the adult stage. Neoteny is thus an evolutionary concept, a telescoping of the life cycle so that the adult stage is entirely eliminated. This also happens in the Larvacea in the Tunicata, which appear to be larvae but can reproduce bisexually and never metamorphose.

It would be beneficial to the understanding of these processes if in all cases the term paedogenesis were to be used for the process of reproduction (whether one includes all or only sexual) in a larva, and neoteny to refer only to the evolutionary process that produced a sexually mature larva.

A further instance should be cited because it has been erroneously described as parthenogenetic paedogenesis. The reproduction of larvae of some Trematoda involves a sporocyst from which emerge rediae, from which either more rediae or cercariae emerge. These were once believed to arise from unfertilized eggs, but no one has described any oogenesis. It seems certain that the successive generations of larvae are simply products of the splitting of an original germ ball and its successors. This has recently been called polyembryony, but it is very different from ordinary polyembryony in other animals and is here called successive polyembryony. In each larval stage, the germ ball breaks up to produce daughter balls which each produce one of the next stage larvae (see "Asexual Reproduction" in Chapter 2).

REFERENCES

Balfour, F. M., *A Treatise on Comparative Embryology,* 2 volumes, Macmillan, London, 1885.
Beklemishev, W. N., *Principles of Comparative Anatomy of Invertebrates,* 2 volumes, University of Chicago Press, Chicago, 1969.
Brønsted, H. V., *Planarian Regeneration,* Pergamon Press, Oxford, 1969.

Counce, S. J. and Waddington, C. H., Eds., *Developmental Systems: Insecta,* 2 volumes, Academic Press, London, 1972.

Frost, S. W., *Insect Life and Insect Natural History,* Dover, New York, 1959.

Gray, P., Ed., *The Encyclopedia of the Biological Sciences,* Reinhold, New York, 1961.

Hyman, L. H., *The Invertebrates,* McGraw-Hill, New York, volumes 1 (1940), 2 (1951a), 3 (1951b), 4 (1955), 5 (1959), 6 (1967).

Imms, A. D., *A General Textbook of Entomology,* 8th ed., Methuen, London, 1951.

Kaestner, A., *Invertebrate Zoology,* volumes 1 (1967), 2 (1968), 3 (1970), Interscience, New York.

Kerkut, G. A., *Implications of Evolution,* Pergamon Press, Oxford, 1960.

Kume M. and Dan, K., *Invertebrate Embryology,* NOLIT, Belgrade, 1968.

Marshall, A. J., *Parker & Haswell, A Text-Book of Zoology,* Vol. 2, ed. 7, Macmillan, London, 1964.

Raven, C. P., *An Outline of Developmental Physiology,* Pergamon Press, London, 1959.

Ubaghs, G., General characteristics of the echinoderms, in *Chemical Zoology,* Florkin, M. and Scheer, B. T., Eds., Academic Press, New York, 1969.

Chapter 7

LIFE CYCLES

TABLE OF CONTENTS

I.   The Adult Stage 160
     A.   Definitions 160
     B.   Adulthood Difficulties 161

II. Life Cycle Features 161
     A.   Normal Features 161
     B.   Start of Life History 161
     C.   Life History Diversity 162
     D.   Metagenesis 164
     E.   Composite Life Cycle Diagrams 165
     F.   Molting 166
     G.   Growth 169
     H.   Eutely 171
     I.   Dormancy 173
     J.   Regeneration 175
     K.   Senescence 177

III. Theory of Recapitulation 178

References 179

I. THE ADULT STAGE

A. Definitions

One of the biological ideas that is so familiar that one scarcely sees any need to define is "adult". Adults of *Homo sapiens* may occasionally have a problem about when a teenager becomes an adult, and some arbitrary age may be set. Biologically and medically, an individual becomes an adult when the reproductive organs reach functioning condition. There are few exceptions.

In other animals a variety of difficulties arise in this definition. Many individuals of adult size and form never become sexually reproductive. A wide variety of reproductive processes take place in obviously immature forms, although these are usually asexual. Some obvious larvae become sexually mature without assuming any of the features expected in an adult (see "Neoteny and Paedogenesis" in Chapter 6).

In many animals the word "adult" is simply not appropriate. For example, in one hydrozoan species the polyp form may reproduce sexually, but in neighboring species the polyp asexually produces a medusa, which will reproduce sexually. It is not possible to specify either polyp or medusa as the exclusive adult stage in all Coelenterata. If "adult" is defined as the sexually reproducing stage, then many species never reach adulthood. If it is defined as the terminal phase of the life cycle, then it is possible to say that most species do produce some adults, but many individuals in many species find their terminal phase as an embryo or a larva.

There are various terms applied to adults in different groups. For example:

1. Adult — the final developmental stage of a life cycle, usually the stage in which maximum size is attained and in which reproduction occurs (especially sexual, which rarely occurs elsewhere)
2. Epitoke — in a few Polychaeta, this is a sexually reproducing form (see Chapter 3)
3. Female — a sexually mature individual that produces only ova (or pseudova)
4. Gamont — the gamete-producing individual in Protozoa
5. Hermaphrodite — a sexually mature individual that produces both ova and spermatozoa
6. Imago — the sexually mature adult in Arthropoda
7. Male — a sexually mature individual that produces only spermatozoa
8. Medusa — the free-swimming form of Coelenterata, always sexual; may or may not alternate with a polyp
9. Neuter — a mature individual that does not have organs of either sex
10. Person — the part of a massive sponge associated with one osculum
11. Polyp — the vase-like attached form of Coelenterata, may be sexual or not; see medusa
12. Zooid — one individual, usually in a colony, in Graptozoa, Bryozoa, and Pterobranchia

It is impossible to separate the organs and processes of one stage, such as the adult, from the development that produced them. Nevertheless, in this book, the processes and structures of the adult are the subject of Chapters 12 to 20 and are therefore not discussed under "Development". Reproduction by adults is treated with that of all other stages under "Origin of Individuals" (Part II). Nevertheless, it is not intended to remove the adult stage from the life cycle, where it is usually the most obvious stage and can often be said to be biologically the goal of all reproduction and development. Features of the adult stage are dealt with in these chapters on development in such matters as growth, dormancy, polymorphism, regeneration, and life cycles.

B. Adulthood Difficulties

It is often forgotten that adulthood is not *invariably* the result of a development of the "normal" type. In the asteroid genus *Linckia*, for instance, a new adult may develop from an arm broken off in a form of division or fragmentation, and the new individual (the separated arm) is virtually fully adult upon separation; it undergoes a development consisting only of regeneration of the missing parts. Thus, some of the organs of the new individual do not arise by the usual development.

The most obvious case of discontinuity occurs in the pupa of holometabolous Insecta. Here, all ordinary larval organs are resorbed in the pupa, and the adult organs develop anew from imaginal discs on the inside of the body wall. There is, in these cases, no real continuity between a certain organ of the adult and the larval organ from which it would otherwise have developed.

Another difficulty arises when the life history includes several larval stages (hypermetamorphosis), decreasing the chance of continuity. Furthermore, in cases of life cycles composed of several life histories (see "Cycles of Development" in Chapter 5), the various individuals may be so different as to raise questions of continuity.

II. LIFE CYCLE FEATURES

A. Normal Features

Although there are omissions or interpolations in many animal life cycles, there is a common sequence that can be taken as the normal cycle. The egg, whether fertilized or merely activated, divides by what is called cleavage into a mass of cells that becomes the embryo. In the early embryo the germ layers are formed and the archenteron is produced. The eventual body cavities appear, and the appropriate organs develop. The late embryo changes into a larva, usually motile, which frequently is a feeding stage. The larva may pass for a time through a resting stage, before changing into the adult form. These changes may not be abrupt, so that the stages are merged or indistinguishable. The diversity in some of these occurrences is tabulated in Chapters 5 and 6.

The most interesting feature of all this is the frequency with which this "normal" cycle is either bypassed or drastically altered. The cycle is not necessarily the same for all members of a single species, and the diversity in cycles in some large classes is approximately as great as in the entire animal kingdom.

Very few of the features listed in the "normal" cycle can be used to classify major groups. This is because any of the features can be omitted, any part of the sequence can be interrupted by "unusual" processes, and a given animal form may be attained in one group by as many as ten parallel, but drastically different pathways (see Figures 8 to 15 in a later paragraph).

B. Start of Life History

The old question of which came first, the chicken or the egg, is easily "solved" here by merely describing complete ontogenies from egg to adult, without taking any interest in the historical origin of the cycle. The question of whether development starts with reproduction (gamete production) or with fertilization might be harder to settle, mainly because of familiarity with vertebrates and cliches that have been widespread. Reproduction may be the end goal of life, but that set of processes, like all the others in metabolism, are merely a prelude to liberation (and perhaps delivery) of gametes. A new life history begins only when a new individual is formed at fertilization, activation, or asexual separation. Reproduction may have occurred during that life history or may not; in fact, it may have been biologically impossible. Each life cycle ends with production of a duplicate of the original individual. It will have involved reproduction if it involves more than one individual in the sequence.

Reproduction is therefore a diverse group of processes resulting in new individuals, the processes occurring at almost any time in a normal life cycle, according to the species involved. Reproduction is always the start of a new life history (or several), but it is not itself necessarily the start of a new cycle. It is herein dealt with under "Origin of Individuals" in Part II.

As suggested in both Chapters 4 and 5, there may be confusion in the usages of "life history" and "life cycle".

To avoid this, an effort is made here to use *life history* only to refer to the sequence of the development of one individual and *life cycle* for the sum of the life histories that are required to produce a duplicate of the first individual. To refer to all the sequences (histories or cycles) found in one species, one would use "composite of species cycles".

Thus, life history refers to the life of one individual, from its origin to the end of its separate life. Life cycle refers to the entire sequence of events from an individual of one sort (such as a polyp) on to the production of a second individual (the medusa) and around to the polyp again — thus two life histories. Together they make up the life cycle of that species.

There are at least five stages at which a new individual may arise. These are zygote (or apozygote or agamete), blastomere, embryo, larva, and adult. The life of a new individual may start at any of these points:

1. Development from a fertilized egg
2. Development from an activated ovum
3. Development from an agamete
4. Development from a blastomere from a cleaving zygote (polyembryony)
5. Development from a multicellular fragment of a cleaving zygote/embryo (also polyembryony)
6. Development from an embryo formed by fusion of many blastomeres from several zygotes
7. Production as an adult by budding from an adult
8. Production by regeneration of a fragment of an adult
9. Growth from a multicellular gemmule
10. Production as a larva by budding from a larva
11. Production as a larva (juvenile) by frustulation (fragmentation) from an adult

These origins may be arranged into four groups, thus:

1. Unicellular reproductive body or fragment   1—4
2. Proliferation of cells into a mass that can separate from the embryo   5, 7, 9,
    or larva or adult   10
3. Proliferation from an embryo formed by fusion of several zygotes   6
4. Regeneration of a fragment of the adult   8, 11

After a new individual comes into existence there are only three ways in which it can cease to exist (come to the end of its separate existence):

1. Death
2. Division into two (or more), both of which are new
3. Fusion of two to form one new one

C. Life History Diversity

A new individual may come into existence in any of the five stages under "Start of Life History" above. A zygote may immediately divide into two (or more) cells that each act like a zygote; the first zygote is a very short-lived individual. (In these formulae Z stands for zygote, AZ for apozygote, E for embryo, L for larva, and A for adult; subscript numerals identify successive stages of larvae.)

$$Z \text{---} Z_1 \quad\quad \text{(all cases of polyembryony)}$$
$$\searrow Z_1$$

An adult may divide into two, as in fragmentation of many worms or polyps.

$$A \text{---} A_1 \quad\quad \text{(Rhynchocoela)}$$
$$\searrow A_1$$

Of course, most animals begin life as a zygote or apozygote and live to death.

$Z \text{---} E \text{---} L \text{---} A$ (Amphineura with trochophore)

$Z \text{---} E \text{---} L \text{---} P \text{---} A$ (holometabolous Insecta)

$Z \text{---} E \text{---} L_1 \text{---} L_2 \text{---} L_3 \text{---} L_4 \text{---} A$ (Trematoda)

$AZ \text{---} E \text{---} L \text{---} A$ (Turbellaria)

$AZ \text{---} E \text{---} L \text{---} P \text{---} A$ (holometabolous Insecta)

$AZ \text{---} E \text{---} L_1 \text{---} L_2 \text{---} L_3 \text{---} A$ (Crustacea)

Some begin life as an embryo or larva, by either budding or fragmentation.

$E \text{---} L \text{---} A$ (budding Bryozoa)

$L \text{---} A$ (Hydrozoa)

These are only the beginning of the diversity. In each of these examples the reproducing stage disappears as it changes into the next stage. More often the original stage continues to exist and may then start other cycles in the same or different manner (see Figure 5).

Change of Form. The very expressions "life cycle" and "life history" imply that there is change through time. The change could be continuous or itself cyclical, in steps. The change may be external, rapid, and visible, or internal, slow, and hidden. In many asexually produced animals, the only life history changes are regeneration and senescence; the first rapid, brief, and evident, the second gradual, slight, and almost undetectable.

It is said that "Change of form is continuous throughout the whole of the life-history of every metazoan", but if this refers to individuals, it is a gross overstatement. For example, when an individual *Hydra* develops by budding from an adult, the new individual is itself immediately adult. In many forms of asexual reproduction there is little development and no real change of form; growth and senescence occur, but imperceptibly. Again, in the case of insects with complete metamorphosis, the stages — egg, larva, pupa, adult — are each relatively unchanging; the life cycle changes are not continuous but episodic.

Thus, the quotation would be more accurate if it read: Most animals undergo continous change from beginning to death, but some animals change almost not at all during life, and some change repeatedly and suddenly only after periods of little visible change.

Life cycles can be grouped under a reasonable number of headings, but the distribution of these among the phyla of animals is too nearly random to be meaningful. In this book the diversity of the sequences of reproduction have been illustrated in Chapter 4, and some of the diversities at various points in development are discussed in Chapters 5 and 6. One cannot usefully do more with the endlessly diverse series of combinations of events.

Terms sometimes used with reference to life history include: autobiology, the study of the life history of an individual; ontogeny, the life history of the individual; and phenology, the study of life history events as correlated with season and weather.

D. Metagenesis

Alternation of generations is part of the life cycle rather than of the life history, because it takes two individuals to make an alternation. In animals it is usually the alternation of a sexual phase with an asexual one; in plants and a few Protozoa, the alternation is of a diploid phase with a haploid phase (see description below). In animals, a variety of "alternations" occur, in some of which the two or more kinds of individuals are produced successively. There is no easy way to distinguish these from ordinary development, where one individual passes through several forms, produced by successive metamorphoses.

Whereas meta*morphosis* involves successive changes of form in one life history, meta*genesis* involves a sequence of separate individuals of different form or nature within the life cycle (the one sequence). This sequence may be fixed and invariable (obligate) or it may be occasional and unpredictable (facultative). The term is seldom defined, but *metagenesis* is the occurrence in a species of obligately successive individuals of two or more structural or functional types. It is surprising to find that this concept is difficult to separate from life history (of which it is part) and from life cycle (which it may complicate by forming offshoots). For example:

$$\text{zygote - - - larva - - - polyp} \quad\text{------}\quad \text{polyp}$$
$$|$$
$$\text{medusa - - - zygote}$$

The types of metagenesis in animals are diverse, but all together they form just one of the kinds of polymorphism cited in Chapter 9. Not only can the "generations" be related to the form of reproduction, but they can be functional types with or without reproductive capability. They may be environmentally controlled, environmentally produced, or they may be of poorly understood processes that maintain them as variants in the genotype pool. To illustrate alternations one should start with the plant type, which is the best understood.

It is usually believed that neither Metazoa nor Protozoa show the well-known form of alternation of generations of plants. This is (1) sexual production of a sporophyte which will then (2) asexually produce the gametophyte. It is true that no stage in Protozoa or animals is called a sporophyte, but the name is of less importance than the fact that the stage is haploid; thus the alternation is essentially of a diploid and a haploid "generation". Although such an alternation does not occur in Metazoa, it does occur in a few Protozoa and not among those sometimes thought of as actual plants — the Phytomonadina.

The three forms of alternation in organisms are cited by Grell (1973) under terms not usually used in zoology. The plant type is cited as (2):

1. Diplo-homophasic alternation — the gametes represent the only haploid phase; all reproduction is in the diploid phase (Heliozoa, Ciliata)
2. Heterophasic alternation — sexual reproduction is in the diploid phase, asexual (agamogony) in the haploid (Foraminifera only; plants)
3. Haplo-homophasic alternation — only the zygote is diploid, immediately followed by meiosis; the asexual reproduction is by fission (Sporozoa)

It will be seen that Metazoa fall into group (1), but care must be exercised to recognize that ameiotic parthenogenesis forms an exception (see Chapter 4).

There are only three types of metagenesis, all involving confusion situations. They can be diagrammed by the use of the following symbols: A = "adult", A_P = polyp, A_M = medusa, A_H = haploid, A_D = diploid, A_{AT} = atoke, A_{EP} = epitoke, Z = zygote, --- = develops into, and — = produces.

1. Polyp-medusa. The standard example of metagenesis is such an animal as *Obelia*. An asexual polyp produces a sexual medusa, whose gametes produce a polyp again. *Obelia* is a colony, but it would not be necessary for polyps to remain attached to produce an alternation. Both polyp and medusa are considered to be adults (certainly neither one fits the definition of a larva), and there often are even two successive forms of polyp in the cycle. The real difficulty arises when we realize that there are species in which the first polyps produced will reproduce asexually and later ones sexually, with no medusa stage. There are a few cases in which the medusa stage may bud other medusae.

$$Z \cdots A_P — A_M — Z$$

2. In Protozoa, the Foraminifera undergo an alternation of type (2) in the list above. Two shell types are produced sequentially. The organism forming first is haploid and is called a megalosphere, and it produces gametes by mitosis; the second is the result of the union of two gametes and is the diploid zygote or microsphere organism. It will undergo meiosis to produce agametes that will grow into a new megalosphere generation. In this group there are many variations of the cycles, so much so that one writer (Farmer, 1980) wrote: "Thus many reproductive avenues are available to the protozoa — some straight and narrow, others appearing impossibly complex." This type of alternations is called either haploid-diploid or megalosphere-microsphere.

$$Z \cdots A_H \cdots A_D \cdots Z$$

3. A developmental sequence apparently never cited as an alternation is that found in those cases of epitoky in which the separated epitoke regenerates the head and becomes a distinct individual. The atoke is asexual, the epitoke sexual. Neither is a larva.

$$Z \cdots A_{At} \cdots A_{Ep} \cdots Z$$

E. Composite Life Cycle Diagrams

The following eight diagrams are selected to show the diversity of life cycles in certain phyla or classes. Each one shows the pathways that may be followed by the individuals of the various species in that group, from the simple dioecious Merostomata with no apomictic reproduction and no highly divergent larvae, to the fantastically diverse Hydrozoa with hermaphroditism, parthenogenesis, a variety of larvae, and a variety of asexual processes, capable of a variety of additional combinations not even shown in the diagram (Figures 8 to 15).

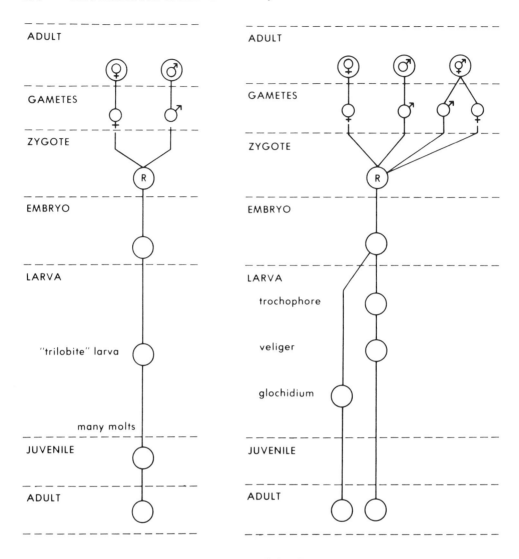

FIGURE 8.   The single dioecious pathway used by all species in the Merostomata.

FIGURE 9.   The two dioecious and two monoecious pathways used by the species of Bivalvia.

FIGURES 8 to 15.   Composite diagrams of the reproductive pathways of the species in various groups. In these diagrams the large circles are individuals, sometimes with sex shown. Gametes are shown by sex symbols not in circles. R indicates that there has just been reproduction of some sort and this is a new individual. An apozygote is indicated by apo-. Each pathway includes only such forms as shown by a circle in the appropriate tier (all from Blackwelder and Shepherd, 1981).

F. Molting

This word is used in different groups for four rather different processes. In birds and mammals it is the periodic shedding of feathers and hair formed by the epidermis and, in the case of feathers, with participation of a mesenchymal dermal pulp.

In reptiles and amphibians the keratinized outer layer of the epidermis may slough off continuously in fragments or periodically in a single piece (as in snakes).

In such Ciliata as *Blepharisma undulans*, there is a process of molting in which the pellicle is lost but the cilia remain.

In all other animals that molt, it is the cuticle (or exoskeleton) that is periodically

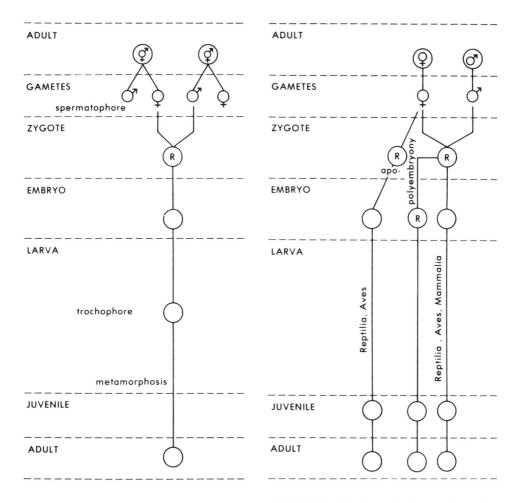

FIGURE 10. The single dioecious pathway of
the hermaphroditic species of Myzostomida.

FIGURE 11. The three dioecious pathways of the
species of higher Vertebrata. Polyembryony occurs
occasionally in Mammalia but may also occur elsewhere in the phylum.

shed. In these animals the process is usually called *ecdysis.* A new cuticle is secreted by
the epidermis under the old one before each molt. By means of folds and overlappings,
the new cuticle may actually be larger than the old, allowing for growth of the animal.
In some instances, segments are added to the body before each molt (see "Anamorphosis" in Chapter 6).

Molting is known to occur in the following groups only. Where number of molts is
cited, this is the number normally occurring in the life cycle:

Ciliata, as cited above
Kinorhyncha, the entire cuticle is shed intact, including the lining of the proctodaeum
Nematoda, four molts, including the entire cuticle and the linings of the buccal cap-
sule, pharynx, rectum, and vagina
Gordioidea, reported to keep the larval cuticle into the adult stage, but "the proboscis
stylets and hooks and their accompanying epidermis and musculature degenerate and
are lost at the molt" (Hyman, 1951)
Priapuloidea, one molt in the form of shedding of the lorica
Tardigrada, four to six molts, which may be in response to unfavorable environmental
conditions; the claws and the lining of the rectum are shed with the cuticle

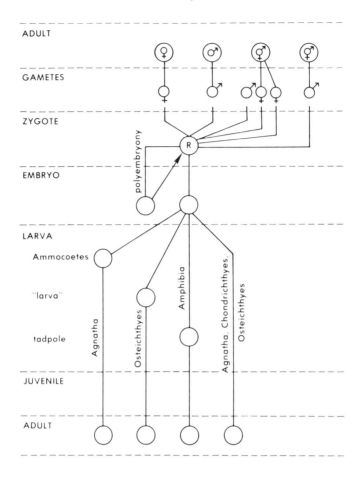

FIGURE 12.   The many pathways followed by species of lower Vertebrata. Polyembryony produces cells which function as zygotes. The four
developmental pathways involve different types of larvae (or none).

Pentastomida, the chitinous cuticle is shed periodically during larval development;
adults molt periodically

Annelida, in most books no molting is mentioned, although some epidermal structures
of the larva are said to be ephemeral. Vorontsova and Liosner (1960) state that "the
cuticle of the annelids is periodically shed and renewed by the superficial layer of the
epithelial cells"

Onychophora, the juvenile molts once; the adult of *Peripatopsis* molts every 6 to 7
days during its life of 6 to 7 years

Arthropoda, molts occur repeatedly in most larvae and many adults, 1 to 25 times; the
cuticle, its appendages, the lining of the tracheae and of the fore- and hind-intestine
are shed; the number of larval molts may be related to sex determination

Larvacea, the so-called "house" secreted by the epidermis is gelatinous and frequently
shed, as often as every few hours; it is not certain whether this is a cuticle in the usual
sense

Vertebrata, as cited above.

The terms that have been applied to molting processes and periods include:

1.   Diecdysis — the period between the end of one metecdysis and the beginning of
the next proecdysis; in Crustacea

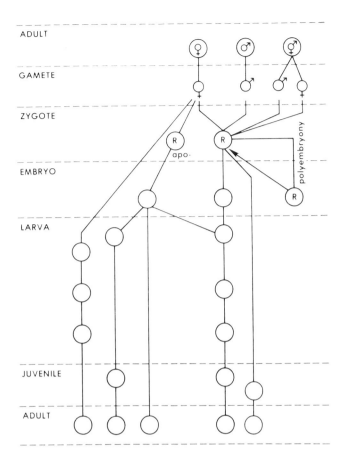

FIGURE 13. The many pathways followed by species of Insecta, in their diverse larval development. Polyembryony produces a second generation of zygotes. In some cases (not shown), the females may be of two types, producing different sexes or different body forms. This diagram is thus not as elaborate as the actual facts.

2. Ecdysis — periodic shedding of the cuticle; same as molting
3. Instar — the insect during a stadium
4. Intermolt — the period between molts
5. Metecdysis — the molting recovery period, when the animal is still soft; in Crustacea
6. Molt — (a) the act of shedding the entire cuticle or exoskeleton; (b) the periodic loss of epidermal structures such as hair and feathers
7. Molting — periodic shedding of the cuticle
8. Proecdysis — a period of preparation for the molt, in Crustacea
9. Shedding (of feathers, hair, or epidermal fragments) — molting in Vertebrata
10. Stadium (pl. stadia) — the period between two successive molts

G. Growth

"Cells grow; so do tissues, organs, whole organisms, and animal populations" (Scharrer and Scharrer, 1963). Growth is one of those subjects that are usually referred to with such a sweeping generalization as, "The most universal feature of all life is, of course, growth" or "Growth in organisms is chiefly by multiplication of cells". Neither of these statements is really true. Growth is sometimes effectively restricted to brief parts of the life cycle; in many animals growth is never visible, because it all takes

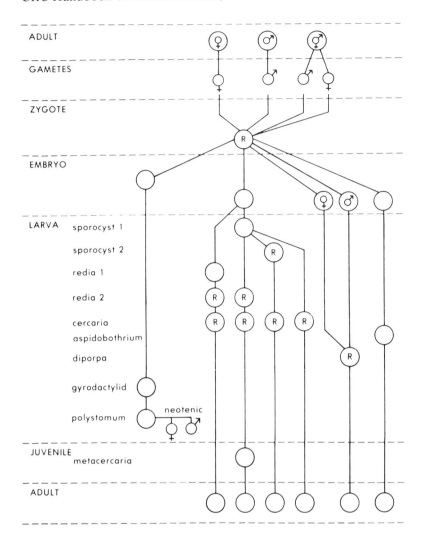

FIGURE 14.   The many pathways followed by species of the group of parasites comprising the Trematoda. Because the zygote may be from self-fertilization, the later pathways may all be dual (not shown). Here many of the larvae also reproduce (asexually) and neoteny occurs.

place at any early stage. In a variety of groups, all growth takes place after multiplication of cells has ceased.

A better definition of *growth* is this: "Lasting increase in volume is the chief criterion of growth. It may be achieved through increase in cell number, or cell volume, or some combination of the two" (Milne and Milne, 1959). In the few animals where postembryonic growth consists solely in the increase of cell volume, the condition is called eutely (see below).

Increase in size is *positive growth*. Except in the cases of eutely, the growth is always accompanied by differentiation of cells and morphogenetic movements. *Negative growth* is decrease in the size of the animal or organ. This can be by reduction in the number of cells or by reduction in the size of the cells, but in any case the total volume of protoplasm may be greatly reduced. This was described by Carter (1951) thus: "We must therefore distinguish (1) negative growth (reduction in the size of the body); (2) resorption (loss of structure in one or more organs, which may lead to their disappearance and (3) dedifferentiation of the whole body (complete loss of specific form)."

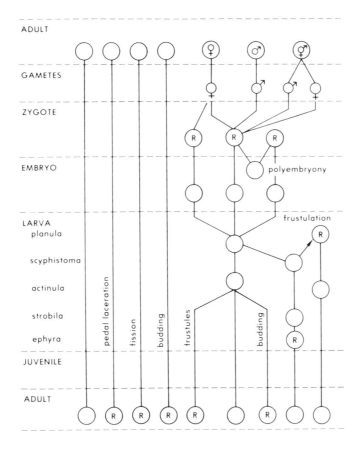

FIGURE 15. The many and diverse pathways followed by the species of Hydrozoa. First, on the left, the theoretically possible reconstitution of an individual from separated cells (as in Porifera), and three processes that can produce new individuals without sex of any sort and even with no real development. These same processes mixed with the cross- and self-fertilized cycles produce a diversity even greater than shown. This is probably the most diverse class of animals in this respect.

Although a small amount of "negative growth" can probably take place in any animal, a few can undergo drastic forms of this, as described (for example) under reduction and anabiosis in the section on dormancy below.

In the Vertebrata a distinction is made between determinate growth, which implies a steady increase in size up to maturity, after which the process essentially ceases for the remainder of life, and indeterminate growth, in which there is continuous increase in size throughout life. These are exemplified by mammals and fishes, respectively.

H. Eutely

In many embryology books it seems to be stated as a principle that all growth is by multiplication of cells. This may be because this is probably true in all vertebrates. However, among invertebrates there are several groups in which the rule fails completely, because of the condition called eutely.

The definitions of eutely are not uniform. It is substantially synonymous with *cell constancy*, which is the condition in which there are a constant number (and arrangement) of cells in the organs of mature animals in a given species. It is also cited as the condition in which an animal retains the same number of nuclei in the adult throughout its life, except perhaps in the gonad, and which therefore grows only by increase in the cytoplasmic mass.

Implicit in these definitions of eutely and cell constancy are several ideas: (1) that the adult has no cell divisions (except perhaps in the gonads) during adult life; (2) that it is the nuclei that are important, because some tissues are syncytial; and (3) that all postembryonic growth is thus by increase in size of the cells already existing.

The definition by Hyman (1951) seems to reflect all the facts well: "The property of nuclear constancy or eutely (is that), except in the gonads, the number of nuclei in the various tissues and organs attained during larval development remains fixed through life, so that size increase results entirely from cytoplasmic augmentation without nuclear division." Because in some animals the nuclear constancy is only in certain organs, it is preferable to restrict the term cell constancy to cases in which only individual organs show this condition, and use the term eutely for animals in which the entire body shows constancy.

The list of completely eutelic animals contains some surprises:

1. Orthonectida (Kerkut, 1960)
2. Rhombozoa (Kerkut, 1960)
3. Monoblastozoa — not known but likely
4. Trematoda — miracidium larva (Hyman, 1959)
5. Acanthocephala (Hyman, 1951b)
6. Rotifera (Hyman, 1951b)
7. Gastrotricha (Hyman, 1951b)
8. Kinorhyncha (Hyman, 1951b)
9. Nematoda (Hyman, 1951b)
10. Gordioidea (Hyman, 1951b)
11. Nectonematoidea (Hyman, 1951b)
12. Priapuloidea (Hyman, 1951b)
13. Tardigrada (Kaestner, 1968)

In addition to these, there are several groups in which it is said that the constancy applies only to certain organs. To this situation, Hegner (1933) applied the somewhat inappropriate expression *partial constancy*, but the distinction made above seems preferable. Cell constancy (defined as within some particular organ) occurs in these groups:

1. Turbellaria (Hegner and Engemann, 1968)
2. Trematoda (Hegner and Engemann, 1968)
3. Annelida (Hegner and Engemann, 1968)
4. Arthropoda — ommatidia of compound eyes (Hegner and Engemann, 1968)
5. Insecta — salivary glands of *Drosophila* (Demerec, 1965)
6. Insecta — germ cells of *Miastor* (Hegner and Engemann, 1968)
7. Tunicata — (Hegner and Engemann, 1968)

In most of these records (except for the Aschelminthes groups and Mesozoa and Tardigrada), there is not sufficient detail to clarify the situation. The most unexpected occurrence, which is clear and unequivocal, is that of the Tardigrada. These are usually not placed near the Aschelminthes, although there are several other striking similarities between the two groups.

I. Dormancy

Some summary statements about development or life history imply that development is continuous from activation of the egg or separation of the bud or fragment until death. Inasmuch as metabolism does continue and the developmental processes are in a strict sense irreversible, the implication is justified. In another sense, however, development is in many animals delayed at certain points by the slowing down or virtual cessation of metabolism and therefore of the entire cycle. There may also be degeneration of tissues.

The most general term for this slowing of the developmental rate seems to be *dormancy*. It occurs in many ways which differ widely in their place in the cycle, their duration, the extent of suspension of metabolism, the nature of any preparation for the dormancy, its cause, and the purpose served. (Some dormancy terms, such as anabiosis, have been used in both general and specific senses; some others overlap in meaning or usage.) Dormancy includes at least the following:

1. Aestivation — dormancy during a warm or dry season (Gastropoda, Oligochaeta, Insecta, Pisces, Reptilia)
2. Anabiosis — in general, arrested development or suspended animation, cyclic, seasonal, or occasional; existence in a resting stage, often involving dehydration or dedifferentiation of tissues, reduction in size, or encystment (see below)
3. Arrested development — see Quiescence
4. Asphyxy — state of inactivity due to lack of oxygen; lasting no more than a few days (Tardigrada)
5. Asthenobiosis — either the condition of an inactive larva before pupation or auto-intoxication (Insecta)
6. Death-feigning — see Thanatosis
7. Dedifferentiation — reversal in the differentiation of tissues that has already taken place
8. Desiccation — inactive state occurring under abnormally dry conditions (Rotifera, Nematoda, s.Gastropoda, Tardigrada, Insecta)
9. Diapause — a period of suspended development or growth, characterized by inactivity and greatly decreased metabolism (s.Gastropoda, s.Crustacea, s.Insecta)
10. Diurnation — dormancy during the daytime
11. Dormant egg — see Resting eggs
12. Egg dormancy — occurrence of specially resistant eggs to survive periods of desiccation (Rotifera; Crustacea: Cladocera, Phyllopoda, Copepoda)
13. Encystment — the process of becoming enclosed in a protective capsule (Protozoa, s.Rhynchocoela, "and a few small Metazoa")
14. Estivation — see Aestivation
15. Gemmulation — formation of many resistant bodies for survival in difficult periods; because of the large number produced, this can also be a reproductive process (Porifera, gemmules and sorites; Scyphozoa, podocysts in scyphistoma larvae; Bryozoa, hibernacula and statoblasts)
16. Hibernation — dormancy during the winter, but especially if accompanied by sharp drop in body temperature, see also "Lethargy of Carnivores" (#19)
17. Inanition — type of dormancy induced by starvation (Turbellaria)
18. Kinetopause — cessation of activity; includes rest, sleep, death feigning, aestivation, hibernation, and death
19. Lethargy of carnivores — winter rigidity, usually mistermed hibernation (s.Amphibia, s.Reptilia, s.Mammalia)
20. Playing dead — ceasing all movement; see also Thanatosis (#28) (s.Insecta)
21. Pupation — occurrence of an inactive and encysted stage during which the larval tissues and organs are converted into those of the adult (Insecta)
22. Quiescence — cessation of development during unfavorable conditions; arrested development (Oligochaeta, Insecta)

23. Reduction bodies — term rather loosely used for gemmulation, encystment, and various forms of anabiosis
24. Resting, dormant, and winter eggs — fertilized eggs that will over-winter before hatching (s.Coelenterata, s.Turbellaria, s.Tardigrada, s.Crustacea, s.Rotifera, s.Gastrotricha, s.Rhynchocoela, s.Oligochaeta)
25. Sleep — the periodic state during which the activity of the nervous system is reduced and recuperation of its powers takes place
26. Statoblast formation — see Gemmulation
27. Suspended animation — popular term for anabiosis
28. Thanatosis — feigning death or "playing dead"; a protective device of some Insecta
29. Torpidity — a condition physiologically resembling hibernation (Aves)
30. Torpor — general term for dormancy, sluggishness, or suspended animation
31. Winter eggs — see Resting eggs (# 24)
32. Winter rigidity — see Lethargy of carnivores (# 19)

Many of these conditions are included under the more technical term *anabiosis*, which may be defined as existence in a resting stage with great decrease in metabolism: often involving dehydration, dedifferentiation of tissues, reduction in size, or encystment. Some examples are

1. Protozoa — many Protozoa can encyst (see paragraph below)
2. Porifera — a process akin to encystment is here called gemmulation (see Chapter 3)
3. Platyhelminthes — Turbellaria (in starving condition they may get smaller and simplified in structure)
4. Rotifera — extreme desiccation can be withstood, but they are incapable of any regeneration
5. Bryozoa — degeneration of polypides is constant to form a mass called a brown body in each, with almost all organs disappearing; this brown body may produce a polypide again either by regeneration or by being used as food
6. Tardigrada — under desiccation, metabolism becomes very low, water is lost, and there may be degeneration of organs and encystment

Some protozoan species encyst to survive unfavorable conditions, such as exhaustion of food supply, desiccation of the habitat, and putrefaction in the medium. In other species encystment is part of asexual reproduction, as they divide only within a cyst (s.Flagellata, s.Ciliata). In many parasitic species, the stages that are transmitted to another host are usually enclosed in a resistant cyst (s.Sarcodina, m.Sporozoa).

The encystment of the trophozoite of *Lophomonas blattarum* proceeds as follows: it ceases to feed, extrudes the remains of previous food, becomes rounded and inactive; the whole organism becomes dedifferentiated, resorbing such organelles as flagella and axostyle; it then secretes substances which become solidified into a resistant wall — the cyst.

J. Regeneration

There is a curious difference in the way regeneration is defined for vertebrates and for invertebrates. For the former it is described as "replacement of lost parts"; for the invertebrates it is "restoration of a complete functioning individual from some part of the parent body other than the egg."

Regeneration is neither a single nor a simple process which can be tabulated as present or absent. The processes of regeneration are mostly the same as those of early development. This reminds one that regeneration is not a feature of the adult alone; many larvae and even embryos can regenerate to some degree.

Furthermore, it is often impossible to separate regeneration from asexual reproduction. No fragmentation of any sort, even budding, is possible without regeneration of some parts. The processes of preparation for splitting, or even the making of the bud, are the same as regeneration. One of the few books on the comparative features of these processes emphasizes the similarity through its title, *Asexual Propagation and Regeneration* (Vorontsova and Liosner, 1960).

There is a reasonable tendency on the part of zoologists to think of replacement of aging cells or tissues as a metabolic process of normal living, and of regeneration as the replacement of cells, tissues, or structures that were accidentally lost. No matter how reasonable this may seem in an individual case, it represents merely a momentary forgetfulness of the continuing nature of body processes and the use of some of these in regeneration. Much of regeneration is merely the extension of normal processes.

There are three activities of animals that utilize these normal metabolic processes. One is the continuing normal replacement of cells and structures. Second is the entirely normal duplication or replacement involved in asexual reproduction. Third are the occasional reparative processes that are needed to restore completeness to a more or less drastically impaired individual.

The individual's regenerative powers may vary from ability to restore a complete individual from a fragment consisting of only a few cells to the ability merely to heal a wound by reorganizing existing tissues. This was expressed by Weiss (1939), thus: "In some forms regenerative power is enormous, while in others it is almost nil. On the whole, one gains the impression that regenerative capacity tends to vary inversely as the scale of organization." These abilities in different animal groups can be indicated thus:

Porifera. Many sponges can regenerate from minute fragments or reconstitute themselves from a pile of completely separated cells. They can regenerate from gemmules.

Coelenterata. Many can regenerate from minute fragments and some can reconstitute themselves as do sponges. They can replace lost parts and may retrogress with dedifferentiation, followed by regeneration involving redifferentiation.

Turbellaria. Some can regenerate from small fragments. Multiple fragmentation is frequently possible. Temporary dedifferentiation is possible in some.

Rhynchocoela. Can regenerate entire proboscis and other parts. Said to be able to regenerate from a 1-mm piece cut from the center of the body.

Rotifera. Other Aschelminthes apparently cannot regenerate at all, or even heal wounds. This is because cell division ceases at an early age (eutely).

Bryozoa. Seem to have high powers because they can regress by dedifferentiation and can readily bud new individuals.

Phoronida. Said to be capable of regression; they probably do bud, although this may not be frequent.

Mollusca. In some Gastropoda an ovary can be regenerated by its duct; it is said that appendages can be regenerated.

Annelida. Regenerative power is usually high; fragmentation is common; schizometamery occurs in some cases of epitoky, with small fragments from the middle of the worm regenerating readily. In leeches, the capacity is said to be small.

Arthropoda. In Crustacea some appendages are gradually regenerated at later molts. In insects some appendages can be regenerated.

Echinodermata. Many starfish practice autotomy (self-mutilation) under certain conditions; the two fragments may be as much as half the body; in just one genus *(Linckia)* a large fragment will regenerate, so that two individuals result. In Holothurioidea a most extensive regeneration is required by the drastic autotomy when "the viscera" are discarded through the mouth.

Pterobranchia. These apparently can dedifferentiate like some lower animals and then reconstitute the tissues.

Tunicata. These also may dedifferentiate under adverse conditions. They also bud extensively and may produce buds that fuse in pairs.

Vertebrata. Lower vertebrates may regenerate limbs, tails, eyes, or fins. In higher forms regeneration is limited to wound healing, although this may involve large areas of epidermis, as well as blood vessels and parts of nerves.

Regeneration is as complicated a process as development itself. The following quotations will present some of the thought-provoking ideas involved.

"A brief consideration of regenerative processes will disclose that they are fundamentally of the same nature and follow the same principles as ontogenetic processes" (Weiss, 1939).

"The capacity for regeneration is, therefore, not a novel and secondarily acquired adeptness of the organism at meeting later accidents by adequate repairs, but is simply a residue of the original capacities for growth, organization, and differentiation through which the individual was first formed. Hence, the extent of regenerative capacity is limited by the extent to which formative capacities survive the ontogenetic phase" (Weiss, 1939).

In an earlier section it was noted that the early formation and differentiation of the embryo is not under control of any nervous system, because none has yet been formed. Yet, "it is interesting that the presence of the nervous system is absolutely necessary for the regeneration process (in vertebrates)" (Needham, 1942).

"The repair of lost parts can be accomplished in two ways: by internal reorganization and transformation of old tissues without addition of new growth or by outgrowth of new tissue from the cut surface in the form of a regeneration bud or blastema" (Hamburger, 1942).

"As a general rule, the tissue which forms any organ in regeneration is derived mainly from similar tissue in the parent body . . . But this is not always so" (Carter, 1951).

"In order that an organ may regenerate, the following conditions, among others, must be fulfilled. There must be a *stimulus* to provoke renewed formative activity. There must be *cellular material* with a sufficient store of *potencies* to produce all the histological differentiations necessary. There must again be *organizing factors* to make the right differentiations appear in the right places, to cause the proper alignments, movements, and functional transformations of the cells, to direct the growth of the reconstituted parts with the proper proportions, and to control the resumption of functional activity in joint cooperation with the old parts. Finally, there must be an adequate *supply of food* and other vital necessities" (Weiss, 1939). An example of failure of the potencies is the crustacean which cannot regenerate an eye, but grows in its place an antenna.

Some of the features of regeneration are suggested by these terms:

1. Archihiston — the mesenchyme, said to be, above all else, the tissue that has regenerative powers
2. Blastema — an area of undifferentiated cells, or at least ones with potency for differentiation
3. Compensatory hypertrophy — indirect regeneration by means of extra growth of a partner organ
4. Epimorphosis — the part of restitution which is by new tissue which grows out from the cut surface

5.   Heterochely — an instance of compensatory hypertrophy, in which a small chela enlarges to compensate for the small size of the regenerated one
6.   Heteromorphosis — the formation, in regeneration, of an organ different from the one lost
7.   Homoeosis — the same as heteromorphosis, when a serial homologue is regenerated
8.   Hormonal control — in Arthropoda and Vertebrata, regeneration may be controlled in part by hormones
9.   Morphallaxis — restitution by the transformation and shifting of material, not by growth
10.   Re-association — separated cells of some sponges can re-associate to form a new and smaller sponge
11.   Reconstitution — the same as re-association, in sponges
12.   Regeneration — the re-creation of cells, tissues, or organs which have been lost by degeneration, dedifferentiation, or autotomy, or the formation of tissues and organs missing from separated fragments
13.   Regulation — the processes of returning to a stable organization when the original one has been disturbed

Some writers suggest that loss of capacity to regenerate is related to evolutionary level of complexity, that regenerative capacity progressively declines with the increased degree of differentiation and the advancing grade of evolution of the animals. There is surely some truth to this, as all examples of high regenerative power are from the lowest groups and most arthropods and vertebrates have limited powers. The generalization has little real meaning, however, as many simple animals cannot regenerate at all and some "higher animals" have very considerable regenerative powers.

K. Senescence

Aging and senescence are words of very similar meaning. *Aging* can be merely the passing of time in the later parts of an animal's life; *senescense* is the occurrence of degeneration of various sorts during that time. Almost everything written on the subject is in reference to humans as a part of *gerontology*, the study of aging. An exception appears in the article on gerontology by Shock in *The Encyclopedia of the Biological Sciences* (1961) where the following appears: "Biological gerontology is concerned with the ability of the organism or one of its parts to adapt to its environment as a consequence of the genetically or developmentally determined progressive and essentially irreversible diminution of adaptive capacity with the passage of time. As the animal ages, there is a decrease in its ability to withstand the stresses to which it is subjected. The ultimate event is the death of the organism."

Only one aspect of aging might be subject to tabulation: the total length of life. It turns out that only in a relatively few species is there any likelihood of a "natural" death, for nearly all individuals of most species fall prey to predators of some sort.

Aging is simply the final aspect of the general phenomenon of development. It involves a gradual loss of versatility in the parts of the organism; by some writers it is said to start at sexual maturity and by others at the time of fertilization.

It is possible to think of aging of the whole individual, but this aging occurs only in the aging of its parts, its cells. No matter how healthy the rest of the body, the failure of one essential part will be fatal to the whole.

Aside from aging and senescence, which culminate in *senility* (failure of nonessential capacities), there is only one term relevant here. This is *moribund*, which means in a dying state, on the point of death.

III. THEORY OF RECAPITULATION

Although it is beyond the basic purpose of this book to challenge or discuss the broad concepts and theories that have been a feature of zoology for a century, it seems appropriate to point out some of the problems that larval diversity presents to one who expects to see the ancestor mirrored in a developmental stage.

Larvae are organisms and as such they are subject to the same selective pressures as other animals. Their structure will be the result of a combination of factors, including: (1) their genetic make-up, (2) specializations required for their own immediate existence, (3) specializations required to produce adults that are differently specialized, and (4) factors linked to (2) or (3) and being temporarily carried along in the slow processes of evolution. Of these four, the first may appear to be the most basic, but in reality it appears to have the least visible effect.

In groups of what are believed to be closely related animals, there can be great diversity in the early stages. It is possible to produce an adult of a given species by more than one route. Larval stages can be bypassed and evidently have sometimes been eliminated entirely from the cycle.

Planula-like larvae have been developed more than once in different groups. They are so simple that it is impossible to say whether they show any influence of a common ancestor. There are phyla thought to be related by ancestry (Mollusca, Sipunculoidea, Annelida) because they all have trochophore larvae, and yet there are other phyla (e.g., Calyssozoa) with larvae substantially similar to trochophores that are passed off as entirely distinct merely by giving them another name. The trochophore form is not so peculiar as to force us to think it could not have evolved twice independently.

This is not to say that no ancestral features could be seen in a larva. It merely emphasizes that "great caution must be exercised in the interpretation of larvae" (Hyman, 1951). The entire life cycle is subject to evolutionary change. There seems to be no feature of animals that does not occur in a diversity such as to make conclusions on common ancestry extremely hazardous.

There is one place in the animal kingdom in which skepticism of recapitulation is less necessary. This is the phylum Vertebrata, in which there is unusual unity in nearly all respects. This group is sometimes said to be no more diverse in its six or eight classes all together than some single classes in Arthropoda, for instance. There are great similarities in the development of vertebrates, and conclusions on ancestry can sometimes be convincing.

For those who include the vertebrates in a more inclusive group called Chordata, the problems are much greater, and conclusions have often been unjustified. There seem to be no instances where recapitulation in development is convincing evidence of close relationship between two phyla.

REFERENCES

Beklemishev, W. N., *Principles of Comparative Anatomy of Invertebrates,* 2 volumes. University of Chicago Press, Chicago, 1969.

Bronsted, H. V., *Planarian Regeneration,* Pergamon Press, Oxford, 1969.

Carter, G. S., *A General Zoology of the Invertebrates,* 3rd ed., Sidgwick & Jackson, London, 1951.

Counce, S. J. and Waddington, C. H., Eds., *Developmental Systems: Insecta,* 2 volumes. Academic Press, London, 1972.

Demerec, M., *Biology of Drosophila,* Hafner, New York, 1965.

Farmer, J. N., *The Protozoa: Introduction to Protozoology,* C. V. Mosby, St. Louis, 1980.

Frost, S. W., *Insect Life and Insect Natural History,* Dover, New York, 1959.

Gray, P., Ed., *The Encyclopedia of the Biological Sciences,* Reinhold, New York, 1961.

Grell, K. G., *Protozoology,* Springer-Verlag, Berlin, 1973.

Hamburger, V., *A Manual of Experimental Embryology,* University of Chicago Press, Chicago, 1942.

Hegner, R. W., *Invertebrate Zoology,* Macmillan, New York, 1933.

Hegner, R. W. and Engemann, J. C., *Invertebrate Zoology,* 2nd ed., Macmillan, New York, 1968.

Hyman, L. H., *The Invertebrates,* McGraw-Hill, New York, volumes 1 (1940), 2 (1951a), 3 (1951b), 4 (1955), 5 (1959), 6 (1967).

Imms, A. D., *A General Textbook of Entomology,* 8th ed., Methuen, London, 1951.

Kaestner, A., *Invertebrate Zoology,* volumes 1 (1967), 2 (1968), 3 (1970), Interscience, New York.

Kerkut, G. A., *Implications of Evolution,* Pergamon Press, Oxford, 1960.

Marshall, A. J., *Parker & Haswell, A Text-Book of Zoology,* Vol. 2, 7th ed., Macmillan, London, 1964.

Milne, L. J. and Milne, M. J., *Animal Life,* 3rd ed., Prentice Hall, New York, 1959.

Needham, J., *Biochemistry and Morphogenesis,* Cambridge University Press, London, 1942.

Scharrer, E. and Scharrer, B., *Neuroendocrinology,* Columbia University Press, New York, 1963.

Shock, N. W., Gerontology, in *The Encyclopedia of the Biological Sciences,* Gray, P., Ed., Reinhold, New York, 1961.

Vorontsova, M. A. and Liosner, L. D., *Asexual Propagation and Regeneration,* Pergamon Press, London, 1960.

Waddington, C. H., *Principles of Embryology,* Macmillan, New York, 1956.

Weiss, P., *Principles of Development,* Henry Holt, New York, 1939.

Part IV
Adult Individuals

PROLOGUE TO STRUCTURE VS. FUNCTION

Diversity in structure and function of adults is produced by the diversity of development, and of course, the diversities of both are produced by the diversity of genotypes. Because all vertebrates have much the same complement of organs, it is often assumed that all animals have the same systems that perform similar functions. There are indeed some similarities, but the extent of the differences is often forgotten.

Excretory systems seldom work with a blood vessel system. Arthropod breathing is totally different from that of mammals, and most other animals breathe no air at all. Body support is provided by widely differing mechanisms, and so on.

Structures can usually be readily compared from group to group, but functions of these organs are more difficult to compare. Comparison at the biochemical level is actually comparison of the structure of the molecules, not of their activity.

Chapter 8

INTRODUCTION TO STRUCTURE AND FUNCTION

TABLE OF CONTENTS

I.   Why Treat Adults Separately? 186

II.   Physiology vs. Anatomy 186

III. Structure vs. Function 187
      A.   Definitions.. 187
      B.   Structure 188
      C.   Biochemicals 188
      D.   Functions 191
      E.   Metabolism... 191

References 192

I. WHY TREAT ADULTS SEPARATELY?

Most people think of the adult stage as reasonably identifiable and distinct from the early parts of the developmental sequence known as embryo, larva, or juvenile. When the entire animal kingdom as considered, the situation becomes somewhat confused. Almost a majority of animals arise by processes not involving the usual zygote-to-adult sequence. In some an embryo (or even a zygote) may reproduce; in other groups the forms that look like larvae are actually "adults" — the final and definitive stage. Many quite definite larvae do reproduce, some even sexually.

It is a deliberate goal of this book to point out that an individual is such from the time of activation of an ovum or separation of a fragment, until its death, i.e., through its entire development. Development is here defined (in the only way that can be justified), as the entire life of the individual from inception to death. This sequence (the life history) is continuous; although it is in a state of constant development in many respects, there is no place to draw an exact line between "the developmental stages" and "adulthood", because the adult is itself one of those stages. In spite of this, it is found helpful to discuss adults principally in sections different from the earlier developmental stages. In many cases the processes in the earlier stages, e.g., excretion, are similar to those of the adults. Where this is so, they will not be discussed separately. Where they are unique, as in cleavage of the zygote, gastrulation, morphogenesis, or in the larva, they are described under the appropriate developmental stage, in Part III, "Development of Individuals."

The word "death" is used to include all forms of the termination of life of an individual. The forms are listed in detail in Chapter 24.

Adult animals, in this section called simply "animals", can be studied at several levels of organization. One can study the whole individual as a functioning unit with a specific, although changing, form and structure. One can study the organs and tissues of which it is composed. These are themselves composed of cells, whose permanence and ubiquity make them a prime level for attention. Another level of organization includes chemistry in the study of organisms identifying the molecules and their reactions that constitute living protoplasm. Turning in the opposite direction, an animal may develop into a colony, which is a level of organization and function above the individual. Beyond this, both organisms and colonies exist in complex populations and communities (biota), where the importance of the individual is even more reduced.

Individuals will be dealt with here as adults at the levels of biochemistry, cytology, and histology, as well as gross form, structure, and function. These features of the individuals in the stages before the adult are dealt with in Part III when comparative data are available. Colonies and their colony functions are dealt with in Part VI. Populations and communities are not dealt with as such but would find a place in Part V (Behavior).

II. PHYSIOLOGY VS. ANATOMY

The word physiology has been defined in so many ways, and usually in such esoteric manner, that one hesitates to use it at all in a formal way. It has been defined as the study of life, as the study of animal evolution, and as "the visualization of life in terms of groupings and displacements of ultimate particles." These do not seem to be useful definitions in a book on comparative biology.

In this book, *physiology* is used to refer to the study of the functions (or processes or operations) of cells, tissues, organs, and organ systems. The functions of protoplasm would be included also, except that comparative information is not sufficiently available. The logical next higher level, the functions and activities of whole individuals and populations, are herein treated under "Behavior" (Part V).

A comparative zoologist is interested in how each given process is performed by the different organs of different animals. This is in some books restricted to their *normal* operation. It is here assumed that an organ *can* do anything that it *does* do under any set of circumstances, and so at levels below the individual there would logically be interest even in what would be called pathological, abnormal, or experimental function. In reality so little comparative information on pathology is available on a widespread basis among animals that this book will only rarely be able to deal with anything other than normal functions.

Some writers state that physiologists need concern themselves only with the life functions of *well-known* organisms. This limitation is here entirely rejected, because the lesser-known groups are biologically just as important and often are more interesting than the well-known groups. So far as possible, this book will deal with the functions of all animals.

Anatomy is a word which held a distinguished position in the early days of zoology. It later came to imply internal structure and especially dissection. In some groups of animals it is used exclusively for the internal machinery, the organs particularly. In this book there is little need for the word anatomy in the sense of dissection, nor to make a distinction between external and internal machinery.

In the older system, the external structure was called morphology. As discussed in the introduction to this book (and also in the next section), morphology is here restricted to its inherent meaning, the study of form, which is, of course, largely a matter of external features.

It therefore seems appropriate to use "structure" when referring to the physical features of animals and "function" when referring to the processes occurring among those structures (and, indeed, responsible for their existence); morphology will be used to refer to various aspects of form (symmetry, cephalization, etc.).

III. STRUCTURE VS. FUNCTION

A. Definitions

A duality in much of biology is shown by the statements made about the relation between structure and function.

"Physiological differences . . . underlie visible differences in structure."

"A specific function can only be the expression of a specific structure."

Obviously these two are both aspects of what is called life. They are indistinguishable. Most functions are possible only where there is an existing structure. The structure is there only because of a previous function that produced it. There is no start to such a circle, and in a continuous helix of infinite length (the sequence of loops or generations) there is again no starting point, so function and structure go on indefinitely in complete interdependence. It is possible to preserve some aspects of structure after obvious function ceases, and most structure is more readily visible than most functions. For these reasons structures are herein dealt with first and functions second, with no implications intended of their relative importance to biology.

Every organism, at every stage in its life, is an integrated unit of structure and function. All of its structures are the consequences of various processes or reactions, and every process, function, or reaction occurs only because there is an appropriate structure there for it to act upon. What is sometimes called the "biology" of organisms includes everything that can be known about their physiology and their structure; these are included at all levels from atoms and molecules through organs and individuals to populations.

The terms structure and function are commonly used in confusingly diverse contexts. Without attempting to redefine them into a rigid system, *structure* will generally be used for the material product of physical, chemical, and biological processes; *function* (which is often appropriately replaced by *process*) will be used for the (largely chemical) reactions that produce the structures; *activity* for the things done by individuals as a unit or by major parts of the individual for its benefit as a unit, e.g., locomotion performed by appendages; and *morphology* for the resulting overall features of the individuals, such as shape, size, and arrangement.

B. Structure

Structure, as the term is used in this book, is the physical construction of bodies or parts of bodies of animals. The concept can be applied at many levels:

Atoms	Tissues	Populations
Molecules	Organs	Communities
Organelles	Individuals	Biota
Cells	Colonies	

There may even be intermediates between these, such as molecular complexes, protoplasm, syncytia, and organ systems, all of which also show structure. Structure is a feature, at most of the above levels, in each stage in the development of an animal. Thus, the egg has molecular and cellular structure, whereas the larva has tissues and organs.

Atoms and molecules are the province of biochemistry, a subject which is highly relevant to a survey of animal diversity, but for which the data have not been organized comparatively to the extent required for tabulation. A few features of biochemical nature are tentatively listed below.

Organelles and cells are treated together in Chapter 10. Many modern aspects of cell biology do not appear there simply because they are not yet comparative. Cilia and a few unique organelles such as nematocysts are the only organelles so far well enough known to be tabulated across many groups. Some other features of cells are also presented.

Tissues, organs, and organ systems are the subjects of Chapters 11 to 20. Organs and systems can always be treated as structures, but their functions are more difficult to tabulate.

Individuals are included in this book in three places. All reproduction (Chapters 2 to 4) is by individuals and also all development (Chapters 5 to 7). A sampling of activities of whole animals is given in Chapters 21 and 22.

Colonies are the subject of Chapter 23, where they are treated briefly but in much the same way as individuals. Indeed, they often are individuals, at a higher level of integration.

Populations, communities, and biotas are aggregates of individuals. They are not usually included herein because their features are difficult to adapt to comparative presentation.

C. Biochemicals

Physiology and biochemistry have grown together in recent years as more physiologists study the chemical processes of life, but comparative aspects are often forgotten. Yet much of the field of cellular physiology is actually the study of the structure of molecules. This can be studied comparatively by examining the distribution of both inorganic and complex biochemical compounds in different animals. A few of these are tabulated here, and others are cited under "Blood Pigments", "Hardpart Composition", and "Muscle Phosphagens", in Chapters 15, 18, and 20, respectively.

There are more than a dozen organic compounds that are classed as structural materials, although they are mostly not important constituents of skeletons. Their distribution is shown below. The general chemical nature of these is known, but each is a group of similar biochemical compounds in which there is often diversity among animals.

Arthropodin. This is a water-soluble protein in the chitin of Arthropoda (see Sclerotin).

Cellulose. It was once believed that cellulose is restricted to plants, in which it is the chief constituent of cell walls. In animals it has now been reported in at least these groups:

1.   Protozoa — coverings of various Sarcodina and Flagellata
2.   Acanthocephala — fertilization membrane
3.   Insecta — silk of Lepidoptera
4.   Tunicata — in the tunic as tunicin
5.   Mammalia — connective tissue

"It would be unwise, as yet, to conclude that cellulose is not a general component of connective tissue in all animals" (Brown, 1975).

Chitin. Chitin is a substance or class of substances that is widespread among animals. It is a polysaccharide similar to cellulose but includes nitrogen; it may be bound with protein as a glycoprotein. It is reported in many groups and denied in some of those, as indicated:

1.   Protozoa — shells of Foraminifera, thecae of Ciliata
2.   Porifera — gemmules
3.   Graptozoa — perisarc, but also denied
4.   Conularida — calyx, described as chitinophosphatic
5.   Hydrozoa — periderm
6.   Scyphozoa — podocyst capsule, periderm
7.   Anthozoa — periderm
8.   Turbellaria — lining of copulatory bursa
9.   Acanthocephala — eggshell
10. Nematoda — egg membrane
11. Priapuloidea — cuticle
12. Calyssozoa — operculum
13. Bryozoa — cuticle, operculum, statoblasts, larval shells
14. Phoronida — tube or ectocyst
15. Brachiopoda — shell of *Lingula*, pedicle
16. Mollusca — shells of Amphineura and Bivalvia, radula and jaws of Gastropoda, questionably the dorsal shield of Cephalopoda
17. Echiuroidea — spines
18. Annelida — jaws, setae, tubes, digestive tract lining
19. Pentastomida — body wall
20. Onychophora — body wall
21. Arthropoda — exoskeleton, intestinal tract lining, eggshell, tracheae; of all classes
22. Chaetognatha — hooks or spines
23. Pogonophora — tubes

Collagen. "Collagen has been detected in almost all classes of multicellular animals from sponges to mammals" (Brown, 1975). It is a principal component of much fibrous tissue. No reference has been found to it in Protozoa.

Conchiolin. This is described as an albuminoid. It apparently occurs in all shelled Mollusca, where it is mixed with the calcareous material of the shell.

Elastin. This is a relative of collagen, which occurs with it in connective tissue fibers of Vertebrata, at least.

Fibroin. The chief protein of silk, this occurs in Arachnida, Diplopoda, and Insecta (see also Sericin).

Gorgonin. This forms certain fibers in the mesogloea of Anthozoa.

Hemicellulose. See Ophryoscolecin.

Keratin. This is the intracellular structural protein in skin of some Vertebrata and in feathers and hair. A keratinoid is cited in the cuticle of Nematoda.

Matricin. A fibroid occurring in the body wall of Nematoda.

Mucopolysaccharides. These are polysaccharides conjugated to proteins. They occur in various connective tissue fibers, in cartilage and bone, in mesogloea, in jaws, in mucus, in vitelline membranes, in eggshells, in cuticles, in tests and shells, and in cyst walls. Found very widely from Protozoa to Mammalia.

Onuphin. Apparently a glycoprotein, in tubes of some Polychaeta.

Ophryoscolecin. A neutral polysaccharide of Ciliata; also called hemicellulose.

Paraglycogen. This is a component of the "skeletal" plates of some Ciliata.

Pseudochitin. See Tectin.

Resilin. An elastic protein in joint cuticle of some Arthropoda.

Reticulin. A mucopolysaccharide in reticular connective tissue fibers; in Vertebrata at least.

Sclerotin. A water-insoluble protein that hardens the chitinous cuticles of Arthropoda. Reported in eggshells and metacercarial cysts of Trematoda (see Arthropodin).

Sericin. A silk gelatin which joins with fibroin in the silk of Arthropoda.

Spiculin. The organic material of the core of siliceous spicules in Porifera.

Spongin. A collagen-type fiber in Porifera.

Tectin. A mucus-like glycoprotein secreted by Protozoa such as the Testacida; also called Pseudochitin.

Tunicin. Tunicin is a polysaccharide cellulose found in the tunic of Tunicata. An essentially similar substance forms the fibers of some connective tissue in Vertebrata (see Hall and Saxl, 1961).

No comment on the biochemicals of animals would be complete if proteins were omitted. They are not the only major molecules of living things, but they are the most distinctive. Chemically they can be defined as molecules of very high molecular weight consisting of peptide-linked amino acids. They are carbon-chain molecules whose side chains are chemically reactive. Held together by a variety of chemical bonds, they can be modified and reconstructed under the influence of systems of enzymes (which are themselves proteins).

The possible combinations of the 20 or so common amino acids are at least 10^{48}. Even with perhaps 2 million kinds of organisms known, the room for diversity among proteins is limitless. As written by Cameron (1956), "we can be reasonably sure that the proteins of each species of animal differ from those of every other species; it is probable that this is true even for individuals of a species."

The diversity of biochemistry among animals was recognized years ago and was well described by Baldwin in 1963: "Many biochemists have been surprised, not so much by the fact that there are differences between groups of animals, and even sometimes between two species in a single genus, as by the fact that there are not *more* of these differences. Of course, on reflection this must obviously be a rather short-sighted view, for many more differences must undoubtedly exist than have yet been discovered. The reason once again is that comparative biochemistry has not in the past been comparative enough and has discovered only a mere handful of the innumerable differences that must certainly exist between one animal and the rest."

D. Functions

There is no clear-cut way to separate life functions into cell functions, tissue functions, etc. The individual functions of some cells are distinct, and when, for instance, all the cells of an epidermis take part in formation of a cuticle, it is easy to label this as a function of this epithelial tissue. It is possible to deal with each function separately, without concern for the level at which it occurs. The latter approach has the advantage of being more familiar in physiology, where the activity and its resulting changes in the system are more likely to be the focus of interest than the fact that they occur in cells rather than in multicellular organs. Nevertheless, a compromise is here used, in which the functions that can be clearly ascribed to cells and tissues will be described first, followed by the principal organ functions.

There is almost no limit to the number of functions found in animals. One could continue to increase the number indefinitely by subdividing. Respiration is a function, but breathing air is also a function at another level. The oxygen in the air is transferred to blood (a function) for transport to the tissues (another function), and so on. As a result, as many of the well-known general functions as possible will be treated in this book, followed by the more restricted functions that do not fit under any of the major headings. Many times the word "process" will be used instead of "function".

In reality there is little that can be compared at the level of biochemical reactions. Some of the processes seem to be universal in protoplasm, such as the Krebs citric acid cycle, glycolysis, phosphorylation, and the use of DNA as a genetic information carrier, but the absence of diversity among these in different groups of animals cannot be assumed. In oxygen transfer there is diversity in the respiratory pigments employed. In muscle metabolism there is diversity in the phosphagens employed. It seems that in all of these there is increasing diversity known, so that our inability to cite variation in some particular process does not give any confidence that variation does not exist.

E. Metabolism

Even the briefest reference to the functions covered by the science of physiology would be inadequate if there were no mention of metabolism. In its simplest definition this refers to "the exchanges of matter and energy in living organisms" (Scheer, 1953), although other definitions are legion. Furthermore, "the wide range of metabolic changes in organisms do not take place by themselves but are brought about by the action of substances called enzymes" (Sinnott and Wilson, 1955).

The current view of the unity of life was long ago expressed by Goddard (1945) thus: "The essential similarity in the (metabolic) mechanisms from organism to organism is, however, striking and leads to a real unification of our knowledge." Nevertheless, there is known to be diversity in the food utilized, in the immediate source of that food, in the processes of liberating energy, in the structures produced by the processes, and in the specific processes utilized and the enzymes which catalyze them. All cells require nutrients, but these vary from carbon dioxide plus water to complex proteins. All cells require energy; in most it is obtained by aerobic processes, in some by anaerobic processes. All cells produce cell wastes, but these wastes differ considerably.

Metabolism is often separated into *anabolism*, the sum of all metabolic processes involved in building up new protoplasm, and *catabolism*, the sum of the processes involved in the breakdown of protoplasm.

Response to Stimulus is discussed in Chapter 17 ("Nervous and Endocrine System").

Movement is discussed in Chapter 20 ("Miscellaneous Organ Functions").

Reproduction is discussed primarily in the chapters of Part II ("The Origin of Individuals").

REFERENCES

Anthony, C. O., *Basic Concepts in Anatomy and Physiology,* C. V. Mosby, St. Louis, 1974.

Baldwin, E., Comparative biochemistry and the lower metazoa, in *The Lower Metazoa,* Dougherty, E. C., Ed., University of California Press, Berkeley, 1963, chap. 22.

Brown, C. H., *Structural Materials in Animals,* Halsted Press, New York, 1975.

Cameron, T. W. M., *Parasites and Parasitism,* John Wiley & Sons, New York, 1956.

Goddard, D. R., The respiration of cells and tissues, in *Physical Chemistry of Cells and Tissues,* Hoeber, R., Ed., P. Blakiston & Sons, Philadelphia, 1945, sect. 6.

Hall, D. A. and Saxl, H., Studies of human and tunicate cellulose and of their relation to reticulum, *Proc. R. Soc. London Ser.* B:, 155, 202, 1961.

Scheer, B. T., *General Physiology,* John Wiley & Sons, New York, 1953.

Sinnott, E. W. and Wilson, K. S., *Botany: Principles and Problems,* 5th ed., McGraw-Hill, New York, 1955.

Chapter 9

MORPHOLOGY

TABLE OF CONTENTS

I.   Introduction 194

II.   Symmetry 194
       A.   Historical Notes 194
       B.   Forms of Symmetry 195
       C.   Changes of Form 198
       D.   Axes 198
       E.   Polarity 200

III.   Body Arrangement 200
       A.   The Diversity 200
       B.   Cephalization 201
       C.   Repetition 201
             1.   Syzygy 202
             2.   Chains 202
             3.   Strobilation 202
             4.   Pseudometamerism 202
             5.   Segmentation 202
             6.   Regionation 205
       D.   Polymorphism 206
             1.   Forms of Polymorphism 206
             2.   Developmental Polymorphism 206
             3.   Sexual Polymorphism 207
             4.   Colonial Polymorphism 207
             5.   Social Polymorphism, Castes 207
             6.   Seasonal Polymorphism 208
             7.   Other Polymorphism 208

IV.   Size 210

V.   Shape 211

VI.   Transparency 212

References 212

I. INTRODUCTION

Morphology is properly the study of form. This term is here used to cover not only shape but arrangement and size as well. The word has often been used for external structure, in distinction from anatomy which is used for internal structure. There is no possibility of separating external structure from internal, and anatomy or structure are here used for both. Morphology will then be reserved for questions of shape, gross arrangement of both exterior and interior, repetition of parts, symmetry, and polarity. Such topics as individuality vs. coloniality, polymorphism, and cellularity are ancillary to such a morphology.

In this chapter the diversities in body arrangement are emphasized but without much use of the symmetry/polarity concepts that were a century ago borrowed from crystallography. Repetition of parts and existence of polymorphic forms are also discussed. Colonies can be treated in the same manner as individuals in these matters, but they are the subject of a special chapter in Part VI. Cellularity is discussed under CELLS in Chapter 10. Two quotations from Beklemishev (1963) put morphology in perspective in the life of organisms: "An organism is constantly changing, it is a morpho-process, and morphology deals with all stages of its life cycle", and again, "A genuine comparative morphology must be based on a comparison of life-cycles." These comparisons make up a large part of this book, usually reduced to comparisons of organs or systems. The actual life histories are illustrated in Chapter 7 and a different sort of sequence (reproductive) in Chapter 4.

The general features of morphology are tabulated for the phyla in Table 12.

II. SYMMETRY

A. Historical Notes

For more than 100 years zoologists have described animals under a series of terms, borrowed from crystallography, that indicated arrangement with reference to imaginary planes or axes. Bilateral, radial, biradial, spherical, universal, and asymmetrical were the descriptive words most commonly used. It is not now clear why these terms were applied to animals, which never have the regularity of form described as "symmetry" in crystals, but they were apparently thought to be descriptive of basic form in animals.

It is true that in a superficial view some animals are star-shaped, some cylindrical, and some with two "sides" that are mirror images. It is also true that some zoologists thought they saw some phylogenetic significance to the forms, with the arrangements proceeding from spherical (some Protozoa) to radial (Coelenterata) to biradial (Ctenophora) to bilateral (all higher animals). This seemed to lend support to the accepted pathway of evolution.

What is now difficult to understand is the blindness of these writers to the inconsistencies of the scheme. In the coelenterate *Obelia gelatinosa*, one type of individual, the feeding hydranth, is reasonably but indefinitely radial; the reproductive individuals (gonangia) are less obviously radial, the medusa individuals are clearly tetramerous, the ovum is spherical, and the planula larva is bilateral.

In most echinoderms of the class Asteroidea, the adult is reasonably radial in gross form (pentaradiate), but the larva is even more clearly bilateral. Is there any reason to think that the arrangement of the larva is less significant biologically than that of the adult?

In the echinoderm class Holothurioidea, the same external pentaradiate arrangement appears, but the animal is so much elongated orally/aborally that it becomes clearly bilateral like many of the mud-dwelling worms.

The Portuguese man-o'-war is clearly bilateral. This again is symmetry of the colony. The individuals in the colony may be radial, bilateral, or asymmetrical, yet it belongs to a group that is classed as radial.

What good does it do to say, as many textbooks do, that a *Hydra* and a starfish are both radially symmetrical? Their forms actually have nothing in common. If it is implied that they are therefore related, the implication is wrong. If it is implied that they have reached the same level of evolution, it is again wrong. In fact, in stating that *Hydra* is radial, one would be wrong, because the word symmetry implies matching parts, and hydras exist as matching parts only by accident. In stating that starfish are radial, one is also wrong, because they are demonstrably the result of the twisting of a bilateral larva, with the suppression of one side, and some evidence of bilaterality is seen even in some adults.

In any case, the only practical value that could be served by these symmetry terms is to concisely convey to the mind their overall shape. Here one asks what is conveyed by saying that the following are all bilateral: tapeworm, bryozoan, snail, earthworm, barnacle, butterfly, starfish, tunicate, and mammal? These have almost nothing in common: some are cup-shaped, some lack a head-end altogether, some are twisted beyond recognition, and some have almost no paired structures. Some coelenterates (supposedly radial) can be divided into two similar pieces (bilateral) with much more accuracy than a snail, for example (see Figure 16).

If the terms do not usefully describe the shape or arrangement of the animals, they are useless. In fact they are misleading; the authors contend that they are highly misleading. They represent nothing but the hope of early naturalists that living things could be dealt with in the simple systems of inanimate objects, an idea carried along by the evolutionists who hoped to find in the patterns of regularity some supporting evidence for their theories of phylogeny. In reality, although the system never gave any real support to any phylogeny, its abandonment will not in any way damage the modern conceptual scheme of evolution.

Animals are simply too diverse to be grouped in such a simple system. The bilaterality of a mollusk and of a brachiopod, for example, are completely different in the light of the animal as a whole and its way of life. The bilaterality of a rhynchocoel and that of an earthworm compare as poorly as a simple circle and the inside view of half a grapefruit.

It must also be noted that none of the "symmetrical" arrangements are exact. There are inaccuracies, or the organs may take different shapes. In fact, in most groups there are individuals that show little of the expected symmetry, and real symmetry may be mixed with asymmetry. For example: "In certain Plecoptera (Insecta) it may be noted that an individual may so lack uniformity that the wings of the right side are quite different from those of the left" (Chamberlin, 1952).

B. Forms of Symmetry

The early systems of the use of symmetry in describing animals appear to have principally used radial and bilateral. *Radial* implied arrangement around an axis, and *bilateral* implied mirror images on each side of a plane. At that time it was said that Porifera, Coelenterata, Ctenophora, and Echinodermata were radial and all others were bilateral.

As zoologists became more familiar with the many forms that animals take, this simple system seemed to have too many flaws. Many coelenterates had a strong appearance of bilaterality, and all echinoderms were seen to be radial only because of the twisting of a bilateral larva with suppression of one side. Porifera did not really fit the word radial, and Nematoda had little bilaterality and a strong triradiate influence. So further terms were added: *spherical, biradial,* and *asymmetrical.*

Table 12
THE OCCURRENCE OF GENERAL MORPHOLOGICAL FEATURES

A	General shape	Cephali-zation	Symmetry planes	Around an axis	Segmen-tation
Porifera	Vase/multiple	None	Indefinite	Vaguely	None
Mesozoa	Short cylinder	Very slight	1	No	None
Coelenterata	Bell	None	0/1/2/4/many	Yes/partly	None
Ctenophora	Sphere/bell	None	2	Partly	None
Platyhelminthes	Flatworm	Slight	1	No	None
Acanthocephala	Short tube	Slight	1	No	None
Rhynchocoela	Long tube	Moderate	1	No	None
Rotifera	Bilateral	Moderate	1	No	None
Kinorhyncha	Bilateral	Moderate	1	No	Body wall
Priapuloidea	Short cylinder	Moderate	1	No	None
Nematoda	Long tube	Moderate	1	No	None
Gordioidea	Long tube	Slight	1	No	None
Calyssozoa	Stalked cup	None	1	No	None
Bryozoa	Cup	None	?1	No	None
Phoronida	Long tube	Moderate	1	No	None
Brachiopoda	Bilateral	None	1	No	None
Mollusca	Bilateral Twisted Indefinite	Slight None	1	No	None
Sipunculoidea	Short tube	Moderate	1	No	None
Echiuroidea	Short tube	Slight	1	No	None
Tardigrada	Bilateral	Moderate	1	No	Yes
Myzostomida	Bilateral	Slight	1	No	None
Annelida	Long tube	Moderate	1	No	Clear
Dinophiloidea	Bilateral	Slight	1	No	None
Pentastomoidea	Worm-like	Slight	1	No	None
Onychophora	Bilateral	Much	1		Clear
Arthropoda	Bilateral	Very much	1	No	Clear
Chaetognatha	Bilateral	Much	1	No	None
Pogonophora	Long tube	Slight	1	No	None
Echinodermata	Star	None	5 (or 1)	Yes	None
Enteropneusta	Bilateral	Moderate	1	No	None
Pterobranchia	Bilateral	Moderate	1	No	None
Tunicata	Modified cup	None	?1	No	None
Cephalochordata	Bilateral	Much	1	No	Internally
Vertebrata	Bilateral	Much	1	No	Internally

Obvious faults still appeared, and it became necessary to refer to Anthozoa as *tetra-merous* and to Echinodermata as *pentamerous*. Writers who carefully analyzed symmetry found it necessary to add other terms: *discoidal, trabal, pontal, bifrontal,* and *dorsiventral,* each with two forms. It was recognized that other descriptive devices could be more useful, including specification of cephalization, regionation, segmentation, and changes of "symmetry" during development. Nearly all textbooks still describe symmetry forms, but the student cannot see much meaning to them. In reality it serves no useful purpose to state that a bivalved mollusk and a bivalved brachiopod are both bilaterally symmetrical. In the mollusk the shells are identical (mirror images) and one is on each side. In the brachiopods the shells are not identical and one is beneath, the other on top, each of them split in two by the symmetry plane. It is hard to see how these concepts can aid the student in understanding the shape and arrangement of animals and in the significance of these features in comparative zoology.

Terms that have been used in connection with symmetry in animals include the following, taken from several systems:

Table 12 (continued)
THE OCCURRENCE OF GENERAL MORPHOLOGICAL FEATURES

B	General habitat	Digestive tract	Paired organs	Internal cavities
Porifera	Sessile Colonial	None	None	Spongiocoel
Mesozoa	Parasitic	None	None	None
Coelenterata	Sessile Floating Motile Floating colony Sessile tubicolous	GVC	Very few	GVC
Ctenophora	Floating Motile	GVC	Very few	None
Platyhelminthes	Motile Parasitic	GVC	Moderate	GVC
Acanthocephala	Parasitic	None	Few	None
Rhynchocoela	Motile	Complete, straight	Few	None
Rotifera	Sessile Motile	Complete, straight	Few	Pseudocoel
Gastrotricha	Motile Sessile	Complete, straight	Few	Pseudocoel
Kinorhyncha	Motile	Complete, straight	Few	Pseudocoel
Priapuloidea	Motile	Complete, straight	Very few	Coelom
Nematoda	Motile Parasitic	Complete, straight	Few	Pseudocoel
Gordioidea	Motile, larva parasitic	Degenerate	Very few	Pseudocoel
Calyssozoa	Stalked colony	Complete, U-shaped	None	Pseudocoel
Bryozoa	Sessile Colonial	Complete, U-shaped	Very few	None
Phoronida	Tubicolous	Complete, U-shaped	Few	Coelom
Brachiopoda	Sessile	Complete, J-shaped Incomplete	Moderate	Coelom
Mollusca	Motile	Complete, J-shaped Twisted, straight	Few	?Coelom
Sipunculoidea	Motile	Complete, U-shaped	Few	Coelom
Echiuroidea	Motile	Complete, twisted	Few	Coelom
Tardigrada	Motile	Complete, straight	Moderate	Coelom, haemocoel
Myzostomida	Parasitic	Complete, straight	Few	Coelom
Annelida	Motile Tubicolous	Complete, straight Branched colony	Many Many	Coelom Coelom
Dinophiloidea	Motile	Complete or none	Moderate	Coelom
Pentastomoidea	Parasitic	Complete, straight	Few	?Coelom
Onychophora	Motile	Complete, straight	Conspicuous	Coelom + haemocoel
Arthropoda	Motile	Complete, straight	Conspicuous	Coelom + haemocoel
Chaetognatha	Motile	Complete, straight	Moderate	Coelom
Pogonophora	Tubicolous	None	Many	Coelom
Echinodermata	Sessile Floating Motile	Complete Incomplete, U- shaped, twisted Branched	None	Coelom
Enteropneusta	Tubicolous	Complete, straight	Few	Coelom
Pterobranchia	Sessile colony	Complete, straight	Few	Coelom
Tunicata	Sessile Sessile colony	Complete, U-shaped	Few	Coelom
Cephalochordata	Motile	Complete, straight	Conspicuous	Coelom
Vertebrata	Motile	Complete, straight Complete, twisted	Conspicuous	Coelom

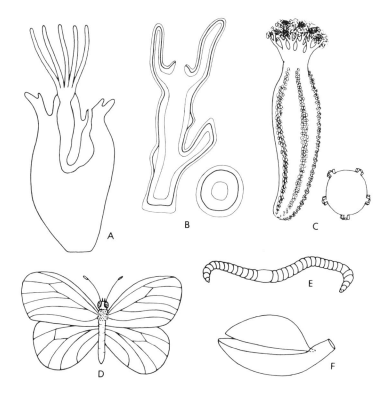

FIGURE 16.   Some of the symmetry forms of animals. All but C are bilateral; C is classed as radial. A, bryozoan; B, hydroid; C, holothurian; D, insect; E, earthworm; F, lamp shell.

1.   Actinomere — one radial section in radial symmetry
2.   Anaxonic — without symmetry
3.   Antimeres — left and right halves in bilateral symmetry
4.   Asymmetrical — without symmetry
5.   Bifrontal symmetry — same as bilateral
6.   Bilateral symmetry — consisting of mirror images along the anterior/posterior median plane
7.   Biradial symmetry — having two planes of symmetry at right angles to each other (more descriptively called bi-bilateral)
8.   Discoidal symmetry — having an isopolar main axis, with or without local differentiations
9.   Dissymmetry — absence or defect of symmetry
10.   Homaxial apolar — same as spherical
11.   Monaxial heteropolar — same as radial
12.   Monosymmetry — same as bilateral symmetry
13.   Multilateral symmetry — same as radial
14.   Octoradiate — in eight similar parts around an axis
15.   Pentamerous — having five similar parts around a central axis
16.   Pentaradiate — in five similar parts around an axis
17.   Polysymmetry — same as radial symmetry
18.   Pontal symmetry — with an isopolar main axis and a heteropolar secondary axis
19.   Promorphology — the study of symmetry in animals
20.   Quinqueradiate — in five similar parts around an axis

21. Radial symmetry — having the parts arranged around a central axis (which is usually heteropolar)
22. Radiobilateral — combination of radial and bilateral
23. Spherical symmetry — spherical, with all radii alike
24. Spiral symmetry — either same as radial, or asymmetrical and twisted like a screw
25. Tetramerous — having four similar parts around a central axis
26. Tetraradial — in four similar parts around an axis (also used as a form of bilateral)
27. Trabal symmetry — having two isopolar axes
28. Triverted symmetry — form of asymmetry
29. Universal symmetry — same as spherical
30. Univerted symmetry — same as bilateral

C. Changes of Form

Having attained a clear-cut form of some sort, it is possible for an animal, developing and changing constantly as it is, to produce a drastic change in that form. Two instances of this occur in well-known circumstances.

Gastropoda. The embryo and early larva of snails are clearly bilaterally symmetrical, but this is suddenly modified by a rapid rotation of part of the body in the process known as *torsion*, resulting in a partly asymmetrical body. Further twisting to fit the body into a spiral shell, although unrelated to torsion, does produce further dissymmetry and further obscures the original bilaterality.

The advantage in torsion appears to be in the adult, where the respiratory currents of water are facilitated. Among Gastropoda which have reduced the shell or lost it altogether, as in some Opisthobranchiata, the torsion has been lost or reduced in a process known as *detorsion*. It is thus seen that in gastropods as a group there are three different processes that twist the body, because the spiral shell often requires a considerable and quite different distortion of the originally bilateral larva.

Echinodermata. As mentioned above, the larvae of echinoderms are among the most obviously bilateral animals, and yet the adults have often been cited as radial. Externally the adults seem to consist of five similar parts arranged around an axis, but they always have important features that do not fit: madreporite, stone canal, anus, and axial complex; these combine with the bilaterality of the larva to weaken or destroy the supposed radiality.

Although the word torsion is not usually applied here, one side of the larva grows rapidly and nearly surrounds the other side, producing a circular object completely different from the larva. This is called *rotation*, but it involves unequal growth, resorption of some organs, and formation of entirely new structures. There are few forms of metamorphosis more drastic than this.

Less obvious and very different changes of form may occur in Porifera, where a substantial inversion of the embryo occurs in a few species; in Coelenterata, where a bilateral planula becomes a radial adult; and in Annelida, where formation of an epitoke region may occur.

It can only be concluded that the symmetry classes of the textbooks are either completely useless and actually misleading, or that they are really based on some other features and do not relate to any actual symmetry in the crystallographic sense. If the latter is true, zoologists would be well advised to adopt a terminology that shows the actual basis for the classes. Some of the possible ways of grouping animals by form are discussed below, but there is no simple system that will replace the symmetry concept used in the textbooks.

D. Axes

It is possible to describe objects by the number of axes and their polarity. An axis of an animal is said to be an imaginary straight line through the body around which organs or parts are arranged, with each end being called a pole. For instance, a mammal would have three axes, head to tail (or anterior or posterior), left to right, and top to bottom (dorsal to ventral). However, very few animals can be fitted to a straight line, and others have no useful poles. Furthermore, a clam has the same axes and polarities as a mammal, and so do some coral polyps. This system has not proven useful as a primary description of animal form in its known diversity.

E. Polarity

Polarity is simply the existence of opposites that can be distinguished; they are at opposite ends of an axis and are called poles. The opposite poles may be similar (homopolar or isopolar) or different (heteropolar). A sphere or circle has no poles (no polarity), but an oval has poles (is polarized). Animals can be polarized by having a head end (cephalization) or an elongate form. A spherical ovum may be polarized by the eccentric placement of the nucleus, by the position of the cleavage spindle, by a micropyle, or by the sperm-entry point.

The only animals that are not polarized are centro- or alecithal zygotes (having a central nucleus) and gemmules and reduction bodies of homogeneous structure.

Polarity has been usefully cited in describing the development of ova, but it does not help in the description of the form of adult animals.

III. BODY ARRANGEMENT

A. The Diversity

Instead of 5 main body arrangements among animals, often cited as radial, biradial, bilateral, spherical, and asymmetrical, there are at least 16 distinct constructions that are not clearly related, and several others also seem to require separate listing. These can be only very roughly grouped, except that there are four arrangements so different from what is found in most other animals that each stands alone (the dagger indicates an extinct group):

Unique arrangements

1. One-celled — Protozoa, all fertilized eggs
2. No internal cavity, no distinct organs — Mesozoa
3. No digestive cavity; permeated by water channels — Porifera, †Receptaculitida, †Cyathospongia
4. Short cylinder of one layer of cells — Monoblastozoa

Animals essentially cup-, or vase-, or bell-shaped, sometimes elongated

5. No complete planes of symmetry — †Graptozoa
6. Blind coelenteron, one or more planes of symmetry — Coelenterata, Siphonophora, Ctenophora
7. Tubular intestinal tract, pentaradiate — Echinodermata
8. Intestinal tract tubular and recurved, no segmentation, no head — Calyssozoa, Bryozoa, Phoronida, Sipunculoidea, Tunicata
9. No digestive tract, no segmentation, no head — Pogonophora

Flattened body or at least not tubular, no definite head, not segmented

10. Blind GVC or no digestive cavity — Platyhelminthes

11. Intestine tubular or lobed, no shell — Rhynchocoela, Rotifera, Gastrotricha, Kinorhyncha, Tardigrada, Myzostomida, Pentastomida, Chaetognatha
12. Dorsal and ventral shells — Brachiopoda
13. With shells or not, but never dorsal and ventral; intestine coiled or looped — Mollusca

Tubular body, not segmented, but with a recognizable head end

14. Acanthocephala, Nematoda, Gordioidea, Priapuloidea, Echiuroidea, Enteropneusta, Pterobranchia

Segmented, usually obviously so

15. No definite head — Annelida
16. Definite head — Onychophora, Arthropoda, Cephalochordata, Vertebrata

B. Cephalization

Many animals are locomotory, moving about to escape enemies, to capture food, and to find mates. All of these activities involve the use of sense organs, and most animals show a concentration of their sense organs at one end of the body, where they can direct the locomotion. For these same animals it is customary to take in food near the front end and to eliminate wastes at the rear, with front and rear determined by the principal direction of body movement. The combination of functions at the head end thus gives that end a special importance; this type of body organization is called *cephalization.*

The heads of animals may be no more alike than is implied by the concentration of functions. In such animals as snails the head is scarcely recognizable as a region or structure. In such segmented animals as earthworms, the head is again almost indistinguishable from the body; however, in such other segmented animals as insects, six or so of the segments may be united into a sensory and feeding region that is structurally clearly distinct from the rest of the body. In vertebrates, the sensory concentration is also accompanied by great concentration of the nervous system in the head, even though no segmentation is visible.

Cephalization is absent in adult echinoderms, in coelenterates, sponges, and bryozoans. It may be developed in varying degree, as in turbellarians (sensory only), tapeworms (attachment only), holothurians (secondarily shown by the mouth end), and lancelets (where the nervous and feeding concentrations are considerable, but no exterior evidence occurs).

C. Repetition

When looking at the body as a whole, there are several ways in which an organism may consist of serially arranged parts, whether these are identical or not:

1. Syzygy — as in the gregarine Sporozoa, produced by union of individuals (usually only two) into a chain
2. Chains — made by incomplete budding or fragmentation, as in some Annelida
3. Strobilation — the formation of a chain by subdivision of a basal region, as in larvae of Scyphozoa, in tapeworms, and in Annelida
4. Pseudometamerism — serial arrangement of organs, such as gut diverticula and gonads, in many Platyhelminthes, Monoplacophora, and Amphineura
5. Segmentation (metamerism) — the serial repetition of mesodermal body parts within one individual, as in Annelida and Arthropoda, especially

The customary citing of Annelida and Arthropoda as segmented (or metameric) is an example of the confusion of meanings in the terms of body arrangement. The body parts of annelids are separated from each other by septae into compartments in which some organs (gonads and nephridia) are repeated in each and other organs (digestive tract) pass through all. The bodies of most arthropods are not divided into compartments, even though some subdivision may be seen in the embryo, and nearly all internal organs (except body wall muscles, nerves, and tracheae) are independent of any body wall subdivision. The Annelida could well be distinguished as metameric: having distinct regions repeated serially. The segmentation of the Arthropoda is then shown by the arrangement of the central nervous system, the tracheae, and the body wall.

It must be noted that in (1), (2), and (3) of the listing above the multiple object is or may be a series of attached individuals, not one animal consisting of linear body parts. These two cases of repetition, involving several individuals or parts of one, are not always distinguished. The former is not relevant here but will be briefly cited so that the cases will be recognized. (See Chapter 23 for further discussion of connected individuals.)

1. Syzygy

This strange association of two or more individuals in a chain is not really relevant to the subject of Repetition of parts. It is a reproductive device not unrelated to sexual reproduction. In Chapter 23 it is discussed as producing noncolonies — aggregations of individuals not qualifying as colonies.

2. Chains

Chains of individuals are formed in syzygy and in some strobilation, as in (1) and (3). Syzygy always involves the union of separate individuals and so is not a matter of repetition of parts. Strobilation sometimes produces new individuals that become separate (as in Scyphozoa), sometimes serial gonophores (organs) which may form a chain (Cestoda), or a series of gonophores which promptly break away so that no chain is formed (as in a few Polychaeta). In other Polychaeta there may be incomplete separation of individuals formed end to end, and these produce chains that may be branched. Among all these none constitute repetition in the usual sense.

3. Strobilation

This is described as a multiplicative process in Chapter 2. It occurs in five widely separated phyla (Protozoa, Coelenterata, Platyhelminthes, Annelida, Tunicata). The chain may consist of separate individuals, in which case it would be a form of reproduction and therefore not appropriate to the present discussion, or it may consist of multiple compartments with duplicated organs, so that the whole is still just one individual, as in tapeworms.

4. Pseudometamerism

This is described as a tendency toward repetition of parts and the spreading of systems throughout the body, as shown by a branching "intestine", and numerous gonads and/or excretory organs. This is thought to suggest a segmented condition, but the absence of compartmentalization of the body shows that it is not segmentation. The situation in such different groups as Turbellaria, Kinorhyncha, and Monoplacophora are so diverse that this term has no definable parameters.

5. Segmentation

Many animals are segmented. This word implies a body divided in some way into a series of more or less similar sections called segments. This may or may not involve repetition of some organs in each segment. There are few subjects in zoology so confused by the terms that have been employed.

The relevant facts appear to be these: Many members of the Annelida show clear segmentation throughout the body, with septae between the segments and some organs duplicated in each. In some species, especially Hirudinea, the segmentation is not obvious. Normally the coelom is fully compartmentalized. The segments are many, generally 33 or more, and nearly all alike.

The Onychophora are sometimes omitted in listing the phyla of segmented animals, but this seems to be because they are considered an insignificant group in this regard. They have paired appendages, a ladder-type nervous system, a coelom reduced to the cavities of the gonads. The legs vary from 14 to 43 pairs, and the leg "segments" are all alike, leaving the head region without repetitions.

The Arthropoda apparently all show "segmentation" in the embryo, but in the adults of some it is not evident. The coelom is reduced, as in Onychophora, and "segments" are not separated by septae. There may be repetition of appendages and their muscles, as in Myriapoda, and the nervous system may show a ladder arrangement, but there is little repetition of organs. The body wall usually shows segmentation as a series of sclerotized rings. The segments are rarely over two dozen, usually about 12, and they are usually diverse among themselves.

In the Vertebrata segmentation occurs almost exclusively in muscles of the body wall and in the central nervous system. There are no segmental divisions of the coelom and no repeated organs along the body other than muscles, nerves, and spinal column. No series of similar "segments" is seen.

It is universally stated that annelid and arthropod segmentation is the same, in spite of the drastic difference in coeloms. It is also universally stated that segmentation of vertebrates is different from the others. Direct support for these statements seems never to be given, it apparently being assumed to be true because Vertebrata are for other reasons believed to be independently derived from some ancestors other than the annulates.

The use of distinct terms for these three types of segmentation would have helped to keep the situation clear. There are several terms that could have been used: segmentation, metamerism, and oligomery, but it is curious to find the first two used as synonymous and then united as metameric segmentation. Only oligomery is still distinctive, where it might describe the Arthropoda and Vertebrata, but it is seldom used.

All that is clear from this is that (1) Annelida have a very clear type of extensive segmentation with coelomic compartmentalization, (2) Onychophora have a surface segmentation with similar "segments" but no body cavity subdivision, (3) Arthropoda have small numbers of surface segments with no body cavity subdivision, and (4) Vertebrata have an invisible "segmentation" in trunk muscles and nervous system, with no compartmentalization of the coelom and with a fixed number of "segments".

Terms that have been applied to these features of repetition include (see also later section on regionation):

1. Heteronomous segmentation — that in which there is some dissimilarity and specialization among the body segments
2. Homonomous segmentation — that in which there is relative similarity among the body segments
3. Locomotory metamerism — a theoretical explanation of the cause of repetition as due to locomotory needs
4. Mesodermal segmentation — that which shows up in tissues derived from mesoderm
5. Metameric segmentation — same as segmentation

6. Metamerism — same as segmentation, but sometimes used to cover all longitudinal division
7. Oligomery — segmentation with only a few compartments
8. Pseudometamerism — defined as serial arrangment of such organs as intestinal diverticula and gonads, suggesting division of the body into segments, but without meeting the mesodermal criterion of segmentation
9. Segmentation — longitudinal repetition of similar parts in an animal body, usually assumed to be shown by the nervous system and mesodermal tissue, such as muscles
10. Strobilation — formation of a strobilus (a chain of either individuals or organs) by partitioning of an original individual and growth of the new parts
11. Superficial segmentation — that which shows up only in surface features; usually called annulation; not by itself evidence of segmentation

When there is any such duplication of body parts, the parts may be designated by such terms as these:

1. Arthromere — segment in Arthropoda
2. Corm — linearly arranged parts of some crustacean appendages
3. Metamere — same as segment
4. Polyisomere — one of several identical parts
5. Proglottid — serial structure in a tapeworm chain that carries a complete set of gonads; here regarded as simply a detachable organ (gonophore)
6. Segment — one of the linearly arranged body subdivisions in segmented animals
7. Somite — (1) same as segment; (2) one of a series of linearly arranged masses of mesoderm along the neural tube in vertebrate embryos
8. Zonite — (1) sometimes used for a body segment of a milliped, one of many very similar ones; (2) body division of kinorhynchs

Repetitions can thus occur in several forms, including these:

1. A long series of closely similar body areas separated by a septum, with some organs repeated in each area: tapeworms, in which the "segments" (proglottids) remain connected only temporarily, and earthworms and other annelids, in which the similar segments are permanent and numerous
2. Many diverse segments, usually less than two dozen, arranged in a fairly small number of regions, not regularly separated by septa nor with repeated internal organs, but shown by muscle arrangement and the ganglia of the central nervous system and usually by exterior annulation (Onychophora, Arthropoda)
3. No repetition except having three or five pairs of embryonic coelomic cavities, not appearing to be annulated (Bryozoa, Phoronida, Brachiopoda, Pogonophora, Echinodermata, Hemichordata)
4. Segmentation not visible externally, but many segments not all alike are suggested by body wall musculature, skeleton, and central nervous system (Cephalochordata, Vertebrata)
5. Some surface indications of repetition of parts but seen to be limited to cuticle, sometimes the body wall musculature, and even the nervous system (Acanthocephala, s.Rotifera, Kinorhyncha, Priapuloidea, s.Nematoda, Hirudinea, Pentastomida)

Thus, segmentation is diverse in expression, and by no single feature can it be certainly distinguished in adult animals. A substantial further diversity occurs among unquestionably segmented animals in their manner of development. In many, the number of segments is fixed in embryology and remains constant throughout life. There seems to be no good term to specify this condition, although in Insecta this special meaning has sometimes been given to the term metamorphosis (to contrast with anamorphosis). Metamorphosis, however, is already used in this very group for a much more fundamental developmental process. When an animal adds segments after its embryology is completed (always at molts), the term *anamorphosis* is applied. This latter occurs in many Annelida and in several groups of Arthropoda (Trilobita, Pycnogonida, some Crustacea, many Myriapoda, and a few Insecta (Protura) (see Beklemishev, 1963).

Quite obviously segmentation is not a feature that can be used by the student of zoology to express a consistent picture of any but the most clearly segmented groups, those which are called the annulates (Annulata: the Annelida, Onychophora, and Arthropoda). Curiously, this very term (annulation) is the one used to describe such supposedly not segmented animals as Kinorhyncha or the extra surface grooves found on such actually segmented ones as Hirudinea.

The drawing of phylogenetic conclusions is always a risky business, and segmentation does not appear to be a dependable feature at the phylum level.

It has sometimes been argued that tapeworms also are segmented (for example, Hyman, 1951). In this volume, we believe that the proglottids of tapeworms are simply gonophores comparable to some epitokes in Polychaeta. They are essentially compartments capable of becoming separated from the chain and continuing to live long enough to perform their reproductive function. To include tapeworms as segmented animals alongside the Annelida is as unjustified as to treat the strobilus of Scyphozoa as segmented.

A discussion of many features of repetition is found in Beklemishev (1969), where the term metamerism is used in the broadest sense. He finds "metamerism" in these groups (with comments added): (1) Protozoa — Flagellata: Dinoflagellata and Hypermastigina; Sarcodina: Foraminifera and Radiolaria; Sporozoa: Gregarinida; Ciliata: *Anoplophrya*); (2) Coelenterata — Hydrozoa: *Staurocoryne*; strobili of Scyphozoa; Anthozoa: *Gonactinia*; also in some colonies of Siphonophora; (3) Platyhelminthes — Turbellaria: *Procerodes lobata*; Cestoda: most species; (4) Rhynchocoela — many species; (5) Acanthocephala — purely external; (6) Rotifera — especially in some Bdelloidea; (7) Gastrotricha — especially in Macrodasyoidea; (8) Kinorhyncha — all species; (9) Nematoda — especially in *Desmoscolex*; (10) Gordioidea — some larvae; (11) Mollusca — Monoplacophora, Amphineura, Gastropoda, Bivalvia such as *Nucula*; Cephalopoda: embryos of Dibranchiata; (12) Myzostomida — ectodermal structures only; (13) Tardigrada — all species, e.g., *Batillipes*; (14) Dinophiloidea — shown by a ladder-type central nervous system; (15) Annelida — oligomerous, polymerous, and heteronomous; (16) Pentastomida — all species, e.g., *Railletiella*; (17) Onychophora — all species; (18) Arthropoda — all species; (19) Echinodermata — only along each arm of Ophiuroidea.

Beklemishev excludes all "Chordata" from his discussion but does incidentally mention metamerism at least in Cephalochordata. It is readily seen that this list includes many animals that are not usually thought of as segmented. However, it illustrates the difficulty of definition of such words as segmentation and metamerism as well as the diversity of animal body arrangement.

6. Regionation

The segments of the polymerous animals (Annelida) are almost all very much alike. In each of the oligomerous Arthropoda the segments are of various sorts; they are often grouped into recognizable regions called *tagmata*. Each region is a *tagma*, and the condition of such regionation of segments is *tagmosis*. For example:

1.   Cephalothorax and abdomen — in Crustacea
2.   Head, thorax, abdomen — in Insecta
3.   Prosoma, mesosoma, metasoma — in some Arachnida
4.   Prosoma, opisthosoma — in some Arachnida

Some other segmented animals appear to consist of several regions, but these are of a different nature and do not concern us here.

D. Polymorphism
1. Forms of Polymorphism

It is necessary to point out, in discussing animal form, that virtually no species of animal exists in just one body form at all times and under all circumstances. Many kinds of animals normally appear in more than one structural form. These multiple forms are called *polymorphs*, which are individuals differing in some obvious way. Among these are those called polyps and medusae, males and females where clearly different, the different individuals within some colonies, the castes of social insects, and the successive forms of most life cycles (e.g., egg, larva, adult). These forms can all be studied as to symmetry, polarity, and arrangement, and so are included above.

The word polymorphism has been defined in various ways, apparently because of different conditions in the special groups of each writer. For example, in the Coelenterata polymorphism is shown by polyp and medusa. In Siphonophora it is shown by colonies with several types of individuals. In freshwater Rotifera and Crustacea there are cyclical changes of form *(cyclomorphosis)*. In Insecta there is an extreme difference between male and female. The workers on some of these groups have defined the word to exclude all developmental forms because they are not simultaneous. In others the sexual forms are rejected because external sex differences in these groups are not obvious.

The forms of polymorphism are listed here with the broadest possible definition; the reader can then select which part he chooses to denote by that word, knowing the nature of the other forms.

One of the last of an earlier generation of biology textbooks has a clear definition in the broad sense: "When the variation within a species is marked, when the different forms are not connected by intermediate gradations, and when they can be correlated with some other factor or condition, then the species is called polymorphic and is said to exhibit polymorphism . . . sexual, geographical, climatic, seasonal, social" (Wolcott, 1946). In recent works the word polymorphism is usually used to denote only such multiple forms as occur in Coelenterata and colonial species of other groups. The word has also been given different meanings in genetics and in biochemistry.

The ways in which some species of animals may appear in various forms are many and difficult to classify:

1.   The sexes may be substantially different
2.   In colonies there may be specialized individuals very different from the norm
3.   There may be two or more forms of one sex in each population, with no intermediates
4.   Developmental stages usually are so different as to qualify as distinct forms
5.   Environmental factors may induce a series of forms sequentially, as in cyclomorphosis

2. Developmental Polymorphism

Many animals begin life as a fertilized egg and then pass through developmental stages to become adults. The stages may be merely embryo and juvenile, as in humans, or they may be embryo, larva, pupa, as in some insects, or they may be a series of several different larval forms, as in tapeworms and flukes. If these stages are distinctly different, the sequence may be called polymorphism, best distinguished as sequential polymorphism.

There are at least two dozen different types of larvae in the animal kingdom. Without exception these are bilateral to some degree, never radial. There are frequently two or more larval types in the life cycle of one species, and there are hundreds of different life cycles. Some of this diversity is cited in Part III, "Development".

3. Sexual Polymorphism

When males and females are noticeably different externally, we say there is sexual dimorphism. It is sometimes forgotten that there are other species in which there are also hermaphroditic individuals or also neuter individuals. These give rise to the possibility of more than two sexual morphs, and existing combinations are listed in Chapter 4 under "Sexuality".

Terms used for special forms of sexual polymorphism, or for the individual forms, include:

1. Alary polymorphism — in insects, where some individuals are winged and some are not; may be correlated with sex
2. Dichromism — having two color phases, corresponding to the sexes
3. Dimorphism — having males and females visibly different (for an extreme case, see Herpyllobiidae, Copepoda, Crustacea, in Markewitch, 1976)
4. First form male — an instar in development of certain crayfish during which the first pleopods are specialized for transferring spermatozoa; the second form male lacks this specialization
5. Free martin — a sterile female member of twins of unlike sexes in cattle; produced by the hormone effects of the male in the placental circulation
6. Pollard — any hornless male in a species of animal which is normally horned
7. Trimorphism — having individuals of three castes, as in the honeybee (this word could also be reasonably applied to the many species in which besides male and females, there are neuters or hermaphrodites)

4. Colonial Polymorphism

In colonial animals there are commonly several types of individuals in each colony. These are a variety of sorts, suggested in the list.

Of the six phyla that include definite and permanent colonies, three have the individuals of several types (polymorphic):

1. †Graptozoa — autothecae, bithecae (possibly = females and males)
2. Coelenterata — polyps: hydranths (feeding) and gonangia (reproductive, asexual) and medusae
3. Siphonophora — gastrozooids (digestive), dactylozooids (grasping), gonozooids (reproductive, asexual), nectophores (swimming bells), phyllozooids (bracts, protective), gonophores (?), pneumatophore (float)
4. Bryozoa — gonozooids (feeding), kenozooids (undifferentiated, stolons, etc.), avicularia (protective, often resembling a bird's head), vibracula (protective, bristle-like), nannozooids (dwarfs)

5. Social Polymorphism

Castes — in three groups of insects belonging to two orders, the individual termites, ants, or bees in the social species can be distinguished by external features as belonging to one of the following castes:

Ants	Termites	Bees, wasps
Queens	Reproductives (m and f)	Females
Males	Short-winged reproductives	Workers
Workers	Workers	Drones (males)
	Soldiers (29 forms, including nasuti)	
	Repletes	

The caste systems in these three groups did not evolve from one source but are surely independently evolved in each. The similarly named castes correspond only in function. Within the Isoptera (termites) there is diversity in the number of castes formed, the structural specialization of each, and in details of behavior.

6. Seasonal Polymorphism

Cyclomorphosis is a cyclic change in body form, such as the distinct head shapes found in Cladocera (Crustacea). These are clearly controlled by environmental influences but are produced in the same manner as developmental changes. Something of the sort occurs in some Rotifera.

7. Other Polymorphism

In hydrozoan coelenterates, some species occur in two adult forms, the polyps and the medusae. These are part of the life cycle, but neither one can be judged to be a larva, and neither changes into the other, as do developmental stages.

Many insects show multiple form; some are related to life cycle or to seasons or to unknown factors. For example, in several beetles some males may have very much larger mandibles or horns, with no intermediates. These seem almost akin to castes, but there is usually no known difference in function.

Terms that have been used include *poecilogeny*, the occurrence in some Diptera where two types of larvae are formed, one to become normally sexual, the other to reproduce parthenogenetically; *phases*, such as color phases, winged phases, etc; *diphygenesis*, producing two types of embryos, as in some Dicyemida.

Several methods have been used to classify the situations that can be called polymorphism. For example, one may cite cases of sexual dimorphism, developmental polymorphism, seasonal polymorphism, allometry, color phases, castes, and colonial polymorphism, but it appears most informative to combine several features into a seven-part system, under which the numerous kinds of polymorphism can be arranged. Some animals show more than one of the types of polymorphism, as indicated in the parentheses. Definitions are given later.

Simultaneously in a population (I)

1. Sexual
2. Castes
3. Color phases
4. Egg types (see also no. 12)
5. Body forms (polyp/medusa) (see also no. 19)
6. Allometry (polypheism) (see also no. 8)
7. Developmental (see also no. 14)

Simultaneously in the life cycle of a species (II)

8. Allometry (see also no. 6)
9. Poecilogeny

Simultaneously in a colony (III)

10. Colonial

Sequentially in a population (IV)

11. Cyclomorphosis (seasonal change) (see also no. 15)
12. Egg types (seasonal changes) (see also no. 4)
13. Metagenesis (see also no. 17)

Sequentially in the life history of an individual (V)

14. Developmental (heteromorphic, pleiomorphic, polyeidic) (see also no. 7)
15. Cyclomorphosis (see also no. 11)
16. Sex reversal

Sequentially in the life cycle of a species (VI)

17. Metagenesis (heterogony) (see also no. 13)
18. Diphygenesis
19. Body forms (e.g., polyp/medusa) (see also no. 5)

Sequentially in a colony (VII)

20. Chaining of individuals

It will be seen at once that the multiplicity of body form is too diverse to be cleanly classified even into as many as 7 classes. At least 6 of the 14 types above have to be listed in 2 places. The various technical terms used to express polymorphism can be briefly defined and exemplified.

1. Allometry — condition of having large and small forms together, as in some horned beetles
2. Castes — the differing forms assumed among social insects, sometimes produced by controlled feeding
3. Chaining — formation of multiple colonies, end to end, as in Siphonophora
4. Cyclomorphosis — seasonal changes in body form, as in some freshwater Crustacea
5. Dichromism — condition of appearing in two color phases, but usually correlated with sexual dimorphism, as in many birds
6. Dimorphism — the existence of two body forms in a species, especially male and female or winged and nonwinged insects
7. Diphygenesis — production of two types of embryos, in some Dicyemida (Mesozoa)
8. Heterogamy — same as metagenesis
9. Heteromorphic — having different forms in the life history of the individual, such as egg, larva, adult
10. Metagenesis — alternation of generations; the basis for restriction varies in different groups, but alternation of sexual and asexual "generations" is usually implied

11.   Phases — the two or more different forms, such as two color phases in the ermine
12.   Pleiomorphic — having several forms in the life history of the individual, such as egg, larva, adult
13.   Poecilogeny — a type of dimorphism in the larvae of certain Diptera (Insecta), normal and paedogenetic
14.   Polyeidic — passing through a succession of forms in the life history; see Heteromorphic
15.   Polymorphic — existing in more than two body forms; defined to include only simultaneous, adult, or all forms of all sorts (as herein)
16.   Polyphenism — the exhibition of several aspects by an individual; especially developmental polymorphism
17.   Trimorphism — in Foraminifera, the phenomenon of producing tests of three types; a form of phasic polymorphism; or having three castes (s.Insecta)

These forms can all be studied as to symmetry, polarity, and arrangement. In fact, all the various aspects of morphology are to be studied in each of the polymorphs. It has been our purpose to describe organs and processes of each form, but separate discussions of these are seldom found in the literature.

Among the successive polymorphs of a species, there may be a complete change of form. For example:

1.   Egg, embryo, larva, adult — in many marine groups
2.   Egg, embryo, larva, pupa, adult — in many Insecta
3.   Egg, embryo, larva I, larva II, adult — in some Crustacea and Echinodermata
4.   Egg, embryo, larva — in Larvacea, where no adult ever appears

IV. SIZE

It is common to think of some animals as large (whales, for example) and others as small (protozoans). One forgets that every whale starts life as a single cell (zygote), no larger than many protozoans. It would not be incorrect to say that at some given moment (especially just after the breeding season) a particular whale (still embryonic) may be no larger than the average invertebrate, and by no means a very large animal. Nearly all sexually produced individuals of all species then range in size during their lifetime from the minute size of the zygote to the ordinary size of the adult. Although the largest animals are truly the whales, the group of the smallest will include the zygote stage of the whales as well as of myriads of other animals.

This large animal could be described as having a size range from one (its initial size) to many million times (its largest size). In contrast to this an asexually produced individual formed by splitting might range in size only from one (its initial size) to twice that (its regenerated full size). The difference between these two size ranges is tremendous.

Aside from these developmental size ranges, the smallest animals are no doubt Protozoa, which may be as small as 1 μm in diameter. Aside from these the smallest animals are probably those which form part of the interstitial fauna (the psammon), whose members live in water films between grains of sand. These are well within the range of the size of Protozoa and include some species in each of the following groups: Ciliata, Sarcodina (Foraminifera), Hydrozoa, Gnathostomuloidea, Turbellaria, Rhynchocoela, Rotifera, Gastrotricha, Nematoda, Bryozoa, Gastropoda, Polychaeta, Archiannelida, Tardigrada, Arachnida (Acarina), Crustacea, Insecta (Collembola).

V. SHAPE

It is interesting to recall the unusual shapes that sometimes are found among animals and their parts. It is probable that the most common shape overall is the cylinder, forming worm bodies, the digestive tracts, all blood vessels and ducts, many cells, and even the tubular fibrils of which cilia are composed. Hexagons are theoretically common, at least in the cross section of some of the cylinders, because crowded cells tend to assume the shape that gives the largest possible area of contact (epithelial cells, honeycomb, etc.). Spheres are also common among ova and eggs, although many are ovoid; some Protozoa, including many Radiolaria, all Heliozoa, and a few Flagellata and Suctoria, are basically spherical. The most perfect form of this is found in such a radiolarian as *Hexacontium*, where there are three perforated concentric spheres tied together by radiating spines and with the nucleus in the center.

Taking consideration of all levels of organization, the most frequently encountered definite shape other than the spheres, cylinders, and hexagons turns out to be spirals or *helices*. There is much notice given in modern biology to the double helix of the DNA molecule. The stalk of colloblast or lasso cells in Ctenophora is a contractile spiral filament — as is the stalk of some sessile Ciliata.

Many muscle fibers are described as striated as cross-striated, with the striations at right angles to the axis of the fiber. However, in some Mollusca, Annelida, Crinoidea, and Tunicata there are said to be spirally arranged striations.

The tracheae of Insecta are lined with spiral thickenings or intimas that keep the tube from being flattened without destroying its elasticity. In many Brachiopoda there is a spiral lophophore on each side of the dorsal valve; each is usually supported by a corresponding spiral brachidium. The lophophore is covered with tentacles and is primarily a device for filter feeding.

The temporary "stomach" of Pogonophora is formed by coiling the tentacle or tentacles into a tight coil, leaving a cavity down the center of the spiral. The entire intestinal tract in both Sipunculoidea and Echiuroidea is not only looped back toward the mouth but is also loosely twisted into a double spiral. In *Amphioxus*, there is a mucus rope of food in the intestine; "here strong cilia twist the string into a tight spiral coil and rotate it under moderate tension" (Morton, 1967). Again, one species of the fish genus *Heterodontus* has a conical egg case with two spiralling flaps.

The entire skeleton (test) of members of one of the extinct classes of Echinodermata (Helicoplacoidea) is spirally arranged, as the name of the class indicates. There are spiral shells in Foraminifera, Gastropoda, and Cephalopoda. Although the torsion of Gastropoda is unrelated to the spiralling of the shell, it is essentially helical although it turns only 180°. The extinct bryozoan *Archimedes* produced colonies that were built on a spiral axis, with a leaf-like frond that was spiralled around it.

Many orb-weaving spiders put down their strands of silk in a continuous spiral out from the center. The diagrams of life cycles of all animals that are usually drawn as circles are, of course, spirals, because they do not go to the same starting point but merely to a comparable but new individual that is the start of a new cycle.

A variation on the helix is found in the action of the stalk muscle of Vorticellidae (Ciliata), as described by Grell (1973); in shortening, the stalk may either coil to a helix or be bent angularly into a zigzag depending on the species. (The latter is evidently a two-dimensional version of the helix.)

Serial rings may be split diagonally down one face, with the ends overlapping in a manner called *imbrication*. This occurs in *Rhabdopleura* in the Pterobranchia, the extinct Graptozoa, and in Polychaeta (*Harmothoë*).

VI. TRANSPARENCY

In the ocean, light is one of the basic necessities of life. It can also be a lethal factor by making organisms visible to predators. It may then be advantageous for a floating animal to be transparent and colorless. Transparency is merely the absence of structures or materials that interfere with the passage of light.

Pelagic animals commonly are invisible in seawater, and are often presumed to benefit from this feature. For example, the ctenophore *Pleurobranchia* is so transparent that it can be illustrated in books only by darkening at least some of its parts. The Chaetognatha also are described as so transparent as to be invisible until stained. Such animals are principally eaten by filter feeders, who do not need to see their prey.

It is said that pelagic larvae of most groups are transparent. For example, the phyllosome larva of *Palinurus*, the spiny lobster, "is among the most remarkable of all crustacean forms. It is flat as a piece of paper and as transparent as glass" (Hardy, 1956). Actually, it is not quite the same as glass, because it can be detected in sunlight by its shadow, which is due to the difference in light refraction by the larva and the seawater.

Plankton in general, defined as consisting of the aquatic plants and animals of small size, is unexpectedly transparent. Diatoms form 90% of the plankton organisms, and even they are largely transparent because their skeletons are made of silica (glass). The larvae and other microscopic animals are usually almost invisible in the water. A drop of seawater may look entirely clear to the naked eye, yet under the microscope be seen to swarm with tiny organisms.

Even in freshwater, transparency can be an advantage to an animal in eluding predators. Crustaceans especially tend to be transparent, even some cave-dwelling crayfishes several inches long.

REFERENCES

Beklemishev, W. N., On the relationships of the Turbellaria to other groups of the animal kingdom, in *The Lower Metazoa,* Dougherty, E. C., Ed., University of California Press, Berkeley, 1963, 16.

Beklemishev, W. N., *Principles of Comparative Anatomy of Invertebrates,* Vol. 1., *Promorphology,* University of Chicago Press, Chicago, 1969.

Bonner, J. T., *Morphogenesis: An Essay on Development,* Princeton University Press, Princeton, N.J., 1952.

Chamberlin, W. J., *Entomological Nomenclature and Literature,* Wm. C. Brown, Dubuque, 1952.

Frey-Wyssling, A., *Submicroscopic Morphology of Protoplasm and Its Derivatives,* American Elsevier, New York, 1948.

Grell, K. G., *Protozoology,* Springer-Verlag, Heidelberg, 1973.

Hardy, A. C., *The Open Sea: The World of Plankton,* Collins, London, 1956.

Hyman, L. H., *The Invertebrates,* Vol. 2, McGraw-Hill, New York, 1951.

Lwoff, A., *Biological Order,* Massachusetts Institute of Technology Press, Cambridge, 1962.

Morton, J. E., *Guts: Form and Function of Digestive System,* St. Martin's Press, New York, 1967.

Schoute, J. C., *Biomorphology in General,* North-Holland, Amsterdam, 1949.

Wolcott, R. H., *Animal Biology,* 3rd ed., McGraw-Hill, New York, 1946.

Chapter 10

CELLS

TABLE OF CONTENTS

I.   Introduction..214

II.   Protoplasm..214
      A.   Protoplasmic Diversity...214
      B.   Protoplasmic Functions..215
      C.   Chemical Diversity 215

III. Cells...215
      A.   The Cell Theory..215
      B.   Cell Origins..216
      C.   Cell Structure 216
           1.   Cell Shape 216
           2.   Cell Components..217
                a.   Organelles 217
                b.   Cilia and Flagella 217
                c.   Nucleus..221
                d.   Cell Inclusions...221
                e.   Cell Secretions...222
                f.   Spicules..222
                g.   Setae 222
                h.   Outer Coverings...223
                i.   Skeletons..223
                j.   Trichocysts 223
                k.   Nematocysts...223
      D.   Cell Oddities 223
      E.   Cell Functions 224
           1.   Phagocytosis 225
           2.   Spicule Formation 225
           3.   Transport by Cells..226
           4.   Cell Division 226
           5.   Cell Motility..228
           6.   Protozoan Cell Functions...229
      F.   Cell Types 229
           1.   Unique Cells 230
           2.   Universality of Cell Types 232
           3.   Gametes, Zygotes, and Blastomeres.............................232

References 233

I. INTRODUCTION

A cell is a mass of protoplasm under the control of a nucleus and surrounded by a limiting membrane. This statement is not put in the form of a definition, because there are exceptions to both of the specifications. There are cells without nuclei, either temporarily or permanently, and there are masses of protoplasm, otherwise cell-like, that lack the surrounding membrane. Both of these exceptions occur widely in the animal kingdom, although organisms entirely without nuclei in their cells occur only in the simplest plants, and ones entirely without cell walls occur only in the shadowland between plants and Protozoa, in the Mycetozoa or slime molds.

The nature of cells and the cellularity of animals was briefly discussed in Chapter 1. The present chapter deals with the diversity of cells, which may differ in the following ways:

1.   Size
2.   Shape
3.   Components (the protoplasm, inclusions, organelles, membranes)
4.   Interconnections
5.   Functions performed for the animal (reception and transmission of stimuli, food and energy metabolism, secretion, excretion, contraction, reproduction)
6.   Motility
7.   Location
8.   Beginning and end of existence

Because protoplasm is the one truly universal feature of cells, it will be discussed first, but it should be noted that it is "universal" only because all cells consist of protoplasm by definition.

II. PROTOPLASM

A. Protoplasmic Diversity

"All living things are characterized by the presence of a complex substance called *protoplasm*." This statement, which has sometimes been labeled as an axiom or principle of biology, exemplifies a common fallacy. The living materials of all organisms are covered by the term protoplasm (in spite of great differences in components and composition and despite the fact that not all of these materials have been examined), and it is then asserted that protoplasm is universal in organisms and that this shows that all organisms are related. It is universal because biologists use that word for the living materials of all organisms, not because they have found these materials to be of such uniform nature in organisms that they can reasonably be covered by one word. The use of this word in such an all-encompassing manner is necessary and helpful, but one must not lose sight of the fact that the word does not show much about the nature of the living material in different organisms.

Protoplasm is immensely diverse. It could not be otherwise. "There could be but one kind of organism if all protoplasm were exactly alike." It has evolved to produce at least 2 million distinct kinds of organisms, each with thousands of types of molecules. It has been calculated that a single cell (a human liver cell, for example) contains at least 230 trillion molecules, of which many are composed of thousands of atoms apiece. In living protoplasm, all of these are in constant chemical activity, undergoing changes of structure and arrangement, and recombining in new ways.

It has sometimes been held that all protoplasm as we know it must have had a common origin, because its molecules metabolize by means of such recognizable sequences as glycolysis, the Krebs citric acid cycle, and the electron-transfer system. These are accomplished in different ways in different cells. The individual chemical reactions are responses to properties of the reacting molecules, not of the protoplasm. Perhaps all protoplasm did arise from one occurrence, but widespread presence of these cycles is not good evidence of anything except that some of the molecules of all known protoplasm are of the same general types.

Unfortunately, the exact composition of protoplasm in different organisms and the sequences of reactions that occur are not well enough known to permit one to compare them through the groups of the animal kingdom. It is probably lack of detailed comparative knowledge at this level that has led so many writers to imply that all protoplasm is alike, except for the genes. We could not have diversity of cells and individuals and species without diversity of the protoplasm.

B. Protoplasmic Functions

Protoplasm performs certain functions irrespective of the cell or whole organism. These include breakdown and synthesis of molecules, differentiation into organelles, release and utilization of energy in molecular bonds, and production and employment of catalysts (enzymes). There is great diversity among these processes, as well as some chemical unity, but little at this level can yet be treated comparatively.

C. Chemical Diversity

Some general biology books imply that there is great unity in the chemical basis of the different forms of life and groups of organisms. At the same time it is held that there is biochemical uniqueness in all kinds of organisms if not actually in all individuals. It is a trend of these times to stress the similarities and to emphasize the unity of life. There is some evidence that this emphasis on unity is overdone, or at least that the very considerable diversity is not adequately recognized. Directly comparative data on biochemistry among animals is very hard to find. Much has been discovered and published about substances and reactions, but this knowledge involves so few kinds of animals that comparison or tabulation or groups is usually impossible.

It should theoretically be possible to list the component types of molecules in each type of cell in each group of animal. This proves to be far beyond the reach of present-day knowledge. It is acknowledged that differences exist between cell types and also between different animal groups, but the nature of the difference is seldom elucidated.

Although it is reported that major biochemical cycles are similar in many animal groups, it is also admitted that there are differences. These differences are not commonly specified, but they are the key to a comparative approach.

Some comparative data on a reasonably broad scale has been accumulated on these substances: the blood pigments involved in oxygen transport, the nitrogenous waste products, the hydrogen acceptors in muscle metabolism, and the organic and inorganic materials of hard-parts. It will apparently be a long time before many other aspects of biochemistry of animal molecules can be so tabulated for any substantial number of groups.

Of the biochemical diversities, blood pigments are tabulated in this book under "Respiration" (Chapter 15), waste products under "Excretion" (Chapter 16), hard-part substances under "Integuments" (Chapter 18), and hydrogen acceptors under "Muscles" (Chapter 20).

III. CELLS

A. The Cell Theory

It has been said that a major characteristic of protoplasm is that it never exists in bulk but always in cells. "All living cells in nature are surrounded by one or another kind of extraneous membrane or jelly-like coating...delicate or tough, thin or thick, soft or hard, elastic or rigid, viscous or plastic." To these generalizations there are many exceptions occurring from Protozoa to Mammalia. These exceptions are masses of protoplasm, otherwise like cells, that lack the bounding membrane. If, in place of the word cell, one uses a term such as *energid* this difficulty is minimized. An energid is a nucleus surrounded by the cytoplasm which it directly controls, with or without a cell membrane.

It was long ago speculated that all organisms would be found to consist of cells. This hypothesis has been called the Cell Theory. Many books treat this as a proven law. It is sometimes stated thus: "Each organism, whether plant or animal, is made up of one or more cells together with any products of these cells." This is true so far as known if "cell" is defined as above to include those without any bounding membrane; however, this is a fact, not a theory. The Cell Theory is one of the historically important ideas of biology, but it is no longer a theory. It should not be called a law because there are exceptions.

Most of the exceptions are in syncytial tissues of Metazoa, which will be cited in the next chapter. In the sarcodine Protozoa the Mycetozoa consist of relatively large masses of protoplasm with many nuclei but without intervening cell membranes. Examination of these apparent exceptions shows that the situation is more complex than usually stated, even where such features are being discussed:

Individuals that are multinucleate (plasmodia)

1. Formed by fusion of myxamoebae and fission of the "zygote" (s.Mycetozoa)
2. Developmental stages temporarily multinucleate by incomplete fission (Sporozoa)

Tissues of Metazoa where intervening cell membranes are lacking (syncytia)

3. Formed by fusion of cells (reported by several authors without examples)
4. Formed by incomplete cell division (syncytia in both embryonic and adult tissues)

B. Cell Origins

"It is a fundamental biological statement that *every cell originates from a cell* (by cell division)." This simple generalization does not take account of the obvious exception that each zygote is a cell but one formed by fusion of two cells, the gametes. These are usually ovum and spermatozoon, but sometimes indistinguishable iso- or hologametes.

Examples of other cells formed by fusion of cells are cited in Chapter 4. Beyond such exceptions, it does seem to be true that cells arise from pre-existing cells by cell division, but it may escape notice that "cell division" is not a single process (see discussion in a later section).

It is true, of course, that the cells of a metazoan animal are all the product of cell divisions, even if fusions have intervened or even if the "cells" are not separated by membranes. When one speaks of "cell division" in general, it can usually be understood that nuclear division is of basic importance, and several things can interfere with cytoplasmic division.

C. Cell Structure
1. Cell Shape

The shape of individual cells is usually determined by the crowding of them into a tissue or organ, but many exceptions occur. Some of the common shapes are

1. Roughly hexagonal plates (squamous epithelium)
2. Roughly cuboidal (epithelium of glands and ducts)
3. Roughly hexagonal cylinders (columnar epithelium)
4. Spherical (many ova)
5. Dendritic (nerve cells)
6. Aciculate (muscle cells)
7. Doughnut-shaped (pore cells of Porifera)
8. Amoeboid (amoebae and amoebocytes)
9. Biconcave discs (red blood cells of Mammalia)
10. Hollow bulbs (flame cells)
11. Hollow cylinders (gullet of Nectonematoidea)
12. Spheres with a cone-shaped collar (choanocytes and Choanoflagellata)
13. Intermediates and all conceivable combinations

2. Cell Components

The usual cell consists of a mass of cytoplasm surrounding a nucleus and bounded by a cell membrane, but this is not an adequate summation of the structure or contents of a cell. It is not intended here to describe the microscopic structure of any cells but to show their diversity, and for this purpose the various structures, contents, and products of cells in general are listed here. No cell includes all of these, and the varying combinations are endless among the cells of animals and protozoans.

The organized structures of cells may consist of either living protoplasm or nonliving secretions of protoplasm. The former are called organelles and the latter cell products.

a. Organelles (Living Parts of Protoplasm)

The "structures" formed in cells are of almost endless diversity. This is suggested by the following list, and a few of these organelles are discussed below: plasma membrane (plasmalemma), centrioles, endoplasmic reticulum, Golgi bodies, lysosomes, microtubules, mitochondria, myofibrils, Nissl substance, plastids, ribosomes, vacuoles, cilia, haptonema, pseudopodia, brush borders, cytopharynx, cytopyge, polar capsules, pigment, trichocysts, nucleus, and nuclear organelles such as nuclear envelope, chromatin granules (or chromosomes), and nucleolus.

b. Cilia and Flagella

Many cells, both protozoan and metazoan, have the surface cytoplasm extended into slender vibratile processes called cilia or flagella (or derivatives of these). Cilia are usually short and numerous on a single cell. Flagella are long and usually present singly or as a pair on each cell. Some other hair-like organelles present the typical ciliary structure of two central fibrils surrounded by a ring of nine fibrils. As listed by Sleigh (1962), these include:

1. Neck between rods and cones in vertebrate eyes
2. Internal flagellum of eyespot in a phytoflagellate
3. Scolopale organs of s.Insecta
4. Plate organs of antenna of honeybee
5. Cnidocils of nematocyst in *Hydra*
6. Stalks of some peritrich Ciliata

Among the normal cilia and flagella one finds one of the few substantial uniformities of structure, occurring very widely. These consist of nine longitudinal fiber pairs in a circle around two central fibers.

There do seem to be cilium-like structures that do not have this structure (e.g., the microvilli of the brush border of many epithelial cells), but it is astonishing how little diversity occurs in these ubiquitous ciliary organelles. There have been a few cases of unusual ciliary structure in the older literature but usually forgotten. For example, the flagellum of some bacteria is said to have only the inner fibers (one or two). However, enough examples of unusual structure have been described in recent years to lead one to expect that a considerable diversity will eventually be known.

The nine sets of peripheral fibers (in reality these are microtubules) usually occur in pairs. In the ciliate *Epistylis anastatica* they are single; in the flagellae of *Trichonympha* they are in triads. Lentz (1966) reports ciliary structures in sensory cells of *Hydra* with "more than the usual two fibers" in the center. In the crustacean *Astacus* the statocyst "hairs" are cilia with a 9 + 0 arrangement (a circle of nine with none in center). Among the gregarine protozoans, Prensier et al. (1980) report that in *Lecudina tuzetae* the tail of the microgamete is a flagellum of 6 + 0 pairs and in *Diplauxis hatti* the tail has a 3 + 0 pair arrangement (see also other diversity in the discussion of the Nematoda below.)

There is little doubt that much further diversity in this structure will be discovered, as ciliary structures are re-examined with modern equipment, but much diversity of other sorts is already well known. First in size — as cilia are always short in relation to cell diameter and flagella are always correspondingly long. Second, in quantity — cilia are always numerous and flagella rarely more than one or two per cell. (The exceptions are found in the Protozoa, where individuals in several orders of Flagellata may have from few to many long flagella; and in the isogametes of the foraminiferan *Discorbis* which all have three flagella.) Third, in mode of movement — cilia move in one plane beating in one direction (sometimes reversible), whereas flagella generally move in a corkscrew manner. (The flagellum may extend back along the protozoan body to form an organelle that is called an undulating membrane.) Fourth, there may be multiple ciliary structures: (1) the stalks of some Ciliata formed from modified cilia; (2) rows of cilia beating synchronously or in sequence forming *velums* in Ciliata and in many aquatic larvae; (3) the cilia in the rows completely fused, as in many Ciliata, resulting in a *membranelle* or a *ciliary undulating membrane,* which differ in having double or single rows of cilia; (4) a plate made of fused cilia forming the *ctenes* that occur in eight rows on the surface of Ctenophora; (5) *cirri* consisting of a cone of fused cilia, as in *Euplotes;* (6) *rigid cilia* said to occur at the anterior end of some larvae of Bryozoa; (7) macrocilia in Ctenophora, which consist of 2000 to 3000 shafts fused, each with the usual 9 + 2 pattern; (8) in Rotifera, a *corona* of cilia around the mouth, sometimes with these cilia compounded into cirri, membranelles, or styles; and (9) in sensory organs of many animals, modified cilia forming rods or fibers whose function is unknown and unguessed.

Ciliary structures also vary in the type of movement, which can be

1.   Funnel-shaped circling (apparently primitive uncontrolled)
2.   Rhythmic forward beat and relaxed recovery stroke (in one plane but sometimes reversible)
3.   Spiral wave from the base to the tip
4.   Spiral wave from the tip to the base
5.   Wave of undulating membrane
6.   Simultaneous beating of cilia in membranelles

In functional arrangement there are several types of ciliary structures:

1.   Isolated flagellum, beating continuously: choanocyte and solenocyte
2.   Isolated or paired flagella, beating at random

3. Isolated or paired flagella, beating in coordination with others
4. Areas of cilia, beating in coordination: epidermal cells and flame cells
5. Cirri, tufts of fused cilia, movable in any direction
6. Undulating membranes of cilia, composed of a row of cilia more or less united; usually longer than a membranelle
7. Membranelle, a double lamella of cilia completely fused; usually shorter than an undulating membrane
8. Flagellar undulating membrane, an expanded flagellum lying along the body of the protozoan

Available information on the occurrence of cilia and flagella is tabulated in Table 13.

As cell organelles, cilia or flagella can occur on almost any cells, but there are regions, organs, and cells which do not have either, and some groups of animals are almost devoid of both. Cilia or flagella commonly occur:

1. On exterior surfaces, for locomotion or feeding currents
2. On surfaces that line body cavities
3. Inside hollow organs, especially where materials are to be moved
4. Inside hollow cells, such as flame cells and solenocytes
5. On motile gametes, most spermatozoa but rarely ova
6. In ducts, for producing current
7. In sense organs, where they are usually nonvibratile and may serve tactile or other functions

Among the body regions and organs which are not usually ciliated are the following:

1. Epidermis that secretes a cuticle or exoskeleton
2. Unusual epidermis, partly syncytial, in flukes and Cestoda
3. External surfaces of animals with dry "skin", where cilia could not operate
4. Many cell types: muscle, nerve, and amoeboid cells

One must note that the word cilia (or sometimes alternatively the word flagella) may be used in a general sense to refer to all such structures, long or short, simple or compound. The context must show whether the broad or the restricted meaning is intended.

In many books it has been noted that cilia (in the broad sense) do not occur in the two phyla Nematoda and Arthropoda. (Together these total over 85% of the animal kingdom!) The supposedly related groups Gordioidea and Kinorhyncha and Tardigrada and Pentastomida were usually supposed to share this feature with the two major phyla. It is sometimes recognized that all four of these minor groups do have internal cilia or ciliary structures, so the two major groups are then restored to their unique position. Most recently it has been recognized that Nematoda also have some internal ciliary structures, and the Arthropoda have both cilia and ciliary "fibers" in several groups, as well as some spermatozoan tails. These groups are discussed below.

The first edition of one excellent invertebrate textbook (now in its fourth edition) wrote of the Kinorhyncha that they "differ from both rotifers and gastrotrichs in their complete lack of cilia". In the second edition, this was corrected to read "in their lack of external cilia", because it was recognized that the excretory system had flame bulbs and that there were cilia in a pair of renal glands, not to mention a flagellar spermatozoan tail.

The Nematoda have no flame cells, and their spermatozoa are said to have no tail.

Table 13

OCCURRENCE OF CILIA AND FLAGELLA

	Cilia		Flagella	
	External	Internal	External	Internal
Protozoa	L, A		A, S	
Porifera	0		E, L, A, S	L, A
Mesozoa	L, A	0	0	0
Monoblastozoa	L, A	A	0	0
Coelenterata	L		A, S	A
Ctenophora	L, A	A	0	0
Gnathostomuloidea	E, A		S	0
Platyhelminthes	L, A	A	S	0
Rhynchocoela	L, A	L, A	S	0
Acanthocephala	A	A	0	0
Rotifera	A	A	S	0
Gastrotricha	A	A	0	A
Kinorhyncha		A	S	
Nematoda	0	0	0	0
Gordioidea	0	0	0	0
Priapuloidea		A	0	A
Calyssozoa	L, A	A	0	0
Bryozoa	L, A	A	S	0
Phoronida	L, A	A		0
Brachiopoda	L, A	A		0
Mollusca	L, A	A	S	0
Sipunculoidea	L, A	A		0
Echiuroidea	L, A	A		0
Tardigrada	0	0	0	0
Myzostomida	L, A	A	0	0
Pentastomida	0	0	0	0
Annelida	E, L, A	A	S	0
Dinophiloidea	A	A	S	0
Onychophora		A		0
Arthropoda	0	0	S	0
Chaetognatha	A	A		0
Pogonophora	L, A	A	S	0
Echinodermata	L, A	A		0
Pterobranchia	L, A	A	0	0
Enteropneusta	L, A	A	S	0
Tunicata	A	A		0
Cephalochordata	L, A	A		A
Vertebrata	L	A	S	0

Note: A, adult; E, embryo; L, larva; S, spermatozoa (flagellated spermatozoa occur in nearly all groups except those in which they are denied by an 0, meaning none at any state).

The electron microscope has revealed ciliary structures in sense organs of many species. Among these ciliary fibers there are no basal bodies and the microtubule pair numbers are highly unusual: $10 + 1$ to $10 + 4$, $9 + 4$, $8 + 4$, $8 + 2$, $5 + 0$ to $10 + 2$, and 20 single tubules arranged randomly. A supposed discovery of cilia in the intestine is now known to be an error; the structures are microvilli.

The Gordioidea are supposedly closely related to the Nematoda. They have no excretory organs and few sense organs. We know of no records of ciliary structures among the few species, but it is likely that they occur as in the Nematoda.

The Tardigrada are confidently reported to have no ciliary structures, as are the

Pentastomida. They both have a few sense organs that may show ciliary structures, but so far these small groups have not shown any cilia. Spermatozoa are not mentioned in this regard.

Arthropoda were long thought to have no cilia at all. The first report of cilia uncovered for this book was in the Crustacea, where one writer described a ciliated epithelium as if it was normal and well known. Then it became known that some spermatozoa had flagellar tails. Some statocyst "hairs" were determined to be cilia, and then fibrils in several types of sense organs in all groups were found to be ciliary. Many spermatozoa in Insecta have flagellar tails, and it is now necessary to summarize the presence of cilia in Arthropoda as probably restricted to sense organs and spermatozoa, although the group is obviously capable of producing cilia if they are needed.

Thus there is no longer much to be gained by citing the groups that lack cilia. If such groups do in fact exist, it is accidental, due to a combination of cuticle on the outside and lack of flame cells and nephridia on the inside. Even then there is usually doubt about the spermatozoa, in which any tail is always a flagellum.

In addition, of course, cilia are frequently arranged in grooves, bands, trochi, velums, etc., in both Protozoa and Metazoa, especially on larvae.

Cilia, flagella, and their compound organelles serve a wide variety of functions: locomotion by swimming or creeping (both in Protozoa and Metazoa: Rotifera, Turbellaria, and most spermatozoa), or by "walking" on cirri (as in some Ciliata); food capture (in both subkingdoms); production of water currents around the organism; flow of fluids in ducts and cavities; support (stalks of Ciliata); movement of solid objects, either food or unwanted detritus; as fibers, presumably of supportive nature (in the eye of Insecta and Aves); sensing, at least as tactile structures but also present in many sense organs; and no doubt others.

c. Nucleus

The nucleus is the most prominent organelle of most cells. It is considered the control center for all metabolism and the source of the hereditary information. Nuclei differ markedly in at least these ways:

1. Whether there is one, two, or many per cell (or none)
2. Whether they are moved about in the cell or remain fixed
3. The number of chromosomes (or amount of chromatin)
4. The actual genes on the chromosomes
5. The number and condition of nucleoli
6. Whether it is ever involved in karyogamy, or nuclear fusion
7. It may be penetrated by other structures such as a skeleton

Although interesting differences occur among nuclei, there is little comparative data for the various groups. Some of the differences are found in the nuclear part of cell division, mitosis and karyokinesis, described in a later paragraph. In Ciliata there are always two types of nuclei (not alike in structure or function), and in other classes there are also species with multiple nuclei. The nuclear components are variously listed by different authors but consist primarily of nucleoli and chromatin in a nucleoplasm or nuclear sap. These occur in various forms and combinations.

d. Cell Inclusions

A variety of unexpected things exist inside cells, most of which are neither part of the living tissue nor formal secretions of it. Some of these are called "inclusions", and others have not been grouped under any general term:

1. Crystals of guanine (in iridocytes of Pisces)
2. Stored materials: (a) fat, as energy reserve, in Insecta and Mammalia, (b) nitrogenous wastes for recycling, especially in Insecta
3. Water, especially in Protozoa
5. Intracellular parasites: (a) Nematoda, (b) Protozoa (some even intranuclear), (c) microorganisms such as Bacteria
6. Intracellular symbionts: (a) zooxanthellae (flagellates inside Foraminifera and Radiolaria), and (b) zoochlorellae (algae in s.Ciliata and cells of Coelenterata)
7. Tracheoles, in some Insecta
8. Blood capillaries, in pinnule cells of Pogonophora
9. Cells, within the axoblasts of Mesozoa, which will become new larvae
10. An extra nucleus, both fertilized, in gynandromorphs of the silkworm

e. Cell Secretions

Cells produce materials for a variety of purposes. For example:

1. Materials to aid in a cell or individual function, such as locomotion (mucus), digestion (enzymes), attachment (adhesives)
2. Wastes, such as water, ammonia, carbon dioxide
3. Defensive materials (poisons, trichocysts, nematocysts)
4. Chemical messengers (hormones and pheromones)

Most of these are given off by the cell, which is what is usually understood by the word secretion. However, the same processes of elaboration may result in materials that remain part of or associated with the cell, and these cannot be excluded here. These latter include:

1. Substances to form strengthening objects (spicules, skeletons)
2. Defensive coverings (tests, loricas, shells)
3. Structures useful to the multicellular individual (cuticles, skeletons, spicules, setae)
4. Stored nutrients (yolk, fat)
5. Pigments

A few of these features can be discussed comparatively to show that there is endless diversity even beyond the selective presence suggested above.

f. Spicules

These are of great variety and diverse composition in Porifera. They may occur also in Anthozoa, Brachiopoda, and Echinodermata, always in mesenchyme or connective tissues, where they are secreted by one or a few amoebocytes. Especially in the Porifera they are extremely diverse in shape, being aciculate, triaxon, star-, anchor-, C-, and dumbbell-shaped, and a variety of intermediates. These are discussed in Chapter 18, where their chemical compositions are also listed.

g. Setae

Setae are said to be present in Echiuroidea, Annelida, Arthropoda, and Onychophora. In all of these, they are said to be each produced by a single cell, perhaps with some assistance from surrounding cells. They are not always clearly distinct from some spines in other phyla. These are cited in Chapter 18, where some of the numerous shapes of setae in Annelida and Arthropoda are illustrated.

h. Outer Coverings

Many terms have been loosely applied to the hard external coverings of animals. Some of these can be distinguished in some cases, but no fixed definitions or classification of the forms has been possible. The word *pellicle* is applied to a secretion of the plasmalemma; it is not particularly hard. More definite hard coverings are variously termed tests, loricas, thecae, or shells, all of which are loosely attached to the cell. In shape these coverings are endlessly diverse. Only a few special shapes are distinctive of groups: chambers in a spiral are common in Foraminifera; serially chambered forms occur in Dinoflagellata; spheres are common in Heliozoa, but rare elsewhere; flask-shapes are common in Tintinnida, but occur elsewhere also; crown- or bell-shaped forms are common in Radiolaria. Although there may be protoplasm outside of these cases, they are often treated as external secretions.

Tests are found in the order Testacea in the Sarcodina. They are covering sacs usually with one opening for the pseudopodia and are made of chitin or pseudochitin sometimes thickened with foreign bodies or siliceous scales formed internally.

Loricas are flask- or vase-like coverings formed in some Ciliata and some Flagellata. In the former is the group Tintinnida, where they are chitinous, often with foreign materials. In the flagellate subclass Phytomastigina there may be a lorica of cellulose, but in others this covering may be little more than a cellulose membrane.

Theca is the term sometimes used in Dinoflagellata for the cellulose envelope, which is elsewhere called a lorica.

Shells occur especially in Foraminifera, where they are calcareous or siliceous and may have inclusions such as sponge spicules. (This word and also test are also used in Dinoflagellata, but because these are of cellulose the term lorica seems preferable.)

i. Skeletons

These may be partly internal as in Radiolaria, simple, or highly complex but usually basically spherical. They may consist of silica or strontium sulfate. This term is sometimes used to include all the hard coverings of Protozoa, the types being not always distinguishable.

j. Trichocysts

These are "explosive" organelles in the ectoplasm, which can be stimulated to extrude long filaments for anchoring or capturing food. They are common in Ciliata but occur also in Dinoflagellata.

k. Nematocysts

These are formed in specialized cells (cnidoblasts or nematocytes) of most Coelenterata and possibly a few Ctenophora. They are also clearly described in two genera of Dinoflagellata (*Nematodinium* and *Polykrikos*). Although the latter resemble some coelenterate nematocysts, they are formed by a tiny area of cell surface, whereas in Coelenterata each is formed by an entire cell (cnidoblast). It seems inappropriate to refer to all these by the same term.

D. Cell Oddities

In addition to diversities already cited, there are developments in a few cells that seem highly unexpected. For example:

1.   Hollow cells (excretory funnels of some Annelids)
2.   Tubular cells (oesophagus of Nectonematoidea)
3.   Protoplasmic bridges (strands between cells across the incurrent canals in Porifera)

4.   Nematocyst darts (Coelenterata)
5.   Cells within cells (germinal cells of Mesozoa)
6.   Cells containing a complete loop of a blood capillary (Pogonophora, tentacular villi)

E. Cell Functions

The functions performed by cells should be easy to list; they would be related to the common beliefs that the cell is the unit of structure and of function. As discussed in Chapter 1, the statements that cells are the fundamental units of all aspects of life are mostly sterile platitudes. They seemed to fit with ideas of evolution, but students have never gotten any real meaning from them. In reality, the functions of cells merge on the one hand with those of protoplasm and on the other with those of tissues and organs (and in the case of Protozoa, with those of whole individuals and even colonies).

In reality, if one tried to list the specific things that are done by cells, the list would be nearly endless. These things seem to segregate into three groups: (A) the things that nearly all cells do most of the time, such as metabolism of food; (B) the special things that certain specialized cells do, such as production of a certain substance by a gland cell; and (C) the things that cells do as part of tissues, organs, and individuals, such as response to stimulus, in which a single cell receiving a stimulus rarely accomplishes any final result.

Some of the common functions of the cells in these three categories are listed here:

The widespread general activities of cells

1.   Cell multiplication by division, mitosis
2.   Maintenance of the genome, for passing the genes to future generations of cells (and thus to individuals)
3.   Conversion of "food" materials into new protoplasm
4.   Excretion of waste products of metabolism

The specific functions of specialized cells

5.   Differentiation into new types, by embryonic cells and certain ones that retain such potencies
6.   Phagocytosis
7.   Secretion of specifc substances such as hormones, digestive enzymes, yolk, and silk
8.   Formation of spicules, bone, and other hard-parts
9.   Transport of materials (erythrocytes) or wastes (amoebocytes) or spermatozoa (also amoebocytes or synergids)
10.   Gametogenesis, meiotic division

The participation of cells in the more general activities of tissues and organs

11.   Response to stimulus
12.   Storage of fat or nitrogenous wastes
13.   Maintenance of turgor and thus body shape
14.   Contraction and other changes of shape, to produce movement, including locomotion
15.   Secretion in general, as of cuticle or saliva
16.   Producing light
17.   Participation in digestion and absorption

Most of these are discussed in later paragraphs and chapters. A few can be exemplified here, including phagocytosis, spicule formation, and transport by amoebocytes.

1. Phagocytosis

The engulfing of particles by cells is very common; it is accomplished by temporary cytoplasmic extensions. It is paralleled by *pinocytosis,*which is the taking in of droplets of liquid. Both of these are aspects of *endocytosis*, the engulfing activities by which materials are brought into cells.

The cells that engulf particles are known as *phagocytes:* they collect wastes, debris, and microorganisms. They may be amoebocytes free in the body fluid or in almost any tissue, or stationary in the walls of vessels, or as epithelial cells lining the digestive tract. They can form phagocytic organs in the pericardial spaces or lymphogenous organs in blood sinuses.

It is said that amoeboid phagocytes are found in the tissues of all metazoans, but the location of such cells in the body is reportedly diverse. They are reported in the blood of Oligochaeta, Crustacea (the corpuscles), Insecta (granular leukocytes), and Vertebrata (leukocytes) and in the lymph fluids of Aves and Mammalia. They may be in the coelom in Hirudinea (coelomic corpuscles) and in Echinodermata (coelomocytes). They may be in the digestive organs in Hydrozoa, Turbellaria, and Bivalvia. They may be in the reproductive system of Crustacea, where follicle cells may phagocytize the oocytes. They may occur among the microgloeal cells of the central nervous system. They are represented by the Kupffer cells of the liver, bone marrow, spleen, and lymph nodes in Mammalia. They may specialize in excretion under the name of athrocytes or nephrophagocytes. They may function in development, as in the metamorphic breakdown of tissues in Insecta and in the development of larval Amphibia.

Phagocytosis occurs, of course, in Protozoa, in some of which it is the feeding method. Besides the groups cited above, phagocytes are reported in Porifera, Rhynchochoela, Nematoda, Cephalopoda, and Tunicata, at least.

2. Spicule Formation

Amoebocytes in sponges give a view of the astonishing capabilities of single cells to form spicules. It is not intended to give here even a summary of the diversity of spicules, which may be calcareous, siliceous, or organic, nor to compare the formation of these three types. It will be enough to suggest the activities of and the cooperation between the individual cells, which in the Calcarea are called *scleroblasts*.

The calcareous spicules are formed of calcium carbonate in its calcite form, and this material is obtained by the cell (or the sponge) from the surrounding seawater. In the case of a simple needle-like spicule, the formation is described in Hyman (1940) thus: ''The spicule begins between the two nuclei . . . of a binucleate scleroblast probably arising by the incomplete division of an ordinary scleroblast. The calcium carbonate is believed to be laid down around an organic axial thread (which is located) between the two nuclei. (The latter) draw apart as the spicule lengthens until the cell separates into two.'' The two cells move along the spicule adding additional layers.

In more elaborate spicules with several radiating arms there may be several scleroblasts cooperating in the formation. In every case the resulting spicule is formed in the exact shape typical of that species. The idea of cooperation between cells is an intriguing one but without explanation. In some cases the exact duplication of angles may be due in part to the crystal structure of calcite, but this will not account for the many intricate forms consistently produced. A few of the forms attained are shown in Figure 17.

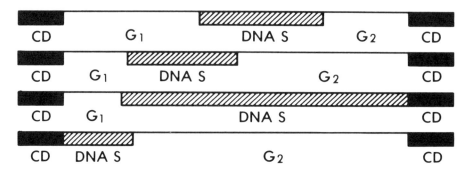

FIGURE 17.   The varying part of the cell cycle in which DNA is synthesized in various Protozoa. CD is the period of cell division; G₁ and G₂ are periods before and after DNA synthesis (Gap); DNA S is the period of DNA synthesis. (Adapted from Sleigh, 1923.)

3. Transport by Cells

Most motile cells can be considered to be transporting materials, and these materials are highly diverse. For example:

Materials needed elsewhere

1. Amoebocytes carrying food, in most animals
2. Erythrocytes carrying oxygen, in Vertebrata

Wastes being removed

3. Nephrocytes, in Insecta and Tunicata
4. Coelomocytes, in Echinodermata

Cell products

5. Amphidisk spicules being transported for incorporation into a developing gemmule, in Porifera
6. Buds being carried by phorocytes on the surface of Thaliacea

Other cells

7. Spermatozoa carried from exterior to ovum by amoebocytes, in Porifera
8. Spermatozoa carried to ovum by synergid cell, in Chaetognatha

4. Cell Division

A great deal is known about cell division and genetics of animals, but only of *certain* animals. No real basis is available for comparing these processes from phylum to phylum. There is diversity, and some of this is indicated below, but the extent of diversity is not yet known. When there appears to be no diversity, one must recognize that the sample is probably inadequate to justify any definite statement to that effect.

A common but not universal feature of cells is the ability to divide. It is usually implied that cell division is always much the same, involving a process called *mitosis,* in which the genetic material which has been duplicated is divided between the two daughter cells.

"The phenomena of cell reproduction, while showing innumerable minor variations, present the same general features of spindle formation, chromosome movement and division, and participation of kinetic elements or centrioles through all of the great phyla of animals'' (Andrew, 1959).

There are, however, both several varieties of mitosis and instances (cells) in which division is amitotic. *Amitosis* is any division in which mitotic activity (spindle formation and separation of duplicated chromosomes) does not occur. It is sometimes implicit that mitosis can be contrasted with a form of cell division called *meiosis*. However, meiosis is the process of formation of gametes, and although its two divisions result in reduction in the number of chromosomes (from two sets to one), the actual division of the cell at each stage is mitotic in nature. These two can be realistically contrasted only if mitosis is defined as that process of nuclear division which produces two new cells both with chromosome complements identical to the original cell.

Nonmitotic or unusual division of cells is more common than one would conclude from Andrew's statement. For example, amitosis may occur in some cells of the following:

1. Vertebrate decidua
2. Embryonic envelopes
3. Periblast of meroblastic ova
4. Accessory nutritive cells connected with the developing germ cells
5. Mammalian cartilage
6. Ciliate and suctorian macronuclei
7. Pathological tissue

Although meiosis is usually thought of as very distinct from mitosis and could be added to this list, there really is no such thing as meiotic division, merely a meiotic pattern of mitotic divisions.

In spite of these, mitosis is nearly universal in animal cells, but ''the mitotic cycle is not so fixed or so invariable as people imagine . . . there are a large number of different mechanisms of mitosis'' (Kerkut, 1965). Among these processes of mitotic cell division are those called:

1. Achromosomal mitosis — cleavage in the total absence of a nucleus
2. Anastral mitosis — mitosis without formation of asters
3. Catenar mitosis — with a large number of asters but not spindles
4. Cryptomitosis — mitosis in which chromosomes are not evident on the achromatic figure
5. Entomitosis — division of the chromosomes within the bounds of the nucleus, thus resulting in polyploidy
6. Eumitosis — mitosis involving a complete series of mitotic figures
7. Haplomitosis — in euglenoid Protozoa, mitosis in which the entire endosome acts as a centriole
8. Heterotype mitosis — a form of reduction division
9. Homotype mitosis — the normal form of mitosis
10. Irregular mitosis — abnormal cleavage, such as that of non-nucleated ova
11. Meiotic mitosis — same as meiosis
12. Mesomitosis — mitosis in which the endosome furnishes the chromosomes but not the centriole
13. Metamitosis — complete mitosis
14. Monocentric mitosis — the form in which the chromosomes are doubled but remain in a single nucleus
15. Multipolar mitosis — mitosis involving several spindles and several centrosomes; in some Protozoa and some fish egg syncytia

16. Paramitosis — mitosis with abnormal chromosome behavior, especially in Protozoa
17. Promitosis — mitosis in which both centrioles and chromosomes come from the endosome
18. Somatic mitosis — mitosis of same cells as distinguished from reproductive cells

The occurrence of these processes, although ranging from Protozoa to Vertebrata, is not sufficiently available for tabulation.

It is sometimes implied that all cells can divide. This is a gross exaggeration. Examples of cells which cannot or do not divide are

1. Gametes, in all groups
2. Nerve cells in Vertebrata
3. Erythrocytes in Mammalia
4. All cells in adults of the phyla with eutely (Acanthocephala, Rotifera, Gastrotricha, Kinorhyncha, Priapuloidea, Nematoda, Gordioidea, Tardigrada)

It is sometimes stated that "cells typically tend to divide into equal parts", but there are many exceptions. For example:

1. In oogenesis, two successive divisions each normally produce by an unequal division a polar body (cell) which is very much smaller than the ovum
2. Fertilized eggs which cleave transversely, rather than meridionally (through the poles) at the first cleavage, may divide equally (through the equator) or unequally (above the equator or below it)
3. Later cleavages may also be unequal
4. Budding of protozoan cells

A functional diversity that has recently become available for comparative study is the varying amount of time in the life cycle of protozoans during which synthesis of DNA occurs.

When the cell requires additional DNA to duplicate its chromosomes, this synthesis takes place at a particular time in the cell cycle, this time varying with the species. This can be diagrammed using the period of nuclear division as a starting point. In Figure 17 it can be seen that the diversity in this timing sequence is as great as is possible: either immediately preceding division, immediately following it, or occurring somewhere between.

5. Cell Motility

There are three rather different forms of motility of animal cells. The first is the imperceptibly slow movement of a cell or a group of cells with respect to neighboring cells or tissues. These are the *morphogenetic movements*, common in developing embryos and occurring also in restorative realignments at any age. These movements are not called locomotion, partly because of their slowness and partly because the movement may not be entirely from internal actions.

The second type is passive but more rapid: *floating* in body fluids that are in movement. This is also not locomotion by the cells because of their lack of active propulsion. Examples are blood corpuscles, coelomocytes, etc.

The third type occurs only in single cells and is *locomotion*. These propulsive mechanisms occur in animal cells:

1. Ciliary propulsion (some Protozoa)

2. Flagellar propulsion (some Protozoa, spermatozoa in most phyla)
3. Amoeboid movement (some Protozoa, spermatozoa or ova in a few groups, amoebocytes in many animals, including *diapedesis*, the process by which the white cell squeezes through the wall of a capillary)

6. Protozoan Cell Functions

Some protozoologists emphasize that Protozoa are complete organisms, not merely cells. This is true, but protozoans are also cells and show the basic features of cells. These include the general functions necessary to all protoplasm, which are present by definition, as we say that all living things are composed of protoplasm, and that protoplasm performs all these basic functions, and that Protozoa are living organisms. Ergo, Protozoa perform the basic functions. But *in comparison to* "the higher animals", they perform them through simple processes and to a limited extent. Protozoa are complete organisms, but they also are far simpler than Metazoa. It is often true also that the protozoan cell is more elaborate and performs more functions than most individual Metazoan cells, chiefly because there is no division of labor.

The behavior of protozoan cells, as that of whole animals, is treated with that of Metazoa in the section on behavior (Part V).

F. Cell Types

Cells illustrate well the dual viewpoint of unity and diversity. Basic cell types are found throughout the animal kingdom, but many unique cell types occur in almost every animal group, performing unique functions or variations of widespread functions.

The common types of cell, those that occur widely in animals or are well known in a few groups, include:

Solitary cells

1. Single-cell organisms (at any stage of life cycle)
2. Agametes
3. Gametes

Tissue cells

4. Epithelial cells
5. Epidermal cells
6. Muscle cells
7. Connective tissue cells
8. Nerve cells
9. Gland cells
10. Storage cells
11. Phagocytes
12. Amoebocytes (including leukocytes, lymphocytes, coelomocytes, etc.)
13. Blastomeres

Single-celled organs

14. Glandular cells
15. Sensory cells
16. Pigment cells

It will be seen, however, that these are simply general names for classes of cells, usually functional classes. For example, the epidermal or glandular cells of different organisms are often very different in structure, location, etc.   Many cell types are very widely distributed among the phyla and some are surely found in all (e.g., gametes, epithelial, muscle, nerve, etc.). This is hard to demonstrate for two reasons: the same name (amoebocyte, corpuscle) may be applied to cells with different functions in different groups or a name may be so general as to denote only its major function and not any peculiarities of its form or activity (as in coelomocytes).

There are no doubt increasing numbers of cell types as one goes up the scale to the higher animals, but even this is difficult to demonstrate. In the Porifera ten cell types are listed, with one of these (amoebocytes) occurring as five subtypes. In Coelenterata about 6 specialized types are added, but in most groups no list is available, and the cells are usually referred to by class names (e.g., epithelial, muscle, nerve, gland cells) without communication of any differences.

There certainly are similarities here among all groups, but the amount of any diversity is hidden by terminology and by interest in general function rather than in any peculiarities of structure.

1. Unique Cells

Many cells, in invertebrates especially, are highly unusual and may even identify a particular group of animals. They may be so distinct from all other cells as to amount to a special cell class, in which they stand alone. Among these the following may be cited:

In Porifera

1. Pinacocytes — contractile epidermal cells
2. Porocytes — tubular cells with a central canal, pore cells
3. Thesocytes — amoeboid food storage cells
4. Scleroblasts — spicule-secreting cells
5. Choanocytes — flagellated collar cells
6. Archaeocytes — undifferentiated embryonic cells for regeneration

In Mesozoa

7. Cells-within-a-cell — a "germinal" cell which contains two free nuclear cells and one axoblast-like germ cell

In Coelenterata

8. Epitheliomuscular — long-branched supporting cells
9. Glandulomuscular — combination gland and muscle cells
10. Cnidocytes or nematocytes — cells with stinging nematocysts, of many types
11. Flagellated epithelial cells — in epidermis and gastrodermis
12. Palpocils — epidermal sensory nerve cells
13. Phorocytes — nurse cells containing the egg and later the embryo

In Ctenophora

14. Colloblasts — lasso cells

In Platyhelminthes

15. Rhabdite gland cells — secreting rod-like structures in the epidermis

16. Flame cells — hollow excretory cells
17. Granular clubs — gastrodermal gland cells
18. Rheoreceptive cells — each with many sensory bristles, sensitive to water currents
19. Athrocytes — large cells wrapped around excretory tubes and apparently excretory in function

In Rhynchocoela

20. Packet-gland cells — clusters with a common gland duct
21. Spindle cells — fusiform amoebocytes in the blood

In Nectonematoidea (Gordioidea)

22. Tubular cell — forming the oesophagus

In Priapuloidea

23. Solenocytes — hollow excretory cells with an "internal" flagellum

In Nematoda

24. Renettes — very large cells, sometimes paired, forming complete excretory systems
25. Pseudocoelocytes — branched or stellate mesenchymal cells

In Annelida

26. Eleocytes — free chloragogen cells in the coelom*

In Insecta

27. Nephrocytes — binucleate cells free in the haemocoel, probably waste storage cells
28. Oenocytes — enzyme-secreting cells in the haemocoel
29. Duct cells — hollow, forming the ducts of some labial glands
30. Thigmocytes — blood cells that aid in coagulation

In Pogonophora

31. Pinnules — much elongated epidermal cells forming a fringe row along each tentacle and each containing a blood capillary loop

In Vertebrata

32. Mormyomasts — electroreceptors in lateral line of fishes
33. Chloride cells — epithelial cells of fishes, excreting chlorides
34. Biconcave erythrocytes — enucleate red blood corpuscles of mammals

A few of these types actually consist of numerous subtypes, so that the diversity is

---

* Often spelled chlorogogen or chloragogue. This word is from the Greek *chloros* and *agoge*. In uniting these the chloros is reduced to chlor- and a connective -o- is not needed. Thus chloragogen is the correct form, as shown in major dictionaries and encyclopedias as well as in most works on annelids. (The form chloragogue is also used.)

even greater than shown. For example, there are 16 or so kinds of nematocysts, several types of flame cells, and a great diversity of erythrocytes.

2. Universality of Cell Types

If one uses sufficiently general terms and definitions, it is possible to show that some sorts of cells are nearly universal in animals. If, for example, one cites as "muscles" all contractile cells, it would then be correct to say that virtually all animals have cells of the muscle type. In reality, contractile cells are of several very different types, and even among unquestioned muscle cells in the strictest sense there are diversities of several sorts as will be shown in the section on movement in Chapter 20.

Nearly all animals have some amoeboid cells that are motile. In general they are similar in structure, but they may be diverse in function. Some produce skeletons, some are phagocytic, some transport materials in the body, some are capable of differentiation into other cell types for replacement. Thus, although they are among the least specialized cells of the animal body, there can be substantial diversity.

Epithelial cells by their nature form an enclosing membrane, but they may differ strikingly in cell shape. They may be elongate columnar cells, flattened and thin plate-like cells tending to be hexagonal in shape, referred to as squamous, or of an intermediate shape called cuboidal. In Cestoda and Trematoda, the epidermal cells are unusual, being greatly elongate with the nuclei at their inner end buried in mesenchyme and their outer cytoplasm broadly joined in a syncytium.

3. Gametes, Zygotes, and Blastomeres

In listing either cell or tissue types in animals, it is generally forgotten that some of the most widespread cell types in animals are (1) the ova, (2) the flagellate spermatozoa, (3) the zygotes resulting from fertilization or activation, and (4) the blastomeres which result from the early divisions of the zygote.

The ova are visually more uniform than most cell types, but their genic contents are, of course, endlessly diverse. Spermatozoa are cited along with ova, although they are not nearly so common because of widespread parthenogenesis. Gametes are herein considered to be fragments of the parent, not new individuals. Their diversity is discussed under "Gametes" in Chapter 3.

The word zygote is usually used loosely enough to cover two sorts of new individuals: (1) the product of the fusion of two gametes in fertilization and (2) the product of activation of a parthenogenetic ovum. The latter is properly called an apozygote. All animals produced sexually (either bi- or unisexually) have this type of cell as the beginning stage of their life.

Blastomeres are the cells formed by cleavage of a zygote. They are visibly much alike, even in very different animals. Blastomeres are almost ubiquitous, occurring in all animals formed (1) from a zygote produced by fertilization of an ovum, (2) from an apozygote produced by activation of an ovum without fertilization, and (3) from an isolated blastomere produced by polyembryony. Only animals that are entirely a-sexual are completely without this type of cell.

One must remember that in every species there is unique potentiality in all four of these widespread cell types that will produce all the tissues of the body of that particular species.

REFERENCES

Andrew, W., *Textbook of Comparative Histology*, Oxford University Press, New York, 1959.

Grell, K. G., *Protozoology*, Springer-Verlag, Berlin, 1973.

Hyman, L. H., *The Invertebrates*, Vol. 1, McGraw-Hill, New York, 1940.

Kerkut, G. A., *Implications of Evolution*, Pergamon Press, New York, 1965.

Kudo, R. R., *Protozoology*, 5th ed., Charles C Thomas, Springfield, Ill., 1966.

Lentz, T. L., *The Cell Biology of Hydra*, W. B. Saunders, Philadelphia, 1966.

Prensier, G., Vivier, E., Goldstein, S., and Schrevel, J., Motile flagellum with a "3 + 0" ultrastructure, *Science*, 207, 1493, 1980.

Satir, P., How cilia move, *Sci. Am.*, 231(4), 44, 1974.

Seifriz, W., *Protoplasm*, McGraw-Hill, New York, 1936.

Sleigh, M. A., *Biology of Cilia and Flagella*, Pergamon Press, Oxford, 1962.

Sleigh, M., *The Biology of Protozoa*, American Elsevier, New York, 1973.

Wilson, E. B., *The Cell in Development and Heredity*, 3rd ed., Macmillan, New York, 1953.

Chapter 11

TISSUES

TABLE OF CONTENTS

I. Cells in Aggregation 236

II. Tissues 236
    A. Definition 236
    B. Embryonic Tissues 237
    C. Larval Tissues 237
    D. Adult Tissues 238
        1. Perspective 238
        2. Structure and Function of Tissues 239
            a. Connective Tissue 240
            b. Muscle Tissue 240
            c. Blood 241
            d. Chloragogen Tissue 241
        3. Syncytial Tissues 243
        4. Number of Basic Tissue Layers 244

III. Tissue Products 245

References 246

I. CELLS IN AGGREGATION

Cells do not usually exist in isolation. In only two situations do they occur as separate entities, not attached to neighboring cells nor in body fluids. These are the solitary Protozoa, such as an *Amoeba* or a *Paramecium,* and the reproductive bodies (gametes, agametes, and zygotes). In all other circumstances cells are associated with other cells in tissues and organs or in body fluids.

Many cells are combined into *organs,* each of which is a group of cells, sometimes also including materials or structures produced by them. Most organs consist of several kinds of cells, and they are then described as being composed of various tissues. The tissues serve different functions that contribute to the activity of that organ. From this viewpoint, the word *tissue* refers to the type of cells, e.g., nervous tissue or connective tissue; the cells of some tissues are very similar in the animals of different groups. This usage of the term tissue, as a type of cell similar in structure and function, is now widespread in textbooks.

In the days of the rise of comparative anatomy and the blossoming of the field of cytology, which then meant merely the study of cells, it was seen that in addition to the functional union of cells into organs, they sometimes were present in large formless masses or sheets that could scarcely be called organs. These also were called tissues — cells organized into functioning masses that did not quite qualify as organs. There is thus, at the present time, a duality of this term that has sometimes been even further confused by the use of the word tissue for the germ layers of the embryo.

It is possible that the first of these usages, as a type of cell in an organ, is replacing the second in current books, but it seems to be necessary here to deal directly with the groups of similar cells that function together as tissues that are not clearly organs or parts of organs. Therefore this type of tissue is discussed as a separate level of integration between the cell and the organ, or between the cell and the individual. The tissues included here are epidermis, blood, chloragogen tissue, and such connective and muscle tissue as do not form parts of organs.

It must be emphasized that there is no sharp distinction between any of these terms or their definitions. Single cells may be part of either an organ, a tissue, or both. The organ may be no more than a single cell. The tissue may be a separately operating mass of cells not circumscribed as an organ. Thus, a functioning structure may be (1) a single cell, or (2) a functioning group of similar cells (a tissue), or (3) a circumscribed mass consisting of several types of tissues (an organ).

II. TISSUES

A. Definition

Tissues are functional groups of cells in which one particular type of cell or fiber predominates; the masses are usually without fixed form or composition and consist of cells (or syncytia) with cell products and the surrounding tissue fluids. Usually the tissues are organized into organs and organ systems. Physiologically a tissue may be looked upon as a region of specialized metabolism.

In reality there is no logical way to separate tissues from single cells, if the latter perform a complete function comparable to that of a tissue. It is said that muscle tissue stores glycogen, yet in reality it is all stored inside the individual cells. Many secretory cells are scattered among other cells and do not form a compact tissue; they operate as independent cells. Many organs are described as consisting of various tissues, but some are so simple as to consist of cells of only one tissue, and these cells may be so reduced in number as to be single-celled organs. Thus, tissues are not really distinguishable from cells on the one hand or from organs on the other.

Because isolated tissues are not circumscribed like organs and are therefore less definite, it is not usually possible to deal with them comparatively to the extent one can with cells or organs. However, tissues occur throughout the life history, and some features of them can be compared. In general three developmental periods are involved, thus:

1. Embryonic tissues — from the first cleavage, which starts the formation of the blastoderm, to the completion of the formation of the primary germ layers
2. Larval tissues — the primary germ layers and any tissues of the immature forms which do not last over into the adult
3. Adult tissues — those present after metamorphosis

B. Embryonic Tissues

There are layers of cells in early embryonic development, but they have generally not been called tissues:

1. Blastoderm — the cells formed by cleavage of the egg before differentiation of primary germ layers, may be a layer around a cavity or a solid mass of cells (see coeloblastula and stereoblastula in Chapter 5)
2. Chordamesoderm — in vertebrates, the mass of cells which will become both the notochord and the mesoderm
3. Coenoblast — same as Blastoderm
4. Ectoderm — in embryos of all animals except sponges, the outer layer after the first inner layer is formed
5. Ectomesoderm — mesoderm elements derived from ectoderm
6. Endoderm — the inner layer or mass that forms the archenteron
7. Endomesoderm — mesoderm elements derived from endoderm
8. Germplasm — tissue consisting of or destined to become the reproductive cells or gametes
9. Mesoblast — same as Mesoderm
10. Mesoderm — the intermediate layer formed from ectoderm or endoderm or both, or even from the blastoderm
11. Somatoplasm (soma) — all the tissues other than the germplasm
12. Trophoblast — same as Endoderm

All these terms are properly applied only to embryos, never to tissues of adult animals (except with reference to their development).

In spite of this list, there are only four important tissue layers in early embryos: blastoderm; its derivatives at the time of gastrulation, ectoderm and endoderm; and the derivative of these latter, either one or both, mesoderm. Ecto-, endo-, and mesoderm are often called the primary germ layers, but from the embryological viewpoint, ecto- and endoderm arise by differentiation from the blastoderm (thus secondary), and mesoderm forms from either ectoderm or endoderm or both, or even from the blastoderm itself. Thus, blastoderm is always the first germ layer, so there may all together be up to four embryonic layers.

In reality, all these germ layers are of somewhat different nature than the complex and permanent tissues of the adult. Their purpose is to differentiate into the many later tissues, and thus organs, rather than to perform a specific continuing function.

The many diversities in the functions, sequences, and potentialities of the germ layers were discussed in Part III ("Development of Individuals").

C. Larval Tissues

Tissues of larvae can be distinguished from tissues of adults only in two rather similar circumstances: (A) when the structure does not survive into the adult — a purely larval feature, and (B) when larval structures of adult type (such as a digestive tract) are broken down and replaced at metamorphosis, as during the pupal stage of Insecta. The former is treated in Chapter 12 under the heading of "Organs", because tissues probably never disappear entirely.

At metamorphosis, many animals merely produce new features rapidly and become adult. Many insects, however, enter a pupal stage in which nearly all tissues, internal and external, are broken down and replaced by new adult tissues which have already been developing separately inside the larva. Thus, in these animals, no adult organ develops directly from the corresponding organ of the larva, and indeed, there is no traceable continuity of tissues or even of cells. (This means only that there is no continuity through the larval tissues. It is sometimes possible to show the embryonic origin of an adult tissue back to early cleavage stages by experimentally manipulating the embryo.)

It is usually taken for granted that the tissues and organs of the adult are formed by a long process of development in which each can be traced back continuously to embryonic structures. In the vertebrates this is usually true, as, for example, the adult intestinal tract is a direct gradual development from the archenteron (primitive gut) of the gastrula. However, in the majority of animals the archenteron does not develop into the adult intestinal tract or any part of it. This perhaps startling statement is true only because the Insecta are 75% of the animal kingdom and most of them undergo a metamorphosis so drastic that virtually all larval organs disintegrate, including the digestive tract. Thus, the adult organs are formed anew, in the pupal stage, albeit from cells traceable to the early embryo. A variety of other animals also may replace some of their larval organs with new ones in the adult.

From this it would seem to follow that the functioning of adult and larval organs in any one species may not be the same. This is presumably what led one writer to state that the general principles underlying the relation of embryonic to adult function have yet to be enunciated.

In any case, the tissues of the larva are classified here with those of the adult, in spite of the fact that in trematodes and some insects they really are a sort of side issue that does not lead to the adult.

D. Adult Tissues
1. Perspective
As seen above, adult tissues and structures are not automatically derived from the corresponding larval tissues. Some of the ways in which they form are

1.   Continuous development from corresponding larval tissues
2.   New and independent formation after metamorphosis; in Insecta this is from imaginal discs, that have similar potentialities to those of embryonic tissues; in Trematoda it is from successive fragments from an embryonic germ ball
3.   New differentiation of tissues in regeneration or asexual reproduction
4.   Restoration of cells and tissues after anabiosis
5.   Reconstitution of sponge tissues after cell separation by bolting cloth (something very similar to this occurs in natural conditions, when certain gemmules "hatch" by extruding a stream of cells; these will rearrange themselves into a new sponge)

It is easy to forget that there are tissues that are fluid (blood, lymph, haemolymph, coelomic fluid) as well as the ones which are stationary (epithelial, connective, nerve, muscle, glandular, etc.). It is also difficult to separate a tissue from a nonliving structure secreted by it, and in our discussions it will be assumed that a "tissue" includes its secreted structures. The following list includes cell aggregates commonly called tissues (but see also below a list of the mesenchyme terms):

1. Adipose tissue — of fat-storing cells
2. Areolar tissue — loose connective tissue beneath an epithelium
3. Blood — a fluid connective tissue that transports dissolved gases and materials
4. Bone — calcified connective tissue
5. Botryoidal tissue — mesenchyme cells in coelom of Hirudinea
6. Cartilage — connective tissue containing collagen, principally in the skeleton
7. Chloragogen tissue — a multipurpose tissue that fills the typhlosoles of Oligochaeta
8. Chondroid tissue — a cartilage-like tissue in the proboscis of Enteropneusta
9. Coenenchyme — a tissue connecting polyps in s.Coelenterata
10. Collenchyme — scattered mesenchyme cells in gelatinous material
11. Connective tissue — tissues of mesodermal origin that bind and connect other tissues
12. Epithelium — any tissue that covers or lines an organ or cavity
13. Germplasm — the gametes and the line of cells that give rise to them
14. Glandular tissue — masses of cells specialized for secretion
15. Lymphatic tissue — a stroma with fibers and lymphocytes
16. Mesenchyme — connective tissue with gelatinous matrix, in invertebrates and in embryos of vertebrates
17. Mesogloea — the intermediate jelly-like layer in Coelenterata, with or without cells and fibers
18. Muscle tissue — the contractile cells of most animals
19. Myeloid tissue — the bone marrow
20. Nervous tissue — the cells that are designed to conduct impulses
21. Notochordal tissue — the large vacuolated cells of the notochord
22. Parenchyma — usually a spongy mass of mesenchyme cells between organs
23. Recticular tissue — an open network of cells in lymph organs
24. Vascular tissue — the conducting vessels, usually those carrying blood

Of the tissues listed, only four (called here massive tissues) are dealt with in the present chapter: connective tissue, muscle tissue, blood, and chloragogen tissue. Of the remainder, most are descriptive terms for the types of cell aggregates of which organs are constructed. A few can be both, such as muscle tissue in large sheets or as separate muscles (organs) and integument, which is usually a mixture of tissues but not isolated into organs. Some are merely the tissues of a certain organ, such as notochordal tissue, heart tissue, and liver tissue.

2. Structure and Function of Tissues

Each massive tissue is composed of similar cells and has a definite structure. These form several structural types, such as epithelium, connective tissue, blood, etc. Other tissues often form part of organs, which also have a definite structure, but tissues by themselves are without definite shape and size, because if they possessed these attributes they would be considered organs. There are some borderline cases, however, such as the tissues that form the various integuments of animals, which not only have no definite shape and size but do function much as organs. Integuments are so extensive compared to other organs that they may be treated as an organ system (see Chapter 18).

There are several other tissues that do not form clearly into organs but which themselves perform clear-cut functions in the body. Most obvious among these are the layers of muscle, the blood, the mesenchyme, and the chloragogen tissue.

Connective tissue is often involved in the structure of organs. Where it does not form organs, it must be treated as a distinct tissue or as several distinct tissues. Blood, although usually treated as a form of connective tissue, is so unusual in its fluid structure that it may seem out of place under tissues. This results in it being dealt with in this book under "Circulatory Systems" (Chapter 14) and under "Respiratory Fluids" in Chapter 15, as well as briefly in the present chapter.

a. Connective Tissue

Connective tissue occurs in three somewhat different situations: (1) as stroma or framework in organs of many types, (2) as sheets that bind such organs as muscles, and (3) forming the support of most organs and the structures that support the body.

The terms applied to connective tissue in general are diverse among the animal groups. The following incomplete list will illustrate the terms in what has been called mesenchymology (with some overlap of a previous list):

1. Botryoidal tissue — a form of mesenchyme in Hirudinea
2. Coenenchyme — tissue in the space between the thecae of coral polyps
3. Collenchyme — an embryonic tissue of cells in a gelatinous matrix
4. Ectomesenchyme — embryonic tissue derived from ectoderm
5. Glia — see Neuroglia
6. Interstitial tissue — this specifies merely whatever occupies small spaces between cells
7. Mesenchyme — unspecialized connective tissue, often gelatinous; in invertebrates and in embryos of vertebrates
8. Mesogloea — a transparent gelatinous matrix found in the walls of sponges and between epidermis and gastrodermis in Coelenterata and Ctenophora
9. Neuroglia — the connective tissue of the nervous system; sometimes written simply as glia
10. Parenchyma — any loose connective tissue
11. Perithelium — connective tissue cells associated with capillaries, in Vertebrata

It is not feasible to tabulate the occurrence of each of these features in the animal kingdom largely because most of the terms are used loosely and in diverse ways. Words such as connective tissue are used for such a variety of cell aggregates that the word itself comes to hide the existing diversity.

Sometimes cited under the broad heading of Connective Tissue are blood, bone, cartilage, etc. Blood is dealt with here and in Chapter 14. Bone is cited under "Support" (Chapter 20) but is dealt with in the chapter on unique organ systems (Chapter 19).

b. Muscle Tissue

The principal muscles that form a clear-cut tissue are the body wall muscles that exist in distinct layers. Among vertebrates, the skin is usually described as consisting of epidermis and dermis; the muscle layers beneath are included in the more inclusive term body wall. Thus, in all animals that have a body cavity, the body wall is usually taken as including all tissues from the surface inward to the body cavity (or to its epithelium). It is generally described as consisting of epidermis (and its cuticle) and the layers of body wall muscles, but in the vertebrates there is also a dermis between these. In most invertebrates there are one or more layers of muscle tissue in the body wall, lying beneath the epidermis. In forms that lack a clear body cavity (Mollusca), there may be no muscle layers. One coelomate group (Echinodermata) has a thick layer of dermis between the epidermis and the muscle layers (as in Vertebrata).

In the different groups there may be one, two, or three layers, showing great diversity in the direction of their fibers:

1. None — (Porifera, Mesozoa, Monoblastozoa, Hydrozoa, Scyphozoa, Ctenophora, Temnocephaloidea, Gymnolaemata, Inarticulata, Bivalvia, Crinoidea, Ophiuroidea, Echinoidea)
2. Longitudinal/circular — (Anthozoa, Saccosomatida)
3. Circular/diagonal/longitudinal — (Turbellaria, s.Trematoda, s.Solenogastres, S.Sipunculoidea, s.Hirudinea)
4. Circular/longitudinal/diagonal — (s.Trematoda, Echiuroidea)
5. Fibers variously mixed — (in some areas of s.Cestoda, Rotifera, Gastrotricha, Kinorhyncha, s.Solenogastres, Amphineura, Myzostomida, Ascidiacea)
6. Circular/longitudinal — (Cestoda, Acanthocephala, Priapulida, Phylactolaemata, Phoronida, s.Solenogastres, s.Sipunculoidea, Oligochaeta, s.Hirudinea, Onychophora, Pogonophora, Asteroidea, Holothurioidea, Enteropneusta)
7. Longitudinal only — (Nematoda, both classes of Gordioidea, Calyssozoa, Articulata, Archiannelida, Chaetognatha, Pterobranchia)
8. Circular only — (Dinophiloidea, Thaliacea)

The Arthropoda have extensive muscles between segments of the body. These are not usually listed as part of the body wall. In Cephalochordata and Vertebrata there are segmentally arranged myomeres; these are here assumed to be individual muscle organs rather than a single extensive tissue.

These occurrences can be rearranged to show the distribution of the sequences in the animal phyla. In these 30 phyla, 6 show more than one arrangement (Table 14).

There does not appear to be any feature of these layers that can be used in classification of the groups.

c. Blood

Blood is a tissue, but as a tissue with a fluid matrix it is very different from most other tissues in any animal. When restricted to animals having a vascular system, blood usually is vital to respiration. It also carries nutrients, frequently carries waste products to the excretory system, and carries some of the chemical messengers for the endocrine system.

The bloods of various animals have little in common except their fluidity. In some, cells are numerous, but in others they are few. Some carry respiratory pigments, but many do not. A variety of other fluids in body spaces (coelom, haemocoel) may be called blood, and it is difficult to define the word either to include or exclude them. These are sometimes called coelomic fluid and haemolymph, respectively.

In the vertebrates, blood is carried in the vessels of the circulatory system. In other animals the vessels may be incomplete, allowing the blood to fill body cavities. In still others there may be no blood vessels, and the fluid is in spaces only. Even in the higher vertebrates, there is a large amount of lymph, a fluid similar to blood but lacking red corpuscles and not restricted to the vessels.

To be called blood in animals in general, a fluid apparently need have only one feature, floating amoeboid cells. It may contain pigments such as haemoglobin, either in the plasma or in some of the floating cells. Many of the pigments function in transport of oxygen, but some do not (see Chapter 15).

d. Chloragogen Tissue

In Annelida only, there exists an extensive tissue that, more than most others, is diverse in its functions. In this it is similar to the liver (an organ) in higher vertebrates,

Table 14
THE BODY WALL MUSCLE LAYERS

	None	l only	lc	c only	cl	cld	cdl	Mixed fibers
Monoblastozoa	0							
Mesozoa	0							
Porifera	0							
Coelenterata								
Hydrozoa	0							
Scyphozoa	0							
Anthozoa			X					
Ctenophora	0							
Platyhelminthes								
Temnocephaloidea	0							
Turbellaria							X	
Trematoda						S	S	
Cestoda					S			S
Rhynchocoela[a]								
Acanthocephala					X			
Rotifera								X
Gastrotricha								X
Kinorhyncha								X
Nematoda		X						
Gordioidea		X						
Priapuloidea					X			
Calyssozoa		X						
Bryozoa								
Gymnolaemata	0							
Phylactolaemata					X			
Phoronida					X			
Brachiopoda								
Articulata		X						
Inarticulata	0							
Mollusca								
Solenogastres					S		S	S
Amphineura								X
Gastropoda		?	?	?	?	?	?	?
Bivalvia		X						
Scaphopoda		?	?	?	?	?	?	?
Cephalopoda		?	?	?	?	?	?	?
Sipunculoidea					S		S	
Echiuroidea								
Echiurida						X		
Saccosomatida				X				
Myzostomida								
Tardigrada								X
Annelida								B
Archiannelida		X						
Polychaeta		S			S		S	
Oligochaeta					X			
Hirudinea					S		S	
Dinophiloidea				X				
Onychophora					X			
Arthropoda	—	—	—	—	—	—	—	—
Chaetognatha		X						
Pogonophora					X			
Echinodermata								
Crinoidea	0							
Asteroidea					X			

Table 14 (continued)
THE BODY WALL MUSCLE LAYERS

	None	l only	lc	c only	cl	cld	cdl	Mixed fibers
Ophiuroidea	0							
Echinoidea	0							
Holothurioidea					X			
Enteropneusta					X			
Pterobranchia		X						
Tunicata								
Ascidiacea								X
Thaliacea				X				
Cephalochordata	—	—	—	—	—	—	—	
Vertebrata	—	—	—	—	—	—	—	

Note: Headings: l, longitudinal; c, circular; d, diagonal; from the outside. 0, none; X, occurs; S, in some species; B, muscle bands — muscle arrangement not comparable.

[a] In Rhynchocoela, the layers may be cdl, cdlc, lcl, or nearly absent.

and some of the functions are also similar. Perhaps its main function is in intermediary metabolism, but it may also synthesize glycogen and fat (which it may store), form waste products such as ammonia and urea, remove excess silicates from the materials absorbed from the digestive tract, participate in haemoglobin synthesis, and produce phagocytic coelomocytes (the counterpart of leukocytes in vertebrate blood).

This tissue surrounds the intestine and some of the blood vessels. It is said to be derived from the coelomic peritoneum. There is some evidence that it passes food reserves through the coelom to other parts of the body, in which case the wandering cells are called eleocytes.

In the Oligochaeta, this tissue, sometimes spelled chloragogue, fills the large typhlosole fold that hangs in the intestine. It thus can be quite an extensive tissue, as well as highly diverse in function.

3. Syncytial Tissues

Syncytia form the major exception to the common generalization that all animal tissues consist of cells. Syncytia are tissues in which the cells are not separated by membranes. Syncytia are widespread in the animal kingdom and may involve most tissues in a few animals and in many embryos. They may occur in (at least) epidermis, parenchyma (mesenchyme), muscles, coelomic and intestinal epithelia, retinal cells, ovaries, and gemmules. It is usually not admitted that such tissues are widespread in the animal kingdom, but at least the following sometimes occur:

1. Porifera — in some gemmules, such as those of *Callyspongia diffusa*
2. Coelenterata — epidermis, early embryo (*Renilla*)
3. Ctenophora — epidermis in some
4. Platyhelminthes — some mesenchyme, some epidermis, some gastrodermis in Turbellaria (many tissues in some Acoela), and epidermis in Trematoda and Cestoda
5. Rhynchocoela — parenchyma
6. Acanthocephala — epidermis, cement glands, some muscles, early embryos from 12-cell stage

7. Rotifera — epidermis, some muscles, most tissues
8. Gastrotricha — epidermis
9. Kinorhyncha — epidermis
10. Nematoda — epidermis, excretory ducts
11. Priapulida — "central mass" of larva
12. Phoronida — coelomic peritoneum
13. Annelida — digestive tract epithelium of some Hirudinea
14. Arthropoda — Crustacea: in certain parasitic forms all tissues except the mucosa of the intestinal tract, the ovary, and the coelomocytes; Insecta: epithelium of some tracheal gills, some intestinal musculature, parts of ovaries, most early embryos
15. Echinodermata — calcigenous cells in the endoskeleton
16. Vertebrata — retina of the eye in some, striated and cardiac muscle, some bone tissues

As reported in the previous chapter, there have been statements that some syncytia are formed by fusion of cells with disappearance of intervening membranes. No clear examples are reported. All other syncytia are produced by failure of the new cell membranes to be formed after nuclear division. Both syncytia and plasmodia can be related to cellularity by citing the functional units as energids rather than as cells (see "Cells", Chapter 10).

4. Number of Basic Tissue Layers

All animals except sponges are said to be either diploblastic (consisting of tissues derived from two germ layers, ectoderm and endoderm) or triploblastic (tissues derived from three germ layers, adding mesoderm). For this purpose the Coelenterata and sometimes the Ctenophora are said to be diploblastic, and all others from Platyhelminthes on as triploblastic.

This is really a meaningless distinction, because probably all coelenterates have some material between the two major layers, including some cells. There is no way to define "tissue" that will exclude these materials, especially as in many coelenterates and all ctenophores the cells are so numerous as to form a mesogloeal tissue as definite as the parenchyma of some Turbellaria.

It is lately coming to be admitted that these animals are actually triploblastic, with some diversity in the number of cells and in the extent of the spaces occupied. The intermediate tissues contain intercellular fluid. In some coelenterates this fluid merely has fewer cells.

However, this is not the end of the story of primary germ or tissue layers. Although some respected students of invertebrates refer to the sponges as cellular but without tissues, in reality two perfectly good tissue layers do occur (epidermis and choanoderm), and there is even an intermediate layer (mesogloea) that contains cells and fluid. The tissues are simpler than in higher animals, but they are still tissues. Porifera, too, are therefore essentially triploblastic (see "Problems of Sponge Embryology" in Chapter 5).

This leaves two often-neglected groups, the Mesozoa and the Monoblastozoa. The Mesozoa have a layer of outside cells around a single axial cell or a small group of interior cells. These surely form two simple tissues, especially as one is an epidermis of sorts and the other is reproductive. These then are the only diploblastic animals.

The Monoblastozoa consists of a single species, so little known that it may be a larva. *Salinella salve* is said to consist of a single layer of cells forming a cylinder, with cilia both inside and out. The inside tube was apparently a digestive tract, and the animal was thus monoblastic.

One further germ layer condition has been cited. In the peculiar parasites called tapeworms, the epidermis was formerly thought to have been lost in development; because the animal never has any digestive tract at any time in its life history, it could be seen as effectively composed entirely of mesoderm tissues. In this view even the "cuticle" on the outside was said to be secreted by the mesenchyme, which would be a unique arrangement among animals. It is recently recognized that there is no cuticle, and an epidermis of unusual structure is actually present. The tapeworms therefore have tissues derived from both ectoderm and mesoderm. This unusual body wall (which is also found in Trematoda) has recently been termed tegument.

It is thus possible to tabulate the germ layer occurrences among Metazoa:

Monoblastic

1. Monoblastozoa

Diploblastic

2. Mesozoa

Triploblastic

3. With three actual layers (Porifera, Coelenterata, and all others not listed above or below)
4. Losing all trace of endoderm tissues in the adult (Pogonophora)
5. With no clear endoderm forming in the embryo or later (Cestoda)
6. Lacking endoderm because none was present in the bud from which it arose (Bryozoan avicularia and vibracula)

III. TISSUE PRODUCTS

Some of the extracellular objects produced by living things are clearly produced by single cells (setae, for example, or by organs (eggshells by the ootype), but some are produced over large areas and seem to be more appropriately cited as products of massive tissues.

Secretions or products that would be attributed to tissues rather than to cells or organs would be those structures in sheets over many cells, such as the cuticle, or those requiring the work of many cells not isolated as an identifiable organ, such as bone. These include all the so-called frame substances, the intercellular fluids, and nearly all nonliving materials of any animal body.

The products may be chemically anything that living cells can produce, such as carbohydrate, protein, calcium phosphate, pearl, chitin, silk, etc. The following are examples of tissue products that are solid: periderm (perisarc) of Hydrozoa, thecae, calyces, loricae, zooecia, shells, cuticles and most other chitinous objects, tubes for worms, cases for insect larvae, tests of echinoids, tunics of tunicates, and bone in vertebrates. Some other objects are more obviously secretions of organs or cells. They include jaws of Mollusca and Annelida, and the various hardparts of vertebrates, such as teeth, hair, feathers, nails, antlers, horns, and beaks.

Some of the major tissue products (both solid and fluid) are listed here for each phylum; the so-called hard-parts are described in more detail in Chapter 20:

1. Protozoa — (not possible because tissues cannot exist)
2. Porifera — spicules and other skeletons, always made by groups of similar cells

3. Mesozoa — (none except possibly intercellular fluid)
4. Monoblastozoa — (none known)
5. Coelenterata — perisarc, coral (calcareous or horny or glassy)
6. Ctenophora — (none)
7. Platyhelminthes — epidermal basement membrane, mesenchymal pigment, hooks, spines
8. Rhynchocoela — rhynchocoel fluid
9. Acanthocephala — cuticle, spines, lacunar fluid
10. Rotifera — cuticle, trophi, gelatinous envelope, pseudocoel fluid
11. Gastrotricha — cuticle, spines
12. Kinorhyncha — cuticle, bristles, pseudocoel fluid
13. Priapuloidea — cuticle, basement membrane, mid-gut cuticle, coelomic membrane
14. Nematoda — cuticle, bristles, spicules, stylets, pseudocoel fluid
15. Gordioidea — cuticle, pseudocoel fluid
16. Calyssozoa — cuticle, spines
17. Bryozoa — zooecium, coelomic fluid, spines, coelomic spicules, cuticle, spines, basement membrane
18. Phoronida — tube, basement membrane, coelomic fluid, blood plasma
19. Brachiopoda — shell, coelomic fluid, blood (which has no cells)
20. Mollusca — shell, blood plasma
21. Sipunculoidea — cuticle, coelomic fluid
22. Echiuroidea — cuticle, coelomic fluid, blood plasma
23. Tardigrada — cuticle, haemocoel fluid
24. Myzostomida — (none)
25. Annelida — tube, cuticle, spines, coelomic fluid, blood plasma
26. Pentastomida — cuticle
27. Onychophora — cuticle, haemocoel fluid
28. Arthropoda — exoskeleton, setae, haemocoel fluid
29. Chaetognatha — cuticle, spines, basement membrane, "coelomic" fluid
30. Pogonophora — tube, cuticle, coelomic fluid, blood plasma
31. Enteropneusta — basement membrane, coelomic fluid, buccal basement membrane, blood (which has no cells)
32. Pterobranchia — coenoecium, basement membrane, coelomic fluid
33. Tunicata — tunic, blood plasma
34. Cephalochordata — blood (which has no cells)
35. Vertebrata — mucus, bone, cartilage, blood and lymph plasma, scales, feathers, hair, etc.

In the sense used here, chitin is a major tissue product when it forms cuticles. It is, of course, a product of the cells. Because chitin occurs almost exclusively in the outer layers of animals, its distribution in the animal kingdom is tabulated under "Biochemicals", in Chapter 8.

REFERENCES

Andrews, W., *Textbook of Comparative Histology,* Oxford University Press, New York, 1959.
Bremer, J. L. and Weatherford, H. L., *A Text-Book of Histology Arranged Upon an Embryological Basis,* 6th ed., Blakiston, Philadelphia, 1944.
Clark, W. E. L., *The Tissues of the Body,* 6th ed., Oxford University Press, Oxford, 1971.
Holmes, R. L., *Living Tissues: An Introduction to Functional Histology,* Pergamon Press, New York, 1965.
McLean, F. C. and Urist, M. R., *Bone: An Introduction to the Physiology of Skeletal Tissue,* University of Chicago Press, Chicago, 1955.

Chapter 12

ORGANS AND ORGAN SYSTEMS

TABLE OF CONTENTS

I.   Organs 248
     A.   Definitions 248
     B.   Organs vs. Tissues 248
     C.   Organs vs. Organ Systems 249
     D.   Unicellular Organs 249
     E.   Movement of Organs 250
     F.   Organ Functions 251
     G.   Detached Organs 251
     H.   Body Openings 253
     I.   Unique Organs 253

II. Organ Systems 254
     A.   Discussion 254
     B.   Six System Functions 257
          1.   Coverage 257
          2.   Alimentation 257
          3.   Translocation 258
               a.   Transport Devices 258
               b.   Tube Systems 259
          4.   Respiration 260
          5.   Expulsion 261
          6.   Control 262
          7.   Enclosure 263

References 263

I. ORGANS

A. Definitions

Animals are composed principally of cells (and cell products) arranged into layers or into organs (structurally and functionally discrete units). The layers may consist of one, two, or several types of cell. The cells may be replaced with a syncytium. The discrete organs may consist of many or a few cells, and an organ may contain several types of cells. All of these diversities are relevant to a definition of the term organ, but current definitions do not attempt to cover this range, thus leaving important features of animals unclassified.

The usual definitions of an organ include: "A discrete mass of cells of specific function." "A structure composed of tissues, having specific functions, and structurally distinct from adjacent structures." "A body part usually composed of several tissues grouped together into a structural and functional unit." "Any part of an animal performing some definite function; a group of cells or tissues acting as a unit for some special purpose." The only requirements common to these definitions are that the structure be discrete and that it have a specific function. In some circumstances the term organ is applied rather loosely. It may include all structures, spaces, and openings of the body. However, in nearly all definitions, the term is restricted to the ordinary multicellular organs, leaving out altogether single cells, syncytial structures, and detached bodies, all of which function as organs. The latter not only do not qualify under the usual definition of organ but are left without any place in the cell-tissue-organs system.

An *organ* is a structure that performs at least one specific function by itself, irrespective or whether it is unicellular, syncytial, or multicellular. Furthermore, it may be part of a group of structures performing a series or complex of functions, in which case such a group of organs clearly form an organ system.

The relation between cells, tissues, organs, and organ systems is suggested in Figure 18.

B. Organs vs. Tissues

The complexity of tissues and the degree of their integration into organs are both very high in what we usually call "the higher animals", such as the arthropods and the vertebrates. Some of the simpler animals have quite complex organs, (witness the Aristotle's lantern in sea urchins, the buccal apparatus of snails, etc.), but it is generally true that "the lower animals" have simpler tissues and less highly developed organs.

It is currently common to say that the phylum Porifera altogether lacks tissues and organs and thus stands apart from all other animals. This was recognized by Hyman (1940) in describing these animals as being "at the cellular grade of construction", rather than at the tissue grade. This is really quite hard to justify. There is an epidermis and the radial canals are lined with a choanoderm consisting of collar cells mixed with pore cells; both of these are functional tissues, though simple ones. It is even a little hard to justify the common implication that the water channels do not form an organ system, since they are well organized, serve a definite purpose, consist of many parts, and are adequately integrated in operation. They are herein treated as a system in Chapter 19 (under "Spongiocoel as a System").

With the exception of Protozoa, whose cells do not form tissues and organs, the latter are here assumed to be present in all animals except in the earliest stages of development of the embryo.

It must be noted that although some textbooks imply that tissues exist only as components of organs, there are a few tissues of the body that do not seem to be part of organs. Of these, four (connective tissue, blood, muscle layers, and chloragogen tissue) were discussed in Chapter 11, and a fifth (epidermis) is included in Chapter 18. The embryonic germ layers also seem to be of the nature of tissues (see Chapter 5).

C. Organs vs. Organ Systems

As with organs, it is unreasonable to limit an organ system to a group of two or more organs. It is conceivable that a single organ or even a single cell might operate so completely by itself in some minute animal that it could be called a system. An animal with one flame bulb, as occurs in some flatworms (Catenulida), might actually have an excretory system consisting of just one organ. In such a case the entire system might consist of just one cell, as its duct may be part of the same cell.

It is sometimes assumed that all organs of animals are parts of a few organ systems. This effort always fails when one gets to the organs for special functions, because of such questions as these: Where does one classify organs for producing color, electricity, or sound? Where are attachment organs to be dealt with, or flotation devices? Is there an easy place to describe storage organs or pumping organs or mechanisms for autotomy or organs for care of the young? As a result one finds in the usages of the term organ system either a few systems with a lot of extra organs or a great many systems showing a great range of complexity. This parallels the situation cited under ORGANS above.

Because five or six organ systems can be recognized in most animals, and a few unique ones rarely, these clear-cut systems are treated separately in Chapters 13 to 19.

Classification or formal grouping of the remaining miscellaneous organs is difficult and indecisive; they are treated individually (in Chapter 20) merely as special organs performing special functions. Emphasis will be placed on the function, with the various organ types listed.

All of these diversities in five levels of integration (cell, tissue, organ, system, individual) turn out to represent only part of the diversity in organization of cells in animals. Cells may be united into tissues, but they may instead form whole individuals (Protozoa or zygotes), they may perform isolated functions and yet not usually be admitted to be organs, or they may be gametes that are separated from the "parent" but are not yet individuals.

Similarly, tissues may combine to form organs, but they may instead form whole individuals (Mesozoa), be separate from organs as tissue layers (e.g., epidermis), or form structures not usually called organs (such as proglottids or motile excretory urns). Organs may be combined into systems or they may remain isolated as gland cells in almost any animal or a solitary flame bulb in some Turbellaria (see Figure 18).

The presence of gametes in this diagram of organization of living cells into individuals raises the next question of whether organs must be multicellular.

D. Unicellular Organs

In virtually all texts it is implied that organs must be multicellular and must consist of cells or more than one tissue. If one finds a discrete body performing a specific function, why should one say it is an organ if it has many sensory cells and many neutrons and refuse to call it an organ if it has only one sensory cell and one neuron? Or just one secretory cell alone?

A pertinent example is found in structures which assist the spermatozoa to find the ova inside the female. When impregnation is into the body cavity, there may be a synergid structure to carry the spermatozoon through the female tissues. In the Porifera this is a single amoebocyte. In the Chaetognatha it consists of two special cells. In the Myzostomida it consists of a syncytial carrier. Are not these all organs with a very specific structure and function?

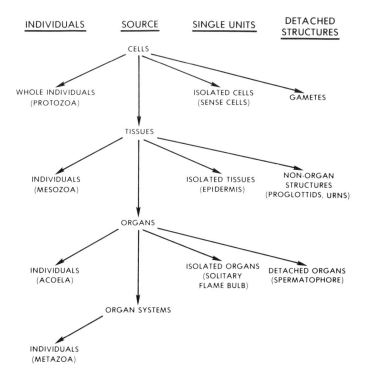

FIGURE 18.   Diagram of relations between cells, tissues, organs, and individuals.

There are many isolated cells that function in the same manner as multicellular organs. For example, the collar cells (choanocytes) of sponges capture food; this is usually a function of elaborate organs of capture, perhaps aided by other organs of detection and locomotion. There are many single cells that perform such a complete function comparable to that of a multicellular organ, and it is therefore necessary to admit that there are unicellular organs.

There is nothing gained by saying that the sensory system of an animal consists of sense organs *and* sense cells. They are all organs, either complex or simple. There is no meaningful place to draw the line between organs and cells, when they perform similar functions in equal isolation.

The rejection of this artificial distinction results in acceptance as organs of all cellular or syncytial structures that are a discrete and functional unit. Many single cells meet these stipulations and are entirely comparable to multicellular organs.

E. Movement of Organs

Movement is not one of the functions usually ascribed to organs, but there are a variety of organ movements in nearly all animals. As organs are herein defined, we would list the contraction of individual muscles and the resulting movement of appendages such as legs, tentacles, and probosces; the amoeboid movement through the body of syncytial gametophores; the swimming of urns and amoebocytes in the body fluids; the slow creeping of bud-carrying cells over the surface of Ascidiacea; and the swimming of detached epitokes and sporosacs. To these must be added morphogenetic movements during development, during which the relative position of organs may be changed. In Insecta, the oxygen-permeable tips of tracheoles may move many times their diameter to reach cells that need the oxygen.

Among single cells regarded as unicellular organs, movement becomes clearly locomotion by amoeboid movement or by ciliary or flagellar propulsion. All of these occur
both in Protozoa and in Metazoa.

Other examples of organ movement are cited under "Movement" in Chapter 20,
where movement is dealt with both as the result of action of a neighboring structure
and as locomotion.

F. Organ Functions

Organs perform numerous functions that are discrete and definite. There is no sure
way to define an organ, but this word is here taken to include all structures, spaces,
openings, cells that perform complete functions of the same sort as multicellular organs, and all detached parts of a body that remain alive.

In this book these functions are treated at several levels: cell, tissue, organ, organ
system, and whole individual. At the organ and organ system level, the functions will
be cited in three places:

1. Those of the major organ systems in Chapters 13 to 18
2. Those of the unique organ systems in Chapter 19
3. Those of the miscellaneous organs in Chapter 20

It is sometimes stated as a principle that "no part of the body functions independently". There are some apparent exceptions:

1. Detached proglottids (Cestoda)
2. Epitokes (Polychaeta)
3. Hectocotyl (Cephalopoda)
4. Gametes (all sexual animals)
5. Gemmules and statoblasts (Porifera, Bryozoa)
6. Buds

Whether or not these structures should be called organs rather than fragments of the
whole animal is debatable. It may not be correct to say that they function independently, but the control of the body over individual organs varies, with some principally
connected by earlier metabolic needs and others at all times under the control of other
organs.

G. Detached Organs

The presence in the diagram of "detached organs" leads to another difficulty, never
solved in histology books. Such books are nearly always oriented to the tissues and
organs of *Homo sapiens*; they find no difficulty in dealing with organs that are always
multicellular and a permanent part of the body. These "organs" are then supplemented, without comment, by unicellular sensory cells, unicellular glands, gametes,
proglottids, spermatophores, etc. It is not said whether these are organs, or what they
are.

Whatever is decided to be the disposition of the unicellular "organs", there is no
way to define organ to exclude an excretory urn (in Sipunculoidea) which may be
attached in the coelom or may detach and float about, continuing to perform its function. Even a proglottid or an epitoke would qualify as an organ before separation; why
not afterwards?

When it is claimed that no part functions independently, the emphasis on the integration of all parts of the organism is sometimes treated as a truism. There are, however, interesting exceptions, among both internal and external liberations.

Proglottids. In some Cestoda the detached proglottids continue to live for some time, maturing the eggs and protecting them, the same functions they serve when they are attached to the chain. Do they cease to be organs at the moment when they become detached?

Epitokes. In many marine Polychaeta, the part of the body containing the gonads separates and swims away. Sometimes it regenerates the missing head and becomes a new individual, but sometimes it remains a headless fragment while performing the functions of locomotion and spawning.

Gonophores. In a few Hydrozoa (especially some siphonophores), the gonads are in gonophore structures that become detached; they live a free existence only briefly before liberating their gametes, because they have no digestive system.

Sporosacs. In other colonial Hydrozoa the gonads are in sporosacs on the hydranth stems; they may be ciliated and become free to swim separately. Sporosacs are evidently a special type of gonophore. (The latter word covers also structures which separate to become medusae.)

Gametophores. Spermatophores and oophores are listed in at least 10 phyla in Chapter 3.

Hectocotyls. In Cephalopoda such as squids, cuttlefish, and octopuses, one of the arms may be modified for carrying spermatozoa; in some octopods, the arm may break off during spermatozoan transfer and remain in the mantle cavity of the female to liberate its gametes.

Buds, fragments, frustules. These frequently form distinct organs before they break away to become new individuals.

Gemmules, podocysts, sorites, statoblasts, hibernacula. These are also organs, before they become separate individuals.

Eudoxids. Some siphonophore colonies produce sections called eudoxids that will break off to form new colonies; if the persons of the "colony" are considered to be organs, then these would be also.

Transplanted testis. As described in Chapter 4, in some Crustacea these organs are liberated from the male and function for the life of the female that receives them.

In addition to the excretory urns of Sipunculoidea that may become free in the coelom and continue their activities, there are, in Acanthocephala, ovaries which may break up into ovarian balls free in the coelom. If the ovaries are organs, can the ovarian balls be denied that status?

One who is persuaded to treat all of these as organs, rather than leave a wide variety of structures out of the system, will find in the following list some of the unexpected organs that are usually not so listed:

1.   Buds — before separation or start of independent function (in many groups)
2.   Proglottids — even when detached (Cestoda)
3.   Epitokes — that do not regenerate into a new individual (s.Annelida)
4.   Gametes — (all sexual animals)
5.   Gametophores — (spermatophores and oophores in several phyla)
6.   Gemmules — before development starts (Porifera)
7.   Gonophores — (s. Hydrozoa)
8.   Hectocotyl — (Cephalopoda)
9.   Sporosacs — (s.Hydrozoa)

10. Statoblasts — before development starts (Bryozoa)
11. Transplanted cells — nematocysts (Turbellaria, Rhynchocoela, Gastropoda, etc.)
12. Transplanted organs — (Crustacea, Vertebrata)

H. Body Openings

To class openings into the body as organs may seem a little far-fetched, yet they are structures performing specific functions and so cannot clearly be distinguished from organs. They may open into alimentary or breathing spaces, into the body cavity itself, or only into some organ near the surface, such as a duct.

Alimentary openings are those that take food into the digestive tract or expel digestive tract wastes. These include mouth and anus, sometimes combined into a single proctostome. There may be one or more anal pores in animals with a proctostome, and other variations occur (these are detailed under "Openings into Digestive Tracts", in Chapter 13).

Respiratory openings may pass either air or water, depending upon whether the animal breathes air or extracts oxygen from the surrounding water. These may be pores, spiracles, nares, mouth, or anus. The air-breathing openings are listed in Chapter 15. Water-admitting openings include:

1. Ostia — (Porifera)
2. Siphons — (Mollusca)
3. Mouth — in animals with pharyngeal gills (Enteropneusta, s.Pterobranchia, Tunicata, Cephalochordata, Pisces); with foregut (s.Crustacea)
4. Anus — with hindgut (s.aquatic Oligochaeta, s.Crustacea, Crinoidea, Holothurioidea)
5. Bursal slits — (Ophiuroidea)
6. Nares — (m.Vertebrata)

Reproductive openings are of several sorts, for release of gametes, zygotes, or embryos, and for entrance of spermatozoa or the organ carrying them. Some of these openings are permanent and specialized for the purpose; some are permanent pores involved also in excretion or other functions; some are temporary holes which promptly close over (see Tables 15, 16, and 17).

I. Unique Organs

Unique organs are rather common, but they often cannot be distinguished by the terms applied to them. There are numerous unique glands, innumerable dermal structures such as hair, feathers, setae, combs, etc. Some specific unique organs with unusual functions are these:

1. Ovejector — used in the expulsion of the eggs (Nematoda)
2. Funnel or siphon — for directing the jet-propulsion stream (Cephalopoda)
3. Pectines and Racquet organs — with sense organs (Scorpionida and Solpugida in Arachnida)
4. Wing of chitin — for flight (Insecta)
5. Pedicellariae — tiny jaw-like structures used for capture and protection (Asteroidea)
6. Aristotle's lantern — a five-part jaw system (Echinoidea)
7. Podia — the tube-feet, for locomotion and feeding (Echinodermata)
8. Feathers — complex epidermal and mesodermal "scales" (Aves)
9. Hair — simple epidermal thread-like organs (Mammalia)

Table 15

THE DUCTS FOR EXIT OF SPERMATOZOA FROM THE MALE

| | Gonopores from | | Opening with other functions | |
	Temporary epidermal	Reproductive organs	Digestive tract	Excretory system
Porifera				
Coelenterata	Rupture		Proctostome	
Ctenophora	X		Proctostome	
Platyhelminthes	X			
Rhynchocoela	X		Anus	
Acanthocephala	X			X
Rotifera	X			
Gastrotricha	X			
Kinorhyncha	X			
Priapuloidea	X			X
Nematoda			Cloaca/rectum	
Gordioidea	X		Cloaca	
Calyssozoa	X			
Bryozoa	0			
Phoronida		X		X
Brachiopoda	0			
Mollusca	X			X/0
Sipunculoidea				X
Echiuroidea				X
Tardigrada			X	
Myzostomida	X			
Annelida		X		
Dinophiloidea				
Onychophora	X			
Arthropoda	X			
Chaetognatha		X		
Pogonophora				
Echinodermata	X			
Enteropneusta	X			
Pterobranchia				
Tunicata			Cloaca	
Cephalochordata		X	Mouth	
Vertebrata	X			

Note: X indicates the nature of the pore; 0 indicates that no such organ or pathway exists.

II. ORGAN SYSTEMS

A. Discussion

The expression "organ system" is widely used as a level of integration between organ and individual. In applying this concept to the diverse mechanisms of animals, the idea that it will help to explain the features of animals has some validity within any one group being studied, but when it is applied to animals in general, it runs into numerous minor problems and proves to be more confusing than helpful. It cannot be entirely avoided, if only because of its familiarity in textbooks and its helpfulness in dividing a book into chapters.

Organ systems are groups of organs integrated into a functional whole for the accomplishment of a major function or group of functions. It must be noted that in another sense really separate "systems" do not exist in animals. The term is merely a way of systematizing the maze of interacting functions and structures. It is completely arbitrary what will be called a system and what will not.

Table 16
THE DUCTS FOR ENTRANCE OF SPERMATOZOA INTO
THE FEMALE

	Permanent gonopores into		Temporary openings	With other functions
	Reproductive organs	Body cavity		
Porifera				Ostia
Coelenterata				
Ctenophora				
Platyhelminthes	X	X		
Rhynchocoela	X/0			
Acanthocephala	X			
Rotifera			X	
Gastrotricha	X/0			
Kinorhyncha	X			
Priapuloidea				
Nematoda	X			
Gordioidea				Anus
Calyssozoa				
Bryozoa	0			
Phoronida				
Brachiopoda	0			
Mollusca				
Sipunculoidea	0			
Echiuroidea	0			
Tardigrada				
Myzostomida				
Annelida	0	X		
Dinophiloidea				
Onychophora			X	
Arthropoda	X/0			
Chaetognatha	X			
Pogonophora				
Echinodermata	0			
Enteropneusta	0			
Pterobranchia				
Tunicata	0			
Cephalochordata				
Vertebrata	X/0			

Note: X, occurs; 0, none; no information available for others.

Each so-called organ system is merely one or more organs integrated to perform the various aspects of its function. There is much diversity in how such systems are listed in different books, but the universally cited systems, from the vertebrate viewpoint are

1. Digestive (intestinal tract)
2. Respiratory (breathing)
3. Excretory (kidneys)
4. Circulatory (oxygen-carrying blood in vessels)
5. Reproductive (gonads, glands, ducts, and copulatory mechanisms)
6. Nervous (sense organs, brain, nerves)

To these are often added:

Table 17
THE OPENINGS FOR EXIT OF OVA (OR EMBRYO) FROM THE FEMALE

	Gonopore reproductive organ	(Permanent) Body cavity	(Temporary)	Openings with other functions	
				Digestive tract	Excretory system
Porifera				Osculum	
Coelenterata			Epidermal rupture	Proctostome	
Ctenophora				Proctostome	
Platyhelminthes	X		Rupture	Proctostome	
Rhynchocoela			Rupture/pore		
Acanthocephala	X				
Rotifera				Cloaca	
Gastrotricha	X				
Kinorhyncha	X				
Priapulida	X				X
Nematoda	X				
Gordioidea	X			Cloaca	
Calyssozoa	X				
Bryozoa		X			
Phoronida					X
Brachiopoda					X
Mollusca	X			Cloaca	X
Sipunculoidea					X
Echiuroidea					X
Tardigrada				X	
Myzostomida	X			Cloaca	
Annelida		X			X
Dinophiloidea	X				
Onychophora	X				
Arthropoda	X				
Chaetognatha	X				
Pogonophora	X				
Echinodermata	X				
Enteropneusta	X				
Pterobranchia	X				
Tunicata				Cloaca	
Cephalochordata		X		Mouth	
Vertebrata	X	X			

7. Endocrine (isolated endocrine glands)
8. Muscle (all muscles of the body)
9. Support (bones, ligaments, cartilage)

These are reasonably effective when applied to vertebrates, but when these phrases are applied to invertebrates also, they become so general as to obscure what are great differences in function and structure. It is then necessary to add descriptive phrases (as above), as there is little similarity between an intestinal tract and a gastrovascular cavity, or between a vertebrate kidney and a flame-cell system.

There is not one of these systems that is represented in all animals. An astonishing number of animals have no digestive system of any sort, and although reproduction must occur in most, there are more than a few animals with no system of reproductive organs. On the other hand, some animals have real organ systems that are unique to them (see Chapter 19).

These difficulties can be exemplified: (1) The neat concept of a respiratory system in vertebrates becomes confused when extended to a holothurian or any skin-breathing animal; the system label begins to fail. (2) One of the most universal functional assemblages of cells and tissues is not usually called a system but merely "the integument". (3) Most animals have a reproductive system, but these range from one male (or one female) system per individual, to two (one of each sex) per individual, to many complete systems (of one or both sexes) per individual (as in tapeworms). Is it logical to call all these together "a system"? (4) What if the system is merely a budding zone?

There is thus no way to define organ system that gives reasonable satisfaction in all groups and enables the classification of all organs. The systems cited here are the best substantiated of those that have been used elsewhere. It is here concluded that it is ineffectual to carry the universal organ system concept beyond the six most obvious and widespread and the six unique systems. Although this book tries to deal with all functions, many of them seem to be quite isolated from any real system, and they are herein treated together in Chapter 20, "Miscellaneous Organ Functions".

It is almost universal to list reproductive system among the regular systems. In Vertebrata this is quite reasonable. In animals as a whole, there is such a variety of reproductive processes and organs in both sexual and asexual reproduction that there is no such thing as "a reproductive system". A compromise is made here by setting reproduction off as a special section headed "The Origin of Individuals" (Chapters 2 to 4).

There are no real functions of an organ system separate from those of the organs which compose it. The system merely completes and unifies the functions of the organs and their appurtenant structures such as ducts and openings.

B. Six System Functions

1. Coverage

The six functions or function complexes which are the subject of the following chapters are these:

1. Alimentation — ingestion + digestion + assimilation (Chapter 13)
2. Translocation — in tubes or otherwise (Chapter 14)
3. Respiration — gaseous exchange (Chapter 15)
4. Expulsion — of all metabolic waste materials or products (Chapter 16)
5. Control — both nervous and chemical (Chapter 17)
6. Enclosure — of the body as a whole (Chapter 18)

Each of these functions has many points of contact or overlap with others, and as indicated most of the terms cover a group of mechanisms sharing some features. For example, digestive systems, even in the broad sense, are only one of the devices by which animals can obtain food, where we would also list provision of yolk and absorption (by parasites) from the host. The broadest term would be alimentation. When a system is discussed individually, one may lose sight of its position in the broader field, thus losing perspective. To enable one to deal with even a few systems separately without this loss of perspective, it is suggested here that both the broader ways of looking at functions and the areas of overlap should be kept in mind.

2. Alimentation

In the broadest sense, the function of the digestive system is reasonably clear-cut, to provide nutrients for all processes. This includes the intake of food, its digestion, its assimilation, and elimination of undigested wastes. There is overlap with other systems in several ways: (1) food must be captured and brought to the mouth by locomotory and manipulative functions of the body and its appendages; (2) the digestive tract is likely to be involved in respiration, circulation, and excretion, (3) it sometimes is directly involved in locomotion; and (4) it occasionally has a function in reproduction.

The digestive system is usually defined as concerned with the uptake of food, which is itself defined as materials for metabolism. Strangely, however, it usually does not include such things as oxygen and water. There is thus a somewhat more inclusive field of which feeding is just one part. This can be labeled as intake of substances or ingestion.

Here we have to note that many animals take into their digestive tracts materials that they do not digest. These are all ingested, and we may therefore use the word *ingesta* for all materials that are eaten. From the ingesta, each animal will digest what it can, and it is this latter material that we will call *food*. The ingesta thus may contain some or much matter that cannot be digested and will therefore be egested, i.e., eliminated. Included under this term ingesta are many things not normally intended by the word food: soil that may contain food, water for metabolism or that may contain food, stones that may be used in a food-grinding organ, spermatozoa that will then be used to fertilize ova, and even air. Thus, the subject of the intake of food is only part of the subject of ingestion.

3. Translocation

It is commonplace to think of a circulatory system as a system of vessels using blood to carry materials to and from the tissues. There are several groups that have such a system: Vertebrata, Crustacea, Annelida, Pogonophora, and even Rhynchocoela. However, the function of material transport in the animal body is not limited to tube systems, and there are many systems of ducts that do not perform the vertebrate function of oxygen and food transport. Both of these are outlined here, with examples.

a. Transport Devices

Most circulation in animals is of liquids in a system of tubes or channels. Tube systems are of several sorts and perform a variety of transport functions other than real circulation, a word which implies a circular flow returning to the starting point. Before one can deal with circulation in the latter sense, one must put into perspective all of the transport mechanisms of animals. The following occur:

1.   Cyclosis, within individual cells
2.   Cell to cell through the cell membranes (universal in Metazoa but supplemented by other methods)
3.   Through hollow cells (porocytes of Porifera, and many fine ducts in Metzaoa)
4.   Among cells, in intercellular spaces
5.   In open channels among the tissues (for water movement, as in Porifera)
6.   Through interconnecting lacunae among tissues
7.   In large body cavities, such as the coelom
8.   Carried by migrating cells, such as amoebocytes and phorocytes
9.   Through special tube systems, such as tracheae or blood vessels
10. Through combinations, such as (7) and (9) together (dorsal vessel and haemocoel, in Insecta)

It must not be thought that these operate alone. Most animals utilize several of them, and complex animals probably use them all.

The structures involved in the above list of transport mechanisms are extremely varied. The following may be cited, mostly to be treated in later chapters:

1.   Flagellated passages, for water in sponges

2.   Spaces lined with epithelium for fluids such as lymph and coelomic fluids, also with floating cells
3.   Tracheae carrying air or oxygen
4.   Vessels containing blood with floating cells

Transport by cell. A curious transport occurs in some Thaliacea, as described by Beklemishev (1969): "On the ventral side the oozooid of *Doliolum* has a filamentous stolon, which at an early stage begins to bud off minute 'pre-buds'. At the base of the stolon numerous small amoeboid cells, *phorocytes*, are clustered: they lie along the stolon and immediately grasp the pre-buds as they separate off. The phorocytes carry the pre-buds in twos or threes to the dorsal outgrowth of the mother   . . .   and there deposit them in regular order."

Water channels in sponges are largely spaces left between the layers of choanocytes. These water channels form the simplest of organ systems, varying from a single cavity to complex branching channels. There are organs to control the intake of water, through the ostia, and its outgo, through one osculum or several. Pore cells control the passage from one chamber to another, and the flagella provide power for a continuous unidirectional movement. These are further described in Chapter 19, "Unique Organ Systems".

Body spaces vary from mere intercellular spaces of minute dimensions to large coeloms. Those that concern us here are spaces surrounded by the tissue called epithelium, which are represented in vertebrates by lymph passages and in many animals by the coelom. The coelom is often described as if it were a large cavity with internal organs lying or suspended within it; this gives an impression of spaciousness that is seldom justified. Most coeloms exist only theoretically, being fairly small spaces around and between the organs. Each exists by virtue of the epithelium that lines it.

Another body space that is extensive is the haemocoel of Arthropoda. This has nothing to do with the coelom, also present in these animals, but is a derivative of the early embryonic blastocoel. Here it is simply the space between tissues of ectodermal and those of endodermal origin.

Tracheae are air tubes found only in Arthropoda and Onychophora. They are discussed among the unique organ systems of Chapter 19. The very different tracheae of Vertebrata are described in Chapter 15.

Blood vessels are, strictly speaking, the true vascular tissue, although that term is used in some recent general textbooks to include also the "tissues" moving inside the vessels. The vessels are here treated as part of the circulatory systems (Chapter 14), but the blood is treated as a tissue (Chapter 11).

b. Tube Systems

Although not all transport methods employ a system of tubes, many do so. One must not forget, however, that there are a variety of tube systems that do not circulate blood. The tubes are always used for the transport of something within the body, but many of them are not considered to be part of a circulatory system. For perspective, all the tube systems are outlined here, even though they are discussed in several different chapters.

The tube systems of animals are of several sorts, serving widely different purposes. Although there is no place to draw the line between a tube system and a tubular organ, or between a tube long enough to be obvious and one so short as to be merely a passage between adjacent organs, we can illustrate some of the obvious ones:

1.   Open water canals — for circulation of seawater containing food, oxygen, spermatozoa, etc. (Porifera)

2. Closed water tubes — for hydrostatic pressure to manipulate tube feet; water vascular system (Echinodermata)
3. Air passages — for respiration; tracheal system, branching tubes to take air (or rarely molecular oxygen) direct to the tissues (Onychophora, Arthropoda)
4. Blood vessels — to transport such materials as nutrients, oxygen, hormones, waste products (Rhynchocoela, Phoronida, Mollusca, Annelida, Arthropoda, Pogonophora, Tunicata, Cephalochordada, Vertebrata)
5. Excretory tube systems — for elimination of the waste products of metabolism and of osmoregulation: (a) flame cell tube systems, including those without the flame (Platyhelminthes, Rhynchocoela, Rotifera, Nematoda, Cephalochordata), (b) nephridial systems, open tubes to drain coelomic wastes (Phoronida, Brachiopoda, Mollusca, Sipunculoidea, Echiuroidea, Annelida, Onychophora), (c) Malpighian tubules, closed at the inner end but bathed in blood (Arthropoda), and (d) kidney tubules, ureter, and urethra (Vertebrata)
6. Digestive tubes — including many intestinal tracts: (a) radial canals, actually branches of a gastrovascular cavity (Coelenterata), (b) digestive canals, replacing a GVC and without openings other than the mouth, and rarely a few anal pores (Ctenophora); (c) intestinal tracts, tubular and open at both ends, mouth and anus (Rhynchocoela, Rotifera, Gastrotricha, Nematoda, Bryozoa, Phoronida, Mollusca, Sipunculoidea, Echiuroidea, Annelida, Onychophora, Arthropoda, Chaetognatha, s.Echinodermata, Tunicata, Enteropneusta, Pterobranchia, Cephalochordata, Vertebrata); and (d) intestinal tracts, tubular but without anus (Brachiopoda)
7. Reproductive ducts — from the gonads to carry away the gametes; in most animals there are oviducts or sperm ducts, but in only a few are these so long and complex as to be distinctive tube systems (Nematoda, where the coiled oviduct or sperm duct is one of the most obvious features in the body cavity)
8. Neural tubes — (Vertebrata)

These tube systems thus serve a variety of functions, including hydraulics, respiration, feeding, excretion, and reproduction, but the nature of the systems is much more diverse than their general functions. In addition to the fact that they may be produced from ectoderm, endoderm, mesoderm, or combinations of these, they are of diverse construction (see descriptions in later sections);

1. Passages through a series of cells, as in the flame bulb systems
2. Passage through a single elongate tubular cell
3. Passages lined with gastrodermal cells
4. Passages lined with cells of mesodermal origin
5. Passages lined with epidermis (and sometimes cuticle)

The open water channels are unique in the Porifera, where the channels serve a variety of functions. The closed water vascular system in Echinodermata is unique in form and origin, but there are other hydraulic devices such as the use of blood pressure in arteries or the use of body cavity fluids to extend such organs as probosces.

This list of tube systems does not list all the systems described as circulatory, because some of the latter do not operate in tubes. If a circulatory system is defined as consisting of all the organs and tissues associated with movement of materials within the body, it would include many other devices than just tubes.

4. Respiration

Although respiration is a universal life process, many animals do not have a respiratory system. Where one exists it functions in concert with other systems. It delivers oxygen to the blood or to the tissue cells themselves and removes carbon dioxide. It may have a physical connection with the digestive tract, and part of its oxygen-supplying function may be usurped by the digestive tract in providing oxygen from metabolism. It seems to be the most highly specialized system, dealing principally with the two inorganic molecules oxygen and carbon dioxide.

5. Expulsion

The removal of waste products of metabolism is just one of the functions involved in removal of materials from a living body. These removals are diverse and are dealt with in a variety of places in this book. They may be listed in several ways, and there is appended to the lists some immaterial emissions. (There seems to be no commonly understood term for this broad concept. Elimination would be used, except for its common employment for just one of the processes: expulsion of undigested residues from the digestive tract.)

In the life of every animal there are a wide variety of materials given off under various circumstances. These may be parts of the body, undigested "food", excess water, metabolic by-products, or materials elaborated for some exterior use. The list is almost endless, but the diversity may be suggested by the following:

1. Body parts — fragments, moulted cuticles, gametes, spermatophores, proglottids, extrusomes
2. Metabolic materials — water, carbon dioxide, and nitrogenous wastes of protein metabolism
3. Incidental inclusions — digestive wastes, water
4. Secretions — to the outside, for all external purposes
5. Nonsubstances — light, heat, sound, electricity

The materials may be listed by the purpose for which the elimination is performed:

1. Reproduction — fragments, buds, gametes, spermatophores, zygotes, embryos, larvae
2. Excretion — wastes, metabolic by-products
3. Elimination — of digestive wastes and bacterial decomposition products
4. Development — molted materials, egg cases, capsules, lost teeth, spines, hair, feathers, cuticle
5. Behavior — silk, poisons, mucus, enzymes, cement, nematocyst darts, flotation gas, food for others, autotomized parts, pheromones, emanations, shells, "houses"
6. Emission of nonsubstances — light, heat, sound, electricity

These expulsions are discussed in appropriate parts of this book, for which consult the index.

Most of the listed substances require no explanation, but in Protozoa the term *extrusome* has been applied (Grell, 1973) to all things given off. Eight terms are applied to these substances or their ejectors:

1. Cnidocysts — similar to nematocysts (Dinoflagellata)
2. Ejectisomes — of unknown function (Flagellata)
3. Haptocysts — a balloon for penetrating (Suctoria)
4. Kinetocysts — movable along the axopods but of unknown function (Sarcodina: Heliozoa)

5.   Mucocysts — protective mucus (Flagellata)
6.   Pexicysts — threads for anchoring prey (Ciliata)
7.   Toxicysts — a paralyzing toxin (Ciliata: Gymnostomata)
8.   Trichocysts — firing a thread (Ciliata, Flagellata)

This subject is one of those involved in a large area of overlap. In three widely separated phyla (Acanthocephala, Priapuloidea, and Vertebrata) the excretory organs and the reproductive organs are so intimately associated that the combination has been called a urogenital (or urinogenital) system. There is, however, almost no amalgamation of functions; the association is largely through use of common ducts. They are treated separately herein.

6. Controls

All activities are limited by conditions of the physical environment such as temperature, light, pH, and pressure. Beyond this, control of processes is required in living systems at all levels and through a wide variety of means. There must be control of every chemical reaction, coordination of all metabolic functions, and control of behavior (from within or from without). The control may arise from within the organism (even if the initial stimulus was from outside) or from outside, and in the latter case the influence may be air- or water-borne or parasitic.

Control of metabolism

1.   By enzymes
2.   By nervous stimulation of organs
3.   By hormones

Control of behavior from within the individual

4.   By nervous stimulation of muscles, organs, appendages, etc.
5.   By hormones acting on metabolic processes

Control of behavior from outside of the individual

6.   By pheromones, airborne
7.   By water-borne chemicals, such as seminal fluid in the sea (Sipunculoidea, Echinoidea)
8.   By parasitic control (see Behavior): (a) control of ant by fluke cercaria in suboesophageal ganglion, (b) control of amphipod by cystacanth of acanthocephalan, or (c) control of fish by fluke metacercaria in the eye lens

Control of processes is thus principally effected by inherent enzyme systems, nerve impulses, hormones from within, and pheromones from without. Of these, the distribution of enzyme systems is too little known, or too uniform, to be tabulated for diversity; nerve impulse mechanisms are discussed in Chapter 17, under "Nervous System"; hormonal control is also discussed in Chapter 17 under "Hormones", and pheromonal and parasitic control under "Exploitation" in Chapter 22.

The two major control systems, nerves and hormones, are not as distinct as once imagined. Although at some times they seem rather different, it is now understood that although some aspects of hormonal control are mediated by the circulatory system, there are aspects of nerve transmission that are closely similar to hormone action. Furthermore, although the best known sources of chemical messengers are endocrine glands, other sources are neurosecretory cells, especially in the brain. Thus, there are two ways in which the hormone type of control is intimately involved with the nervous system, and this is the justification for their combination in a single system in one chapter (Chapter 17).

7. Enclosure

One of the necessary features of all individuals and most organs is containment. This is the function of the tissue called epithelium, which covers most structures and lines most cavities. On the outside of metazoan animals this tissue is called epidermis. As the lining of cavities such as coelom it is sometimes called endothelium. Both epidermis and gastrodermis in coelenterates are epithelia.

The coverings of internal organs and spaces may be mentioned when discussing those features individually. Outer body coverings are dealt with in Chapter 18, "Integuments".

REFERENCES

Beklemishev, W. N., *Principles of Comparative Anatomy of Invertebrates,* 2 volumes, University of Chicago Press, Chicago, 1969.

Clark, W. E. L., *The Tissues of the Body,* 6th ed., Oxford University Press, London, 1971.

Grell, K. G., *Protozoology,* Springer-Verlag, Heidelberg, 1973.

Hyman, L. H., *The Invertebrates,* Vol. 1, McGraw-Hill, New York, 1940.

Rudnick, D., Organogeny, in *The Encyclopedia of the Biological Sciences,* Gray, P., Ed., Reinhold, New York, 1961, 716.

Willier, B. H., Weiss, P. A., and Hamburger, V., *Analysis of Development,* W. B. Saunders, Philadelphia, 1955.

Chapter 13

DIGESTIVE SYSTEM

TABLE OF CONTENTS

I.   The Digestive System 266
     A.   Introduction... 266
     B.   Utilization of Food 266

II. Food and Feeding... 267
     A.   Ingestion 267
     B.   Food Types.. 267
     C.   Feeding 269
     D.   General Feeding or Nutrition Types... 269

III. Structures and Functions... 273
     A.   Basic Function.. 273
     B.   Features of Protozoan Nourishment 273
     C.   Metazoan Digestive Tracts.. 274
     D.   Openings into Digestive Tracts 275
     E.   Features of the Coelenteron 276
          1.   General Features 276
          2.   Organs of the Coelenteron.. 277
     F.   Features of the GVC 277
          1.   Gastrovascular Cavity 277
          2.   Organs of the GVC 278
     G.   Features of the Intestinal Tract... 278
          1.   The Tract 278
          2.   Organs of the Intestinal Tract 279
     H.   Unusual Features 284
     I.   Functions of the Tract 286
     J.   Miscellaneous Aspects of Digestive Systems................................. 288
          1.   Site of Digestion 288
          2.   Increasing the Surface 288
          3.   Nutriments for Ovum and Zygote 289
          4.   Embryonic Origin.. 290

References 291

I. THE DIGESTIVE SYSTEM

A. Introduction

Of all aspects of the biology of animals, the one which at first glance seems to be most uniform is the utilization of food. Food must be taken into the body, broken down into usable molecules, and absorbed into the tissues and cells of the body. These processes of feeding and digesting are usually performed by a group of organs integrated into a *digestive system.*

A system as widespread and essential as this one should not be hard to define. It is collectively all the organs concerned with ingestion, digestion, absorption, and elimination. It is substantially synonymous with *digestive tract* (but not necessarily with *intestinal tract*). Some difficulties do arise when it comes to organs that may help in feeding or in capture of food.

The system thus includes the hollow organs of the digestive tract, the associated glands, and the nonliving objects produced by some parts of it. The term *enteron* is approximately synonymous with digestive tract, but it is usually restricted to the embryonic system and adult parts derived from endoderm; in many animals (especially insects) large parts of the digestive tract are of ectodermal origin and in some the entire tract arises from mesoderm. The word *gut* has been used both as synonymous with digestive tract and as equivalent to *intestine.* Its relationship to "guts", the vertebrate internal organs as a whole, is unfortunate. For both reasons it would be best not used as a technical term even though it is well established in the derivatives foregut, midgut, and hindgut.

The most general term is thus digestive tract or system. There are three types of digestive systems, although they are often cited as two. The *coelenteron* of Coelenterata and Ctenophora is sometimes grouped with the *gastrovascular cavity* (GVC) of Platyhelminthes under the latter term. The differences are considerable, and they are here kept as distinct. The third type is the *intestinal tract.*

In addition to these three types of systems, there are many animals with no system at all, either during part of their life or all of it. The means by which they obtain nourishment are cited under "Metazoan Digestive Tracts" below. It is also necessary to include some protozoan organelles, such as food vacuoles, cytopharynx, and cytopyge, under the heading of digestive system, as they may perform the general functions of a multi-organ tract.

B. Utilization of Food

There are two things involved in the utilization of food in the metabolism of organisms. These are processes for the utilization of the food and structures to perform or contain the processes. It is not really possible to separate these in discussion. Some of the general terms must be dealt with first.

It is difficult to know what term related to the intake and use of food is the most general. *Metabolism* is the general term for the chemical conversion of all types of materials into energy and/or new materials. *Intussusception* is the absorption of materials by protoplasm for conversion into more protoplasm. *Nutrition* is defined in ordinary dictionaries as "the sum of the processes by which an animal . . . takes in and utilizes food substances." This is a very general meaning and could serve us here, but unfortunately the word is more commonly used in a medical sense, as the science of the needs for particular nutrients, mostly by humans.

Although *digestion* is often used solely for the processes of chemical breakdown of food, it is sometimes used to include a variety of processes beyond mere breakdown. For this reason the expression "The Utilization of Food" is here preferred to cover all the processes from the entry of food to the elimination of food wastes and to the absorption of the nutrients into the tissues of the body.

Before an animal can take in and utilize food, it must detect the food in its environment, capture it, and convey it to a mouth or other "port of entry". The means of detection are treated under "Sense Receptors" in Chapter 17. The means of food capture are cited in Chapter 21. The means of engulfing the food are tabulated below, followed by an analysis of what are called nutrition types — the general means used for obtaining nutrients by animals with diverse ways of living.

II. FOOD AND FEEDING

A. Ingestion

Food is any substance which upon ingestion or absorption can furnish the body with energy and materials for building body parts.

Feeding, in the broadest sense, is one of the basic activities of all animals. It can be defined as the sum of all the processes involved in taking in and preparing food for digestion. There is great diversity in the materials taken in and the manner of their use in metabolism, but no animal species can continue to exist unless at least some individuals in each generation ingest and metabolize enough food to provide for the succeeding generation.

In addition to food, many animals take into their digestive tracts materials that they cannot digest. All of these are "ingested", and we may therefore use the word *ingesta* for all materials that are eaten. From the ingesta, each animal will utilize what it can, and it is the latter material that we will call food.

The ingesta may also contain matter that cannot be digested and will therefore be eliminated as *egesta*. Included under the term ingesta are many things not normally intended by the word food: soil and water that may contain food, stones that may be used in a food-grinding organ, spermatozoa that are to be used to fertilize ova, and even air.

The word food is sometimes loosely used for all the materials taken in, what is here called the ingesta. As defined above, food more properly consists of all the materials of any sort that are used in metabolism, whether for building materials or for energy. In brief, this will include sources of energy and nutrients (mostly organic molecules), as well as water, oxygen, and required minerals. It is a curious fact that some "food" is not originally taken into the body for nutritional purposes and may never be in the digestive tract. For example, the *excess* gametes, cited under A in the following list, which are already in the reproductive tract, may be absorbed and used as food. This situation is called *hypergamesis*.

In common parlance, the term food does not include oxygen or water. These are customarily dealt with under separate headings, and that custom will be followed here.

B. Food Types

The food itself, which is also part of the ingesta, is unendingly diverse. This can be illustrated by the following partial list of types, with examples:

Animal body materials

1. Entire animals — (many predators)
2. Cell fluids — (s.Nematoda, s.Tardigrada)
3. Muscle and any organs — (many predators)
4. Blood — (Gastropoda: Pyramidellidae, many bloodsucking Insecta, Mammalia: s.bats)

5. Collagen — (Insecta: blowfly larvae)
6. Keratin — (Insecta: clothes moths)
7. Skin cuticle — (Insecta: Mallophaga)

Animal products

8. Excess oocytes, ova, or spermatozoa — (Gastropoda: slugs, Insecta: *Cimex*)
9. Hair — (Insecta: clothes moths)
10. Feathers — (Insecta: clothes moths)
11. Slime — of snails (Insecta: s.ants)
12. Milk — of mammals (their offspring or other mammals)
13. Secretions — from bromatophores; see below (Crustacea: Copepoda)
14. Honey — (s.Insecta, s.Mammalia)
15. Honeydew — (Insecta: ants)
16. Royal jelly — (Insecta: ants)
17. Silk — (Insecta: clothes moths)
18. Beeswax — (Insecta: bee moths, Aves: honey guides)
19. Cuticle — shed at last molt (Onychophora)
20. Excrement — (Oligochaeta, Insecta: s.flies, Mammalia: rabbits)
21. Eggs — (s.Gastropoda, Archiannelida: *Histriodrilus* on lobster eggs, s.Crustacea, Insecta: s.wasp larvae, Aves, Mammalia)
22. Regurgitated food — (Insecta: ant guests, Aves)

Plant tissues and parts

23. Wood — cellulose, see below (Flagellata: *Trichonympha,* Crustacea: an isopod, Bivalvia: *Teredo*, s.Oligochaeta, Insecta: s.beetles)
24. Leaves — (m.Insecta, s.Vertebrata)
25. Fruit — (s.Crustacea, s.Aves, s.Mammalia)
26. Spores and fruiting bodies — (Insecta: ants)
27. Seeds — (s.Insecta, Aves, Mammalia)
28. Cell fluids — s.Tardigrada, Gastropoda: *Sacoglossa*)

Plant products

29. Nectar — (m.Insecta, s.Aves)
30. Sap — (Mammalia: humans)
31. Pollen — (s.Insecta)

Biological molecules

32. Haemoglobin in seawater — (s.Tunicata)
33. Metabolic molecules of host — (m.parasites)
34. Digested food of host — (intestinal parasites)
35. By-products of symbiont metabolism — (Insecta: Isoptera, s.Mammalia)
36. Colloids in ground water — (Insecta: Collembola)
37. Salts as ions — (incidentally in food; by gills of some fishes)

Decomposing organic matter

38. Plants and animals — (Oligochaeta, Insecta: s.fly larvae)
39. Detritus — (many sessile animals)

In the above list is included "wood cellulose". It is sometimes implied that no animals digested wood, and yet there are five examples listed here. Any discrepancy may be due to the fact that wood is 18 to 38% lignin, which is apparently never digested by animals. Of the rest, 40 to 62% is cellulose, which can be broken down by some animals into assimilable sugars. Thus, wood as a whole is not digested, but the major cellulose fraction may be.

Also in the list is "Secretion from bromatophores". In parasitic copepods of the family Lernaeopodidae, the male feeds on the secretion of these female glands that are located between the cephalothorax and the trunk.

For many animals the list is too specific. These are the unselective filter- and deposit-feeders, the ones that ingest whatever comes along, whether digestible or not. These occur in nearly every group of marine animals, from Porifera to Mammalia.

Many of the examples given above are insects, in which group diversity of food is extreme, but many other groups show similar ranges. For example: Hyman (1967) cites for prosobranch Gastropoda that they are "grazers, herbivores, scavengers, carnivores, and mucociliary feeders." Among Protozoa, species may be holophytic (*Volvox globator*) or plant-feeding (*Pelomyxa palustris*) or predaceous (*Peranema trichophorum*), or either predaceous or holophytic as circumstances requires (*Euglena gracilis*).

Nutritional requirements are known in some detail for a few organisms, and the general differences between some groups can be surmised from their manner of living; however, there is simply no truly comparative data available for most groups, and even the existence of much diversity cannot honestly be claimed.

C. Feeding

The most basic division of feeding methods is into (1) those that involve manufacture of "food" from carbon dioxide and water with energy from sunlight (autotrophic), and (2) those that involve feeding on other organisms or their components (heterotrophic). In animals the only known autotrophs are some Flagellata (Phytomastigina) and one ciliate (*Cyclotrichium meunieri*). Other green protozoans or metazoans are believed to harbor photosynthetic algae and to absorb some of their products.

The words feeding and ingestion are both usually associated with animals that possess and use a mouth. Ingestion is herein restricted to such oral admission, but feeding is here used in a general sense to include both oral ingestion and absorption through surfaces. The latter include:

1. Absorption through the general body wall (m.Trematoda, Cestoda, Acanthocephala, Gordioidea, Gastropoda: *Enteroxenus*, s.male Echiuroidea)
2. Absorption by a peduncle or stalk (Crustacea: s.Cirripedia)
3. Transmission between connected polyps or zooids (m.Coelenterata, S.Bryozoa)
4. Absorption through a placenta (embryos of Onychophora, s.Insecta, m.Mammalia)
5. Absorption of yolk through cell membrane, in developing zygotes (in many animals; see list under "Nutriments for Ovum and Zygote").

The terms for feeding and nutrition types in the following lists suggest the many ways by which animals (and plants) obtain food. Some take in selected food whole, with some of these requiring it to be alive, some crush or macerate or tear the food, some absorb liquids only, and some ingest quantities of indigestible material to digest out the included "food".

D. General Feeding or Nutrition Types

There are several systems of terms to describe the nature of animal food, the preferences of animals, and the manner of feeding. There is considerable overlap between these sets, and there are numerous variations in the definition of the terms, especially between zoology and botany. The terms in the various sets (the -trophic, the -phagous, and the -vorous terms) are often intermixed in usage. The duplication, the overlap, and the variety of definitions make it impracticable for one to give a single set of recommended terms. Therefore the following lists contain the terms in use, with the most appropriate definitions found. Because these terms are most often used as adjectives (-trophic or -phagous), they are so listed here, but most of them can also be used as collective nouns (-trophy and -phagy) and as individual nouns (-trop or -trophe and -phage).

The trophic terms. Feeding types are represented by adjectives that may apply either to "nutrition" or to "organism", to the method or to the individual behavior:

1. Amphitrophic — can switch from autotrophic to heterotrophic (s.Flagellata)
2. Autotrophic — "self-feeding" or holophytic (photosynthetic or chemosynthetic); using simple inorganic substances as food, plus a source of energy (microorganisms, plants, and a few Protozoa)
3. Chemautotrophic — same as Chemotrophic
4. Chemotrophic — autotrophic in which the energy is obtained from chemical processes independent of light
5. Ectotrophic — feeding as an ectoparasite
6. Hemotrophic — absorption by the embryo through the placenta
7. Heterotrophic — using complex organic food derived from other animals or plants
8. Metatrophic — existing on organic nutrients only
9. Monotrophic — feeding on only one kind of prey
10. Osmotrophic — taking in energy-rich molecules in solution through the body surface; see saprotrophic
11. Paratrophic — obligately parasitic (holozoic or saprotrophic)
12. Phagotrophic — ingesting solid foods
13. Photoautotrophic — same as phototrophic
14. Phototrophic — autotrophic in which the energy is obtained from light
15. Saprotrophic — absorbing organic molecules

At least four -trophic words have been used to signify that an organism may utilize two or even three of these basic methods: poly-, mixo-, amphi-, and mesotrophic. These words all have other meanings and do not serve well to show that an organism uses two methods. Examples of dual feeding capabilities are

1. Both heterotrophic (such as predatory + saprotrophic)
2. Autotrophic + heterotrophic
3. Autotrophic + predatory + saprotrophic

A more explicit classification of feeding types has been proposed to show both the energy and carbon sources and covers all organisms. The following cumbersome terms are used:

1. Photolithotrophic — light, carbon dioxide
2. Photoorganotrophic — light, organic compounds
3. Chemolithotrophic — inorganic oxidation, carbon dioxide
4. Chemoorganotrophic — organic oxidation, organic compounds

All animals and most Protozoa would herein be chemoorganotrophs. It is doubtful whether such a term system will be widely adopted by zoologists.

Holozoic. Individual organisms can also be described as:

1. Holophytic — producing its organic food internally by photosynthesis or chemosynthesis
2. Holozoic — feeding on already elaborated organic matter

Saprozoic. The term saprotrophic was used above for heterotrophic nutrition involving the absorption of dissolved nutrients.

The terms saprozoic (and even saprophytic) are used by some parasitologists for this same concept (with the emphasis on the difference between "absorption" of molecules (sapro-) and "feeding" on organic matter. However, among other animals, such as insects and fungi, the sapro- terms are used to indicate that the organism feeds on decaying organic matter. In both of these systems the endings -zoic and -phytic specify that the consuming organism is animal or plant, respectively.

Carnivorous. The root -vorous refers to devouring or eating greedily. The following compounds have been used:

1. Carnivorous — eating flesh (animal tissues)
2. Herbivorous — eating plant tissues
3. Insectivorous — eating insects
4. Limivorous — mud-eating (Oligochaeta)
5. Omnivorous — eating a wide variety of food, plant or animal, dead or alive
6. Piscivorous — eating fishes
7. Zoosuccivorous — sucking animal fluids; bloodsucking

Phytophagous. The root -phagous refers to eating. The following compounds have been used (see also next list):

1. Coprophagous — feeding on digestive wastes
2. Microphagous — eating small food particles
3. Myrmecophagous — eating ants
4. Necrophagous — feeding on carrion
5. Phytophagous — eating plant tissues
6. Saprophagous — eating decayed organic materials
7. Zoophagous — feeding on animals

Prey. Among animals the animal- and the plant-feeding habits are both common, and various terms are used to describe the nature of the prey organism:

Feeding on animals

1. Bloodsucking — (s.Hirudinea, s.Insecta, s.Mammalia)
2. Cannibalism — the eating of members of an animal's own species (s.Mammalia)
3. Ectoparasitism — the feeding of a small animal on surface tissues or products of a host (s.Acarina, s.Insecta)
4. Endoparasitism — the feeding on internal cells, tissues, and cell products of a host (Trematoda, s.Crustacea, s.Insecta)
5. Micropredation — killing a much larger animal by eating from within (s.Insecta)
6. Predation — killing and eating other animals, including insectivorous, etc. (m.Vertebrata)

7. Coprophagy — the eating of animal excrement (s.Insecta,s.Aves)
8. Entomophagy — the eating of insects
9. Meliphagy — the eating of honey
10. Necrophagy — the eating of carrion (s.Insecta)
11. Saprophagy — the feeding on decaying organisms (s.Crustacea, s.Insecta)
12. Scavenging — feeding on dead animal material killed by some other animal (s.Aves, s.Mammalia)
13. Tecnophagy — the eating of an animal's own eggs

Feeding on plants

14. Plant-feeding — phytophagous or herbivorous animals
15. Alga-feeding (s.Crustacea)
16. Pollen-feeding (s.Insecta)
17. Sapsucking (s.Insecta, s.Aves)
18. Spore-feeding (s.Insecta)
19. Tissue-chewing (s.Insecta)

Feeding on both plants and animals (the feeding types are not clearly distinct)

20. Detritus-filtering (s.Anthozoa, Endoprocta, Bryozoa, Tunicata)
21. Filter-feeding — unselective as to food type but of controlled size (many marine animals: Porifera to Mammalia)
22. Plankton-filtering (Siphonophora, s.larval Crustacea, s.Pisces, Mammalia: Pinnipedia)
23. Soil-filtering (Oligochaeta)
24. Suspension-feeding, ciliary feeding, selecting from what falls upon it

Ectoparasitism. At lower levels there is again diversity. For example, within ectoparasitism will be found:

1. Feeding on hairs, feathers, etc. (Insecta: Mallophaga)
2. Feeding on skin tissues (Insecta: Mallophaga)
3. Feeding on surface secretions (Insecta: s.crickets and cockroaches on the larvae of s.ants)
4. Sucking blood on or through the surface (s.Hirudinea, s.Arachnida, s.Insecta, s.Mammalia)

Phagocytosis. One widespread form of feeding is not directly covered among the preceding. This is phagocytosis, the engulfing of food particles by individual cells, in the manner of an amoeba. This occurs not only in many protozoans (where it may be called *phagotrophy*), but in most other groups from the collar cells of sponges to some of the cells of the intestinal lining in vertebrates, and also in the walls of blood vessels of the latter. Of course, amoebocytes are ubiquitous in the animal kingdom.

A companion word to phagocytosis is *pinocytosis*, which is the engulfing of fluid by a cell. The fluid may contain nutrients. Thus, pinocytosis differs from *saprotrophy* in that the material is admitted as a membrane-lined vacuole, not as a fluid absorbed directly into the cytoplasm.

In the parasitic insects called Strepsiptera the hymenopterous host's blood is filtered through the delicate cuticle of the female parasite as it lies in the haemocoel of the host.

Some animals do not feed in the larval stage, some not in the adult stage. In early development some animals are nourished through part of their life on nutrients stored as yolk in the ovum or adjacent cells.

Much of the cited diversity in animal feeding is exemplified only in the Arthropoda and Vertebrata. This is partly because most other groups are marine, where plankton and detritus are common, and partly because many of the animals feed by more than one method. Thus, a sea anemone may live largely on detritus but will on occasion capture a fish and eat as a predator. Many also feed on either living or dead prey. Some absorb solutes directly from the surrounding water.

Even in the Arthropoda the diversity is inadequately shown. Crustacea feed on many animals (small and large), many plants (marine and terrestrial), detritus, plankton, microorganisms, dissolved organic material, and no doubt on other nutrient sources. The food of Insecta lacks the marine plankton and detritus aspect but is endlessly diverse on land, including animal prey, all parts of nearly all sorts of plants, decaying matter, microorganisms and their by-products, animal and plant fluids, and in general, virtually anything of an organic nature.

Thus, in spite of the universal necessity of taking in food, there is much diversity in the manner of feeding. This is further accentuated when the structures for ingesting and digesting the food are examined and when the life history stage is considered.

III. STRUCTURES AND FUNCTIONS

A. Basic Function

All digestive tracts consist of organs performing specific functions designed to make the particular food available for metabolism. It is easier to list the organs as separate structures than it is to list the functions as distinct. Therefore, the gross structure of the various tracts is herein followed by brief treatment of the specific functions and the organs that perform them.

All types of digestive systems perform the basic functions in some way. These are selection of food, ingestion, breakdown of the food, absorption of the products, and egestion of unused materials. Thus, the basic purpose of the digestive tract is to prepare foods for incorporation into the metabolic system of the body. In general, this preparation consists of breaking down the structure of the solid food as well as the complex organic molecules it contains.

B. Features of Protozoan Nourishment

The digestive provisions among Protozoa are more diverse than in all the rest of the animal kingdom, including photosynthesis, diffusion, active transport, pinocytosis, phagocytosis, filter-feeding, harboring symbionts that give out nutritional by-products, and no doubt others. They are thus autotrophic or heterotrophic (and in the latter either predaceous or saprotrophic), and a few are both auto- and heterotrophic as the occasion demands. No metazoan species or group approaches this range of food and nutritional mechanisms.

In Metazoa it is easy to make a distinction between feeding and later absorption by the cells. Because the Protozoa feed as single cells, it is not easy to make such a distinction, because the feeding individual and the absorbing cell are the same. This united process will therefore be briefly outlined here instead of in Chapter 21 ("Activities of Individuals").

"Protozoa obtain nourishment in manifold ways" (Kudo, 1966) and these can be grouped as auto- or heterotrophic as in other organisms. The distinction is not sharp because some protozoans can do both, and some or possibly all autotrophic protozoans require intake (in at least minute quantities) of certain organic materials that they cannot synthesize. These are loosely called "growth factors".

In protozoology it is common to separate heterotrophic feeding into two: holozoic (the ingestion of solid food) and saprozoic (here, the absorption of dissolved food).

There are three modes of food uptake, which may be designated thus:

1. Permeation of dissolved substances, involving a variety of processes represented by such terms as diffusion, osmosis, ion transport, and active transport, depending on the nature of the cell membrane, its ionization, the presence of necessary enzymes, and its permeability to the substance in question.
2. *Pinocytosis* of liquids by abscission of vesicles from the membrane into the interior of the cell.
3. *Phagocytosis* is the intake of solid food particles, larger than would be included in the liquids of pinocytosis. This is by cytoplasmic extensions that enclose the object in a food vacuole.

In addition to these named processes, food of protozoans may be taken in by a variety of other methods, often not well understood. An "immobilizing influence" is often involved as well as organelles such as the collars of choanocytes, micropores, a cytostome, cilia, a proboscis, and tentacles.

C. Metazoan Digestive Tracts

One of the most nearly universal features of animals is the digestive tract. At first glance these seem to be much alike in diverse animal groups. Nevertheless, diversity appears at once when we note the animals that completely lack digestive organs:

No Digestive Tract in the Adult

1. All Porifera (intracellular digestion)
2. All Mesozoa (direct absorption; parasitic)
3. Some Coelenterata (fed by other polyps)
4. Some Platyhelminthes (direct absorption; parasitic)
5. All Acanthocephala (direct absorption; parasitic)
6. Some Bryozoa (fed by neighboring zooids)
7. Mollusca: Gastropoda (*Enteroxenus*) absorbs through body wall from its holothurian host
8. Some Echiuroidea (direct absorption; parasitic males)
9. Some Annelida which are epitokes (use reserve nutrients only)
10. Some Arthropoda (direct absorption; some parasitic Crustacea)
11. All Pogonophora, which form a temporary cavity among the tentacles (digestion in this cavity)

Larvae and embryos in some groups may also lack a digestive tract, being fed from yolk in the egg or by direct absorption. Even an archenteron may degenerate, or a digestive tract functional in one stage may disappear in the next (as in some Bryozoa and Echinodermata).

The remaining animals do have digestive cavities of some sort, but the diversity of their form and structure is considerable.

Coelenteron. A cavity, usually large in relation to the body size, filled with water from outside in which food may be present. The cavity may be

1. Sac-like, as in *Hydra*, often also with connecting tubes
2. A sac with septal sheets dividing it incompletely into chambers (Anthozoa)
3. An elaborate system of tubes only (Ctenophora)

Gastrovascular cavity (GVC). A cavity, sac-like or with several or many diverticula, reaching to most parts of the body; even when anal pores are present, it is less freely communicating with the outside, so that contents are mostly food and secretions (Turbellaria and Trematoda).

Intestinal tract. A tubular digestive system (sometimes with diverticula) divided into regions, one of which is an intestine (most animal phyla, Rhynchocoela to Vertebrata). Said to be complete if open from mouth to anus, or incomplete, if not open throughout or lacking either mouth or anus.

D. Openings into Digestive Tracts

In nearly all digestive tracts the opening through which food enters is called the *mouth.* If there is a second opening for egestion, this is the *anus.* Either the mouth or the anus may be multiple (very rarely), but there usually are no other food openings to the digestive tract. When one opening serves both for entry and exit, it is properly termed a *proctostome.* The only other exterior openings of any sort, besides the nares cited below, are involved with the gill slits in the pharynx of Pterobranchia, Enteropneusta, Tunicata, Cephalochordata, and some Vertebrata; these are for passage of respiratory water, not food.

The diversity with respect to openings into (or out of) the digestive tracts of animals is great. The coelentera and gastrovascular cavities are sometimes said to be incomplete, but they are too different from intestinal tracts to be covered by the terms incomplete and complete. They are not tubular with the usual openings; i.e., they do not consist of a passage through the body from mouth to anus. These digestive cavities are not the only ones that do not form an open tube, as many intestinal tracts are incomplete. For example:

Coelenteron

1. (Coelenterata, Siphonophora, Ctenophora)

Gastrovascular cavity

2. (Gnathostomuloidea, Platyhelminthes)

Incomplete intestinal tract

3. Midgut missing (larvae of s.Insecta)
4. Midgut replaced by ligament (Insecta: s.scale insects)
5. Anus not present or not open (s.Rotifera, s.Nematoda, all Gordioidea, all Brachiopoda, s.Gastropoda, s.Crustacea, all Ophiuroidea)
6. Passage blocked from midgut to anus (Insecta: s.Neuroptera)
7. Midgut not connected to the proctodaeum (Insecta: s.Hymenoptera)
8. No mouth; only rudiment of stomach-intestine (s.Rotifera)
9. Stomach not connected to the intestine (Insecta: s.Coccidae and s.larvae of others; Arachnida: *Ixodes*)
10. Intestinal tract present but not functional in feeding, being converted into an air-storage balloon (Insecta: s.Ephemeroptera)

In a broad view, digestive tract openings include the following:

1. Mouth — in all animals except those lacking digestive tract altogether (listed above)
2. Polystomium — many mouths but no anus: (a) in certain medusae of Scyphozoa,

the coelenteron opens through the oral arms, with literally thousands of openings, (b) in certain Turbellaria, there are multiple proboscises (pharynges) each with a mouth

3. Proctostome — functions of mouth and anus in a single opening: (1) coelenteron (Coelenterata, Ctenophora); (b) gastrovascular cavity (s.Platyhelminthes)
4. Oral pore — as a posterior mouth (s.planula larvae of Coelenterata)
5. Nares — in at least one tadpole, the mouth is preoccupied as a holding sucker, and the nostrils are used for the feeding and respiratory current
6. Anus — in all animals except those listed as having incomplete tract: (a) those lacking digestive tract altogether (as listed above), (b) those having a coelenteron or GVC (listed above), and (c) those having an intestine but with no anus (listed above)
7. Anal pores — (a) one or two into gastrovascular cavity (Trematoda), (b) two pores into two of the coelenteron extensions on the aboral surface (Ctenophora), and (c) many pores from radial canals (medusae of Hydrozoa and Scyphozoa)
8. Pore of duct from intestine to dorsal body wall (Hirudinea: Trematobdellidae)
9. Oesophageal or pharyngeal respiratory openings such as gill slits (Pterobranchia, Enteropneusta, Tunicata, Cephalochordata, Vertebrata)

E. Features of the Coelenteron
1. General Features

A coelenteron is found only in those two phyla usually cited as consisting of tissues derived from just two germ layers. This interpretation that there are just two germ layers is rejected here (see Chapter 5), but the coelentera are found only where the body consists mainly of epidermis and gastrodermis (with no highly organized third layer between them). These are the Coelenterata and the Ctenophora.

These cavities are completely different from the intestinal tracts of higher animals, and it is therefore inappropriate to apply to them terms used for regions or organs of the more complicated tracts. The word mouth implies simply an incurrent food opening, so it would be acceptable here, but in the coelenteron regions are sometimes called pharynx, stomach, and intestine although they are merely suggestive of such regions in higher animals. The "pharynx" would be better called gullet, the "stomach" and "intestine" each better called gastric cavity.

The coelenteron is correctly the entire digestive system, from the mouth (or multiple mouths) to the various canal systems and pores; the word is sometimes used for the central cavity alone. The *mouth* is more properly a *proctostome* (a combined mouth and anus). It opens into the major cavity either directly or via a gullet or a cavity in the hypostome or manubrium. The central cavity may itself be a blind pouch with the same shape as the whole animal, a large cavity divided by septa into chambers, a large cavity giving rise to radiating tubes, or a small cavity giving rise to a bilateral tube system.

Even in the comparatively few species of these two phyla diversity continues to appear. The canal or tube system may appear in any of these forms:

1. Four radiating radial canals and a ring canal (s.medusae of Hydrozoa)
2. Many radiating and branching radial canals and a ring canal (medusae of Scyphozoa and s.Hydrozoa)
3. Eight peripheral canals connected to the central cavity by a bilateral system (Tentaculata of the Ctenophora)
4. Gastrodermal canals (solenia) in the stalks or stems of polyps or in colonies (Hydrozoa)
5. Many radiating canals but no ring canal (some Scyphozoa)

6. Numerous small canals throughout the body, arising from the eight meridional canals (Nuda of the Ctenophora)

Although these coelentera are described as blind pouches, they sometimes have terminal pores on the radial canals that seem to serve for egestion of unused particles; each serves in place of an anus. These occur in several groups. In the medusae of some Hydrozoa and Scyphozoa each radial canal has an opening (pore) near the base of the tentacles; in some Ctenophora the aboral canal terminates in an anal pore. The coelenteron is in close contact with most parts of the body, thus distributing nutrients as well as releasing them from food. It is thus a form of gastrovascular cavity, performing both gastric (digestive) and vascular (circulatory) functions.

The lining of the coelenteron is the gastrodermis, a tissue usually of cuboidal or columnar cells in a single layer. The cells are glandular (mucus-secreting), nutritive (absorptive), enzymatic glandular, epitheliomuscular, sensory, and cnidoblasts producing nematocysts (limited to filaments of anthozoans). There may also be symbiotic zoochlorellae or zooxanthellae among these gastrodermal cells.

2. Organs of the Coelenteron

The mouth opens into a gullet (of ectodermal origin) and this into the coelenteron (of endodermal origin). The gullet (sometimes called pharynx) may be very long (as in some Scyphozoa) or very short (as in *Hydra*).

In polyps, the coelenteron is a sac, undivided (Hydrozoa) or divided by hanging sheets or septa (Anthozoa).

In medusae, the coelenteron may be quadrate, with each corner leading into a radial canal that connects to the peripheral circular canal (Hydrozoa), circular with many radial canals to the circular canal (s.Scyphozoa), without the circular canal (s.Scyphozoa), with the main cavity divided into four pockets by four gonads, or other variations.

In the polymorphic Siphonophora feeding is accomplished by the gastrozooids, and digestion is by the gastrodermal cells of the gastrozooids and connecting dactylozooids. In some of the latter there are "apical" pores for removal of undigested material.

In Ctenophora the coelenteron consists of a regular system of endodermal tubes: a central longitudinal tube, two lateral tubes, and four peripheral longitudinal tubes from each lateral tube. The tubes extend along the eight comb rows to the apical (aboral) pole and to the tentacles (when present). There are no distinct digestive regions or organs except the tubes.

F. Features of the GVC

1. Gastrovascular Cavity

A gastrovascular cavity system, differing from the coelenteron principally in arrangement, is found in all Platyhelminthes that have a digestive apparatus. It is a cavity of endodermal origin, with a proctostome (combined mouth and anus). It is sometimes a simple pouch but may have many diverticula which may even be branched, but it consists of only two regions — the pharynx (or proboscis) and the main cavity or GVC (not properly an intestine but sometimes called caecum). The part of the system between the mouth and the caecum may be muscular; it is commonly called pharynx. Although this term probably should be reserved for a region of an *intestinal* tract, the structural similarity leads most writers to use it also in the Platyhelminthes. The tube connecting the "pharynx" with the main cavity (often also tubular) above any branching is sometimes called "oesophagus", although it has no real similarity to the oesophagus in intestinal tracts.

The lining of the GVC is called gastrodermis. It is a single-layered epithelium, often syncytial, but usually consisting of large phagocytic cells and smaller "granular clubs" which probably are secretory. The cells are usually ciliated. (The presence of these phagocytic cells as the major cell type of the gastrodermis is a feature distinguishing this gastrodermis from that in the Coelenterata.)

A GVC occurs only in some flatworms, especially the Platyhelminthes. It is here considered that the groups Nemertodermatida, Xenoturbellida, and Gnathostomuloidea are distinct phyla; they also may have a GVC. Even within the Platyhelminthes diversity appears in several ways:

1.   The GVC may be entirely absent (Turbellaria: Acoela, Cestoda, Cestodaria)
2.   The "mouth", or the opening of the proboscis cavity, may be at any point on the midventral line except at the posterior end (Turbellaria)
3.   There may be multiple proboscises opening into a common cavity, and thus multiple mouths (some Turbellaria such as *Phagocata*)
4.   There may be one or several anal pores (Trematoda, Turbellaria)
5.   There may be no mouth or proctostome in the adult, even though the larval GVC had one (Fecampiidae in the Turbellaria)
6.   The proboscis may be of any of three types in Turbellaria, called simple, bulbous, or plicate
7.   From a ventral mouth the main cavity may be a single pouch or a sac with one anterior and two posterior diverticula, or with few or many branches or lateral expansions of the diverticula (Turbellaria)
8.   From an anterior mouth the cavity is tubular with two elongate posterior sacs, sometimes called "intestinal caeca" (Trematoda)

2. Organs of the GVC

In Turbellaria the GVC (when present) consists of (1) a proboscis (protrusible and not highly muscular) or rarely an anterior muscular pharynx and (2) a sac, simple or branched. The latter is sometimes erroneously called intestine. A short "oesophagus" may connect the proboscis with the GVC. The latter may be a simple sac, have two or three large lobes, or it may be broken up into many slender tubes. The only organs besides the proboscis are separate gland cells.

In Trematoda, the anterior mouth usually opens into a muscular pharynx. From this extends a long caecum, usually branched into two which are sometimes further divided. Although a pharynx is present, there is no justification for calling the posterior extensions by the term intestine. The GVC operates in much the same manner as the coelenteron and has few of the features of an intestine. There is no anus, but in a few Digenea there are one or two anal pores.

G. Features of the Intestinal Tract
1. The Tract

The term intestinal tract should be reserved for the basically tubular digestive systems that have an intestine. Definition of the term intestine requires specification of three aspects: structure, function, and embryonic origin. In structure it is a tube, possibly with diverticula or folds, posterior to the stomach and leading to or toward the anus. In function it is principally digestive and absorptive. It always arises from endoderm in the embryo.

The extent of endodermal derivatives in the digestive tract varies greatly, but the intestine is always endodermal. The oesophagus in the Insecta is of ectodermal origin, whereas the oesophagus in Mollusca or Vertebrata is endodermal. In these groups, such names have been used to represent the structure and function of the organ and its position in the digestive tract as a whole, rather than its embryonic origin.

The posterior part of the intestinal tract may consist of intestine right to the anus, but in many animals (all Arthropoda) there is a substantial "hindgut" that is of ectodermal (proctodaeal) origin and is therefore not truly part of the intestine. In these arthropods the endodermal section may be called midgut, rather than intestine, but the structure, function, and origin make it reasonable to classify it as an intestine.

Some of the diversities of the intestinal tract are related to its arrangement and the means adopted to increase the absorptive surface over the amount in a simple tube. Another diversity has been suggested above as the occasional presence of a digestive tract that is not a continuous tube. There are three circumstances:

1. Lacking mouth opening (only in some embryos and some Rotifera)
2. Lacking connections between the foregut and the hindgut (some insect larvae and adults)
3. Lacking anal opening (s.Rotifera, s.Gastropoda)

Although basically tubular, this shape is obscured in Myzostomida and Hirudinea by paired caeca, usually corresponding with internal segmentation. In Asteroidea, there is a very short intestine with very large glandular caeca in each of the arms (varying from 4 to at least 21).

Where caeca do not occur and the animal is elongate, as in Annelida and many Arthropoda, the surface of the relatively long tube may suffice for absorption. In shorter animals, where considerable bulk occurs relative to the length, other means are found that increase the absorptive surface. The intestine may be much lengthened by convolution or coiling, as in Pelecypoda and Vertebrata. It may be doubled back into U- or J-shape (as in Bryozoa and Cephalopoda) or it may also be twisted like a rope (in Sipunculoidea). In others the inner surface of the tube is increased by numerous small folds or extensions of the walls called villi, sometimes so small as to be termed microvilli. More obvious is the large typhlosole fold, hanging from the top of the tube throughout much of its length, in the diverse groups Bivalvia, Oligochaeta, and Ascidiacea, and the very striking "spiral valve" of some Chondrichthyes (which is not a valve but rather a spiral flap).

2. Organs of the Intestinal Tract

The structures and their functions in the intestinal tract are endlessly diverse. The differences are correlated with the functions performed. Often apparent similarities among groups, such as presence of a proboscis or introvert, is due to the fact that the same term is applied. For example, the proboscises of Turbellaria, Rhynchocoela, Acanthocephala, Priapuloidea, Sipunculoidea, Tardigrada, and Pterobranchia have almost nothing in common. Little comparative data is available that is not obscured by the multiple terms or by the use of one term to cover different things. Of the former, for example, the 20 or more mechanisms for seizing prey range from trichocysts to tentacles to radula to podia to trunks. As example of one of the latter, tentacles occur in Protozoa (part of the cell), Coelenterata (around the mouth), Ctenophora (a pair, like wings on the spherical body), Brachiopoda (inside the shell, along the spiral brachidia on each side), Pogonophora (from one to many, almost more massive than the body), and Annelida (where the feathery tentacles form large retractable fans).

This chapter should cover digestive organs at all stages in the life cycle. Nevertheless, it is inevitable that attention will be given principally to adult organs. It all starts in the embryo, where invaginations form the stomodaeum and the proctodaeum (and sometimes other features too). These are organs, but they are usually without digestive function, being primarily steps in the development of later organs. One exception is reported: In Porifera an early invagination does ingest neighboring cells to make feeding the earliest function of all.

Larvae do feed, in most animals, and a digestive tract is present. It may be an early stage of the adult tract, or it may be a special larval organ that will be resorbed at metamorphosis. An example of the first is the ephyra larva of some Scyphozoa, in which the early digestive tract becomes the adult coelenteron. Of the second, it is necessary only to recall that pupation in many insects destroys the digestive tract completely, replacing it with an entirely new one (perhaps one adapted to a different type of food). A similar replacement of the larval digestive tract occurs in Echinodermata.

An example of the simplest solution to development of a digestive system is found in parasitic Crustacea of the family Monstrillidae, where "At no stage in the life history of these copepods is there any trace of digestive organs, neither mouth, gut, nor anus" (Baer, 1951).

There is no direct way to compare the features of the intestinal tract in the many classes that have one, and yet the substantial diversity must not be left unrecognized. First of all, there is much diversity in the overall arrangement of the tract, whether it is straight from mouth to anus, recurved, coiled, or otherwise unusual. (It has already been noted that it may be entirely absent or partly missing.) In most worm-like animals, where it occurs at all, it is reasonably straight: Rhynchocoela, Nematoda, Gordioidea, Priapuloidea, Solenogastres, Dinophiloidea, Archiannelida, s.Polychaeta, s.Oligochaeta, Pentastomida, Onychophora, m.Arthropoda, Enteropneusta, and Cephalochordata. A few with essentially straight tracts have such extensive diverticula as to seem different: s.Tardigrada, Myzostomida, s.Polychaeta, s.Oligochaeta, Hirudinea, Pycnogonida, Arachnida, s.Insecta, Chaetognatha, Asteroidea, and Ophiuroidea.

The tract is quite commonly recurved (J- or U-shaped), in which the mouth and anus are not at opposite ends of the body: Calyssozoa, Bryozoa, Phoronida, Scaphopoda, Cephalopoda, Sipunculoidea, Merostomata, Crinoidea, Pterobranchia, Plantosphaeroidia, Ascidiacea, Thaliacea, and Larvacea.

The tract is coiled in these groups: Brachiopoda (where it is also recurved), Monoplacophora, Amphineura, Gastropoda, Bivalvia, Echiuroidea, s.Polychaeta, s.Arachnida, s.Crustacea, s.Insecta, Echinoidea, Holothuroidea, and Vertebrata.

There is a basic sequence to the digestive tube that holds in most groups, and from this each section can then be discussed as to diversity:

mouth — oral cavity — pharynx — oesophagus — stomach — intestine — rectum — anus

Mouth. The mouth opening may be at or near the front end of the animal body or at the top of the cup- or vase-shaped body or mid-ventral in such extremely shortened (flattened) animals as starfish. The mouth may be bordered with movable lips that aid in food intake and closure; these may be placed above and below the mouth, as in Vertebrata, or as a circle of 3 to 6 as in Nematoda.

Oral cavity. A cavity behind the mouth may be used for various purposes, such as filtering or mastication. The word mouth is in common parlance often used to include the cavity into which it opens. The term oral cavity or *buccal cavity* is applied if it is between the mouth and the pharynx or oesophagus. In some animals there may be no space between mouth and pharynx, or the pharynx may also be absent so that the mouth leads directly into the oesophagus. The term oral cavity is usually used in Insecta and Vertebrata. Buccal cavity is more likely to be used in Rhynchocoela and other invertebrate groups.

Various modifications of the oral (or buccal) cavity occur. For filtering plankton food from seawater, some Mammalia (whales) have many parallel horny plates of whalebone (baleen) suspended from the upper jaws; these may reach a length of 12 ft. In some Insecta, a so-called *infra-buccal* or *buccal chamber* in the floor of the oral cavity, receives small food particles, squeezes out any juice that is swallowed, and casts out the solid residue through the mouth. It is this buccal cavity through which the radula in many Mollusca extends forward from the pharynx.

The oral cavity sometimes opens into the pharynx (in Gastrotricha, Kinorhyncha, Nematoda, Priapuloidea, Echiuroidea, Myzostomida, s.Annelida, and Vertebrata) or directly into the oesophagus (in Calyssozoa, Phoronida, Brachiopoda, Sipunculoidea, Chaetognatha). In other animals there is no oral cavity, and the mouth may lead almost directly to the stomach as in Pelecypoda and Asteroidea.

In some Nematoda, there is a protrusible *stylet* in the buccal cavity; it is used to puncture plant and animal cells, from which its hollow core permits intake of fluid food (see also odontostyle, under Pharynx, below).

Structures called *jaws* are of many sorts and serve functions such as grasping, perforating, tearing, and grinding. The diverse jaws have little in common, besides their functions with food, except an appropriate hardness and movement by muscles. They may be hollow for sucking fluids or for injecting poison. They are cited in Bivalvia, Cephalopoda, Tardigrada, Polychaeta, Oligochaeta, Hirudinea, Onychophora, Crustacea, most Myriapoda, Insecta, and Vertebrata.

The word *tooth* is used widely among animals for a variety of hard pointed structures; different "teeth" may have nothing in common except this shape, occurring anywhere in or on the body and performing a wide variety of functions. The best known teeth are found in the oral cavity of some Vertebrata. They can be used for a variety of stabbing, crushing, tearing, and chewing functions or to transmit venom.

The teeth of Vertebrata are generally on bones of the jaw, but they can occur in the roof of the mouth, on the tongue, and even in the pharynx. Each is usually formed of three calcified tissues: dentine, enamel, and cement; the core of dentine (around a pulp cavity), enamel on the exposed surface, cement to fasten it in place.

Many fishes have teeth in successive rows so that as they wear out they are replaced from behind. In some coral fishes, the teeth are fused to form a single tooth plate, which aids in breaking the coral. A few fish are toothless.

Amphibians and reptiles usually have a single row of teeth above and below, in the poisonous reptiles some of them may be developed into fangs, which may be movable. Extant birds have no teeth, although several extinct groups of birds had teeth.

Mammals all possess teeth, except for such "primitive" ones as the echidnas. In the platypus, some of the anteaters, and a few whales, embryonic teeth do not persist into the adult.

In some Echinoidea there is a large scraping or chewing apparatus projecting from the mouth and consisting of five "teeth" operated by a complex of ossicles and muscles called the *Aristotle's lantern*. Most drawings show the oesophagus (pharynx) passing up through the center of this organ, with the teeth projecting from the mouth. There is thus a buccal cavity behind the teeth, from which the oesophagus leads.

In most Vertebrata the floor of the oral cavity is extended into a usually freely movable and often protrusible *tongue*, used principally in the capture and manipulation of food.

Pharynx. Behind the mouth and any oral cavity the usual first part of the digestive tube is muscular and functions as a sucking pump to draw fluids into the mouth. In vertebrates the pharynx is not usually muscular. In lower vertebrates it is the cavity from which the gill slits arise. In higher vertebrates it is the chamber formed by the crossing of the respiratory and the digestive tracts, not really serving any digestive function. In invertebrates, where the pharynx arises from the stomodaeum, it may be clearly tripartite with a triangular lumen. This occurs in Gastrotricha, Kinorhyncha, Nematoda (often called oesophagus), and Tardigrada. It can be everted in Priapuloidea, Myzostomida, and some Polychaeta. It is called *mastax* in Rotifera, where it is a grinding organ. In animals with a *radula* (Mollusca), that structure originates in the pharynx and may be protrusible into the oral cavity and out through the mouth. Radula-like organs occur in Onychophora (roof of the buccal cavity) and in some Arachnida: Acarina (on the labrum).

In some Nematoda a stylet is formed in the buccal cavity, but in others it is formed in the pharynx. To distinguish these, Hyman (1951) proposed the term *odontostyle* for the pharyngeal organ. It is sometimes hollow. Elsewhere some Hirudinea have one or two stylets, apparently also from the pharynx. In Tardigrada a pair of stylets in associated with the pharynx.

In Cephalochordata and most Tunicata, there is a longitudinal mid-ventral ciliated groove termed the *endostyle*, running the length of the pharynx, which secretes mucus for use in capture of food particles at the gill slits. These are carried to a dorsal groove and back to the intestine (feeding by a conveyor-belt system).

In chordates, the pharynx arises as a combination of ecto- and endodermal tissues. It is a development of the pharynx which forms the *branchial basket* in animals with respiratory perforations of the digestive tract (pharyngotremy) which produce gill slits (Tunicata, Cephalochordata, lower Vertebrata). In animals with such pharyngeal gills, the food and oxygen enter in water by the mouth and are separated in the pharynx so that food passes to the oesophagus and oxygen to the gill slits. In the groups cited, and in early stages of all Vertebrata, this aquatic respiratory function of the pharynx is present. In air-breathing vertebrates the food passage and the air passage merely cross in the pharynx.

Oesophagus. The slender tube called oesophagus (or sometimes *gullet*) is either short or long, usually not muscular, sometimes ciliated (Sipunculoidea), sometimes lined with cuticle, and may have diverticula (s.Annelida). It is said to be of stomodaeal (ectodermal) origin in Nematoda, Mollusca, Annelida, and Crustacea, but in Hirudinea it is stated to be definitely endodermal, and would thus be part of the midgut. In all Vertebrata the oesophagus is derived from endoderm.

The oesophagus is most often a simple tube connecting to the stomach or midgut, but it may be divided into compartments, such as *crop* and/or *gizzard* in Echiuroidea, Oligochaeta, Hirudinea, Crustacea (gastric mill), Insecta, Reptilia, and Aves. In Insecta the crop is a sac connected to the oesophagus by a duct. In Aves the crop is oesophageal, but the gizzard is part of the stomach.

The carnivorous *Philine* (Gastropoda) crushes shells of small bivalves in an oesophageal gizzard with calcified internal teeth. In Nematoda, the oesophagus (sometimes called pharynx) is unique in being the primary site of secretion of digestive enzymes.

The term *proventriculus* is used in several groups. In earthworms it is equivalent to the crop. In insects it is the gizzard. In birds it is the anterior part of the stomach.

In many Insecta but in no other animals, a chitinous cylindrical peritrophic membrane extends back from the end of the oesophagus, forming a tube which extends far back into the intestine; it is permeable to digested food and thus serves to keep undigested material away from the intestinal wall while passing the solutes for absorption.

Stomach. The stomach and the intestine are usually assumed to be the midgut and thus to be endodermal in origin, but in Rhynchocoela the stomach is said to be part of the foregut. It may be ciliated (Rotifera) and is sometimes not clearly distinguished from the intestine.

With the exception of Agnatha and some Pisces where no stomach exists, the stomach of Vertebrata is unique in being a truly distinct part of the digestive tract where true gastric digestion occurs. It is usually U-shaped, with valves at entry (from oesophagus) and exit (into intestine). It may be extremely distensible, allowing some deepsea fish to swallow other fishes as large as themselves. In Mammalia it may be divided by constrictions into functionally different chambers, such as the four chambers in ruminants.

Glandular diverticula are called *gastric* or *pyloric caeca* (or stomach pouches) or sometimes even *hepatic caeca* when the secretory and digestive functions are combined. Such diverticula occur in many groups, including Gastrotricha, Brachiopoda, Mollusca, Myzostomida, Annelida, Arthropoda, Echinodermata, Enteropneusta, and Vertebrata.

The stomach may also contain a ciliated *style sac* from which projects the *crystalline style*. This is a translucent proteinaceous mass that is revolved by ciliary action, the anterior end rubs against a gastric shield, and gives off carbohydrate-digesting enzymes. It is known only in Mollusca (Monoplacophora, Gastropoda, Bivalvia).

Intestine. The word intestine always refers to tissues derived from endoderm, at least in cases where it persists from embryo to adult. It may be blind (closed at the anal end), have one or more caeca or diverticula, lead directly to the anus or open into a rectum or a cloaca, be combined with the stomach, be muscular or not, have many glands or none, or be divided into subregions (small and large or duodenum, jejunum, ileum, and colon). It is usually the principal site of digestion and absorption.

Like other parts of the digestive tract, the intestine may have diverticula or caeca. These occur in each of these phyla: Rhynchocoela, Nematoda, Myzostomida, Annelida, Arthropoda, Echinodermata, and Vertebrata.

In Oligochaeta the dorsal wall of the intestine is folded down into an elongate suspended *typhlosole*. This greatly increases the absorptive surface of the intestine. A similar structure is reported under the same term in both Mollusca and Tunicata. A so-called "spiral valve" in some fishes seems to serve the same function.

Rectum. When properly identified the rectum is always derived from a proctodaeum. It connects to the posterior end of the intestine and may also receive the discharge of the malpighian tubules (Insecta). It may have caeca or a rectal bladder, and it may be muscular for elimination or for pumping when it has a respiratory function.

Unusual rectal diverticula are found in the Sipunculoidea, where a single diverticulum is found, varying in the different species from small to "enormous", and in Echiuroidea (a pair) of long caeca or anal sacs. In Hirudinea a rectal bladder is cited, but this is merely the distensible rectum itself. This "bladder" is ciliated and is said to be formed from endoderm and thus part of the midgut.

When the rectum serves also for discharge of excretory products or gametes or both, it is called a *cloaca*, defined on the basis of this multiple purpose. It occurs with digestive plus reproductive functions in Rhynchocoela, s.Rotifera, and Nematoda, and with digestive plus excretory in Tardigrada and Myzostomida. It occurs with all three functions in some Rotifera and Vertebrata. The term is also used in some Crustacea and Holothuroidea, where the two functions are digestive elimination and respiration.

Anus. The principal diversities relating to the anus are three: (1) embryonic source, whether by formation of the archenteron or by a later invagination; (2) its presence or absence as a functional opening; and (3) its location on the body. The first is treated in Chapter 5, and the second is tabulated in a previous section of this chapter. The anus may occur terminally on the body, as in Kinorhyncha, Arthropoda, and others; it is ventral and nonterminal in Nematoda and Vertebrata and many others. It is said to be dorsal in the nematode order Desmoscolecida and in the Hirudinea. Through the recurving of the tract, the anus may be at the same end as the mouth as in Calyssozoa (inside lophophore), Bryozoa and Phoronida (outside lophophore), some Sipunculoidea, Crinoidea, some Echinoidea (on oral surface), or it may be ventrally more or less midway of the body, as in some Sipunculoidea, Pterobranchia, Ascidiacea, and Larvacea.

Glands. In all of the foregoing regions there may be glands of various sorts, but the terms for them give more clues to their function than to their origin and possible structural similarity. *Salivary glands*, releasing digestive enzymes in the vicinity of the mouth, are found in Mollusca, Onychophora, Arthropoda, and higher Vertebrata. In some Insecta there is a *salivary pump* for ejection of the saliva into the prey. Such glands are sometimes called *mandibular* or *labial glands* in Insecta, where they may be converted to other purposes.

The functions of the salivary glands have been listed (Morton, 1967) as secretion of various substances:

1.   Amylase (Vertebrata)
2.   Mucoid lubricants but no enzymes (Aves)
3.   Moistening food and lubricating mouthparts and secreting amylase and invertase (in cockroaches)
4.   Neurotoxin (cone shells)
5.   A toxin (Cephalopoda and Arachnida)
6.   Protease (*Octopus*, Arachnida)
7.   Acid to soften cocoon at emergence (honeybee)
8.   Royal jelly, amylase, invertase (honeybee)
9.   Fatty emulsion to work wax used in comb-building (honeybee)
10.   An irritant to stimulate blood flow (*Glossina*)
11.   Anticoagulant (leeches)
12.   Silk (many insects)

Other digestive tract glands occur, called *pharyngeal* or *oesophageal glands* in Nematoda, *gastric glands* as in Rotifera and Polychaeta, and livers in Vertebrata. Some of the diversity of function of the liver in mammals is suggested by Morton (1967);

1.   Secretion of bile (alkaline)
2.   Metabolism of amino acids from the blood (deaminizing and converting)
3.   Storing carbohydrate from the blood as glycogen
4.   Storing fat as such or metabolized
5.   Synthesizing vitamin A from carotene
6.   Phagocytizing foreign matter from blood (cells of Kupffer)
7.   Destroying old red blood cells
8.   Producing new red blood cells (in youth)
9.   Synthesizing prothrombin and fibrinogen
10.   Breaking down toxic substances such as alcohol

The term "liver" is sometimes used for completely different structures, as in Siphonophora, where it is apparently excretory in function. *Hepatopancreas* glands combine the functions of food storage and digestive enzyme secretion in Crustacea. The pancreas of Vertebrata secretes digestive enzymes into the small intestine. There are rectal glands, especially in Vertebrata, where they may open into the cloaca. Their function is usually uncertain, but in fishes they may secrete salt.

H. Unusual Features

Several unique and unexpected organs or features of the digestive tracts of various animals have been cited in this chapter: a buccal "wringing-out" chamber, stylets, the radula, the tongue, the mastax, the endostyle "conveyor-belt", the peritrophic membrane, the crystalline style, the typhlosole, and the spiral "valves". In addition to these, there are a few other specialized features.

Proboscises. Many animals have an extension of the body called a proboscis, although seldom more than one per individual. Some of these are part of the digestive

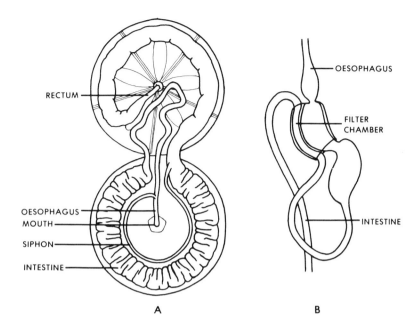

FIGURE 19. Diagrams of intestinal bypass mechanisms. A, echinoid, by a siphon; B, sipunculoid, by a filter chamber.

tract and some are not. Of the latter we can cite Rhynchocoela, Acanthocephala, Echiuroidea, Enteropneusta, and even Mammalia (trunks etc.). The proboscis is clearly an extension of the mouth in these: Turbellaria (where it is sometimes called pharynx and may be multiple), Priapuloidea (presoma), some Hirudinea (pharyngeal), Pycnogonida, and some Insecta (used loosely for the mouth tubes formed by mouth parts). Of these the proboscis is protrusible in Turbellaria; it is eversible in Hirudinea.

Siphons. This word refers here to tubes which parallel the intestine to bypass excess water taken in with the food. Such siphons occur in Echiuroidea, s.Oligochaeta (tube in the typhlosole), s.Polychaeta (Capitellidae), and Echinoidea. The word siphon is used in Cephalopoda and Sipunculoidea for quite different structures (Figure 19).

Filter chambers. In some Insecta (Homoptera) there is a loop of the digestive tract that brings part of the intestine back into contact with the proventriculus. A filtering action into the intestine apparently serves to remove excess water from the plant juice ingested, thus serving much the same function as the siphon above.

No digestive enzymes. In some bloodsucking leeches (Hirudinea), there is no production of proteolytic enzymes. Digestion of the blood corpuscles of its food is by a symbiotic bacterium. An intriguing case is reported without conformation or details. In one species of African monkey, there is said to be no secretion of at least some necessary digestive enzymes by the wall of the stomach. These enzymes are brought to the tract by amoebocytes from some more or less distant source. It is further reported that a similar mechanism is found in one species of Crustacea. Note that this would mean that it occurs in 1 out of roughly 50,000 species of vertebrates and in 1 out of at least 800,000 species of arthropods, so far as known.

Digestion in the legs. The curious marine Pycnogonida (sea spiders) have such a slender and short body that the intestine sends long caeca into each leg, where digestion is intracellular in the intestinal walls.

Feeding without a mouth. Many endoparasites absorb nutrients from their hosts. In many such Copepoda (Crustacea) there are palp-like appendages developed on various parts of the body for "sucking" food. These may be on the head or the thorax, and perhaps elsewhere.

Air-storage stomach. In some short-lived adult Insecta (Ephemeroptera), the digestive tract does not function in alimentation, and in the stomach food is replaced by air, which lessens the specific gravity of the insect. Brooding of embryos and larvae takes place in the stomach of certain New Zealand frogs. Although digestive activity must cease during this activity, it does not seem to be known just how the embryos are introduced into the stomach.

Because the lung and swimbladder of vertebrates are derived from the archenteron (embryonic digestive tract), their respiratory and other functions might be looked for in this list. We consider that these are more appropriate to respiration (Chapter 15).

I. Functions of the Tract

The function of the digestive tract is, of course, to provide nutrients for the entire body. Although the basic chemical needs of all animals are much the same, consisting of carbohydrates, proteins, and fats in various combinations in addition to water, salts, and vitamins, the source of these molecules is very different in different animals, and the processes of digestion vary accordingly.

Strictly speaking, the functions of the digestive tract do not include the detection, mechanical capture, and often the dismembering of the prey. These are treated as functions of the whole individual in Part V, but the diversity of animal structure produces difficulties with this arbitrary separation. For example, in Sipunculoidea, the "proboscis" or introvert is greatly extensible and is used in food capture, with the food taken directly into the mouth, which is at the extremity. The very long anterior proboscis of most of the Rhynchocoela, on the other hand, has no direct connection to the digestive tract, but delivers its captured prey to the mouth near its base. In the latter, digestive tract functions begin when the food is delivered to it, but in the Sipunculoidea the capture is really effected by the extended anterior part of the tract.

The basic function of the digestive tract is covered by the term *alimentation*, which includes collectively the processes of ingestion, digestion, and egestion. There is a tendency in recent books to restrict the meaning of the word digestion to its chemical aspects, but in this section digestion is used to include all the processes between intake of food and elimination of wastes, as well as some exceptional occurrences.

Ingestion involves filtering, swallowing, engulfing (in Protozoa), absorbing (in parasites), phagocytosis, and pinocytosis (by cells) in varying combinations. *Digestion* (as here defined) includes both mechanical and chemical breakdown of food, and to this one must append *absorption* of the digested food into the tissues. *Egestion* normally involves elimination of undigested residue from the "food"; to this residue other waste material discharged into the tract may have been added.

Among all the varied structures forming digestive tracts of endless diversity, there are many functions. Some may be considered primary, part of the basic function of alimentation or nutrition. Others are secondary, performed incidentally by parts of the tract and not directly related to nutrition. The obvious ones can be listed with a few examples.

The primary function of the digestive tract is to nourish the animal. This may involve at least the following: (1) filtering, both to keep out unwanted solids or to take in only solids; (2) maceration, as the word is used in zoology — both mechanical breakdown and preliminary digestion of solid food; (3) secretion of mucus, enzymes, poisons; (4) temporary storage of food; (5) movement of food; (6) final digestion; (7) absorption of nutrients; and (8) egestion of wastes.

In addition to these eight primary functions, there are a few cases of specialized but related functions. For example, the problem of dealing with excess water entering the digestive tract is dealt with in various ways. In some ants there is a receptacle just below the mouth in which solid and viscous food may be held while any fluids are drawn into the pharynx; the solid residue is then thrown out as a pellet. In the Echiuroidea almost the entire length of the intestine (much looped) is paralleled by a second tube, or siphon, apparently designed to pass unwanted fluids around the intestine. A similar bypass tube occurs around the stomach in Echinoidea, about as dissimilar an animal as one could find.

It is quite common for the digestive tract to be involved in functions other than nutrition and therefore also to be modified for those other purposes. Such secondary functions of the intestinal tract include associations with the following:

Respiration

1. Pharyngotremy (gill slits) (Enteropneusta, Tunicata, Cephalochordata, Vertebrata)
2. Rectal respiratory tree (Holothurioidea)
3. Ciliated rectal epithelium (s.Oligochaeta)
4. Digestive gland diverticula into the dorsal cerata (s.Gastropoda)

Excretion

5. Organs empty into digestive tract for elimination: (a) Malpighian tubules (Insecta), and (b) rectal glands (Onychophora)
6. Cells of intestinal epithelium slough off parts with wastes contained (Insecta: Collembola)

Reproduction

7. Channels for passage of egg or spermatozoa to the outside (Gordioidea)
8. Brooding in the mouth (s.Pisces)
9. Brooding in the stomach (s.Amphibia)

Defense

10. Salivary secretions for entanglement (Onychophora)
11. Salivary secretions for poisoning (Arachnida)
12. Teeth for biting or as tusks (Vertebrata)

Water control

13. Siphon tube (Echinoidea, Echiuroidea)
14. Filter chamber, 3 types (Insecta: Homoptera)

Manufacture of substances

15. Wax (Insecta)
16. Regurgitated foods (Insecta)

Hydrostatics

17. Inflation for bursting old exoskeleton (Arthropoda)

Materials produced by some part of the digestive tract for some external use include: mucus, saliva, poisons, repellants (the "tobacco juice" of grasshoppers and the "explosive fluid" of the bombardier beetles), honey, royal jelly, honeydew, anticoagulants, antidessicants (the rectal "spittle" of frog-hoppers), and silk (for cocoons of Neuroptera, secreted by the malpighian tubules through the anus).

J. Miscellaneous Aspects of Digestive Systems
1. Site of Digestion
Although it is easy to think of all digestion as occurring in the digestive tract, of whatever sort, this is an over-simplification. In Protozoa digestion is necessarily intracellular. Even in animals with a special digestive tract, some digestion may be accomplished outside of the body, by ejected enzymes. In the tract itself, digestion may occur via enzymes secreted into the lumen or internally by individual cells in the walls of the cavity. These are performed at varying locations inside and outside of the body, as follows:

Inside cells, in these tissues

1. Epidermis (Porifera)
2. Choanocytes and amoebocytes, by phagocytosis (Porifera)
3. Gastrodermis of coelenteron (Coelenterata, Ctenophora)
4. Gastrodermis of GVC (Platyhelminthes)
5. Wall of intestinal tract (Vertebrata)
6. Botryoidal tissue (Annelida)
7. Reserve food cells in coelom (Tardigrada)
8. Blood, see next paragraph (s.Insecta)

In the digestive tract, by secretion

9. In the coelenteron lumen (Coelenterata, Ctenophora)
10. In the lumen of the GVC (Platyhelminthes)
11. In the lumen of any part of the intestinal tract (in most animals)
12. In the "digestive glands" (Asteroidea)

Outside of the body, from digestive glands

13. Secretions of digestive tract onto the outside food, effecting partial or complete breakdown there (Insecta, Bivalvia, Arachnida)
14. Secretions from epidermal cells: (1) general body surface (juvenile Gordioidea), (2) tentacles (Pogonophora)
15. Enzymes of the host (for internal parasites)
16. Secretions from an everted stomach (Asteroidea)
17. Enzymes injected into prey (Arachnida)

"In the digestive tract (of the pith-eating larva of the noctuid moth *Nonagria*) are found great numbers of motile conidia of a fungus (*Isaria*) which exist among the devoured vegetable fragments. The conidia are always accompanied by a micrococcus which secretes an enzyme capable of dissolving cellulose. . . . The conidia develop and multiply at the expense of the dissolved cellulose and eventually penetrate the walls of the gut, escaping into the blood. Most of them are there attacked by phagocytes and transformed into products which serve to nourish the tissues of the host" (Imms, 1930).

2. Increasing the Surface
Several devices have been evolved to increase the intestinal surface for absorption.

Typhlosole. In earthworms the digestive surface is roughly doubled by the large hanging typhlosole ridge; a similar "typhlosole" is cited in some Bivalvia and Tunicata.

Coiling. Coiling of the intestine greatly increases the length and therefore the surface, as in Mammalia and all those listed under "Organs of the Intestinal Tract", above.

Spiralling. Spiral valves and valves of Kerkring slow the passage of food and increase the absorptive surface in some fishes and in higher vertebrates, respectively.

Villi. Many animals have the intestinal surface broken up into minute extensions, the villi. In the vertebrates these consist of gland-rich epithelium, lymph and blood vessels, basement membrane, muscle tissue, and lymphatic tissue.

3. Nutriments for Ovum and Zygote

Yolk. The most distinctive feature of eggs in general is the food reserve or yolk (also called deutoplasm). The yolk is usually inside the ovum but is sometimes in special nurse cells or yolk cells that may be inside the shell with the egg. Although yolk frequently consists largely of fatty materials, it may also be carbohydrate or protein. As listed by Raven (1961), these three types often occur together in the same class (and sometimes in the same genus), as shown in this list:

1. Carbohydrate yolk, glycogen (Nematoda, Sipunculoidea, Crustacea, Chilopoda, Insecta); other polysaccharides (Sipunculoidea, Pisces)
2. Fatty yolk (Gastropoda, Bivalvia, Cephalopoda, Oligochaeta, Archiannelida, Merostomata, Arachnida, Crustacea, Chilopoda, Insecta, Crinoidea, Asteroidea, Echinoidea, Pisces, Amphibia, Aves, Mammalia)
3. Protein yolk (Gastropoda, Bivalvia, Cephalopoda, Archiannelida, Merostomata, Arachnida, Crustacea, Chilopoda, Insecta, Crinoidea, Asteroidea, Pisces, Reptilia, Mammalia)

The distribution of the yolk in the ovum (or egg) is reflected in the embryonic cleavage pattern, inasmuch as the yolk mass is with difficulty penetrated by a cleavage plane. The amount of yolk is correlated with the length of development before the larva can feed. For example, in the small class Echiuroidea, there is little yolk in the eggs of *Urechis* and much more in those of *Bonellia*.

Egg Yolk Terms. There are terms to specify the relative amount and location of yolk in an ovum. These include the following:

1. Alecithal — without yolk, or with very little (see also microlecithal)
2. Centrolecithal — having much yolk, concentrated at the center, the nucleus frequently lying on the periphery
3. Ectolecithal — (1) with the yolk absent from the center of the egg, where the nucleus lies; (2) same as exolecithal
4. Entolecithal — having the yolk inside the egg, as distinct from exolecithal
5. Exolecithal — having the yolk outside, in yolk cells
6. Homolecithal — with any yolk evenly distributed throughout the cell
7. Isolecithal — having the yolk evenly distributed
8. Medialecithal — having considerable yolk but still capable of holoblastic cleavage
9. Megalecithal — having such large amounts of yolk as to be capable only of meroblastic cleavage (same as telolecithal)
10. Mesolecithal — with moderate amounts of yolk (see medialecithal)
11. Microlecithal — same as alecithal
12. Miolecithal — having small amount of yolk

13.   Telolecithal — with much yolk, capable only of meroblastic cleavage

The various other means of providing nutrients to the embryo include:

1.   Yolk may be outside of the zygote, in special cells such as nurse cells (Porifera, Hydrozoa, Platyhelminthes, Gastropoda, Polychaeta, Hirudinea, Dinophiloidea, Myzostomida, Onychophora, Crustacea, Insecta, and Tunicata where they are called kalymmocytes)
2.   Host tissues may supply nourishment in the case of parasitic zygotes and embryos
3.   Placentae are formed to nourish the developing embryo (Onychophora, s.Insecta, Mammalia)
4.   Excess spermatozoa may be consumed (hypergamesis)
5.   Adelphophagia, consumption of neighboring embryos or unfertilized ova

It is not usually possible to attach the -lecithal terms to groups of animals or even to species, as they overlap and may designate both quantity and position of yolk. In most animals there is either little or much yolk, and it is all inside the ovum and thus later inside the egg. The exceptions to this include these:

1.   Porifera — the yolk is in nurse cells or trophocytes, which accompany the developing egg
2.   Platyhelminthes — there may be little to much yolk in the ovum, it may be in vitelline cells (altered ovocytes) enclosed with the ovum in a capsule, cells or yolk later becoming enclosed in the blastula, or yolk may be obtained by fusing with ovocytes
3.   Rhynchocoela — in the ovum, little or much; "each egg is formed through the aggregation of yolk cells around a germinal vesicle, the whole structure then becoming enclosed by a thin to thick egg membrane"
4.   Brachiopoda — there is much yolk in the ovum in some, where there is brooding, or in others it is in extra ovocytes which later are absorbed
5.   Arthropoda — there may be much yolk in the ovum, or in some Crustacea there are three nutritive cells

4. Embryonic Origin

It is generally assumed that the digestive tract arises from the archenteron, as does the stomodaeum and proctodaeum, thus at least in part from embryonic endoderm. In addition to the usual direct development, as in the starfish, in many asexually produced animals the digestive tract of the new individual is formed as an offshoot of the tract of the parent. In others nearly all organs are formed from undifferentiated cells, or at least from cells which are still capable of differentiation. For example, in frustulation or pedal laceration in Coelenterata, only epidermal cells are included in the new fragment, and the gastrodermis must therefore develop from these.

However, the digestive tract of the adult in many animals has no such tripartite origin and may arise without any cells of endodermal origin. For example, in those other animals which have an indirect development, the digestive tract of the adult has simply developed from that of the larva, and the larval from the archenteron of the embryo. This does happen in some Coelenterata (archenteron to coelenteron), in most Platyhelminthes (archenteron to GVC), and in Mollusca, Echinodermata, Vertebrata, and others (archenteron to intestinal tract).

In most Insecta the embryo develops without any archenteron formed by invagination. The anterior and posterior ends of the tract develop by invagination, but these form only ectodermal stomodaeum and proctodaeum. The embryonic intestine forms between these, long after the mesoderm has been formed. In insects with a complete metamorphosis, the breakdown of organs in the pupal stage also breaks the continuity between larval and adult tracts, with the latter forming anew from imaginal discs.

In Gordioidea the archenteron never develops into a functional digestive tract, although rudiments exist and may have functions other than digestion. In gymnolaemate Bryozoa the larval digestive tract degenerates, and a new one is formed in the adult. In the Phylactolaemata the embryonic tract degenerates, and a new one is formed in the adult.

In Cestoda and Acanthocephala there is no archenteron and therefore no digestive tract. In Pogonophora there is also never any tract, because the endodern is solid and no trace exists of mouth or anus.

To summarize, the digestive tract of the adult may be a continuation of the larval tract or it may form anew at metamorphosis. It may form from original endoderm or from undifferentiated cells at a later stage. It may consist entirely of endodermal tissues or much of it may be formed of invaginated ectoderm.

REFERENCES

Baer, J. C., *Ecology of Animal Parasites*, University of Illinois Press, Chicago, 1951.

Carlson, A. J. and Johnson, V., *The Machinery of the Body*, 4th ed., University of Chicago Press, Chicago, 1954.

Clark, W. E. L., *The Tissues of the Body*, 6th ed., Oxford University Press, Oxford, 1971.

Farmer, J. N., *The Protozoa: Introduction to Protozoology*, C. V. Mosby, St. Louis, 1980.

Hyman, L. H., *The Invertebrates*, 6 volumes, McGraw-Hill, New York, 1940—1967.

Imms, A. D., *A General Textbook of Entomology*, 2nd ed., E. P. Dutton, New York, 1930.

Imms, A. D., *A General Textbook of Entomology*, 8th ed., Methuen, London, 1951.

Jennings, J. B., *Feeding, Digestion and Assimilation in Animals*, Pergamon Press, Oxford, 1965.

Kudo, R. R., *Protozoology*, 5th ed., Charles C Thomas, Springfield, Ill., 1966.

Marshall, A. J., *Parker & Haswell, A Text-Book of Zoology*, Volume 2, 7th ed., Macmillan, London, 1964.

Morton, J., *Guts: The Form and Function of the Digestive System*, St. Martin's Press, New York, 1967.

Raven, C. P., *Oogenesis: The Storage of Developmental Information*, Pergamon Press, New York, 1961.

Chapter 14

CIRCULATORY SYSTEMS

TABLE OF CONTENTS

I.   Introduction 294

II. Circulation 295
     A.   General Functions 295
     B.   Types of Transport 295
          1.   Cyclosis 295
          2.   Transport Between Cells 295
          3.   Movement in Intercellular Spaces 295
          4.   Transport in Body Cavities 296
          5.   Cell Migration 296
          6.   Movement of Fluid in Ducts 297
          7.   Transport in Blood Vessels 297
          8.   Transport in an Open System 299

III. Lymphatic System 299
     A.   Circulation of Lymph 299
     B.   Lymph Organs and Materials 300

IV. Blood Circulation 301
     A.   Organs of Blood Circulation 301
          1.   Vessels 301
          2.   Pumping Mechanisms 303
     B.   Blood 304
     C.   Spleen 304
     D.   Thymus Gland 304

References 305

I. INTRODUCTION

The systems referred to herein as circulatory systems are those involving movement of fluid in tubes, often with the movement extending into the body cavity. The first would be the closed systems, and the latter the open systems.

Transport in the vessels of closed systems is typified by vertebrates, where the fluid is called blood and the principal tubes are called blood vessels, with a pump called a heart. Other closed systems are found in Rhynchocoela, Phoronida, Echiuroidea, Annelida, Pogonophora, and Cephalochordata, besides the Vertebrata. In these six, the vessels and the blood are in general similar, carrying oxygen in plasma or corpuscles by means of haemoglobin, with longitudinal trunks, but with contractile vessels for blood pumping, except in the Vertebrata.

It appears to be appropriate to refer to these six as systems of blood vessels carrying blood. The point is important because such other invertebrates as Arthropoda and Mollusca have vessels and spaces containing rather different fluids sometimes also called blood.

The term blood and blood vessel will therefore be restricted in this chapter and the next to the ones in the six phyla cited above. All others will be cited by the less specific terms circulatory channels and fluids. In other parts of this book, the term blood will often be found in its common but indecisive meaning that tells us only that there are circulatory channels carrying fluids.

Even the universally used expression circulatory system can be misleading if one takes it to mean a system of blood vessels. In sponges it is seawater that circulates. In coelenterates virtually the only circulation is in the digestive cavity. In some coelomate animals the coelomic fluid replaces blood, but the coelom is seldom called a circulatory system. In insects air or oxygen circulates in tubes, and in echinoderms seawater is used throughout the body in a system of hydraulic tubes.

The list of tube systems in Chapter 12 does not contain all the mechanisms described as circulatory, because some of the latter do not operate in tubes. A circulatory system consists of all the cells, organs, fluids, and tissues associated with movement of materials within the body, except, of course, the digestive tract, excretory organs, and other special tubes concerned with entrance or exit of materials instead of their translocation within the organism. The components of such a system will usually include most of the following: a set of channels (tubes or spaces), a fluid, a propelling organ such as a heart (to produce movement of the fluid), tissues to produce any cells involved in the transport, and a source of the circulating fluid.

The fluid in circulation varies considerably in components, functions, and the nature of the channels in which it moves. This has given rise to two terms that are descriptive but not very explicit — closed systems and open systems. These simply tell whether the fluid is continuously in distinct vessels or during part of its circulation is outside of vessels and thus in body spaces. For animals like the insects, with their single dorsal vessel and large haemocoel, the term open system is reasonable, but some other groups (such as mollusks) have more vessels and fewer open spaces and so confuse the term. The best examples of closed systems are in Oligochaeta, Pogonophora, and Vertebrata.

There are a few groups of animals, mostly with very small individuals, in which there are no circulatory systems of special organs. These include: Protozoa, Porifera, Coelenterata, Platyhelminthes, Rotifera, Gastrotricha, Kinorhyncha, Nematoda, Gordioidea, Priapuloidea, Calyssozoa, Bryozoa, Sipunculoidea, s.Echiuroidea, Tardigrada, Myzostomida, Pentastomida, Dinophiloidea, Chaetognatha, and a few Arthropoda.

II. CIRCULATION

A. General Functions

The function of a circulatory system is to transport materials from one place to another inside an individual (and in a few cases also between members of an interconnected colony). In general, however, the word circulation is limited to the function of moving the following:

1. Oxygen from respiratory organs to all tissues
2. Carbon dioxide from the tissues to the respiratory organs (or elsewhere)
3. Nitrogenous wastes from the tissues to the excretory organs
4. Nutrients from the digestive tract to all tissues
5. Hormones to reaction sites, in arthropods and vertebrates at least

It must be emphasized, however, that many circulatory systems perform only part of these functions. Few of the functions are always present, notably the carrying of nutrients and nitrogenous wastes.

The various circulatory systems perform several secondary functions beside the primary one — transport. These include at least:

1. Defense: phagocytosis and antibody activity
2. Temperature regulation
3. Hydraulics: body turgor (maintenance of shape) and organ turgor (inflation)
4. Maintenance of the system

B. Types of Transport

Transport of materials within a living organism, to use the broadest concept of translocation, is provided by a wide variety of processes. Some work within a single cell, some from one cell to another. Some carry materials from organ to organ, some make complete circuits to and from all parts of the body. The broadest list of translocation devices is given in Chapter 12. We briefly mention some of those that are involved in movement of nutrients, oxygen, and metabolic wastes.

1. Cyclosis

The circular flow of cytoplasm within a cell is cyclosis. It was first described in some ciliate Protozoa but is said to be common in cells. It moves vacuoles and cytoplasm along apparently predetermined paths and thus hastens the passage of materials to all parts of the cell, a function that would otherwise have to be performed by the slower process of diffusion. Cyclosis seems to be related to amoeboid movement, in which streaming of the protoplasm is a major factor.

2. Transport Between Cells

This may be by diffusion or by active transport. They involve movement of selected solutes through both membranes. It presumably occurs in all Metazoa, but it is not possible to tabulate whether there is diversity among cells or animals.

3. Movement in Intercellular Spaces

This is generally by diffusion. This is seen in a relatively organized condition in the lacunar system in the body wall of Acanthocephala, in which an unusual situation exists. The Acanthocephala "lack a directional flow circulatory system but possess instead a loose network of tube-like cavities without linings or pumps. These cavities form channels known as the lacunar system which interconnect forming a definite pattern in some species but less so in others . . . there are usually a pair of main longitudinal channels that traverse the length of the body with numerous connections to the remainder of the system (which includes many ring channels)'' (Miller and Dunagan, 1976).

4. Transport in Body Cavities

The chief distribution method employed by multicellular animals that lack a tubular circulatory system is in the body cavity. In most animals with a body cavity that is a pseudocoel or a coelom, there is transport of materials through the spaces by means of a fluid which is in many respects similar to blood and sometimes referred to by that word. This movement is relatively slow and is produced by diffusion and movements caused by body muscles. The body cavity fluid may contain cells such as amoebocytes, and pigment-carrying erythrocytes, but such pigments may be free in the fluid instead. A colorless fluid is usually called lymph, haemolymph, oe coelomic fluid.

At least the following groups have extensive body cavities with fluid that can serve some transport functions, but without tubular circulatory systems:

In the pseudocoel

1.   With numerous amoebocytes (Rotifera, Gastrotricha, Kinorhyncha)
2.   With few amoebocytes (Nematoda, Gordioidea, Calyssozoa)

In the coelom

3.   With coelomocytes (Bryozoa)
4.   With few cells (Chaetognatha, Pterobranchia)
5.   With amoebocytes and red corpuscles (Priapuloidea, Sipunculoidea)

Although all coelomate animals have in the coelomic spaces fluids that perform some transport functions, some of the coelomate animals not already listed also pass some of the blood through the heart and channels of an open system. Here are the Brachiopoda (with coelomocytes), Mollusca, and possibly Enteropneusta. In these there can be no real difference between the ''blood'' in the vessels and the coelomic fluid.

In Onychophora and Arthropoda, there are no real spaces in the coelom and a different cavity, the *haemocoel,* takes over its functions. In a haemocoel system there are a heart and sometimes a few vessels, which open into the extensive body cavity to bathe all organs. This system transports food and wastes but no oxygen, with the latter moving in a completely separate tracheal system. The ''blood'' contains amoebocytes and is more explicitly called haemolymph.

5. Cell Migration

There is transport by cell migration in several ways. First, oxygen is carried in many circulatory systems only in special cells, such as erythrocytes. Here the translocation is passive, so that the cells are usually described as floating. Second, a variety of materials and objects are transported by individual cells or small groups of cells; some are listed here.

In Porifera, a collar cell which captures a spermatozoon may lose its flagellum and collar and then (being essentially an amoebocyte, will carry the spermatozoon to the waiting ovum), or the spermatozoon may be transferred by a normal choanocyte to an amoebocyte for the transport. A single spermatozoon in Chaetognatha is conducted through the tissues by a pair of synergid cells. Other synergids are carriers of masses of spermatozoa through the body cavity of Myzostomida.

In that peculiar phylum Echinodermata only one type of circulation has been described, a *haemal system* or "blood lacunar" system. This is a poorly defined system of small vessels that are presumed to function in circulation, although it is usually admitted that "circulation" is unproved. "Its channels are not definite vessels, as they lack definite walls and have the peculiarity of being enclosed inside coelomic channels" (Hyman, 1955).

In Asteroidea it is said that coelomocytes transport absorbed food along the haemal channels. In this group the coelomocytes can absorb injected poisons and then pass to the exterior by way of the epidermal papillae, to disintegrate outside. In Holothurioidea coelomocytes may carry wastes through the walls of the respiratory trees and thus to the outside. This may also occur through the walls of the intestine. Similar movement of wastes to "exterior" surfaces is reported in Hirudinea.

6. Movement of Fluid in Ducts

This occurs in all but the lowest Metazoa and a few others of small size. It is produced by hydrostatic pressure, muscular contractions (muscles in the duct wall and body wall muscles), or by ciliary beating. Ducts appear first in the radial canals of medusae, the solenia of colonial Coelenterata, and the coelenteron tubes in the Ctenophora, although the water chambers of the Porifera serve a similar function. Some ducts are simple elongated cells pierced by a tube (as in the gullet of Nectonematoidea), and some are simply doughnut-shaped cells (porocytes of Porifera).

7. Transport in Blood Vessels

Although there is sometimes no clear distinction between systems that have (1) "no cavities", (2) extensive coelomic spaces, (3) some vessels with some open spaces, and (4) entirely closed vessel systems, all but (4) have now been exemplified. This last group includes the two best known systems (in Annelida and Vertebrata). The following six phyla have essentially closed systems with a real circulation of blood. It should be remembered that many animals with blood vessel systems also have circulation of other types. For example, in both Oligochaeta and Polychaeta the comparatively spacious coelom provides additional transport in its colorless fluid.

In certain digenetic Trematoda there is a system of mesenchymal vessels variously called a "blood vessel" system, a set of lymph channels, or a lymphatic system. It consists of two to eight longitudinal vessels, not interconnected but with many blind branches. The vessels (probably better termed channels) contain a fluid in which there are floating cells called haemocytoblasts, similar to vertebrate white blood cells. These vessels are supposed to function in the distribution of food, respiratory gases, and excretory products (Hyman, 1951). Whether there can be any real circulation in such blind tubes is open to question, but in sluggish animals a back and forth movement of the fluid might be sufficient.

Rhynchocoela have a closed system consisting of blood vessels and some small lacunae. The latter are not classed as body spaces because they are lined with a delicate endothelium similar to that forming the inner surface of the vessels. There are two or three longitudinal trunks and a few branches. These are in close association with the digestive tract, the rhynchocoel, and the flame-cell excretory system. There are contractile vessels but no single heart. The blood is colorless or colored and may contain haemoglobin in corpuscles. These animals have no general body cavity (acoelous), being classed as acoelomate.

Phoronida have a system of vessels closed except for the haemal plexus on the stomach wall. There are two longitudinal trunks, each ending at the top in an incomplete ring vessel in the lophophore. Here they unite, with valves, so that there is only one vessel in each tentacle in which the blood surges back and forth. The blood comes up in the dorsal vessel and returns by the ventral. The two trunks come together in the plexus on the stomach.

Annelida have a closed system with two longitudinal vessels, one dorsal and one ventral, connected in most segments by commissures that have branches to parapodia and internal organs, and to gills if present. The blood flows forward in the dorsal vessel, back in the ventral, with the flow produced by contractions of the vessels rather than by any definite heart. In earthworms five anterior segments have paired commissural vessels that are often called "hearts", because they are enlarged and contractile. The blood may be colorless, with few amoebocytes, but it usually contains pigments in the plasma — haemoglobin, chlorocruorin, or haemerythrin. There are red corpuscles in some species. There are many variations of the system in the Annelida.

Pogonophora have an amazingly elaborate closed blood vascular system, with red blood that has haemoglobin in the plasma. There are two longitudinal trunks, the full length of the elongate body, communicating with each other by capillaries in the tentacles and again posteriorly by transverse commissures. As there is no digestive tract and the animal lives in a tight tube, all digestion and respiration originate in the tentacles. There is a muscular heart on the ventral vessel. A unique feature of this system in most species is the nature of the relation of the tentacle vessels to the tentacle itself. Each tentacle has on one side a longitudinal (and therefore very long) row of delicate filiform pinnules, described also as villi. Each pinnule is a single cell with its nucleus in the epidermis and the cell greatly elongated and extending out from the surface. In each pinnule, and thus within the cell itself, a capillary from one trunk enters at the bottom, loops at the outer end, and extends back to the base again where it connects to the other trunk. Thus each pinnule appears to have two capillaries joined at the apex.

Cephalochordata have a blood vessel system said to be very similar to that of vertebrates, but there is no heart and the vessels can be called arteries and veins only with some question. The system consists of a dorsal vessel, a ventral vessel, a complex of branchial arteries, and an hepatic portal from intestinal to "liver" capillaries. Oddly, there is no respiratory pigment in the blood and therefore no respiratory function. Although the system is closely similar to that of annelid worms, it differs in that the blood flows forward in the ventral vessel and back in the dorsal, just the reverse of the annelids. There are said to be also lymph spaces, with a fluid similar to the blood.

Vertebrata have a very complex closed blood vessel system, consisting of arteries and veins connected by capillaries and containing red blood propelled by a heart with valves. The system may consist of a single loop, characteristic of fishes, or a double loop, as in higher vertebrates.

The single loop system consists of a heart, arteries to the gills (where there are capillaries to pick up oxygen and give off carbon dioxide), other arteries from the gills to the body organs (where a second set of capillaries will exchange materials), and veins that return the blood to the heart.

The double loop system consists of a dual heart of which the two parts are designated as right and left. The right heart forms the pulmonary loop, with arteries to the lung where capillaries aerate the blood; veins then lead to the left heart, completing the pulmonary loop. From the left heart the systemic loop consists of arteries to all body organs (except lungs) where there again are capillaries for exchange of materials. From there veins return to the right heart, completing the second loop.

The blood carries oxygen, nutrients, and wastes to and from various organs. The oxygen is carried by the pigment haemoglobin, which is in red blood corpuscles; these are called erythrocytes in Vertebrata.

Generally in any closed system of vessels, the arteries and veins must be connected in such a way that the blood at the consuming tissues can return. This is usually accomplished by a network of capillaries between the arteries and the veins and lying in contact with the cells. These capillaries are simply tiny vessels with thin walls through which the metabolites readily pass. In the vertebrates they consist solely of squamous epithelium. In Pogonophora they are said to be a structureless membrane. In most other groups even the existence of capillaries is seldom mentioned.

When a section of vein originates in one capillary bed and leads to another, the vein is called a portal vein and the combination of vein and two sets of capillaries is called a *portal system*. The principal portals are the hepatic and the renal.

Capillaries are usually defined as blood vessels scarcely larger in diameter than an erythrocyte, having a wall consisting of one thin layer of epithelial cells (in Vertebrata called endothelium), and connecting the arteries and veins. At least one peculiar development (beyond the one listed above in Trematoda) occurs: in some Polychaeta, where there are blind contractile vessels projecting into the coelom, their significance is uncertain.

8. Transport in an Open System

Although the very active animals of the Vertebrata have developed an efficient closed system of circulation in blood vessels, the even more active animals of the Arthropoda have an adequate transport system that is basically different in two principal respects. First, it employs few vessels (essentially just a heart) and a large body cavity full of the "blood", here called *haemolymph*. Second, it usually takes little part in the transport of oxygen.

The open circulatory system usually has just one haemolymph vessel, extending most of the length of the body just under the dorsal body wall in the haemocoel. The portion of this tube through the thorax leads to its opening in the head. The portion in the abdomen forms a segmental series of contractile units, each with valves and lateral openings called ostia. These contractile chambers together are called a heart. They drive the haemolymph forward in the tube, admitting other fluid from the haemocoel through the ostia.

Thus, the haemolymph circulates through the haemocoel from the head to the abdomen, where it enters the heart to be pumped forward to the head again. All internal organs and most tissues are constantly bathed in this haemolymph. The obvious tissue exception is the epidermis.

Open systems are not always as simple as this. In some of the aquatic Crustacea, some sinuses and additional vessels pick up haemolymph from the haemocoel and conduct it to the gills and then to the heart. In others, vessels are entirely lacking. Flying insects may have additional hearts to supply the very active muscles of the wings.

III. LYMPHATIC SYSTEM

A. Circulation of Lymph

Circulation in the vertebrates is also accomplished in some vessels and organs not usually thought of as part of the blood vessel system. This is the lymphatic system, which is an extensive system of blind capillaries, thin-walled vessels, no erythrocytes, and much lower circulatory pressure. Because it is a system found only in the Vertebrata, it might be treated in Chapter 10 (Unique Organ Systems). Because it is essentially an alternate pathway to blood circulation and is similar in many aspects of structure and function, it is included here with the blood system.

This system may include the following: (1) many delicate but blind vessels in many parts of the body, (2) a return to the venous system, and (3) most importantly, a fluid (lymph) similar to blood plasma or intercellular fluid.

(A major gland called the spleen is always described as consisting of lymphatic tissue and sometimes said to be one of the lymph glands. Because it has no lymphatic vessels and is a major organ for storage of blood corpuscles [including erythrocytes], it is herein treated as part of the blood system. A second but much smaller gland formed of lymphatic tissue is the thymus. Its function is not circulation, but it serves as an endocrine gland to promote immunological competence of lymph tissues. It is therefore treated herein as an endocrine gland.)

This lymph system may also include the following in one or more groups: (4) lymph nodes in several sites, (5) spacious lymph sinuses around some blood vessels, (6) stomata which are minute communications with the coelom, (7) valves in the lymph vessels to maintain direction of movement, (8) lymph heart along some of the vessels, and (9) large lymph sacs or spaces between the skin and the body.

The functions of the lymph system are diverse. They include:

1. Returning tissue fluid from tissue spaces to the blood
2. Filtering solid particles too large to pass into blood capillaries
3. Manufacturing lymphocytes
4. Destroying old leukocytes
5. Phagocytizing bacteria and particulate wastes
6. Maintaining the fluid balance of tissue cells and extracellular fluid
7. Providing entry for newly made proteins into the blood
8. Absorbing fats from the digestive tract

The lymph system is fairly well developed in some fishes. There may be lateral lymph channels and a caudal lymph heart, but valves and lymph nodes are lacking.

In Amphibia there is an extensive lymph system, with the vessels and sacs ensheathing the blood vessels. The lymph vessels do not have valves, but there may be many complicated lymph hearts, which also act as valves. There are no lymph nodes, but lymph nodules are numerous.

In Reptilia the system is in general similar to that of Amphibia. Lymph nodes occur only in crocodiles. The main vessel forms a sheath around the aorta.

In Aves the extent of the vessels is greater than in the lower vertebrates, and lymph hearts are lacking except in embryos of some. A caudal lymph heart occurs, and relatively simple valves occur in a few species. The nodules show for the first time the germinal or clear centers. The lymph nodes have no special capsule or may be lacking.

In Mammalia lymph hearts are not present, although lymph sacs may occur in the embryo. Valves are numerous in the vessels, and lymph nodes are well developed. The node consists of a peripheral cortex and a central medulla, with a capsule of connective tissue.

Return of the lymph is to various parts of the venous system: (1) in mammals, it is through the thoracic duct near the heart, (2) in fishes and birds there may be a major flow of lymph into the veins in the pelvic region, and (3) entrance in the middle region of the postcava is rare in mammals, but common in urodeles. In all cases one or more entrances occur near the heart (after Romer, 1955).

B. Lymph Organs and Materials

The parts of the vertebrate lymph system have been designated by the following terms:

1. Afferent vessels — those that connect the vessels to the nodes
2. Cisterna chyli (see Thoracic ducts)
3. Lacteals — lymph vessels from the digestive tract, carry the milky chyle or fatty lymph (all classes)

4. Lymph — colorless fluid in lymph sinuses and vessels (all classes)
5. Lymph capillaries — the small blind terminal lymph vessels, very thin-walled
6. Lymph ducts (see Lymph vessels)
7. Lymph follicles — patches of reticular tissue crowded with lymphocytes, in the intestinal wall (Aves)
8. Lymph hearts — flimsy pulsating lymph sacs (s.Pisces, Amphibia, Reptilia, s.Aves)
9. Lymph nodes — spongy masses which strain foreign matter from the lymph and produce lymphocytes (Aves, Mammalia)
10. Lymph nodules — masses of small lymphocytes in the lymph nodes (Mammalia and "other vertebrates")
11. Lymph plexuses — undefined arrangements "in regions where nodes are found" (s.Aves)
12. Lymph sacs (see Lymph sinuses)
13. Lymph sinuses — channels, sacs, the spaces that surround the blood vessels (Amphibia and presumably others)
14. Lymph vessels — in general the relatively large vessels from the large capillaries to the termini on veins near the heart (all classes)
15. Lymphatics — vessels that return fluids from the tissues to the heart (all classes)
16. Lymphoblasts — lymph node cells that are the precursors of lymphocytes (all classes)
17. Lymphocytes — a type of nongranular and nonphagocytic white blood cell, originating in lymphoid tissues but occurring also in blood (all classes)
18. Phagocytes — phagocytic cells in the lymph nodes (Mammalia and probably others)
19. Stomata — minute apertures connecting the lymph sinuses with the coelom (lower Vertebrata)
20. Thoracic ducts — pair of large longitudinal vessels, which collect lymph from the lacteals; may fuse into a cisterna chyli in some fishes and reptiles and most mammals (Pisces, Reptilia, Aves, Mammalia)
21. Valves — structures in lymph vessels where there are no lymph hearts; to direct the flow of lymph (Aves, Mammalia)

The blind vessel system of some Trematoda, cited earlier in this chapter under "Transport in Blood Vessels", is sometimes called a lymph system but without any direct similarity to a vertebrate lymph system.

IV. BLOOD CIRCULATION

A. Organs of Blood Circulation

The organs directly assignable to the "blood" circulatory systems of various animals include vessels, hearts, valves, and glands. To these, must be added (of course) the circulating fluids with their special cells. Of these only the hearts, the vessel arrangements, and the "blood" are cited in detail in enough groups to make comparison useful (Table 18).

1. Vessels

"Blood" vessels are diverse in that some form closed systems, whereas others open into unlined spaces to form open systems. Efficient circulation can be attained in an open system only if a large haemocoel forms the return branch of the system. In these, capillaries are unnecessary because the haemolymph bathes the internal organs and thus reaches most cells directly.

Table 18
CIRCULATORY SYSTEMS

	Present or absent	Open or closed	"Blood"	Hearts, pumps
Porifera	0			0
Mesozoa	0			0
Coelenterata	GVC			0
Ctenophora	GVC			0
Gnathostomuloidea	GVC			0
Platyhelminthes	GVC			0
Rhynchocoela	X	Closed		Contractile vessels
Acanthocephala	X	Lacunar	Nutritive fluid	0
Rotifera	0			0
Gastrotricha	0			0
Kinorhyncha	0			0
Nematoda	0			0
Gordioidea	0			0
Priapuloidea	0			0
Calyssozoa	0			0
Bryozoa	0			0
Phoronida	X	Closed	Blood	Contractile vessels
Brachiopoda	X	Lacunar	Coelomic fluid	Contractile vessels
Mollusca	X	Open/closed	Haemolymph	Heart(s)
Sipunculoidea	?0			0
Echiuroidea	0/X	Closed	Blood	Contractile vessels
Tardigrada	0		Coelomic fluid	0
Myzostomida	0			0
Annelida	0/X	Closed	Blood	"Hearts", contractile vessels
Dinophiloidea	0			0
Pentastomoidea	0			0
Onychophora	X	Open	Haemolymph	Dorsal vessel
Arthropoda	0/X	Open/closed	Haemolymph	Dorsal vessel, APO[a]
Chaetognatha	0		Coelomic fluid	0
Pogonophora	X	Closed	Blood	?Heart
Echinodermata	X	Lacunar	Blood	0
Pterobranchia	X	Closed lacunar	Blood	Heart vesicle
Enteropneusta	X	Closed lacunar	Blood	Contractile vessels
Tunicata	X	Closed lacunar	Blood	Heart
Cephalochordata	X	Closed	Blood	Contractile vessels
Vertebrata	X	Closed	Blood	Chamberile heart

[a]   APO = accessory pulsating organs.

There are diversities in such features as the make-up of the vessel walls, the number of cell layers, and the presence of muscle, but these are too little recorded to be tabulated. In some contractile vessels the propulsion in one direction is made possible by one-way valves, which function in the manner as heart valves. Propulsion may also be achieved by peristaltic constrictions travelling along a vessel, and vessels among body muscles may be constricted by action of those muscles, with valves determining the direction of flow.

Definite systems of blood or haemolymph vessels occur in the following groups. (The expression open system merely implies that there are large blood-filled spaces. These spaces are enclosed by endothelium, so that the system does not merge into the tissue spaces, but is also not entirely enclosed in vessels.)

1.   Rhynchocoela — a closed system except for a plexus in the stomach wall; two longitudinal trunks, one efferent, one afferent; no capillaries

2. Phoronida — a system closed except for a network of sinuses between dorsal and ventral vessels; no capillaries

3. Mollusca — an open system with a few vessels; in Cephalopoda the vessels are more extensive, nearly a closed system

4. Echiuroidea — a simple closed system in most, with two trunks; none in *Urechis*

5. Annelida — a closed system usually, with longitudinal trunks; rarely none

6. Arthropoda — an open system in most with only one or a few vessels, but in some Crustacea the arteries may be well developed

7. Pogonophora — an extensive closed system, with capillaries at least in the tentacles

8. Cephalochordata — an extensive closed system with longitudinal trunks and capillaries but no heart

9. Vertebrata — an extensive closed system of one or two complete circuits (one to the entire body or one each to the lungs and the body tissues), with arteries, veins, capillaries, and a complex heart

2. Pumping Mechanisms

For most circulatory systems to function, they must include some means to propel the fluid in the desired direction in the vessels. There are several mechanisms to do this:

1. Contractile vessels without valves, presumably peristaltic
2. Contractile vessels with valves
3. Contractile vesicle ("heart" or "accessory hearts") without valves (Pogonophora)
4. A pulsating organ with chambers and valves (heart)
5. In addition to the above, movement of body muscles may squeeze the vessels and aid in blood movement

Pumping organs occur in most groups that have a closed system of blood vessels and also in those with a haemocoel. There is considerable diversity, and the term heart has been used for many contractile vessels:

1. Rhynchocoela — contractile vessels
2. Phoronida — contractile vessels
3. Brachiopoda — contractile vesicle or several or none
4. Mollusca — contractile chambered heart in pericardial cavity of an open system; accessory "hearts"
5. Echiuroidea — contractile vessels
6. Annelida — contractile vessels
7. Onychophora — tubular "heart" with serial valves
8. Arthropoda — tubular "heart" with serial valves; accessory pulsating organs in legs, thorax, antennal base
9. Pogonophora — muscular tubular "heart" without valves
10. Tunicata — a pulsating sac in a pericardial cavity of an open system; direction of flow alternates
11. Cephalochordata — contractile vessels, but no heart
12. Vertebrata — chambered heart with valves, in a closed vascular system

Hearts. This term is sometimes used loosely for pumping mechanisms in invertebrates. The best usage seems to be to restrict the term heart to special pumping organs of several chambers and valves which carry blood (i.e., oxygen-bearing fluid). These occur only in the Vertebrata, in a closed system, and in some Mollusca, in an open system.

Axial organ. In most Echinodermata there is an organ below the madreporite called the axial organ (or gland). It is physically involved with both the stone canal and the haemal system. In some, it contains two contractile chambers and a pulsating vessel. Although probably a propelling organ, it seems to serve some function with both the coelomic fluids and the haemal lacunae, possibly one of mixing materials of the two (Ubaghs, 1969).

B. Blood

Familiarity with the blood systems of higher vertebrates may lead one to assume that all animals have blood that carries oxygen to the tissues. In reality, the vast majority of animal species do have circulatory fluids, but these do not carry oxygen in significant amounts. This is true because of the numerical predominance of insects, in which the very different tracheal system carries the oxygen (usually as air directly to all tissues). For the purpose of this section, the term blood is restricted to fluids carrying oxygen.

If blood is to serve an efficient respiratory function, it must contain a respiratory pigment to transport more oxygen than can be carried in the fluid alone. The presence of respiratory pigments and their identity, briefly suggested above, are tabulated in Chapter 15.

It is not easy to distinguish blood from other body fluids, such as coelomic fluid and haemolymph, both because of the diversity of the fluids and because of loose usage of the terms. The following terms have been employed.

Blood, a fluid tissue used for transport of dissolved and other materials such as oxygen, nutrients, and metabolic wastes; always at least partly in a system of vessels and always containing cells of amoeboid type and often cells carrying respiratory pigments. An exception to this is the "blood" of Cephalochordata, which contains no cells of any sort.

Lymph, in Vertebrata, basically blood plasma with various white corpuscles, which is found in lymph vessels and spaces. It is the fluid residue when blood plasma filters out of the capillaries leaving behind the erythrocytes and protein molecules. The lymph re-enters the venous system at various points but especially near the heart.

Haemolymph, a term properly used for the body fluid of Mollusca, Annelida, and Arthropoda; a fluid in tissue and body cavities similar to blood.

Coelomic fluid. This term is used for the fluid in all coelomic spaces. It is seldom described sufficiently to permit comparison between groups. It may contain amoebocytes. In pseudocoelomate animals it is called pseudocoel fluid.

C. Spleen

In all vertebrate classes blood corpuscles are formed, stored, and later destroyed in this organ, which is usually described as composed of lymph tissues. This "gland" and the lymph nodes and bone marrow are the principal sites of haemopoietic (blood-forming) activities.

D. Thymus Gland

This organ is of uncertain function and is often not described as part of the circulatory system. In most vertebrates it is present and arises with the gill pouches in embryology. It was once thought to be haemopoietic during development and to have an endocrine function in control of growth; it is now described as a glandular organ essential to most immunological activities.

REFERENCES

Chapman, G., *The Body Fluids and Their Functions,* St. Martin's Press, New York, 1967.

Clark, W. E. L., *The Tissues of the Body,* 6th ed., Oxford University Press, Oxford, 1971.

Hyman, L. H., *The Invertebrates,* Vol. 2, McGraw-Hill, New York, 1951.

Hyman, L. H., *The Invertebrates,* Vol. 4, McGraw-Hill, New York, 1955.

Marshall, A. J., *Parker & Haswell, A Text-Book of Zoology,* Vol. 2, 7th ed., Macmillan, London, 1964.

Miller, D. M. and Dunagan, T. T., Body wall organization of the Acanthocephalan, *Macracanthorhynchus hirudinaceus:* a Reexamination of the lacunar system, *Proc. Helminthological Soc. Washington,* 43, 99, 1976.

Rateliffe, N. A. and Rowley, A. F., Eds., *Invertebrate Blood Cells,* (2 volumes). Academic Press, London, 1981.

Romer, A. S., *The Vertebrate Body,* 2nd ed., W. B. Saunders, Philadelphia, 1955.

Ubaghs, G., General characteristics of the echinoderms, in *Chemical Zoology,* Vol. 3, Florkin, M. and Scheer, B. T., Eds., Academic Press, New York, 1969, chap. 1.

Chapter 15

RESPIRATION

TABLE OF CONTENTS

I.   Introduction 308

II.   Respiratory Mechanisms 309
        A.   The Organs 309
        B.   Air-Breathing 311
        C.   Devices for Respiratory Exchange 312

III.   Respiratory Organs 314
        A.   The Diversity 314
        B.   Gills 315
        C.   Lungs 317
        D.   Tracheae 318
        E.   Respiratory Trees 319
        F.   Respiratory Terminology 320
        G.   Respiratory Fluids 322
        H.   Oxygen-Carrying Pigments 323

IV.   Associated Functions 323

V.   Systematic Summary of Respiration 324

References 326

I. INTRODUCTION

All animals must have mechanisms to provide needed oxygen and to remove waste carbon dioxide. More than in most body functions, this gas exchange is seldom accomplished by a single organ system. In many groups there is no actual system at all but only cellular mechanisms. The situation here is not unlike that in reproduction, where it is noted that few animals have "a reproductive system", but reproduce in many ways with one, two, or many systems, differing greatly in male and female, and sometimes involving no special organs at all. The result is again a chapter titled by the function rather than by a sometimes nonexistent organ system.

The word *respiration*, whose meaning would be clear enough to most biologists, has in recent decades come to have two different and almost conflicting meanings. Classically, and in all comparative works, respiration by an organism has stood for the intake of oxygen from air or water, and its exchange for waste carbon dioxide from the tissues. The term was thus basically used for the movement of these two gases.

Recently there has been a more biochemical approach. In most works respiration involves only the chemical reactions and cycles by which energy is released in the cells. At this biochemical level respiration in all animals seems to be much alike. This statement is possible because of two things: first, some of the processes and cycles really are the same in different groups; and second, cell biologists have taken little interest in a comparative approach and have investigated only a fraction of existing organisms. Thus, attempts at broad comparison are ineffective at this level.

Respiration is the total of all the physiological processes involved in the intake of oxygen and the release of carbon dioxide. The oxygen is intended for use in energy release; the carbon dioxide is a by-product of the same processes. This is stated at the physiological rather than the biochemical level because the more detailed biochemical processes of respiration do not so far yield much comparative data.

The entire process of respiration is often discussed under the topic of gas exchange. This expression leaves the impression that respiratory organs and the blood that serves them are a two-way street, in which oxygen is brought into the body and carbon dioxide is given off. The idea of an exchange of the two gases is so common that it is a surprise to find that the intake and the outgo may be handled by different mechanisms. Most accounts of respiration describe the entry of oxygen in detail and discuss the processes in which the oxygen is used and from which the carbon dioxide is a by-product, but often there is little detail about the exit of the carbon dioxide.

The waste carbon dioxide may be carried to the respiratory surfaces by the blood as carbonic acid, or may be directly discharged through the general body surface from the intercellular fluids.

Aerobic and anaerobic. The metabolic processes of respiration are generally supposed to be similar in all protoplasm, involving a common sequence of chemical reactions for the release of energy within the cells. This supposition is not entirely correct, because some cells can deviate from the usual sequence in certain circumstances. The usual implication in elementary books is that respiration can be either aerobic (utilizing environmental oxygen) or anaerobic (not utilizing oxygen from air or water). These can be distinguished as oxidative and fermentative respiration, but the biochemical processes are not wholly different. They differ essentially in that fermentative respiration stops short of the Krebs cycle and liberates energy by glycolysis alone.

An environment is said to be aerobic or anaerobic depending on whether or not there is free oxygen present. The organisms present are said to be *aerobes* or *anaerobes* depending on whether they have access to environmental oxygen or not. In the following discussion, cellular respiration is not further involved; thus the environmental or organismic definitions of the words aerobic and anaerobic are the only ones employed here.

It is sometimes said that some animals, such as internal parasites, are anaerobic. This could not be true of blood parasites which have ready access to oxygen; in the case of intestinal parasites, it turns out that they are merely adapted to life with very little environmental oxygen. In some other animals certain cells, such as over-taxed muscle cells, can function under temporarily anaerobic conditions.

So far as could be determined here, only one group of animals contains truly anaerobic individuals, and these are not parasitic. In the mud at the bottom of lakes and seas, where waterlogged soils are often completely devoid of oxygen, there may yet be significant free-living nematode populations. These are obligate anaerobes. They have the fermentative form of energy metabolism, which does not require oxygen. Other species of nematodes, called facultative anaerobes, can live either with or without environmental oxygen, switching from one metabolic pathway to another when the environment changes. In all other animals (the aerobes), the energy metabolism is oxidative and requires molecular oxygen from the environment.

II. RESPIRATORY MECHANISMS

A. The Organs

When a respiratory system is present, it is the sum of the organs directly involved in moving oxygen from the environment to the cells and carbon dioxide from the tissues to the environment. Such a unified system of organs is not always present in animals, and even where one is present it is usually supplemented by other mechanisms of respiratory function. In all such systems or "nonsystems", the essential features with respect to oxygen are these:

1. A source of molecular oxygen (air or water)
2. A transport mechanism for carrying oxygen either to an intermediate interface or to a cell interface
3. A carrier interface, a moist membrane with the carrier fluid for further transport
4. A second transport mechanism, from carrier interface to the cell interface
5. A cell interface, between either the source or the carrier fluid and the cell cytoplasm

With respect to carbon dioxide, the same features are essential but in reverse order. There must be transport from the production site (cell metabolism) to an interface, either an exterior point for gaseous discharge or the site of another metabolic reaction that requires carbon dioxide.

It is very easy to slip into the trap of thinking of all respiration as involving air. There are no major phyla whose members all breathe air, and at least three fourths of all the phyla have only freshwater or marine forms. (In number of species, of course, the air breathing insects swing the total to the air breathing side, because even among the so-called aquatic insects there are many that breathe air.)

An *interface* is always a moist membrane: a body surface, the surface of an internal cavity or vessel, or a cell membrane. The interface at the cell may be with blood or other fluid, another cell, or a tracheal tube. The oxygen is always dissolved in the fluid of the moist membrane of the interface. This oxygen is either in solution in the surrounding water or in air, from which it diffuses into the water film on the interface surface. Thus, in all animals the mechanism of movement of the gases across an interface seems to be diffusion, whether or not there are special organs. Even when there are no such special organs, diffusion will still be involved, for example, across the epidermis of the general body surface. This is called integumentary or *cutaneous respiration*. For example, in Protozoa the diffusion is always through the cell membrane.

Likewise in some species of the following groups, the required oxygen is obtained by direct diffusion from surrounding water, either by each cell itself or by diffusion from neighboring cells: Porifera, Coelenterata, Turbellaria, Nematoda, Rotifera, Bryozoa, a few Annelida, and no doubt others.

In general, an air respiratory mechanism will consist of the organs of breathing (exchange of gases), accessory structures to facilitate breathing, and a transport system to move the oxygen toward, and the carbon dioxide away from, the tissues.

The variety of existing respiratory mechanisms might have been shown here by individual examples, but the mechanisms prove to be so diverse that a few examples will not suffice. An adequate listing requires at least 8 groups and 44 distinct combinations of organs, as follows:

Body surface, variously specialized; WATER

1. General cell surface (Protozoa)
2. General body surface: (a) direct to cells (Porifera, Coelenterata, Ctenophora) and (b) indirect by means of a carrier (Gastropoda, s.Polychaeta, Hirudinea, s.Crustacea, s.Pisces, s.Amphibia)
3. Mantle surface (Mollusca)
4. Parapodial surface (Polychaeta)
5. Vascularized area of carapace (*Mysis* in Crustacea)

Body surface, variously specialized; AIR

6. General body surface (Insecta: Collembola, s.Amphibia)
7. Surface of part of pleopods (s.Crustacea)

Gills; WATER

8. Gills in mantle cavity (Mollusca)
9. Gills on dorsal surface (s.Gastropoda: Nudibranchiata, Polychaeta)
10. Radioles in the fans (Polychaeta)
11. Paired segmental gills (Hirudinea: *Ozobranchus*)
12. Book gills on abdomen (Merostomata)
13. Pleopod filaments (s.Crustacea: Isopoda and Stomatopoda)
14. Coxal gills on thorax (s.Crustacea)
15. Caudal filaments, with blood (larvae and nymphs of s.Insecta)
16. Spiracular gills, with blood (pupae of s.Insecta)
17. Tracheal gills, with molecular oxygen (larvae of s.Insecta) (also listed as no. 38)
18. Dermal branchiae (Asteroidea)
19. Peristomial gills, 5 pairs (s.Echinoidea)
20. Pharyngeal gills (Enteropneusta, Tunicata, Cephalochordata, aquatic Vertebrata)
21. External gills, from the gill bars (larval Amphibia)
22. Cerata, sac-like dorsal gills which may contain diverticula of the intestine (s.Gastropoda)

Gills; AIR

23. Vascularized tufts in branchial cavity (s.terrestrial Crustacea)
24. Pharyngeal gills, when the fish is out of the water (Pisces: *Symbranchus marmoratus*)
25. Extensible "vesicles" (Arachnida: Palpigradi and Amblypygi)

Respiratory chambers; WATER (sometimes as a secondary function)

26. Hindgut (s.aquatic Oligochaeta, s.Crustacea)
27. Foregut and stomach (s.Crustacea)
28. Rectum or cloaca (Crinoidea)
29. Bursae (Ophiuroidea)
30. Respiratory trees (Holothurioidea)

Respiratory chambers; AIR

31. Gill chambers (branchial cavity), vascularized walls (s.Crustacea)
32. Buccal cavity, pharynx, stomach, intestine surface (s.Pisces, s.Amphibia)
33. Lungs in mantle cavity (pulmonate Gastropoda)
34. Pharyngeal diverticulum (s.Pisces: *Amphipnous*)
35. Swim-bladder (open type) (s.Pisces: Holostei)
36. Lungs from the pharynx (s.Pisces, s.Amphibia, Reptilia, Aves, Mammalia)
37. Book lungs (s.Arachnida)

Tracheae; WATER

38. Tracheal gills, with molecular oxygen (also listed as no. 17)

Tracheae: AIR

39. Taking in environmental air; with tracheoles (Insecta)
40. Taking in air trapped or stored underwater (s.aquatic Insecta)
41. Taking in air from self-renewing plastron bubble (s.aquatic Insecta)
42. Receiving molecular oxygen from a moist gill (s.Insecta)
43. Sucking molecular oxygen from submerged plant tissue spaces (s.aquatic Insecta)
44. Taking in environmental air; without tracheoles (Onychophora, s.Arachnida, s.Crustacea: s.Isopoda, Chilopoda, Symphyla, Diplopoda)

It is surprising to find air and water in each of the four categories, body surface, gills, respiratory chambers, and tracheae; because it would usually be assumed that the first two involve only water and the last seldom or never water. This gives emphasis to the generalizations (1) that respiratory processes are more diverse than usually admitted and (2) that the various respiratory organs cannot be fitted into clearly distinct systems.

B. Air-Breathing

Although all but a few organisms take in oxygen, only terrestrial animals breathe. Breathing is the taking of air into an organ from which the oxygen can diffuse through its moist membranes to be transported to the cells of the body. In spite of some diversity, there are only two types of organ that receive this air, lungs and tracheae. In addition, there need to be mechanisms to conduct the air to the transfer cavity, to store it temporarily, and to expel the unused air with the waste carbon dioxide. These four functions are briefly summarized below.

Admission. In the vertebrates, air is admitted only through two sets of openings in the head, either the nares (nostrils) or the mouth. Other organs may produce a suction that pulls the air in, but in some Amphibia air in the closed mouth is squeezed backward into the lung. In the tracheate arthropods, air is admitted by a varying number of lateral pores called spiracles. In arthropods with paired book lungs, there are again spiracles.

Conduction. In terrestrial vertebrates air is transported to the lungs by tubes called tracheae which branch into bronchi. In arthropods the air is conducted from the spiracles to the body cells by tracheae (of very different structure from those in the vertebrates) which usually end in tiny tracheoles.

Storage. The only vertebrates that store air are some of those fishes that possess the converted lung structures called swim-bladders. Sometimes the bladder is open and part of the respiratory system. More often it is closed and serves only as a hydrostatic organ. Expansions of the bronchial or lung spaces may form air sacs, as in birds, but these are not primarily for storage. Air breathing arthropods store air in several ways outside of the body (as bubbles) or inside in air sacs that are expansions of the tracheal tubes.

Expulsion. The expulsion of the used air with its greater carbon dioxide content is through the same passages as its admission, except for occasional alternate use of nostrils and mouth and possible selective use of spiracles in insects.

Air breathing is, of course, not confined to adults. In terrestrial animals even the eggs may need to absorb oxygen for the developing embryo. This is not easy to achieve in an egg that is surrounded by a chorion to prevent desiccation. In many insect eggs there are minute *aeropyles* passing through the plug in the micropyle. These conduct air into the spaces of a meshwork between the egg membranes, from which oxygen can be absorbed and perhaps carbon dioxide given off. Some aquatic insect eggs may have one or more *respiratory horns* projecting above the water. They also have a gas-filled meshwork into which oxygen can diffuse but from which water is excluded. In at least some, this meshwork serves as a *plastron*, with the oxygen entering on one side and being absorbed by the protoplasm on the other. In amniote air breathing vertebrates, the chorion of the embryonated egg has an extension of the circulatory system of the embryo through which gas exchange may take place, either directly from surrounding air or from maternal tissues.

C. Devices for Respiratory Exchange

The following list is intended to summarize the exchange devices throughout the animal kingdom. Note that respiration by diffusion through the general body surface occurs in most soft-bodied animals, even though cited only in those where it is the principal mechanism.

1. Protozoa — diffusion through the surface of the cell
2. Porifera — diffusion from the water into the cells of the outer surface and the canals, and on into all other cells
3. Mesozoa — diffusion from fluids of the host directly into the surface cells
4. Coelenterata — diffusion directly into cells, both epidermal and gastrodermal, and from cell to cell
5. Ctenophora — diffusion into cells, possibly aided by "circulatory" movements within the tubular digestive system
6. Platyhelminthes — diffusion through the integument
7. Rhynchocoela — diffusion through the integument
8. Acanthocephala — diffusion through the integument from host fluids
9. Rotifera — diffusion through the integument
10. Gastrotricha — diffusion through the integument
11. Kinorhyncha — diffusion through the integument
12. Nematoda — diffusion through the integument
13. Gordioidea — diffusion through the integument
14. Priapuloidea — diffusion through the integument
15. Calyssozoa — diffusion through the integument

16. Bryozoa — diffusion through the integument
17. Phoronida — diffusion through the integument
18. Brachiopoda — diffusion through the mantle
19. Mollusca
    a. Monoplacophora — five pairs of gills on the mantle, supplied with blood by a special system of vessels
    b. Solenogastres — gills from anal chamber or cloacal walls
    c. Amphineura — gills in mantle cavity
    d. Gastropoda — a pair of mantle gills (ctenidia) or dorsal gills, usually reduced to a single one; or a vascularized pulmonary sac or lung, of vascularized mantle; or cerata on the dorsal surface
    e. Bivalvia — paired gills (ctenidia) in mantle cavity (in most), plus the general mantle surface
    f. Scaphopoda — no gills, diffusion through the mantle surface
    g. Cephalopoda — paired gills, or diffusion through the general surface, or both
20. Sipunculoidea — diffusion through the integument
21. Echiuroidea — diffusion through the integument
22. Tardigrada — diffusion through the integument
23. Myzostomida — diffusion through the integument
24. Dinophiloidea — diffusion through the integument
25. Annelida — specialized surfaces vascularized
    a. Polychaeta — gills in most, always with diffusion through the integument, the gills on parapodia or dorsum of some segments; radioles of fanworms
    b. Oligochaeta — diffusion through the integument; filamentous or finger-like gills rarely
    c. Archiannelida — diffusion through the integument
    d. Hirudinea — diffusion through the integument; leaf-like gills rarely
26. Pentastomida — diffusion through the integument from host fluids
27. Onychophora — tracheae with many spiracles, without tracheoles
28. Arthropoda — (only Crustacea have vascularized surfaces; only Insecta have tracheoles)
    a. Merostomata — book gills on ventral surface, with partially closed blood vessel system
    b. Pycnogonida — diffusion through the integument
    c. Arachnida — either book lungs or tracheae or neither, the tracheae without taenidia or tracheoles; rarely with vesicles in air
    d. Crustacea — gills usually attached at base of appendages; mantle and cirri in some; integumentary diffusion in all, sometimes exclusively
    e. Chilopoda — tracheal lungs with fans of short tracheae, without tracheoles
    f. Diplopoda — tracheal lungs with numerous short tracheae, without tracheoles
    g. Symphyla — long tracheae, but apparently only into the haemocoel and thus without tracheoles
    h. Pauropoda — usually only diffusion through the integument; rarely with spiracles and tracheae that extend only into the haemocoel, thus having no tracheoles
    i. Insecta — tracheae with tracheoles in most; rarely only diffusion through the integument; abdominal gills on a few aquatic larvae; rectal pumping occurs with rectal gills; caudal filaments on some aquatics; spiracular gills in some
29. Chaetognatha — diffusion through the integument
30. Pogonophora — diffusion through the integument
31. Echinodermata — diffusion through the integument, often in special areas
    a. Crinoidea — general surface, especially the podia

     b. Asteroidea — surface of papulae and podia

     c. Ophiuroidea — five pairs of bursae, invaginations of the dorsal surface

     d. Echinoidea — five pairs of peristomial gills in most, otherwise surface of podia

     e. Holothurioidea — rectal respiratory trees

32. Pterobranchia — pharyngeal gill slits
33. Enteropneusta — pharyngeal gill slits
34. Tunicata — pharyngeal gill slits
35. Cephalochordata — pharyngeal gill slits
36. Vertebrata

     a. Pisces — pharyngeal gill slits and sometimes lungs or open swim-bladder; diffusion through the integument; rarely gills on surface

     b. Amphibia — external gills; lungs; diffusion through the integument

     c. Reptilia — lungs

     d. Aves — lungs

     e. Mammalia — lungs

III. RESPIRATORY ORGANS

A. The Diversity

From the above list it can be seen that these mechanisms do not usually form a system of clear organs integrated to perform a major function. However, organs (or organelles) are often involved, and these can be listed and briefly described even if they do not lend themselves readily to classification as systems.

Air breathing organs and passages

1. Tracheae (Arthropoda)
     a. Spiracles/tracheae/tracheoles (Insecta)
     b. Spiracles/tracheae (Onychophora, Arachnida)
     c. Spiracle/pseudotracheae (Crustacea)
2. Breathing tubes into tracheal system (s.aquatic Insecta)
3. Breathing passages into the lungs; nostrils/pharynx/trachea/bronchi/bronchioles (Vertebrata)

Water-conducting organs

4. Proctostome (Coelenterata)
5. Mantle siphons (s.Mollusca)
6. Mouth/pharynx/gill-slit (Tunicata, Cephalochordata, s.Vertebrata)

Respiratory cavities

7. Respiratory chambers, cribriform organs, and bursae (s.Asteroidea, Ophiuroidea)
8. Buccal cavity (s.Amphibia)
9. Rectal respiratory trees (Holothurioidea)
10. Rectum, with pumping (Crinoidea)
11. Lung/swim-bladder (m.Vertebrata)
12. Book lungs (s.chelicerate Arthropoda)
13. Mantle cavity

Interface organs

14. General body surface (Protozoa, integument of most animals, including Coelenterata, many worms, s.small Arachnida, s.small Amphibia)
15. Specialized areas of body wall, such as mantle (Mollusca) or part of the carapace (Crustacea: *Mysis*)
16. Simple extensions of body surface (dermal branchiae of Echinodermata)
17. External gills with blood in vessels (Mollusca, s.Annelida, s.larval Amphibia)
18. External gills (or gill books) with blood in a haemocoel (s.Crustacea, Merostomata, Arachnida) or gills in book lungs (s.aquatic Insecta)
19. External gills with molecular oxygen in tracheae (s.aquatic Insecta)
20. Pharyngeal gills (Enteropneusta, Pterobranchia, Tunicata, Cephalochordata, aquatic lower Vertebrata)
21. Mantle lungs (pulmonate Gastropoda)
22. Swim-bladder (Pisces)
23. Pharyngeal lungs (air breathing Vertebrata)
24. Tracheoles (Insecta)
25. Pseudotracheae or "tracheal lungs" (Crustacea: Isopoda)

Oxygen-transport organs

26. Body cavity spaces (with pseudocoel fluid or coelomic fluid or rarely blood in haemocoel)
27. Blood vessels (with blood)
28. Tracheae open to outside (with air)
29. Tracheae in gills (with molecular oxygen)

B. Gills

A gill is an extension of the body wall which is specialized to facilitate the diffusion of oxygen into the body and carbon dioxide out. The specialization may be by thinning of the integument, perhaps with reduction in the number of layers of tissues, and with provision for transport. The latter is accomplished by (1) many blood vessels (vascularization), (2) extension of the haemocoel, or (3) tracheal tubes in place of blood vessels.

Gills are of almost endless variety and grade into areas of the body wall which are not organized into distinct respiratory organs. They may be filamentous, folded, lamellar, branched, lobed, or feathery, all of which increase the surface area. They are adaptations for obtaining oxygen that is dissolved in water, and they are therefore usually on exposed outer surfaces or in the path of water currents. There may or may not be a circulatory system in association with the gills, but a gill provides a greater surface for exchange of respiratory gases between the outside and the inside. On the basis of the nature of the internal transport, there are four types of gills:

1. Blood gills with the blood in vessels
2. Blood gills with the blood in a haemocoel
3. Gills with coelomic fluid in extensions of the coelom
4. Tracheal gills, with molecular oxygen in the tracheae

Unquestioned gills occur in some species of nine phyla, including Mollusca, Annelida, Arthropoda, Echinodermata, Pterobranchia, Enteropneusta, Tunicata, Cephalochordata, and Vertebrata. Among these, gills containing blood vessels are by far the most common, occurring in all nine of the phyla, but in the last five of them, the gills usually are the surfaces of the pharyngeal gill slits. These nine phyla may be tabulated thus:

1. Mollusca — vessels in mantle cavity gills in all except Scaphopoda
2. Annelida — vessels in epidermal gills
3. Arthropoda — haemocoel in most, vessels in some Crustacea, tracheae in a few aquatic Insecta
4. Echinodermata — coelom in peristomial gills in Echinoidea and in papulae of Asteroidea
5. Pterobranchia — vessels in gill-slit surfaces
6. Enteropneusta — vessels in gill-slit surfaces
7. Tunicata — vessels in surfaces of branchial basket
8. Cephalochordata — vessels in gill lamellae
9. Vertebrata — gill-slit surfaces in most aquatic species; rarely external gills on some Pisces and Amphibia

In Mollusca, gills are rarely lacking, but they are generally in the mantle cavity or rarely on the dorsal surface. The former may be very large and plate-like, small and leaf-like, dendritic, or thread-like. The number varies from 1 pair (or just 1 gill in Gastropoda after torsion) to at least 26 pairs (in the Amphineura). Lobate dorsal gills called cerata may contain diverticula of the digestive tract (Gastropoda: m.nudibranchs and saccoglossans).

In Annelida, gills occur in all classes except Archiannelida, but only in Polychaeta are they more than exceptional. Here they may be branched tufts, cribriform, spirally branched, thread-like, or arborescent. In textbooks an area of the parapodium is often cited as a gill; this area does not seem sufficiently different from the rest of the body surface to be classed as a gill rather than just a respiratory surface. Although gills are exceptional in Oligochaeta, they may be finger-like, filamentous, or tuft-like. In Hirudinea gills are found only in the Piscicolidae, where they may be branched or leaf-like. It is sometimes implied that the radioles of fan worms can act as gills; there is increased surface, but the main function is food-gathering.

In Arthropoda gills are found in all of the marine, most of the freshwater, and a few terrestrial species. In Merostomata there are 5 sets of plate-like gills, together called book gills, on the venter (actually 5 pairs united); each plate has up to 150 soft gills on its posterior border. Some Crustacea are said to lack gills, but even these nearly always have vascularized parts of the limbs that have sometimes been called gills. In some Insecta, principally in aquatic larvae, there are terminal abdominal gills or gills on the abdomen, thorax, or even head; there may also be gills on the rectal surface. Gills may contain finger-like extensions of the haemocoel containing blood, or tracheae containing molecular oxygen received by diffusion through the gill. These are called blood gills and tracheal gills, respectively, although in these circumstances the blood is more appropriately called haemolymph.

In Echinodermata there usually are no gills. The epidermis lends itself to minor devices to increase the respiratory surface. Although the podia or tube-feet may serve this function, there are many small evaginations called dermal branchiae, each of which contains an extension of the coelom and functions as a simple gill. In addition, in Echinoidea, there may be five pairs of peristomial gills filled with coelomic fluid around the mouth (see also "Respiratory Trees", below).

In Pterobranchia the simplest form of pharyngotremy occurs. There may be only a single pair of gill pores from the pharynx or their place may be taken by a pair of ciliated grooves.

In Enteropneusta the large pharynx has gill slits leading to surface pores, with the walls of this branchial apparatus serving for gas exchange.

In Tunicata a large pharynx has gill slits opening out into an atrial cavity communicating with the outside by a single siphon. The walls of the slits are vascularized and serve as gills.

In Cephalochordata, again, the pharynx wall is perforated by gill slits, with a special blood supply in the gill arches. Actual gills are not present because projecting filaments are lacking.

In Vertebrata gills usually consist of highly vascularized branchial filaments on the walls of gill slits; the slits extend through the pharyngeal wall to the outer surface, channeling water from the mouth over the gills to the outside. These occur in aquatic larvae (Pisces and Amphibia) and in adults of fishes only. One fish, *Symbranchus marmoratus*, is unusual in having gills that function in either water or air. In some Amphibia there may be external gills, which are outgrowths of the body wall near the gill slits.

C. Lungs

The simplest definition is that a lung is an internal chamber that can be filled with air and that is highly vascularized for gas exchange. The word is sometimes restricted to vertebrates, but there are such cavities in other animals which operate in much the same manner. A person wishing to restrict the word to the vertebrate lung can do so by specifying that it must arise from the digestive tract, because the mantle lungs of Mollusca and the book-lungs of Arthropoda do not do so.

Mollusca. In the pulmonate Gastropoda part of the mantle cavity is converted into a "pulmonary sac", opening to the exterior by a pneumostome. There may be folds and even gill-like structures to increase the surface, which is usually vascularized. There seem to be all intermediates between ordinary molluscan mantle cavity gills and the pulmonate mantle cavity lungs, gills within the lungs, or absence of all such structures, in which case the general surface of the mantle and foot serves the respiratory needs.

Arthropoda. In many Arachnida there are paired abdominal invaginations called *book-lungs*. The thin lining cuticle may be folded into delicate laminae which somewhat resemble the book gills of the Merostomata. (Many arachnids also have a tracheal tube system; see below.)

In Crustacea, several groups of terrestrial forms have respiratory chambers that are sometimes called lungs. Of these, one type is the *pseudotrachea,* described under Tracheae. Similar chambers without the "tracheal" tubes growing out occur in some Isopoda (*Oniscus*). In some Decapoda, the branchiostegal wall (of the open chamber usually occupied by gills) is highly vascularized, and a complex series of ridges and villi may be present.

In some Chilopoda (*Scutigera*), there is a spiracle near the posterior edge of each tergite. Each leads into a *tracheal lung* consisting of an atrium with up to 600 short tracheal capillaries, which may branch once or twice. These are bathed by the blood (haemolymph), and they contain air. Thus, oxygen is passed into the blood, which must carry it to the tissues. Kaestner (1968) reports that "Similar organs are found in some spiders", but in his section on spiders it is not clear whether the "tube trachea" of the abdomen is the similar organ.

Vertebrata. Lungs occur in all vertebrate classes except the Agnatha and the Chondrichthyes, but only in the Tetrapoda are the internal surfaces of the lung formed into alveoli. Because the *swim-bladder* is homologous with the lung (i.e., developed from the earlier lung) and is sometimes used as a supplementary respiratory organ, most bony fishes must be included as having lungs in some form. These are well known in the Dipnoi, and are believed to be the ancestors of the Amphibia. As most fishes have swim-bladders and some also have lungs, we can recognize either two or three types of vertebrate lungs: the two being ventilation lungs (all vertebrate lungs and open swim-bladders) and the closed type of swim-bladder; the three types being ventilation lungs (all vertebrate lungs), open swim-bladders into which air can be gulped, and closed swim-bladders which receive their gas only by secretion from the wall. In one teleost,

Amphipnous, the gills are poorly developed and functionally replaced on each side of the body by a vascular sac developed as a diverticulum from the pharynx. These are not always called lungs, but they are similar in function.

The air passages of Vertebrata are not very diverse. In most Tetrapoda they consist of (1) the nostrils or nares, (2) the nasal passages (or all of these replaced by the mouth), (3) the pharynx from which a median ventral opening or glottis leads to an expansion called the larynx (4), a median ventral trachea (5) which branches into two bronchi, (6) one leading to each lung, dividing further into bronchioles (7). These passages serve to conduct the air to the alveoli, where diversity does appear, as suggested below.

The efficiency of a lung depends principally on the extent of the internal surface available for gas exchange, although the air passages could become a limiting factor if an adequate flow of air is not provided.

In fishes with lungs, they (lungs) are of relatively simple internal construction. In some, an opening in the floor of the pharynx leads to the bilobed lung sac alongside the oesophagus. The inner surface of the lung is smooth except for a few furrows. In others, a duct leads from the pharyngeal opening to the lungs which are above the oesophagus (or only one occurs and is directly above). The internal surface is now moderately subdivided into pockets and alveoli.

In most amphibians the lungs are similar to those in fish, with some having the inner surface almost smooth. In others, there appear septa or ridges (containing connective tissue which increase the respiratory surface and give that internal surface a honeycomb appearance.

A few reptiles, supposedly primitive, have lungs that are similar to those of amphibians except for increasing subdivision of the interior surface into alveolar pockets separated by septa. In more advanced reptiles, lizards, turtles, and crocodiles, the lungs have the septa more developed and subdivided so as to give the appearance of a solid but spongy texture. Branches of the bronchi further subdivide and finally reach all the alveoli.

In birds, the lung is much more complex, although relatively small and compact. Out from the lungs extend numerous paired air sacs, which ramify into every major part of the body, even the bones. The lining of these sacs is usually smooth and not highly vascularized, so they are not important for respiration. The lung itself is solid and spongy, not consisting of bags with sacculated walls as in most lower groups. Bird lungs are unique in that there are no "dead end" alveoli. Instead a series of parabronchi loop from the bronchus through the lung tissue and back to the bronchus. From the parabronchi countless tiny air capillaries loop outward in the lung tissue and back again to the parabronchus. Thus, "every passage, large and small, is open at both ends so that there is a true circulation of air" (Romer, 1955).

In Mammalia, the alveoli are numerous and thin-walled, surrounded by a dense network of blood capillaries. This gives a relatively immense respiratory surface.

D. Tracheae

In the arthropodan sense, tracheae are air-filled respiratory tubules, as described in Chapter 19. They extend from the body surface, at an entrance opening called a *spiracle*, to a system of minute *tracheoles* (or simple branches) that extend to each cell. These tubes conduct air from the exterior, or in a few aquatic insects molecular oxygen from a tracheal gill, to the tissues. Some carbon dioxide may pass into the tracheae and so eventually be expelled with the excess air.

Considerable differences in the structure and operation of the active surfaces of tracheae occur, although few textbooks cite such differences. These are described in Chapter 19.

Onychophora. Here the tracheae are short and numerous, extending from the atria behind the very small spiracles. They arise in tufts from each atrium. Each trachea is a simple straight tube that extends directly to one particular tissue. There are no tracheoles and no strengthening spiral taenidium.

Arachnida. In the orders Chelonethida, Solpugida, Ricinulei, Opiliones, and Acarina respiration is by means of tracheae. (These are said to be diverse in origin.) Although the Araneida are sometimes described as having only *book-lungs*, there are many in which tracheae extend from the "lung" and some in which tracheae occur without any "lung". These tracheal tubes appear to have arisen from book-lungs; they apparently do not have the taenidia and do not end in tracheoles.

Crustacea. In a few terrestrial isopods there are tube structures called pseudotracheae from some of the limb exopodites. In these, a spiracle opens into a thin-walled air sac from which extend, into the haemocoel of the appendage, many thin, branching, blind tubules. The air sac is called a tracheal lung. Details of their structure and function are not available, but there are no tracheoles and the tubes end in the haemocoel.

Myriapoda. All classes but Pauropoda are known to have tracheae; these are in clusters arising from a pouch beneath the spiracle. There are no tracheoles and the tubes end in the haemocoel.

Insecta. From each of the spiracles (1 to 11 pairs, usually 10), a trachea extends, usually to be united with longitudinal trunks and frequently connected across the body by commissures. Branches then go into each appendage and to major organs of the viscera. Tracheae are internally supported by the spiral *taenidium*, and tracheoles are present. Tracheae are entirely absent in most Collembola and some Protura, in which all respiration occurs through the integument in general.

Comparative information on the tracheal systems of these eight classes is scant. It appears that tracheoles occur only in the Insecta, and thus the tracheae in the other groups do not reach to the cells but are bathed by the blood in the haemocoel. It would seem reasonable to conclude that in the latter oxygen is carried from the blind tracheae to the tissues by the blood. The blood of many crustaceans and arachnids contains haemocyanin (as well as sometimes haemoglobin), but whether this is the case with the species having relatively simple and short tracheae is not known.

Tracheoles. Although it is universal to cite tracheae as being respiratory organs, the real work of oxygen transfer in Insecta is done by the fine branches called tracheoles. The tracheoles have a thin chitinous lining, but this is not shed at molting. They form an interface with the cell membrane, or actually penetrate into the cell. They have been observed to move as much as 1 mm toward an area of oxygen deficiency. No evidence has been found that tracheoles occur in tracheal systems of any but Insecta.

Spiracles. These are the openings of the tracheal system to the outside and are sometimes called stigmata; thus they are not really respiratory organs. In Onychophora there may be many all over the body. In Insecta there may be up to 11 pairs or as few as a single spiracle, but most have 10 pairs. They may be permanently open or may have a closing mechanism. In the simplest examples, these are mere openings. In some there is merely a slit that can close, and in many there are elaborate closing devices and sieves to keep out all but air.

E. Respiratory Trees

In the Holothurioidea there are internal finely branched caeca of the cloaca, like a gill inverted into the interior. Although the animal is obviously pentaradiate, there are just two of these arborescent sacs, adding to the evidence of bilaterality seen in these animals. The trees are alternately filled with water and emptied by pumping of the rectum (cloaca). Apparently the oxygen is carried to the tissues by the coelomic fluid.

F. Respiratory Terminology

In keeping with the usage in this chapter, the following terms are principally ones that are applied to the respiration of individuals, rather than that of cells.

1. Aerobic — utilizing atmospheric (molecular) oxygen in energy metabolism
2. Air capillaries — the fine branches of the parabronchi that form complete loops (in Aves)
3. Alveolus — the tiny terminal cavity of the bronchiole in the lung tissue, where gas exchange takes place (higher Vertebrata)
4. Anaerobic — not utilizing oxygen in energy metabolism
5. Anoxybiotic — same as anaerobic
6. Blood gill — any gill filled with blood from the haemocoel
7. Book gill — the thin page-like external gill in the gill books of the Merostomata
8. Book-lung — a respiratory organ of page-like plates retracted into a cavity in the body wall
9. Branchiae — (sing. Branchia) the simple protrusions of the surface that serve for respiration, such as dermal branchiae
10. Bronchiole — one of the fine branches of a bronchus, each ending in an alveolus
11. Bronchus — one of the two air tubes into which the trachea divides, in Vertebrata
12. Bursa — respiratory invagination of the dorsal surface in Ophiuroidea
13. Caudal filament — terminal tracheal gill in some aquatic Insecta
14. Cerata — (sing. ceras) the external dorsal gills of nudibranch Gastropoda
15. Coxal gill — respiratory sac on coxae of some Amphipoda (Crustacea)
16. Cribriform organ — area of thin integumental folds between marginal plates in some Asteroidea
17. Ctenidium — comb-like structure of some gills
18. Cutaneous respiration — respiration through the skin without special structures
19. Dermal branchia — minute finger-like projection of body wall involving coelomic epithelium and epidermis, to increase respiratory surface of some Asteroidea
20. Facultative anaerobe — an organism in which respiration can be either aerobic or anaerobic
21. Gill — an organ for aquatic respiration, through the walls of which oxygen passes from the surrounding water; either a thin-walled exterior sac, usually much branched or the filamentous surface of a gill slit (see also book, coxal, peristomial, pharyngeal, rectal, spiracular, and tracheal gills)
22. Gill book — the packet of external page-like gills in Merostomata
23. Gill filaments — slender extensions of any gill surface
24. Gill slit (cleft) — gill-lined opening between the pharynx and the exterior (Vertebrata)
25. Integumentary respiration — respiration through any general body surface
26. Interface — in respiration any membrane through which oxygen or carbon dioxide must pass
27. Larynx — anterior part of vertebrate trachea performing special nonrespiratory functions
28. Lung — vascularized air sac used for respiration, especially in terrestrial Vertebrata where it is usually alveolate
29. Mantle — general respiratory surface of the body, consisting of folds of the body wall of which the exposed areas may function as gills (Brachiopoda, Mollusca)
30. Mantle cavity — any exterior cavity partially surrounded by mantle
31. Nostril (external nares) — external openings into the nasal passages
32. Oxybiotic — same as Aerobic

33. Papulum — see Dermal branchia
34. Parabronchi — the two primary branches of each bronchus in birds
35. Parapodium — flat lateral extension of a segment in Annelida, often vascularized for respiration
36. Peristomial gill — one situated near the mouth; in some Echinoidea
37. Pharyngeal gill — the respiratory surface lining the gill slit in fishes
38. Pharyngotremy — perforation of the walls of the pharynx for the passage of respiratory or feeding water
39. Pharynx — in Vertebrata, the chamber behind the mouth shared by digestive and respiratory systems
40. Plastron — a self-renewing air bubble carried underwater by an insect; air from the bubble is taken into the tracheal system, where its oxygen is absorbed into the cells; the oxygen in the bubble is constantly replaced by diffusion from the surrounding water
41. Pleopod — one of the paired abdominal appendages of certain Crustacea, with respiratory function in some
42. Pneumostome — the entrance to the mantle lung of Gastropoda
43. Pneustic — pertaining to air intake or to spiracle condition
    a. Amphipneustic — having two methods or locations of respiration: (1) gills and lungs (s.Pisces), (2) gills and vascularized body surface (s.Amphibia), (3) with only the prothoracic and the last abdominal spiracles open (a form of hemipneustic in s.larval Diptera)
    b. Apneustic — either having closed spiracles or none
    c. Branchiopneustic — having the spiracles functionally converted into gills (spiracular gills)
    d. Hemipneustic — having some of the spiracles open and some closed (in m.larval Insecta)
    e. Holopneustic — having all the spiracles open
    f. Hypopneustic — having less than the usual number of spiracles
    g. Metapneustic — with only the last pair of abdominal spiracles open; a form of hemipneustic
    h. Peripneustic — with the spiracles lateral and only the prothoracic and abdominal ones open; a form of hemipneustic
    i. Propneustic — with only the prothoracic spiracles open; a form of hemipneustic
44. Pseudotracheae — hollow tuft-like invaginations through the surface of pleopods in some terrestrial Crustacea (Isopoda); also called respiratory sacs
45. Radiole — a feathery process in the fans of some Annelida (fanworms)
46. Rectal gill — gill arising internally from the wall of the rectum or cloaca, sometimes projecting outside (s.Insecta)
47. Respiratory tree — dendritic extension of the rectum or cloaca into the body cavity (Holothurioidea)
48. Siphon — an air or water tube, either from or to the outside; e.g., carrying air in some larval Insecta; carrying feeding and respiratory currents in Mollusca. (Also as an intestinal bypass in Echinoidea)
49. Spiracle — (1) opening in the exoskeleton leading to the tracheae (in m.Arthropoda); (2) respiratory pores in some aquatic vertebrates
50. Spiracular gill — an outgrowth of a spiracle, in some aquatic Arthropoda (branchiopneustic)
51. Stigmata — (sing. stigma) same as spiracles in Arthropoda
52. Swim-bladder — gas-filled sac, sometimes paired, usually above the digestive tract, into which it may open (m.Pisces)

53.   Trachea — (1) in Arthropoda, air tubes from spiracle to all tissues, often branched and interconnected (rarely terminating in the blood); (2) in Vertebrata, air tube from pharynx or larynx to bronchi
54.   Tracheal gill — a gill containing tracheae instead of blood; receives molecular oxygen from surrounding water (Insecta)
55.   Tracheole — minute blind terminal tube of tracheal system, extending to every cell (Insecta)

G. Respiratory Fluids

In some animals, including vertebrates, oxygen reaches the tissues via fluids in which (1) the molecular oxygen is dissolved, (2) free respiratory pigments carry the oxygen, or (3) special cells carry the oxygenated pigments. This fluid is usually called blood. Like so many words in biology, blood is difficult to define, but it is a fluid (the plasma) with floating cells (amoebocytes, erythrocytes, etc.). In the present context the term blood refers to respiratory circulating fluids and their oxygen-carrying pigments (for a more general listing of body fluids, see the section on "Body cavities" in Chapter 20). These respiratory fluids may be in a circulatory tube system, in the general coelomic cavity, or in less definite tissue spaces. The exact components of the fluids are usually not stated. They are variously denoted by the words blood, lymph, haemolymph, and coelomic fluid, as described in Chapter 14. When oxygen is carried in a fluid, it may be either dissolved in the fluid or chemically bound to a carrier pigment. The oxygen-carrying pigment may be either in the plasma or in the circulating cells called corpuscles or erythrocytes (red blood cells).

Many body fluids have no respiratory function. Furthermore some chemical pigments, even ones that can be respiratory, often are situated in tissues other than blood and are not transporters of oxygen; rather they participate in cellular respiration. For example, in Rhynchocoela, haemoglobin (or erythrocruorin) may also occur around the brain and main nerves. It is often impossible to tell of a reported pigment whether or not it is a carrier of oxygen or a participant in cell respiration or both or neither.

Among the fluids which may have a respiratory function are the following:

1.   Blood in vessels (a closed system)
    a.   Rhynchocoela — erythrocytes may be present and may contain haemoglobin, or the latter may be in the plasma
    b.   Phoronida — blood contains corpuscles which contain haemoglobin
    c.   Mollusca — a mostly closed system lacking capillaries but containing blood or haemolymph with haemocyanin or rarely haemoglobin in either corpuscles or plasma; in some, the system is much more open
    d.   Annelida (most) — usually with a closed system, with blood containing haemoglobin, chlorocruorin, or haemerythrin in the plasma
    e.   Arthropoda (a few) — closed system with haemocyanin in the plasma, rarely with haemoglobin in the plasma
    f.   Pogonophora — a closed system with haemoglobin in the plasma
    g.   Vertebrata — a closed system with blood containing haemoglobin in erythrocytes
2.   Blood — (preferably called haemolymph) in noncoelomic open systems with few or no vessels
    a.   Brachiopoda — haemerythrin present in the plasma
    b.   Onychophora — because there are no tracheoles, oxygen is transferred by the haemolymph from the numerous tracheae to the cells
    c.   Arthropoda (rarely) — haemoglobin (erythrocruorin) is occasionally present in the blood plasma (s.Crustacea, larvae of s.Insecta) (in most Arthropoda oxygen is provided by the tracheal system alone)

3. Fluid in body cavities only (pseudocoelic or coelomic)
    a. Nematoda — the pseudocoel fluid and some tissues may contain haemoglobin
    b. Priapulida — haemerythrin occurs in the coelomic fluid
    c. Hirudinea (some) — haemoglobin in the fluid
    d. Echiuroidea — haemoglobin in corpuscles
    e. Echinodermata — possibly by coelomic fluid; in some Holothurioidea there is haemoglobin in coelomic corpuscles

H. Oxygen-Carrying Pigments

When oxygen is transported by respiratory pigments, there four principal ones are utilized: haemoglobin, haemocyanin, haemerythrin, and chlorocruorin. Other pigments in the body are generally not involved in oxygen transport but may be active in cell respiration. These include: myoglobin, pinnaglobin, echinochrome, cytochrome, daphniarubin, haemovanadin, naphthoquinone, anthraquinone, and myohaemerythrin, but their nature, cellular functions, and distribution in the animal kingdom are not sufficiently known for further tabulation here.

Table 19 gives the four widespread circulatory pigments used for oxygen transport. Haemoglobin has sometimes been divided into two.

The peculiarities in the distribution of these substances is even greater than shown above. Not only do some annelids have haemoglobin and some chlorocruorin, but others lack blood pigments entirely. Still others have both at the same time.

The number of hemes per protein molecule also varies. The "basic unit" is one; this occurs in some Mammalia, Pisces, Gastropoda, and at least one plant. Four hemes per molecule are found in *Homo sapiens*, many other Vertebrata, and in Bivalvia. Eight hemes occur in some Reptilia. Many invertebrates have such molecules containing even larger numbers of hemes; for example, 96 in some Polychaeta.

Although some Mollusca and some Arthropoda have haemocyanins, there is a consistent difference in the copper content in the two groups.

In addition to the fact that the blood pigment may vary from species to species within a group, it is also known that "there may be different haemoglobins in one individual at the same time or at successive periods in life" (Fox and Vevers, 1960). There are examples of both in human blood. Similar multiplicity is found in haemocyanins in some Mollusca and in some Crustacea.

It is seen (1) that blood pigments are diverse at several biochemical levels, (2) that haemoglobin, particularly, is widespread in the animal kingdom but often replaced by some other pigment, and (3) that within each class of pigment there may be diversity among animal species. Apparently diversity of pigments does not usually occur between the individuals of a given species, but there may be change from one to another form of the pigment in the life of the individual.

IV. ASSOCIATED FUNCTIONS

Sound production may occur in a larynx between the pharynx and the trachea. Amphibia and Reptilia possess a larynx in which there are simple vocal organs of cartilage and chambers which function as resonators. Hissing is the result of forcing air out through the mouth or nares. In the Mammalia, sound is produced in the larynx by air passing between the vocal cords. Control of the sound lies in the tension on the vocal cords and in movements of the mouth cavity, tongue, and lips. In the class Aves, at the point where the trachea joins the two bronchi, there is usually a small chamber called the syrinx, in which cartilages, muscles, and a tympanum can cause vibrations that are audible as bird songs or cries. In the few birds that are mute, such as the turkey vulture, the syrinx is absent altogether.

Table 19
BLOOD PIGMENTS

	Haemoglobin	Haemocyanin	Chlorocruorin	Haemerythrin	Pigments in other tissues
Porifera		(No blood)			
Mesozoa		(No blood)			
Coelenterata		(No blood)			
Ctenophora		(No blood)			
Platyhelminthes		(No blood)			
Rhynchocoela	X				Haemoglobin
Acanthocephala		(No blood)			
Rotifera		(No blood)			
Gastrotricha		(No blood)			
Kinorhyncha		(No blood)			
Nematoda					Haemoglobin
Gordioidea		(No blood)			
Priapuloidea		(No blood)			
Calyssozoa		(No blood)			
Bryozoa		(No blood)			
Phoronida	X				
Brachiopoda				X	Haemerythrin
Mollusca	X	X			Myoglobin, Pinnaglobin
Sipunculoidea				X	
Echiuroidea	X				
Tardigrada					(None known)
Myzostomida					(None known)
Annelida	X		X		
Dinophiloidea					(None known)
Pentastomoidea					(None known)
Onychophora					(No pigments)
Arthropoda	X	X			
Chaetognatha		(No blood)			
Pogonophora	X				(Or none)
Echinodermata		(No blood)			Haemoglobin, naphtho-quinones
Pterobranchia					(None known)
Enteropneusta					(None known)
Tunicata		(No blood)			Vanadium chromagens
Cephalochordata					(No pigments)
Vertebrata	X				

The respiratory organs may also be involved in production of hormones, maintenance of water balance, and temperature regulation. Comparative data are not available.

V. SYSTEMATIC SUMMARY OF RESPIRATION

The occurrences of respiratory organs, fluids, and pigments are summarized in Table 20. Where two pigments or more are indicated, they may not occur in the location shown on the same line but in one of those listed.

Table 20

DISTRIBUTION OF RESPIRATORY MECHANISMS

	Respiratory system	Major organs	Fluid	Pigment	Location
Protozoa	0	0		Haemoglobin	Cytoplasm
Mesozoa	0	(Surfaces)		0	
Porifera	0	(Surfaces)		0	
Coelenterata	0	(Surfaces)	0	0	
Ctenophora	0	(Surfaces)	0	0	
Gnathostomuloidea	0	(Integument)	0	0	
Platyhelminthes	0	(Integument)	0	0	Tissues
Rhynchocoela	0	(Integument)	Blood	0	Erythrocytes, plasma, rhyncho-coel
Acanthocephala	0	(Integument)	0	0	
Rotifera	0	(Integument)	0	0	
Gastrotricha	0	(Integument)	0	0	
Kinorhyncha	0	(Integument)	0	0	
Nematoda	0	(Integument)	Pseudocoel fluid	0	Pseudocoel
Gordioidea	0	(Integument)	0	0	
Priapuloidea	0	(Integument)	0	Haemerythrin	Coelomic erythrocytes
Calyssozoa	0	(Integument)	0	0	
Bryozoa	0	(Integument)	0	0	
Phoronida	0	(Integument)	0	Haemoglobin	Corpuscles
Brachiopoda	0	(Integument)		Haemerythrin	Coelomocytes
Mollusca	0/X	Gills, lungs, cerata	Blood	Haemoglobin Haemovanadin	Corpuscles plasma
Sipunculoidea	0	(Integument)	Coelomic fluid	Haemerythrin	Erythrocytes
Echiuroidea	0	(Integument)	Coelomic fluid	Haemoglobin	Coelomocytes
Tardigrada	0	(Integument)	0	0	
Myzostomida	0	(Integument)	0	0	
Annelida	0/X	Gills or integument	Blood	Haemoglobin, haemerythrin, chlorocruorin	Blood or coelomic fluid
Dinophiloidea	0	(Integument)	0	0	
Onychophora	X	Tracheae	Blood		
Pentastomida	0	(Integument)	Blood	Haemocyanin	
Arthropoda	0/X	Gills, book-lungs, tracheae	Blood or none	Haemocyanin Haemoglobin Daphniarubin Haematin	Plasma
Chaetognatha	0	(Integument)	0	0	
Pogonophora	0	(Integument)	Blood	Haemoglobin	Blood
Echinodermata	0/X	(Integument), gills or rectal trees	Coelomic fluid	Haemoglobin Chlorocruorin	Coelom
Pterobranchia	X	Gill slits			
Enteropneusta	X	Gill slits	Blood		
Tunicata	X	Gill slits	Blood	0	
Cephalochordata	X	Gill slits	Blood		
Vertebrata	X	Gill slits, lungs, gills	Blood	Haemoglobin	Erythrocytes

Note: 0, None occur; X, a system is present.

REFERENCES

Clark, R. B., *Dynamics in Metazoan Evolution: The Origin of the Coelom and Segments,* Oxford University Press, Oxford, 1964.

Florkin, M., Ed., *Biochemical Evolution,* Academic Press, New York, 1949.

Fox, H. M. and Vevers, G., *The Nature of Animal Colours,* Macmillan, New York, 1960.

Goodwin, T. W., Pigments in Echinodermata, in *Chemical Zoology,* Vol. 3, Florkin, M. and Scheer, B. T., Eds., Academic Press, New York, 1969, chap. 6.

Imms, A. D., *A General Textbook of Entomology,* 8th ed., Methuen, London, 1951.

Kaestner, A., *Invertebrate Zoology,* Vol. 1, Interscience, New York, 1967.

Kaestner, A., *Invertebrate Zoology,* Vol. 2, Interscience, New York, 1968.

Lee, D. L., *The Physiology of Nematodes,* W. H. Freeman, San Francisco, 1965.

Manwell, C., Comparative Physiology: Blood Pigments, *Annu. Rev. Physiol.,* 22, 191, 1960.

Marshall, A. J., *Parker & Haswell, A Text-Book of Zoology,* Vol. 2, 7th ed., Macmillan, London, 1964.

Romer, A. S., *The Vertebrate Body,* 2nd ed., W. B. Saunders, Philadelphia, 1955.

Waterman, T. H., Ed., *The Physiology of Crustacea,* Vol. 1, Academic Press, New York, 1960.

Wilbur, K. M. and Yonge, C. M., Eds., *Physiology of Mollusca,* Academic Press, New York, 1964—1966, 2 volumes.

Wilson, J. A., *Principles of Animal Physiology,* Macmillan, New York, 1972.

Chapter 16

EXCRETION

TABLE OF CONTENTS

I.   Introduction...328

II.   Excretory Organs 329
      A.   The Diversity...329
      B.   Protonephridia 329
      C.   Flame-Cell System 329
      D.   Solenocytes...331
      E.   Nephridial Kidney 331
      F.   Nephridium 331
      G.   Coxal Glands 331
      H.   Malpighian Tubules 331
      I.   Nephron Kidneys or Glomerular Kidneys.............................332
      J.   "Liver" 332
      K.   Lateral Canal System 332
      L.   Renettes 332
      M.   Brown Body...332
      N.   Urns 333
      O.   Nephrocytes 333
      P.   Mycetocytes 333
      Q.   Ciliated Urns or Ciliated Funnels 333
      R.   Glomerulus..333
      S.   Brown Funnels 334
      T.   Chloragogen Tissue 334
      U.   Stomach Epithelium..334
      V.   Terms for Excretory Organs 334

III. Excretory Pores 337

IV.   Diversity by Group 337

V.   Excretory Mechanisms..338
      A.   The Devices 338
      B.   Excretory Pathways 340
      C.   Excreted Substances..340

References 340

I. INTRODUCTION

In Chapter 12 the materials expelled from the body for any reason are summarized. Among these were waste products of metabolism, which include nitrogenous wastes, carbon dioxide, and excess water. Carbon dioxide is principally removed by the respiratory system, and so it is not treated here. Excess water comes from two sources: from metabolism itself in all animals, or in freshwater animals directly from the outside by osmosis. It seems most appropriate to deal with the expulsion of all such water under the heading of "Osmoregulation" (Chapter 20), even though such expulsion often involves the same organs as for metabolic wastes.

In medical use the two words excretion and elimination are often loosely applied to removal of the undigested material in the digestive tract. These terms are best used to distinguish two processes, *excretion* for removal of all chemical wastes of metabolism, and *elimination* for removal of wastes produced in the digestive tract. This latter material is never really inside the animal, only in a tube that passes through. These digestive wastes are not included in this discussion of excretion, which here includes only the nitrogenous substances such as ammonia, urea, and (rarely) amino acids, which have been part of the body proteins.

In the case of metabolic wastes, "removal" merely implies taking them out of the metabolic system, i.e., out of the tissues where they are formed. Wastes are not always removed completely from the body and some "wastes" are later recycled into new uses in the body.

Some of the methods of removal are (1) dissolved wastes may be given off through the body surface by diffusion; (2) wastes may be taken up by phagocytic cells and discharged to the outside or into the digestive tract; (3) wastes may be stored in cells or tissues, either until death of the individual or until these wastes are again needed by the individual and are thus "recycled"; and (4) dissolved wastes may be conducted to the outside by a tube or tube system, from some organ that extracts the waste from the blood or body fluid. The organs utilized in these removals are listed in several ways in the following pages.

In the customary sense, an excretory system consists of the mechanisms associated with the collection, concentration, and removal of nitrogenous wastes from the body. If these mechanisms form an integrated unit, one can call it a system — an excretory system. It is easily seen, however, not only that the excretory mechanisms in animals are highly diverse but that they are often not well organized into a single system. There may be a wide variety of organs, tissues, and cells, not closely connected or integrated, that serve this excretory function. For this reason there is here no list of "excretory systems", but rather careful description of the various organs and mechanisms involved in excretion in the broad sense.

Even so, there are a few excretory mechanisms that are frequently called systems; these are here treated as organs.

1. Flame-cell systems
2. Solenocyte systems
3. Ducts draining the pseudocoel
4. Coelomoducts
5. Nephridial systems
6. Glandular organs (e.g., antennary and coxal glands)
7. Malpighian tubules
8. Glomerulus (proboscis gland)
9. Nephron kidneys

Many of the animals that have one of these systems (often paired or in several pairs) also utilize other mechanisms for excreting wastes. This is why it is so often inappropriate to speak of "*the* excretory system" in some animal.

II. EXCRETORY ORGANS

A. The Diversity

Some excretory organs occur in several phyla or in one large and diverse phylum. Others are of narrower distribution. Among the former are flame cells, solenocytes, nephridial kidneys, nephridia, coxal glands, malpighian tubules, and nephron kidneys. The less widespread organs would then be "liver" of certain medusae and the very different one of endoprocts, lateral canals and renettes of nematodes, brown body of bryozoans, urns of sipunculoids, mycetocytes in a few insects, urns in holothurians, glomerulus of enteropneusts, and nephrocytes of a few insects and of tunicates. Of course, much excretion is through the integument or by organs with additional functions, as shown in the list of respiratory mechanisms.

B. Protonephridia

Before describing the simple excretory organs of such groups as the flatworms, it is necessary to establish the meaning and appropriateness of several terms.

Nearly all books imply that such terms as nephridium and protonephridium are explicit, so one feels that when he knows the nature of a "protonephridium" in one animal, he can accept the term as telling him much about the "protonephridium" in another. This assumption cannot generally be avoided, and conclusions have been based on the fact, for example, that "protonephridia" occur in many phyla. In reality these organs are strikingly diverse among these phyla. This diversity "within the term" is exemplified below, where the term protonephridium is replaced by the terms flame cell, flame bulb, solenocyte, and canal system.

The use of the term protonephridium is sometimes a convenience. It helps to identify a certain group of phyla. It is sometimes overlooked that this "group" consists of Platyhelminthes, Rhynchocoela, Acanthocephala, the five phyla of Aschelminthes, Calyssozoa, Mollusca (larvae), Echiuroidea, Annelida, *and* Cephalochordata. It is hard to find much significance to a term that makes a grouping of such diverse animals. Among these so-called protonephridia there are three types of organs: flame cells (or bulbs), solenocytes, and lateral canals. It is the solenocytes that bring the most far-flung distribution, but flame cells are not far behind (see Figure 20).

There are two reasons for avoiding this term. First, the phyla encompassed form a meaningless group, as implied above. Second, the word implies that the organs are a form of nephridium, but no definition of nephridium will justify this unless it exactly corresponds to excretory organ. Nephridium is seldom if ever used in this broad sense, but is used for a very specific organ of totally different sort.

The general solution to this problem is to be specific whenever possible. Use flame cell (or bulb), solenocyte, or lateral canal system as appropriate, thereby making all statements more explicit and avoiding altogether the misleading term protonephridium. These three types of internally blind tube systems (all nephridia are internally open!) will now be described. All three are basically excretory ducts consisting of comparatively few cells. In spite of all this, there are circumstances in which this is the only term available to encompass the four types of simple excretory systems. At such times the term protonephridium, however inappropriate, may be used merely to enable one to refer to this group of structures.

C. Flame-Cell System

This is any excretory system consisting of one or more ducts each with one or more

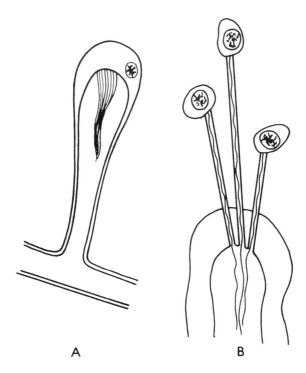

FIGURE 20.   Simple excretory cells. (A) Flame cell, (B) solenocytes.

flame cells. The *flame cell* is an extension of the wall of the excretory duct to form a chamber enclosed by a single cell; it thus forms a bulb. In the blind end of the cavity there is a tuft of cilia, whose movement gives the impression of a flickering flame. The cilia do not extend out of the chamber.

A *flame bulb* is the same as a flame cell except that more than one cell is involved in the enclosing wall. Both expressions are sometimes used loosely to cover both types of extensions, with little or no confusion because the organs are essentially the same. Hyman uses flame bulb as the more general term, whereas in older works the number of cells involved seemed irrelevant so that flame cell was used in all cases.

In the operation of both of these, wastes presumably enter the lumen of the "bulb" via minute pores through the cells, and they leave by the tube (and often additional ducts) to an exterior pore. It is sometimes implied that the "flame" of vibrating cilia drives the wastes down the duct from a hollow cell, but this is, of course, hydrostatically impossible; only osmotic or hydrostatic pressure could drive a fluid out of a closed sac, and the cilia could serve only a mixing function. It now appears from electron microscopy that the cell is perforated, and the influx of wastes would be aided by the action of the flame in driving them into the ducts. The bulbs may be numerous and the ducts very long; when the latter are present, there may be one, two or three pairs running most of the length of the animal. These paired ducts may each have a storage bladder or they may enter a single bladder, before reaching the exterior excretory pore.

It is a curious fact that in Turbellaria at least, the excretory function of flame bulbs is in question. Hyman (1951) reports, "No evidence has been seen of any passage of substances through the flame bulb in any turbellarian. It seems probable that . . . the necessity of eliminating nitrogenous wastes is avoided by converting them into insoluble granules that are held permanently in mesenchyme and in pigment cells." It is possible that here the flame bulbs are osmoregulatory in function rather than excretory.

D. Solenocytes

In some of the bulbs just described, there is no flame of cilia but a single very long flagellum. Such bulbs are called solenocytes; they are more widespread in the animal kingdom than flame cells. The flagellum extends out of the chamber and down the duct to a common duct called a protonephridial tubule. Its undulating motion inside the slender duct can be seen to have a tendency to drive fluid out of the chamber. As in flame cells, however, this would be entirely ineffective if there was not an increasing pressure in the chamber caused by entry of additional fluid through the bulb wall. It is astonishing that Cephalochordata possess solenocytes identical to those of annelids and showing no similarity whatever to organs of either vertebrates or echinoderms. These solenocytes appear to consist of single cells with a hollow interior and a long duct.

E. Nephridial Kidney

Mollusks are usually said to have a kidney, but this is not similar to the vertebrate kidney, so that term is misleading. In its simplest forms it may be little more than a nephridium, consisting of a duct from the coelom to the mantle cavity. In others it becomes a glandular mass in a sac, with or without openings into the pericardial cavity. It is said to be nephridial in nature, but this is usually not obvious.

F. Nephridium

This word has generally been defined as an open excretory duct with a ciliated *nephrostome* in the coelom and a *nephridiopore* to the outside. This definition is entirely adequate, although this structure is sometimes physically united to other coelomic ducts and may then receive other names, such as *nephromixium*, signifying its dual purpose. This nephrostome duct occurs only in coelomate animals and more particularly in segmented ones. It is in some books called a *metanephridium*; we believe this to be an unnecessary word as there is no other kind of nephridium (see Protonephridia above). It is again astonishing to note that the pronephros of larval vertebrates and even a few adults (Pisces) are actually nephridia, with ciliated nephrostomes in the coelom. By not using the term nephridia, the similarity is obscured.

G. Coxal Glands

In several arthropod groups, the only excretory organ is a gland in the base of an appendage. Thus, in crustaceans they are in antennae or maxillae (lying in the haemocoel) and are then called antennary (or green) glands and maxillary glands. In chelicerates, the gland opens at the base of a leg (on the coxa), but such glands are in the haemocoel and are often closely associated with the digestive tract. Guanine is known to be excreted in some cases, but apparently much of the nitrogenous wastes are recycled and not excreted.

H. Malpighian Tubules

In most insects there are organs for excretion in the form of *Malpighian tubules*, which are not open into the haemocoel; these originate from the anterior end of the hindgut and extend throughout the haemocoel. There may be as few as 1 pair or at least as many as 250 tubes. Wastes, selectively absorbed from the haemolymph through the wall of the tubes, may be concentrated by recovery of water and then discharged into the hindgut for elimination.

These tubules are also reported in the myriapods, where they seem to be of similar nature. In some arachnids, even some with coxal glands, similar tubes exist in the haemocoel, and are known to pass at least guanine.

I. Nephron Kidneys or Glomerular Kidneys

Vertebrates have paired kidneys consisting primarily of masses of tubules and glomeruli arranged in functional units called *nephrons*. Arterial blood enters the *glomerulus*, where most of the plasma is extracted and passed through the Bowman's *capsule* into the *excretory tubule*, where all but the wastes are selectively reabsorbed into the blood capillaries surrounding the tubule. The tubule discharges the remainder (wastes) into the "lumen" of the kidney, which in reality is the *pelvis* (terminal enlargement) of the excretory duct (*ureter*).

Three forms of the nephron kidney are formed in sequence in most vertebrates. The *pronephros* is the functional form in some fish and amphibian larvae; the *mesonephros* is the functional kidney in adult fishes and amphibians; the *metanephros* is the kidney in reptiles, birds, and mammals.

J. "Liver"

The so-called "liver" reported in some siphonophores is a mass permeated with gastrodermal canals. The canal walls are filled with guanine crystals, giving rise to the supposition that the organ is excretory. The obvious difficulty of accounting for this "organ" in a colony of attached individuals disappears entirely when this structure is seen to occur only in the genera *Velella* and *Porpita*, which are elsewhere in this book recognized as modified medusae, not colonies. The "liver" is also unusual in medusae, but it is clearly an organ, not an individual. It stores wastes, rather than eliminating them.

The "liver" of Calyssozoa is an area of brown or olive color along the top of the stomach, so colored because of inclusions that seem to be of excretory material. These seem to be waste storage areas in these short-lived animals, which also have a pair of flame bulbs.

K. Lateral Canal System

In nematodes the excretory mechanism is sometimes stated to be a system of lateral canals joined in an H- or U-shaped manner with a median central pore. The tubes are blind internally, having no flame cells or other end organs. Except for this, they seem to operate in the same manner as the flame cell systems, with fluid passing through the walls of the tubes. There is no direct evidence that these tubes are actually excretory in function or, indeed, as to what their function is, although both excretion and osmoregulation are generally cited. These may be associated with renette cells.

L. Renettes

In many marine and a few freshwater nematodes an excretory cell called a renette, either alone or associated with a lateral canal, forms the "excretory" unit. This gland cell (or each of a pair of such cells) is in the pseudocoel and either has a pore to the exterior or is connected into the canal system. An excretory function is assumed but seems to be unproven (see Figure 21).

M. Brown Body

Although sometimes cited as an excretory organ, the brown body of Bryozoa is a residue from the disintegration of the individual (polypide) and contains waste materials accumulated by that individual. It is thus not an organ, but a residue left by a dying polypide.

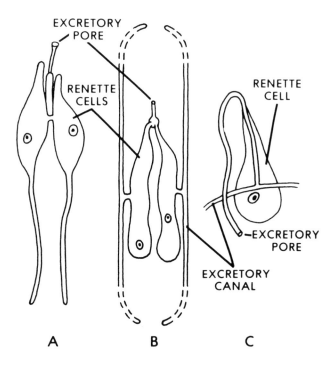

FIGURE 21.   Renette and tubes of three nematodes.

N. Urns
In the coelom of sipunculids there are curious organs called urns. They originate in the coelomic peritoneum but may become free in the coelomic fluid. They are said to swim about in a lively fashion by means of cilia. They accumulate waste materials and are probably eventually eliminated through the nephridia.

O. Nephrocytes
The nephrocytes of Insecta are localized groups of cells, usually near the fat body. These cells are distinctive because they are often binucleate. They take up and store various substances, some of which are excretory in nature, and some of which are apparently further metabolized for use in general anabolism.

P. Mycetocytes
In some Insecta (Homoptera) there are cells called mycetocytes which form an organ called a pseudovitellus or mycetome. The cells contain symbiotic microorganisms which apparently consume waste products; thus, they are believed to be excretory, as at least part of their function.

Q. Ciliated Urns or Ciliated Funnels
In one order of holothurians there are few or many cornucopia-like organs on the mesenteries lining the coelom. The cavity of these urns is filled with coelomocytes (phagocytes), and at least some foreign or waste material is accumulated in these cells. The cells are later passed out through the body wall or united into masses called *brown bodies*. Other echinoderms use such coelomocytes but without the ciliated urns.

R. Glomerulus
Enteropneusts have a possible excretory organ called a glomerulus. The identity of

this term with the glomerulus of the vertebrate nephron was intended to show a relationship between the two, but there is little or no evidence of similarity beyond the
excretory function. This glandular organ is in the proboscis complex in communication
with the dorsal vessel through a sinus, which is surrounded by peritoneal expansions
forming a plexus full of blood. All blood passes through this glomerulus, but the nature of any excretory function is unclear.

S. Brown Funnels

In cephalochordates, the brown funnels (or bodies) are supposed to be excretory
(even though an extensive system of solenocytes is also present). They are at the dorsal
rear of the pharynx and apparently communicate with both the coelom and the atrium.

T. Chloragogen Tissue

The large mass of chloragogen cells surrounding much of the intestine in annelids
forms a special tissue, and its function has been controversial. It now appears that
proponents of an absorptive function and those of an excretory function were both
right, and both functions are performed. In excretion, individual cells appear to gather
waste products, then detach and circulate in the blood or coelomic fluid, eventually
disintegrating in the latter. The wastes are eliminated from the coelom by the nephridia. The chloragoge function is thus not of direct excretion of wastes but of concen-
trating them and transforming them into ammonia or urea which can be eliminated by
the nephridia.

U. Stomach Epithelium

In collembolans the stomach epithelium is active in excretion along with the fat
body, but whereas the cells of the fat body store wastes permanently, the epithelium
accumulates similar concentrations of waste matter only temporarily. In the latter case,
the concentrations accumulate at the inner ends of the cells (along the lumen of the
stomach) and are then periodically pinched off into the stomach cavity. The epithelium
itself is replaced at each molt.

V. Terms for Excretory Organs

The excretory organs are briefly identified here, and their distribution among animals is cited in a later tabulation. Other mechanisms, using organs not primarily or
obviously excretory, are also listed.

1. Amoebocyte — Any amoeboid cell in body fluids or tissues; some perform excre-
    tory functions by phagocytosis; they may be cited also as athrocytes, coelomo-
    cytes, leukocytes, lymphocytes, macrophages, monocytes, phagocytes, etc.
2. Antennary gland — (Antennal or green gland) in Crustacea; each consists of an
    end sac and sometimes a labyrinth in contact with blood vessels, an excretory
    canal and an exit duct, and often a collecting bladder; eliminates ammonia, urea,
    uric acid, and amines in various combinations
3. Athrocyte — An amoebocyte that transports wastes
4. Botryoidal tissues — Clusters of mesenchyme cells enveloping the fore- and hind-
    guts of some annelids
5. Brown body — The remains of the body of a bryozoan; not actually excretory
    but containing some waste materials among the remnants of the degenerating
    individual; in Cephalochordata, this term is applied to a pair of structures above
    the intestine, where excretory function is not certain
6. Bursae — Ten thin-walled pockets from the dorsal surface in Ophiuroidea; prin-
    cipally respiratory but probably supplementing the body surface in excretion

7. Chloragogen tissue — A massive tissue enveloping the intestine in some Annelida; among the various functions are producing and storing some wastes

8. Coelomocyte — See Amoebocyte

9. Coelomoduct — Any open duct from the coelom to the outside; includes nephridia but is often listed separately with other functions, such as discharge of gametes

10. Coxal gland — Glandular vesicle in some Arthropoda, remnant of the coelom; paired in each segment of the haemocoel, or one at the base of each leg of one or more of the leg pairs; sometimes used in a broader sense to include antennary and maxillary glands

11. Excretophores — Glandular bodies in some Annelida, consisting of cells such as athrocytes; in blood vessels or in the coelom; formed from coelomic epithelium and eventually discharged or destroyed by the nephridia

12. Flame bulb — A "protonephridium" in which the expansion of the tube (bulb) is composed of more than one cell, but otherwise identical with flame cells (sometimes used for the bulb regardless of the number of cells involved)

13. Flame cell — A "protonephridum" consisting of a single cell with a hollow interior containing a tuft or "flame" of cilia and elongated into a duct; in a single pair or many, often in clusters of many; in the parenchyma or the pseudocoel (see also Solenocytes)

14. Glomerulus — In Enteropneusta, a mass of blind tubular evaginations from the peritoneum of the proboscis complex is filled with blood and may be an excretory organ (also called proboscis gland); in Vertebrata, see Nephron

15. Green gland — Same as antennary gland

16. Intestinal gland — (Midgut or midintestinal gland); in pulmonate Gastropoda these glands in the wall of the intestine are loaded with granules and concretions, which appear to be stored wastes

17. Keber's organ — Glandular clumps of excretory cells in some Bivalvia

18. Kidney — Highly vascular mass of nephrons that filters wastes from the blood; in Vertebrata only; occurs as pro-, meso-, or metanephros. (An excretory organ in some mollusks should not be called a kidney, because it is basically a nephridium: see Nephridial kidney)

19. Labial glands — In thysanuran Insecta these discharge by means of an excretory duct which opens at the base of the labium

20. Lateral canal — Paired canals in Nematoda, usually joined in H- or U-shape; generally assumed to be protonephridial in nature, but the extent of excretory function is still uncertain

21. Leukocyte — See Amoebocyte

22. Liver — Organs designated by this term and thought to be excretory occur in Siphonophora (a mass permeated with gastrodermal tubes, beneath the float) and in Calyssozoa (a brownish mass of ciliated columnar cells along the stomach); in Vertebrata the liver is a separate organ of many functions, including the deamination of amino acids, resulting in ammonia, which is usually converted into urea or uric acid before excretion

23. Lymphocyte — See Amoebocyte

24. Malpighian tubules — In the Arthropoda long and slender blind tubes arising from the front end of the hindgut, lined with secretory epithelium; lying throughout much of the haemocoel

25. Macrophage — see Amoebocyte

26. Maxillary gland — Similar to antennary gland but in the base of the maxilla

27. Mesonephros — the mid-kidney, functional in both larvae and adults of Pisces and Amphibia (see also Kidney)

28. Metanephridium — See Nephridium
29. Metanephros — The hind-kidney, functional only in adults of Reptilia, Aves, and Mammalia (see also Kidney)
30. Monocyte — See Amoebocyte
31. Mycetocyte — Excretory cells in a few Insecta; with symbiotic microorganisms
32. Nephridial kidney — a glandular excretory organ of mollusks, possibly derived from a nephridium
33. Nephridium — A tubular organ opening from a ciliated nephrostome (funnel) in the coelom (or other body space) and a long convoluted tubule to an external nephridiopore; the tubule may also be associated with blood vessels, sometimes divided into (a) protonephridium, a term to cover various simple systems, such as flame bulbs and solenocytes (however, the term is misleading in that these are not primitive nephridial systems) it is better to be specific, as some of these systems may be of unrelated origin, and (b) metanephridium, this term is unnecessary because it represents the only sort of ciliated coelomoduct; here called simply nephridium
34. Nephrocytes — (Pericardial cells in insects) Cells suspended in chains in the haemocoel; apparently absorb nitrogenous wastes for re-use at the next molt (nephrocyte is used in Echinodermata for athrocytes that transport some wastes to storage sites; it is used in Mollusca for the cells of the inner surface of the nephridial kidney, which accumulate large concretions within vacuoles)
35. Nephron — The functional unit of the kidney in adult vertebrates; consisting of a ball-shaped network of blood vessels (glomerulus) in an invaginated bulb called a Bowman's capsule, which opens through a convoluted tubule into a collecting tubule
36. Organ of Bojanus — This tubular organ of the Bivalvia is sometimes called kidney or nephridium. It is essentially a coelomoduct, if one assumes that the pericardial cavity represents the coelom (see Chapter 20). In any case it leads from the pericardial cavity to the outer surface of the body, being open at both ends; it consists of a glandular part (usually labeled kidney) and a tubular bladder
37. Paranephridial plexus — A system of vessels connecting the flame bulbs with all organs; possibly excretory (in metacercariae of Trematoda)
38. Pericardial cells (See Nephrocyte)
39. Phagocyte (See Amoebocyte)
40. Proboscis gland (See Glomerulus)
41. Pronephros — The "fore-kidney", separately functional only in the larvae of fishes and amphibians (see Kidney)
42. Protonephridia — General term for flame cells, flame bulbs, solenocytes, and nematode canal systems together (an inappropriate term because they are not nephridia)
43. Renette — In Nematoda, a glandular organ consisting of one or two large uninucleate cells provided with a duct to an excretory pore; located in the pseudocoel and sometimes associated with a paired excretory duct system
44. Rosettes — (Cell rosettes) groups of ciliated gastrodermal cells along the canals, around openings into the collenchyme; may be excretory; only in Ctenophora
45. Solenocyte — A multinucleate bulb similar to a flame bulb but having, in place of the flame of cilia, a single long flagellum that projects far down the tube; in a solenocyte system there are generally many of the long tubular bulbs in clusters
46. Urns — In Sipunculoidea, fixed or floating cells in the coelom, often stalked and with other cells attached; the free urns are said to swim actively in the coelomic fluid; they apparently accumulate dead cells and other debris but are not phagocytic; in Holothurioidea: multicellular funnels lined with ciliated epithelium, on

mesenteries in the coelom; accumulate foreign particles and also collect coelomocytes that have themselves phagocytized such particles

III. EXCRETORY PORES

Excretory pores may open at almost any point on the body surface, even on the base of appendages, or into such external cavities as gill chambers. They also may discharge into the oesophagus or into the hindgut. There may be 1, 1 pair, 1 pair in most segments, or as many as 35,000 on each side of the body (as in some Rhynchocoela).

IV. DIVERSITY BY GROUP

Three difficulties interfere with tabulation of the occurrences of the various organs or mechanisms among the phyla and classes. First, many structures reported to be excretory may be involved only in water or ion balance. Second, many organs perform a minor excretory function in addition to their principal function. Third, there are many conflicting reports of the nature of "protonephrida" and "nephridia". Even when the term flame is used (as in Kinorhyncha), it may be evident that the structure is in reality a solenocyte, and the distinction between nephridia and other coelomic ducts is often unclear. Even with these difficulties, the following shows some of the diversity of excretory devices:

1. Protozoa — Cell surface and contractile vacuoles
2. Porifera — Phagocytes discharging to outside and by diffusion from cell to cell
3. Mesozoa — Body surface
4. Coelenterata — Direct diffusion from each cell to the outside; phagocytic mesogloeal cells; in some genera usually placed in Siphonophora, a mass called "liver" permeated with gastrodermal canals
5. Ctenophora — Possibly cell rosettes and body surfaces
6. Platyhelminthes — Flame cell of flame bulb system
   a. Turbellaria — Either system and body surface
   b. Trematoda — Flame cells also in larvae, sometimes with a paranephridial plexus
   c. Cestoda — Flame cells also in larvae
9. Rhynchocoela — Body surface or a tube system or an extensive flame bulb system
10. Acanthocephala — Flame bulb system and body surface
11. Rotifera — Flame bulb system
12. Gastrotricha — Solenocyte system or ventral glands or none
13. Kinorhyncha — Solenocyte system
14. Nematoda — Lateral canal system, renettes, body surface
15. Gordioidea — Body surface only
16. Priapuloidea — Solenocyte system
17. Calyssozoa — Solenocyte system
18. Bryozoa — None, except storage in wall of digestive tract (into brown body), tentacular epithelium
19. Phoronida — Nephridia
20. Brachiopoda — Nephridia and coelomocytes
21. Mollusca — A nephridial kidney which may be a modified coelomoduct; flame cells in trochophore larvae; nephrocytes; storage "glands"; in Bivalvia, a pair of Bojanus' organs or of Keber's organs
22. Sipunculoidea — Nephridia and motile urns
23. Echiuroidea — Nephridia, amoebocytes

24. Myzostomida — Pair of nephridia opening into the hindgut
25. Annelida — Nephridia, sometimes combined with coelomoducts; rarely soleno-cyte system, especially in larvae but sometimes attached to nephridia; excreto-phores (including "heart bodies"), amoebocytes, botryoidal tissue, chloragogen tissue
26. Tardigrada — Blind ducts called Malpighian tubules; or none
27. Pentastomida — Body surface
28. Onychophora — Segmental nephridia
29. Arthropoda — Storage in exoskeleton, plus:
    a. Merostomata — Coxal glands
    b. Arachnida — Coxal glands, stomach and intestine cell storage
    c. Crustacea — A variety of coxal glands, body surface, phagocytes (the inap-propriate word nephridium is sometimes used)
    d. Myriapoda — Malpighian tubules
    e. Insecta — Malpighian tubules, labial and salivary glands, nephrocytes and fat body as storage; midgut epithelial cells (some wastes are absorbed by sym-biotic mycetocytes)
30. Chaetognatha — Presumably general body surface, because excretory organs are lacking
31. Pogonophora — Nephridia
32. Echinodermata — Nephrocytes (phagocytic coelomocytes); general body surface or particular regions:
    a. Crinoidea — Saccules along the ambulacral grooves
    b. Asteroidea — Dermal branchiae and tube feet
    c. Ophiuroidea — Thin walls of the respiratory bursae
    d. Echinoidea — Gills and podia
    e. Holothurioidea — Respiratory trees, digestive tract, or gonads; urns
33. Enteropneusta — Glomerulus (proboscis gland), body surface, coelomocytes
34. Pterobranchia — Probably body surface
35. Tunicata — Nephrocytes and surface of pharyngeal basket
36. Cephalochordata — Solenocyte system and brown bodies
37. Vertebrata — Kidneys (pronephros, mesonephros, or metanephros), body sur-face, liver storage, pigment cell storage, various amoebocytes

V. EXCRETORY MECHANISMS

A. The Devices

The devices for collecting, conducting, and discharging the wastes include these:

Ducts draining the body spaces; open at both ends

1. Coelomoducts or nephridia (Phoronida and many higher groups)

Ducts draining the body spaces, not open internally

2. Cell rosettes (Ctenophora)
3. Flame cell systems (Platyhelminthes, Rhynchocoela, Acanthocephala, Rotifera, trochophore larva of Mollusca)
4. Paired duct system (Rhynchocoela)
5. Lateral canal system (Nematoda)
6. Solenocyte systems (Gastrotricha, Kinorhyncha, Priapuloidea, Calyssozoa, Po-lychaeta, Cephalochordata)

7. Malpighian tubules (Myriapoda, Insecta)
8. Glomerulus (Enteropneusta)
9. Nephron system (Vertebrata)

Glandular organs

10. Glands in base of appendage (s.Arthropoda); (a) antennary (green) glands, (b) maxillary glands, (c) labial glands, and (d) coxal glands
11. Intestinal gland (s.Gastropoda)
12. "Liver" (Hydrozoa: *Vellela* and *Porpita*)
13. Renettes (Nematoda)
14. Ventral glands (s.Gastrotricha)

Phagocytes

15. Amoeboid phagocytes in virtually all groups: amoebocytes, coelomocytes, leukocytes, lymphocytes, macrophages, monocytes, etc.
16. Botryoidal tissue (Hirudinea)
17. Urns (Sipunculoidea, Holothurioidea)
18. Excretophores in mesenchyme (Sipunculoidea, Annelida)

Storage systems

19. Wall of alimentary canal; see also no. 32 below (Bryozoa)
20. Brown body (Bryozoa)
21. Brown funnels (Cephalochordata)
22. Certain vacuolated ectodermal cells (larvae of Gastropoda)
23. Exoskeleton (Arthropoda)
24. Nephrocytes (pericardial cells in Insecta; blood nephrocytes in Ascidiacea)
25. Fat body (Insecta, Vertebrata)

External body surface, without special organ systems

26. General body surface (Protozoa, Mesozoa, Coelenterata, Ctenophora, Platyhelminthes, Rhynchocoela, Acanthocephala, Nematoda, Gordioidea, Pentastomida, Crustacea, Echinodermata, Enteropneusta, Pterobranchia, Vertebrata)
27. Tentacles (Bryozoa)

Internal surfaces

28. Rosette cells in gastrodermis (Ctenophora)
29. "Liver" (Calyssozoa)
30. Chloragogen cells in coelomic epithelium (Oligochaeta, Polychaeta)
31. Stomach epithelium; see no. 20 above (Bryozoa)
32. Intestinal epithelium (Arachnida: Acarina, Insecta: Collembola)

Both external (epidermis) and internal (gastrodermis)

33. (Coelenterata)

Symbiont absorption

34. "Mycetocytes" (Insecta: Homoptera)

B. Excretory Pathways

All excretion is the removal of metabolic wastes in the cells, by diffusion from the cell (1) direct to the outside, (2) into intercellular fluid, (3) into body cavity fluids, or (4) into blood capillaries.

C. Excreted Substances

Among the substances removed from the body of animals, there are four principal excretory types: nitrogenous wastes, carbon dioxide, excess water, and inorganic ions. Water and ions are excreted at least in part for the requirements of osmotic and ionic regulation, rather than as strictly waste products of metabolism, and they are therefore discussed under "Osmoregulation" in Chapter 20. Carbon dioxide elimination is discussed in Chapter 15, "Respiration". In a very general way, the nitrogenous substances excreted by animals appear to be related to the manner of living of the individual, even changing to some extent during its life. Little is known about these materials in many groups, but there is enough to show that there is little correlation with the type of organ.

In most references to excretion in a major group, one or more of the common products are mentioned so that a tabulation shows a very spotty distribution. However, in such a detailed tabulation as that given in the first edition of Prosser (1950), it is seen that virtually all animals excrete one or more of the related nitrogenous compounds ammonia, urea, and uric acid, with only the proportions varying. Purines such as guanine are not so frequently listed, but they are excreted by some Coelenterata, Mollusca, Arthropoda, and Vertebrata, at least (guanine can be converted to uric acid, so it is not an unrelated excretory product).

Animals that excrete primarily ammonia are said to be *ammonotelic*; those that excrete primarily urea are *ureotelic*; those that excrete primarily uric acid are *uricotelic*.

Most excretory organs apparently can remove any of these nitrogenous materials (ammonia, urea, uric acid, guanine). The following are the ones that have been commonly reported as excreted by the major organs:

1. Flame bulbs — uric acid and urea, but information is scanty
2. Lateral canals (of Nematoda) — ammonia, urea, uric acid
3. Nephridial kidneys (of Mollusca) — ammonia, urea, uric acid, guanine
4. Nephridia (in various groups) — ammonia, urea, uric acid
5. Malpighian tubules — ammonia, urea, uric acid, guanine
6. Kidneys (of Vertebrata) — ammonia, urea, uric acid

Although guanine is listed above as sometimes produced in several types of excretory organs, this substance is not as well documented among the groups, because in many books its presence is recorded only by its product uric acid.

The following have been cited as excreted materials: allantoic acid, allantoin, amino acids, ammonia, carbon dioxide, creatinine, creatine, guanine, hippuric acid, ions (K^+, Na^+, H^+, NH_4^+, Cl^-, PO_4^-), leucine, nitrogenous pigments, ornithuric acid, pterines, purines, pyrimidines, trimethyl amino oxide, urea, uric acid, and water.

REFERENCES

Clark, W. E. L., *The Tissues of the Body*, 6th ed., Oxford University Press, Oxford, 1971.

Elias, H. and Mamiszka, C. R., Excretory organs, in Gray, P., Ed., *The Encyclopedia of the Biological Sciences*, Reinhold, New York, 1961.

Hyman, L. H., *The Invertebrates*, Vol. 2, McGraw-Hill, New York, 1951.

Marshall, A. J., *Parker & Haswell, A Text-Book of Zoology*, Vol. 2, 7th ed., Macmillan, London, 1962.

Prosser, C. L., Ed., *Comparative Animal Physiology*, 1st ed., W. B. Saunders, Philadelphia, 1950.

Chapter 17

NERVOUS AND ENDOCRINE SYSTEM

TABLE OF CONTENTS

I.   Introduction 342

II.   Detection of Stimuli 342
      A.   Senses 342
      B.   Sense Receptors 344
           1.   Reception of Stimuli 344
           2.   Photoreception 345
                a.   Detection of Light 345
                b.   Visual Pigments 346
           3.   Chemoreception 346
                a.   Detection of Water-Borne Chemicals 347
                b.   Gustatory Organs 347
                c.   Detection of Airborne Chemicals 347
           4.   Mechanoreception 348
                a.   Detection of Sound and Other Vibrations 348
                b.   Detection of Tactile Stimuli 348
                c.   Detection of Gravity 349
                d.   Proprioception 349
                e.   Miscellaneous Stimuli 350

III. The Nerve Systems 351
      A.   Conducting Devices 351
      B.   Nerve Nets 351
      C.   Centralized Nervous Systems 352
           1.   The Systems 352
           2.   Central Nervous Systems (CNS) 352
           3.   Peripheral Nerve Systems 352
      D.   Neurons 352
      E.   Nerves 354
           1.   Nature of Nerves 354
           2.   Giant Fibers 355
           3.   Impulses and Their Transmission 355
           4.   Synapses 355
           5.   Interneurons 356
      F.   Ganglion and Brain 356
           1.   Ganglia 356
           2.   Vertebrate Brain 357
      G.   Nerve Cords 358
      H.   Circum-Enteric Rings 359

IV.   Chemical Control 359
      A.   Introduction 359
      B.   Chemical Messengers 360
      C.   Endocrinology 362
           1.   Vertebrates vs. Invertebrates 362

2.   Endocrine Glands..362
3.   Hormones 363
       a.   Classification of Hormones 363
       b.   Hormone Functions..364
4.   Effectors...365
D.   Neurosecretions 365
E.   The Message Systems by Phylum 366

References 368

I. INTRODUCTION

A few years ago it seemed to many biologists that there were three systems for controlling organ functions. These were distinguished as sensory, nervous, and endocrine mechanisms. With the discovery of the hormone features of nerve transmission and stimulation, it is today much harder than it was to separate out a nervous system, a receptor system, and an endocrine system. This has led to efforts to combine the three under one system heading. In some books these are gathered under the word control, but this does not seem to stand well among the conventional systems. The term regulatory system has been used, but this is certainly too broad, as it would seem to include many non-nervous mechanisms of regulation of chemical processes as well as water balance, heat, and so forth.

At the present time the endocrine and nerve systems can no longer be separated. Because receptors are always functional partners of the nervous system, it does seem to be reasonable to include them with the nerve system, and we can then speak of the three systems combined as the nervous and endocrine system. (The combination neuroendocrine is not quite appropriate for this combined system because it was invented for and is still widely used for the endocrine functions of the nerves alone — the actual secretion of messenger chemicals by the neurons.)

This combined field of sensory, nervous, and endocrine activity is a very large one. Much is now known and new information is being produced at a rapid rate. Unfortunately, the amount of comparative data between major groups of animals is still small. As a result the amount of diversity shown in this chapter is relatively small, even though differences in detail, especially among nerves, are numerous.

The nervous system in the restricted sense includes all the neurons, the nerves, the nerve connections with the sense organs, and the connections with effector organs such as muscles. It frequently includes several large independent sets of nerves, as well as cords running the length of the body, and in all but the simplest animals includes ganglia, which are masses of nerve cell bodies. This chapter will deal in sequence with the receptors, the nerve systems (in the restricted sense), and the endocrine system (as a mixed effector and transmission system).

II. DETECTION OF STIMULI

A. Senses

The stimulation of the nervous system and the structures that accomplish that stimulation are referred to in several ways. One speaks of *the senses* of sight, hearing, taste, touch, etc. The senses of animals are their abilities to detect influences from the environment (either external or internal).

The senses are sometimes listed as touch, taste, smell, hearing, and vision, to which should be added equilibration. These are the special senses, for which special receptor organs are provided in many animals, sometimes called the primary senses. To these must be added the so-called skin senses: heat, cold, and pain detection, usually sensed by unicellular organs. Internal senses have been termed general senses, because they are apparently not received by special organs but by tissues in general. These general senses include hunger, thirst, internal pain, pressure, and distension, for which no comparative information is available.

The stimuli that produce the senses are of two sorts, probably not really different. The special senses are activated by influences from the environment which produce energy changes upon the receptors. This energy is light, heat, sound, chemicals, etc. The general senses may operate in theoretically similar manner, but energy change is not apparent and receptors have not been discovered.

The special senses thus operate in response to these changes, called *stimuli* (such as chemical, mechanical, thermal, etc.). The *organs of reception* for detection of the stimuli are classed as mechanoreceptors, proprioceptors, chemoreceptors, etc., depending on the nature of the stimulus. It is usually assumed that each receptor responds to just one type of stimulation, giving the animal a sense of that particular sort, but some organs (possibly compound ones) react to several stimuli. For example, the crustacean nauplius eye has been reported to show responses to light, pressure, temperature, pH, X-rays, and ultraviolet light.

In various animals a variety of unusual stimuli may sometimes be received as senses. Examples are unusual parts of the electromagnetic spectrum, such as ultraviolet and infrared light, and atmospheric pressure, humidity, etc. It is not usually possible to identify organs designed for reception of these.

Protoplasm can be sensitive to many stimuli, whether or not it is formed into a receptor and whether or not it can formally pass on awareness of the stimulus to neighboring protoplasm. The stimuli that can be detected include at least the following (with indication of general receptor class, if used):

1. Light — and therefore the absence of light as well as patterns of light and dark (photoreceptors)
2. Heat — above body temperature (thermoreceptors)
3. Cold — below body temperature (thermoreceptors)
4. Touch — (tangoreceptors)
5. Sound — (phonoreceptors)
6. Gravity — equilibrium (statoreceptors)
7. Smell — airborne chemicals (chemoreceptors)
8. Taste — water-borne or solid chemicals (chemoreceptors)
9. Pain, external — (pain receptor)
10. Hunger
11. Thirst
12. Deformation and stress — distension, stretch, pressure (proprioceptors among the mechanoceptors)
13. Position — (proprioceptors)
14. Flow direction — (rheoreceptors)
15. Pain, internal
16. Atmospheric pressure — (baroceptors)
17. Radiation other than visual light — ultraviolet, infrared
18. Salinity — (among chemoreceptors)
19. pH — (among chemoreceptors)
20. Electric fields or current — (electroreceptors)

21.   Humidity
22.   Carbon dioxide

For many of these stimuli there is also no corresponding "sense" term. Even the -reception terms, such as chemoreception, remain rather general and do not serve in comparing between groups. This section is therefore arranged by the nature of the stimulus, as shown by the receptors.

B. Sense Receptors
1. Reception of Stimuli

There are many simple sense receptors in animals, receiving a variety of stimuli. These may be complex multicellular organs or single cells. These frequently have parts that respond to different stimuli, and they are often grouped with other types of receptors in complexes that have received special names. For example, the antennae of insects are spoken of loosely as tactile organs, but they often possess a variety of other receptors such as smell. Again, one speaks of the lateral line system in fishes, yet this complex contains receptors of several types. Both levels are dealt with here, but the basic arrangement will be by the individual stimulus receptor.

According to Prosser (1973): "The basic function of sense organs is to transduce physical stimuli into nerve impulses. Sense organs may be stimulated in three basic ways: chemical, mechanical, or by electric current. Gustatory and olfactory receptors are sensitive to specific chemicals, photoreceptors are stimulated by products of a photochemical reaction, and temperature receptors respond to modulation of chemically controlled spontaneity. Static mechanoreceptors are stimulated by maintained deformation of a membrane, as in some muscle tension receptors and in blood-pressure sensors; dynamic mechanoreceptors are stimulated during the process of deformation, at low frequency as in some tactile endings, or at high frequency as in sound reception. Mechanoreceptors are important for signalling posture, position of appendages, orientation with respect to gravity and acceleration, vibrations of low and high frequency, contact with surfaces, velocity of water and wind, and depth of water. Proprioceptors give information about the relative positions of parts of an animal, and exteroceptors give information about stimuli outside the body. A few kinds of fish have electroreceptors."

It is possible to list sense organs by phylum of animals and show that there is steady increase of complexity. For example, Protozoa and Porifera have none; Platyhelminthes have several types of unicellular receptors as well as light, chemical, and balance organs; Arthropoda have compound eyes that may be very complex and may be highly efficient in certain types of perception; and vertebrates may have the familiar complex retinal eye that can produce a clear image. A closer look will show that some Mollusca have almost no sense organs, whereas others (Cephalopoda) have eyes comparable to those of vertebrates. Echinodermata have almost no multicellular sense organs, and Cephalochordata have virtually no sense organs except for free nerve endings in the skin. Some aquatic animals have excellent eyes, some little more than a light-sensitive skin. Most flying animals do have well-developed senses, as do most active swimmers. It is hard to see much phylogenetic significance to this, as no predator can exist without good detection organs.

If there are surprises among the sense organs of animals, they are few. It is, of course, astonishing to find such very well-developed eyes in Cephalopoda. Although special receptors may not be known, some animals are sensitive to stimuli that seem unusual to us: carbon dioxide in some Insecta, water flow direction in fishes, pH in larvae of Crustacea, X-rays, ultraviolet or infrared light in several groups, temperature change in Insecta, and electricity in some fishes.

Although one is aware of a variety of receptors, and thus senses, in mammals such as humans, and some of these receptors are numerous (e.g., heat and cold receptors in human skin), studies on other animals (particularly Arthropoda) seem to show both a greater variety of sensors and even a larger number (at least per given area). Certainly the diversity of organs to sense a particular type of stimulus is greater in some phyla of invertebrates than it is among the vertebrates.

Many types of sense organs and many specific organs will be listed in later paragraphs, but it should be pointed out that many of these receiving organs are referred to under descriptive terms (such as end organ or sensory cell, and there are some similar terms that do not refer to receptors at all, as eye-spots may be merely circular parts of the color pattern:

1. End organ — general term for the functional termination of a sensory nerve
2. Neurosensory cells — same as sensory nerve cells
3. Non-nervous receptor cells — those exceptional cells in Vertebrata that conduct the stimulus to an axon in the cases of receptors in the acoustico-lateralis system and of the taste buds
4. Sensilla (pl. -ae) — small sense organ, especially a simple epithelial sense organ; usually being a cluster of sensory cells with other types of cells such as pigment or gland cells
5. Sensillum (pl. -a) — one of a variety of receptor complexes in an insect cuticle, consisting of one or many cells
6. Sensory cells — any unicellular receptor; thus cells capable of converting a stimulus into a nerve impulse
7. Sensory nerve cells — nerve cells that send processes to the surface for direct reception of stimuli
8. Sensory nerve endings — the receiving end of the sensory nerve cells; end organ

2. Photoreception

a. Detection of Light

Light is that part of the electromagnetic spectrum that is perceived by animal eyes. It is usually taken to be radiation visible to humans, having wavelengths from 300 to 800 nm. Other parts of the spectrum, such as ultraviolet, may be detectable by some organisms, but wavelengths above 1000 nm do not usually produce any change in the receiving molecules and therefore are not "detected". Radiation of wavelengths much below 300 nm may destroy molecules by breaking covalent bonds. (When expressed in Angstrom units, light is radiation of wavelength from 10^3 to 10^4 Å.)

Response to light (detection of it), in a cellular sense, is the ability of the molecules to absorb the radiant energy that strikes them, which results in changing their own energy levels. The word response, however, is more often used in referring to the reaction of the animal (or part of it) to this received energy. The cellular response is part of the function of the nervous system as a whole. The response of the animal is usually by activity of non-nervous organs.

This reaction of the animal is closely associated with reception and transmission of the stimulus, sometimes being described as a stimulus-response system. In our arrangement of animal functions, most gross response is ascribed to such other systems or organs as muscle and glands.

It is sometimes said that all living organisms have an inherent capacity to receive and respond to light stimulus. Whatever truth there may be to this at the molecular level, there are many animals that show no active reaction to light. These include most internal parasites and the embryos of most animals.

Detection of light by individual animals is normally by special receptor organs, but it may also be by certain cells that are not considered to be such formal receptors. The organs are called *photoreceptors*; they give the animal the sense of vision.

The photoreceptors of many animals are without distinctive names. Although we refer to eye-spots in Protozoa and to compound eyes in Insecta, the light receptors of Mollusca are often simply called eyes, although they are diverse. It is thus not easy to list the photoreceptors of the animal kingdom by type. At least the following terms occur, although there is overlap and synonymy:

1. Eyes, complex
    a. Compound (Arthropoda; the actual receptors are the individual ommatidia)
    b. Double retinal (Bivalvia)
    c. Retinal (Cephalopoda, Vertebrata)
2. Eyes, simple
    a. Stemmata (larval eyes of some holometabolous Insecta)
3. Eye-spots (Annelida)
    a. Eye-spot-flagellum system (Protozoa)
    b. Eye-spots without lenses (Protozoa)
    c. Pigment-spot ocelli (Tunicata)
    d. Stigma (Protozoa)
4. Ocelli (with lenses) (Arthropoda)
    a. Pigment-cup ocelli (Coelenterata, Rhynchocoela, Bivalvia, Sipunculoidea, Chaetognatha, Tunicata)
5. Neurons — some may receive light directly (no examples cited)
6. Skin — dermal light sense (most groups)
    a. Specialized epithelial cells (s.Polychaeta, Hirudinea)
7. Ultraviolet receptors (Turbellaria)

b. Visual Pigments

Photoreceptors are stimulated by the products of a photochemical reaction. This reaction is the result of capture by certain molecules of appropriate energy in the incident light. The reaction is usually by molecules of a chemical called a visual pigment. The receptor is basically a structure that provides an increased area for deposition of this photopigment. A variety of terms are used for the pigments in various animals, but they are apparently all varieties of rhodopsin, a protein conjugated with carotenoid pigments. In the vertebrates there may be different pigments in the rods and cones. For example:

1. Cyanopsin — one of the cone pigments
2. Iodopsin — one of the cone pigments
3. Porphyropsin — the visual pigment in some rods of fishes
4. Retinal — the pigment part of rhodopsin

3. Chemoreception

There are at least five senses that are associated with *chemoreceptors*: taste, smell, and the detection of carbon dioxide, pH, and salinity, but these five are not always clearly distinguished.

Some insects have carbon dioxide receptors on the antennae. The pH of the medium can apparently be detected by some aquatic animals, but special receptor organs seem to be known only in the so-called nauplius eye of *Daphnia* (Crustacea). Salinity is probably included in the chemical aspects detected by a wide variety of sensory neuron receptors.

Chemoreception thus deals with water- and airborne chemicals and the corresponding receptors.

a. Detection of Water-Borne Chemicals

The detection of substances in solution is the function of the organs of taste, but the latter word is apparently used principally in mammals. Chemoreceptors are cited in many animals, but they are not well distinguished or classified.

The ability to detect and respond to dissolved chemicals is reported in Protozoa, Coelenterata, Turbellaria, Rotifera, larval Trematoda, Nematoda, Gordioidea, Bryozoa, Sipunculoidea, Mollusca, Annelida, Arthropoda, Echinodermata, and Vertebrata (at least).

b. Gustatory Organs

Usually thought of as organs of taste, there are identified in a few groups:

1. Hancock's organ, in part (Gastropoda)
2. Osphradium (s.Mollusca)
3. Pre-oral ciliary organ (Enteropneusta)
4. Taste buds (Vertebrata)

In free-living species of Nematoda, there are amphids and phasmids that are believed to be chemoreceptors, although the evidence is meager.

Chemoreceptors are common in insects but most of them detect airborne chemicals.

In Crustacea there are taste endings on mouthparts, antennules, and claws.

These receptors are sometimes called "contact chemical receptors" (see also next section).

c. Detection of Airborne Chemicals

The organs of smell are even less well classified than those of taste. There is really no distinction between the two because airborne chemicals are probably all dissolved in surface moisture before being detected.

Some air-breathing mollusks such as slugs have tentacle-like extensions of the epidermis, called rhinophores, which seem to have an olfactory function.

Some males of Lepidoptera (Insecta) have scent tufts called corema on the abdomen. Other insects have olfactory pits on the palpi or the antennae, where there may be many thousands on each antenna.

Olfactory receptors in Vertebrata are usually neurons themselves connected to microvilli or cilia.

Olfactory organs, usually thought of as organs of smell, are identified in some groups:

1. Ampullacea (Insecta)
2. Basiconica (Insecta)
3. Coremata (sing. corema), scent tufts (Insecta)
4. Hancock's organ, in part (Gastropoda)
5. Hypopharyngeal compound sense organ, in part (Insecta)
6. Placodea (Insecta)
7. Pore plates (Insecta)
8. Rhinophore (s.Mollusca)
9. Sensilla basiconica (Insecta)
10. Sensilla chaetica (Insecta)
11. Sensory pits (Arachnida)

All these are sometimes called "distance chemical receptors", but they would not be distinct from the contact chemical receptors if the chemicals are received on moist surfaces and thus are in solution when detected.

4. Mechanoreception

There is a large group of diverse structures that report on the mechanical relations between parts of the animal and between it and the environment. These are sometimes called the organs of *kinaesthesis*. The senses are equilibrium, proprioception, movement, pressure, vibration (including hearing), stretch, and touch, but for most of them there are no specific -receptor terms. They are cited below under the various stimuli.

Other *mechanoreceptor* types include: (1) movement receptors, including rheoreceptors, the cristae of Cephalopoda that detect acceleration, the labyrinths of Vertebrata, and some detectors in the lateral line system of Pisces; (2) pressure receptors, such as some sensilla in Insecta and the Vater's corpuscle that is said to be a receptor of pressure in some Vertebrata; and (3) nociceptors, detecting distension of organs.

a. Detection of Sound and Other Vibrations

Phonoreceptors or auditory organs are defined as sense organs for detecting vibrations of the surrounding medium. Many animals, perhaps most, react to vibrations, but receptor organs are usually not identified. Only in insects and vertebrates are vibration/sound organs clearly described.

Various tympanic membranes detect vibrations in air in both insects and vertebrates; rarely in the former, appendages such as antennae and cerci (caudal appendages) are said to be sensitive to sound (vibration).

The following organs and descriptive terms have been used:

1. Cerci (Insecta)
2. Chordotonal organ (Insecta)
3. Ears — including tympanum, cochlea, organ of Corti (Vertebrata)
4. Hair sensillum (Insecta, Arachnida)
5. Johnstonian organ (Insecta)
6. Muller's organ (Insecta)
7. Scolophore (Insecta)
8. Scolopophorous organ (Insecta)
9. Siebold's organ (Insecta)
10. Slit sensillum (Arachnida)
11. Subgenual organ (Insecta)
12. Tympanal organs (Insecta)

b. Detection of Tactile Stimuli

Tangoreceptors presumably occur in many animals but they are directly described in Arthropoda and Vertebrata. They are part of the diverse class called mechanoreceptors, which also includes auditory organs and the diverse proprioceptors. The *tangoreceptors* are those responding to contact stimuli, and in the vertebrates they are scarcely more than nerve endings or simple corpuscles, such as Meissner's corpuscles in humans. In Cephalochordata these are represented by tactile sensory cells, which may also occur in other soft-bodied animals.

In informal usage, many movable extensions of the body surface are referred to as tactile organs, including cilia, tentacles, bristles, setae, antennae, palps, and such. These presumably are associated with receptors that detect the movement or deformation of the structure. Tactile bristles occur in Platyhelminthes, Nematoda, Arthropoda, and Chaetognatha (at least).

It is said that the frontal organ of some Turbellaria has both chemo- and tangoreceptor functions.

It seems that little attention has been given to the organs of touch — their structure is seldom discussed. Many of these may be hidden in the frequent references to sense cells and nerve endings, where no reference is made to the nature of the sense involved.

Tangoreceptors (tactile) include the following:

1. Antennae (Crustacea, Myriapoda, Insecta)
2. Antennules (Crustacea)
3. Hancock's organs, in part (Gastropoda)
4. Meissner's corpuscle (Mammalia)
5. Pacinian corpuscles (Mammalia)
6. Palps or palpi (Mollusca, Arthropoda, etc.)
7. Sensory hairs (Crustacea)
8. Touch receptors (Chaetognatha, vertebrate skin)

c. Detection of Gravity

The sense of orientation to gravity is produced by a variety of organs. These are variously referred to as static organs, *gravireceptors,* balance organs, and statoreceptors. They are part of the large and diverse class of receptors called proprioceptors. These detect position of the body with respect to the substrate or position of parts with respect to the rest of the body.

The following terms have been used for the organs that detect gravity (balance organs):

1. Bubble "statocysts" (Insecta)
2. Cordyli — same as Lithostyles
3. Halteres — modified wings of dipterans (Insecta)
4. Johnston's organs — at base of antennae (Insecta)
5. Labyrinths — of inner ear (Vertebrata)
6. Lithocysts (see Statocysts)
7. Lithostyles (Scyphozoa)
8. Otocysts (see Statocysts)
9. Rhopalia (Scyphozoa)
10. Semicircular canals — part of Labyrinths
11. Sense clubs — same as Lithostyles
12. Sphaeridia — probably not a static organ (Echinoidea)
13. Statocyst canals — (statocysts in s.Crustacea)
14. Statocysts (Coelenterata, Ctenophora, Turbellaria, Rhynchocoela, Rotifera, Brachiopoda, Mollusca, Annelida, m.Crustacea, s.Insecta, Holothurioidea, Tunicata)
15. Tentaculocysts — same as Lithostyles

In Ctenophora the statocyst at the aboral pole is a vesicle of modified cilia in the epidermis. From four points in the floor of the cavity extend upward four very long S-curved tufts of cilia, which support a rounded ball of calcareous spherules (the statolith).

In certain Tunicata the statocyst is an ectodermal vesicle containing two sense cells and one cell acting as a statolith.

Many of the so-called static organs in swimming animals are used to detect acceleration, turning, etc. as well as gravity. (See "Lateral Line System" in Chapter 19.) In some Crustacea the term semicircular canals has been applied to the elongated statocysts, but they are not really semicircular and do not operate like those in vertebrates.

d. Proprioception

Many animals can detect deformation and stress of the body. These may be due to any of the following: the pull of gravity (already dealt with), the change in position of parts or appendages, internal muscle movements, movements due to outside mechanical forces such as wind, currents, and movement of substrate, or to internal muscle movements.

A possible proprioceptor has been described in minute detail in an epitheliomuscular cell of a sea anemone. It appears to be adapted to monitoring changes in stretch in the muscle cell. If this is indeed a proprioceptor, counterparts can be expected in other soft-bodied animals that produce muscle movements. Such structures have been expected in annelids, but they have not been identified.

It is in the arthropods that proprioception reaches its peak, because of the jointed exoskeleton and appendages. In many of the body and appendage joints there are organs that signal changes of position. These include various types of sensillae (including some campaniform and slit sensillae) as well as chordotonal organs, Johnston's organs, etc. Some are termed stretch receptors. Many of them monitor position, movement, and pressure.

Hair plates are common in the joints of appendages. Some chordotonal organs in Crustacea are termed myochordotonal organs. CAP (cuticular articulated pegs) organs occur in the joints of some Crustacea. Many of the proprioceptive organs consist in part of ciliary structures, sometimes highly modified.

Special terms have been applied to some supposed proprioceptors, especially among Arthropoda:

1. Apodeme tension receptors (Arthropoda)
2. Campaniform sensilla (Insecta)
3. CAP organs (Crustacea)
4. Chordotonal organs (Insecta)
5. Hair plates (Insecta)
6. Hair sensilla (Insecta)
7. Lyriform organs (Arachnida)
8. Macula (Cephalopoda)
9. Muscle receptor organs (Crustacea)
10. Myochordotonal organs (Crustacea)
11. Sensory cones (Crustacea)
12. Slit sensilla (Crustacea)
13. Stiff cilia (Ciliata)
14. Substellar organs (s.Mollusca)
15. Tuft sensilla (Crustacea)

Such receptors are also common in vertebrates, where they are merely called proprioceptors or referred to descriptively as spindles in the muscles and tendons.

e. Miscellaneous Stimuli

The stimulus detectors described above include most of the obvious receptor organs, at least those organs that are well known and of determined function. In the books that deal with such matters in the different phyla, there are many references to "sense organs" with little or no clue as to their reception capabilities — the nature of the stimulus monitored. Many of them are unicellular.

A few familiar senses are nowhere discussed in relation to any animals except humans. These include senses of pain, hunger, thirst, and the thermoreceptors for heat, cold, and temperature change. Apparently the sensors are unicellular and widely distributed, at least in humans.

Some of the unusual senses follow. On the antennae of such insects as honeybees there are organs sensitive to carbon dioxide. *Rheoreceptors* detect the flow of water past the body in Turbellaria and Pisces. The so-called nauplius eye in Crustacea may respond to ultraviolet light, X-rays, pH, temperature, and pressure. Bees and some Crustacea can detect the polarization of light. Mormyomast cells in the lateral line of fishes may be *electroreceptors.* Humidity is reported to be detected by the *sensilla basiconica* in some Insecta.

III. THE NERVE SYSTEMS

A. Conducting Devices

The system of nerves is the interconnected plexus of neurons by means of which impulses are transmitted from one part of the body to another. Most nerve systems consist of separate neurons and their processes called axons and dendrites, nerve cords consisting of many neurons or their processes, and ganglia consisting of many nerve cell bodies. Critical to operation of these systems are two activities: conduction of impulses along the neuron and excitation of neighboring neurons or other cells across a contact zone called a synapse.

Nerve systems consist either of comparatively simple nerve nets or of systems with centralization in ganglia and brains. The former occur in Coelenterata, Ctenophora, and Enteropneusta, and are present with ganglia in some Mollusca, Echinodermata, and Tunicata. The latter (centralization) occurs in all other animals but varies greatly in its complexity. Thus, the two major types of nerve systems are here called nerve nets and centralized nervous systems.

It was formerly believed that the Protozoa are devoid of conductile organelles that could account for responses to stimuli, and yet coordinated response had been seen for centuries. It was later believed that a neuromotor system existed, at least in ciliates, consisting of interciliary fibrils that connected the basal bodies of the cilia. These were demonstrated by silver staining, but it is now known that they are merely artifacts of the pellicular sculpture.

Porifera are generally believed to have neither sensory nor nerve cells, and yet there are slow reactions to certain stimuli. The lack of reactions by the body as a whole is not mirrored at the cellular level, where reactions similar to those of Protozoa take place. Thus, cells capture food, pores contract and expand, and amoebocytes move through the mesogloea apparently to predetermined targets.

B. Nerve Nets

A nerve net is a system of interconnected nerve cells and fibers without true ganglia. Such a system of neurons may be widely dispersed in the animal, permitting diffuse conduction of impulses. There may be either protoplasmic continuity or synapses between the neurons.

Although nerve nets seem to be a simpler level of organization than a central nervous system (CNS), they show most of the features of nerve action that are found in the centralized systems. These may include synapses (either polarized or not); facilitation, with repeated or combined stimuli required; a wide variety of stimuli detectable; interaction between conducting systems; and true nervous spontaneity in the absence of any known stimulus.

Such nerve nets are always cited in Coelenterata and Ctenophora, but in the latter the evidence is still incomplete. Localized nets also occur in higher animals, where they are often called plexuses. Such nets are reported but also said to be unlikely in Platyhelminthes and Rhynchocoela. Calyssozoa show some evidence of such nets, and Phoronida probably have one. In Mollusca and Echinodermata there are suggestions of limited nets but certainly no general ones. In some hemichordates there is an epidermal nerve net. Plexuses also occur in Tunicata, Cephalochordata, and even Vertebrata. In all of these after the Ctenophora there is also a dominant CNS.

C. Centralized Nervous Systems

1. The Systems

A centralized nervous system is one that includes ganglia and often a brain. Although both of these terms are found in the descriptions of both invertebrates and vertebrates, there are important differences. Although the differences may not represent fundamental changes in evolution, but merely much greater complexity in one, still it is necessary to discuss them separately in certain respects.

Connection from the central system to all parts of the body are by the peripheral system. The latter is principally concerned with transmitting them to the central system and transmitting back impulses to appropriate effectors.

2. Central Nervous Systems (CNS)

All animals with centralized nervous systems have some sort of brain or central concentration of neurons, and they must then also have a peripheral system of some sort to receive stimuli and pass signals to and from the brain. There are ganglia in both systems consisting of masses of neurons. In general, the ganglia of central systems have interneurons, but the ganglia of peripheral systems do not.

In nearly all animals with centralization of nervous control, the brain is located anteriorly in the body and there are one or more nerve cords passing back through the body. In vertebrates this is a single dorsal cord called the spinal cord.

In invertebrates there are always at least two cords, and these are generally ventral or lateral. The nervous tissues may form isolated ganglia, peripheral plexuses, nerve nets, epithelial, stomodaeal, stomatogastric, or enteric systems, etc. In addition to these, there is diversity in such things as neurons, giant fibers, nerve cords, circumenteric nerve rings, cephalization, euthyneury or symmetry of the nervous system, and unusual aggregations of nervous tissue such as stellate ganglia.

A central nervous system, with brain and spinal cord or with a ganglion and one or more nerve cords is found (respectively) in Cephalochordata and Vertebrata and in invertebrates from Platyhelminthes on, but apparently not in Pogonophora, Echinodermata, Enteropneusta, Pterobranchia, and Tunicata.

The brain and the nerve cord are discussed in a later section.

3. Peripheral Nerve Systems

The so-called peripheral system is not a single integrated complex but a series of nerve connections between the sense receptors, the CNS, and the effectors. Each of these thus consists of two parts, transmitting stimuli to a CNS cell and the other transmitting signals from that cell or ones connected to it to an effector. This double structure is duplicated all over the body, so that the "system" actually consists of many of these units performing two separate functions.

All animals with a CNS must possess a peripheral system of some sort, consisting at least of the sensory cells and the motor cells (with their dendrites and axons), but elaborate peripheral systems occur in Mollusca, Annelida, Tunicata (possibly), and the Vertebrata, but apparently not in the Cephalochordata.

In the Vertebrata, parts of the peripheral system have names: the autonomic system to the viscera, which consists of two divisions, the sympathetic, and the parasympathetic.

D. Neurons

It is said that irritability is a universal characteristic of protoplasm. By this it is meant that there is some sort of reaction to certain stimuli. Three activities are required to produce this reaction: reception of the stimulus, conduction of the resulting signal, and appropriate response. The reactivity of the protoplasm of the cells of the nervous system produce activities at the level of the individual or its organs. For this, the most important function is transmission of the signals.

The *nerve cell* has three components: the *dendrite(s)* conducting from the receptor, the *cell body* containing the nucleus, and the *axon(s)* conducting toward effectors. The dendrites conduct signals to the cell body, and the axons conduct signals away from the cell body. All animals react to some stimuli, and transmission of signals has been demonstrated in most.

The specialized cell that performs this transmission is called a *neuron*: a nerve cell with its processes, designed for conduction of nervous impulses and often for neurosecretion.

At this point we must recognize a confusing use of the term nerve, probably a holdover from days when the differences between "nerve", "nerve fiber", and "nerve cell" were not clear. In the most general sense, a nerve is the cellular pathway along which signals can travel from one part of the body to another. The impulse transmission is actually along a nerve process (or a series of them), including dendrites and axons. These two types of processes may occur singly or in bundles in a sheath, in either case being called nerve fibers. A nerve cell is the entire structure including the processes and the soma (nerve body); this is a neuron, which is the term for the functioning cell and all its parts.

The five criteria of neurons in higher animals have been listed as:

1. Having a myelin sheath
2. Containing the Nissl substance
3. Having specialized synapses
4. Having microtubules (neurotubules)
5. Containing neurosecretory granules

Special terms for neurons and their parts and their bundles include these:

1. Axon — a process of a neuron for conduction of impulses over considerable distances; commonly described as conducting away from the nerve cell body in all-or-none fashion, but in invertebrates neither of these stipulations is universal
2. Cell body — that part of the neuron containing the nucleus; also called perikaryon or soma
3. Dendrite — a process specialized for receiving impulses and usually conducting to a cell body
4. Glia (see Neuroglia)
5. Myelin sheath — the covering of the axon
6. Nerve fiber — any neuron process
7. Neurite (see Axon)
8. Neuroglia — covering of non-nervous cells around the axon or axon bundle
9. Neuron — a nerve cell, together with all its processes
   a. Association neuron (see Interneuron)
   b. Bipolar neuron — one having two main processes, one dendritic and one axonic
   c. Internuncial neuron (see Interneuron)
   d. Interneuron — one that connects neurons
   e. Isopolar — having the processes indistinguishable
   f. Heteropolar neuron — one with processes unlike, usually one axon and one dendrite
   g. Motor neuron — one that sends an axon to an effector
   h. Multipolar neuron — one having more than two processes

    i. Sensory neuron — one that sends a dendrite to a sense receptor, and receives signals from that sensor

    j. Unipolar neuron — having only one process, an axon

10.   Node of Ranvier — interruption in the myelination of axons

11.   Perikaryon (see Cell body)

12.   Schwann cell — a cell forming the intimate sheath of one or more peripheral axons

13.   Soma (see Cell body)

Coelenterata are considered to be the simplest animals that possess a true nervous system. It is essentially a net of connected neurons in the epidermis. These primitive neurons, however, lack the first two criteria listed above (myelin sheath and Nissl substance). Instead of synapses, there may be protoplasmic continuity between the neurons. In some colonial Hydrozoa there is a considerable coordination of activity, but there are no nerve fibers between the individuals of the colony.

In Ctenophora a network that is subepidermal but otherwise like that of coelenterates, has been both reported and questioned. It is said that there may be some ganglion cells.

The Platyhelminthes show a variety of sensory neurons. Rhynchocoela and Aschelminthes seem to show no unusual features among their neurons. In Nematoda a few interneurons appear, but of somewhat simple structure.

All groups above those with a coelenteron possess neurons, ganglia often called brains, and nerve cords. It is customary to exempt from this generalization the Vertebrata, because of the vastly more specialized brain; yet there does not seem to be any sharp distinction between the two, except for the single spinal cord.

E. Nerves
1. Nature of Nerves

Neurons are the cells with their processes, axons and dendrites. These processes are usually bound in a myelin sheath and are grouped into bundles called nerves. *Nerves,* then, are (usually myelinated) bundles of neuron fibers. When a nerve (bundle of fibers) enters the CNS, it loses its sheath, each of the neurons forms a synapse with another neuron that traverses part of the CNS, and with others of its bundle now forms a so-called nerve tract which extends between parts of the CNS.

Although neurons are found in Coelenterata and all higher groups, from the Mollusca onward there seem to be no abrupt developments in the evolution of nerves. Wilson (1972) states that "Identifiable nerves (bundles of fibers) are first found in annelids and sipunculids". It must be noted that he deals with Mollusca in a later chapter than the worms, which explains why he thinks the worms were the first to have clear nerves. Other writers place the Mollusca lower in the scale than the annulates, so they would cite the Mollusca as the place where clear nerves arose.

In the sipunculids and higher groups, "ganglion cells are not indiscriminately scattered along nerves as in lower forms" and the nerves in the lower forms are thus not "in the form familiar in higher animals" (Bullock and Horridge, 1965).

Special terms for the nerve bundle and its parts include:

1.   Commissure — a transverse tract of neuron fibers between two parts of the CNS

2.   Connective — a longitudinal tract of neuron fibers between successive ganglia

3.   Neuropile — an area in the CNS consisting of a tangle of fine fibers of axons and dendrites, with no cell bodies

4.   Tract — a bundle of nerve fibers between parts of the CNS

2. Giant Fibers

A giant fiber is a very large, fast-conducting interneuron or motor nerve fiber consisting of one or more axons. This axon may be from a single giant neuron, or it may have been formed by fusion of many cell processes of ordinary unipolar cells. They range from simple conducting fibers to chains with synapses. They function in startle, escape, and grasping reactions, with conduction as much as 1600 times as fast as smaller fibers in the same animal. They are efficient also because one impulse activates muscles of an extensive body area. These so-called giant fibers are apparently of three types: (1) a large axon of a moderately large cell, (2) a moderately large axon from a huge cell; or (3) a large axon resulting from the fusion of axons from many ordinary cells.

Giant fibers are cited in several groups (where known, the types are shown by number): Cestoda (3), Rhynchocoela (2), Phoronida (1,3), Mollusca (Gastropoda, Cephalopoda) (1), Echiuroidea (possibly), Annelida (Polychaeta and Oligochaeta only) (1,3), Onychophora (3 possibly), Arthropoda (Crustacea, Scorpionida, Insecta) (1,2), Pogonophora (possibly), Echinodermata (possibly in Ophiuroidea), Enteropneusta (1), and Vertebrata.

3. Impulses and Their Transmission

All neurons thus far examined are capable of being excited to produce a membrane change called a nerve impulse or action potential. This impulse is conducted along the neuron. Thus, conduction or propagation is the passage of an impulse along the neuron membrane. (The word transmission is reserved for transfer of the impulse from one cell to another.) The impulses are all-or-none and can be repeated from dozens to hundreds of times per second.

These statements are based on properly examined neurons in members of only four phyla: Mollusca, Annelida, Arthropoda, and Vertebrata. There are said to be reasons to believe that other neurons, some of which have only short processes, may not all produce impulses. As information is lacking about the distribution of impulse features among the phyla, it is not useful to deal further with this subject.

As to transmission, there are two methods by which neurons can interact physiologically. These are by protoplasmic bridges and by synapses. Any diversity among the bridges is not available, but they are reported in Coelenterata, Gastropoda, Oligochaeta, Hirudinea, Crustacea, and Pisces (at least).

4. Synapses

The distance between a receptor organ and the appropriate effector organ may be small or large in relation to the body size of the animal. A single neuron may bridge this entire gap, but often the impulse passes from one neuron to another. The nearly universal method of impulse transmission from one neuron to another is by means of a synapse, a functional connection between distinct neurons which have contact or near contact of their membranes.

The fine structure of synapses differ widely as to location (terminal or not), number of contact points (one to three or more), size of the contact area, etc. The junctions may be polarized or not (the transmission is one-way or reversible). The diversity of the mechanisms of synapses is summarized by Bullock and Horridge (1965) thus: "Transmission in different situations and animals is not always accomplished by one and the same mechanism, nor are a large number of different mechanisms employed. Rather it appears likely that there have been developed several closely related and several quite different means of transmitting excitation from one neuron to another or to an effector." At least six biochemicals, as reported by Prosser (1973), illustrate the closely related mechanisms. The quite different mechanisms are the bridges and the synapses.

Synapses do apparently occur in all groups where there are neurons. Differences among synapses are not clearly correlated with the groups of animals, although much diversity does occur.

5. Interneurons

In the reflex arc from receptor to effector via the CNS, there will be sensory neurons conducting impulses inward and motor neurons conducting outward. Inside the CNS these two will be effectively connected by one or a series of interneurons or internuncial neurons. In addition to completing the pathway of the reflex arc and signalling this to other parts of the CNS, interneurons serve other functions such as amplification of incoming signals, inhibition of impulses to motor neurons, and facilitation by overcoming some continuous inhibition.

The distribution of interneurons among animals is seldom mentioned. It may be presumed that they occur wherever ganglia or a CNS occur. The diversities that are to be expected among groups are barely hinted at.

F. Ganglion and Brain
1. Ganglia

One of the places in which different usages in vertebrates and invertebrates give potential for misunderstanding is in the matter of ganglia and brains. Both words are used in both groups, giving the appearance of uniformity.

The ganglia of invertebrates, both peripheral and in the CNS, and the peripheral ganglia of vertebrates, seem to be of one sort. The so-called "ganglia" within the brain of vertebrates are treated as if of a different nature, although clear distinguishing features are not cited. The brain of invertebrates is composed of ganglia, more or less united in the anterior part of the body. The brain of vertebrates is implied to be of a different nature. It is thus appropriate to deal with just two subjects: ganglia (and invertebrate brains formed from them) and the brains of vertebrates.

Ganglia are discrete masses of nerve cells bounded by connective tissue. Both fibers and cell bodies are present. This is the definition generally used for invertebrates. Books on vertebrates often use the term ganglia in referring to cell masses in the brain. It seems to be believed that these are not the same as ganglia in invertebrates or peripheral ganglia of vertebrates, although no clear-cut distinctions have been found.

Omitting the vertebrates for the moment, ganglia thus form at least part of the CNS in all invertebrate phyla that have one. Ganglia are one of the features of a CNS, but because the latter term is indefinite in application, the distribution of ganglia among animals is not clear-cut. They apparently do not occur in any nerve nets, but they do occur in Platyhelminthes in which a simple CNS is usually considered to be present.

In Platyhelminthes, ganglia generally occur, but they are often very simple. They are sometimes called cerebral ganglia. There may be a pair alone, or a pair with a median ganglia, or other combinations, or they may all be loosely united, in which case the word brain has been applied. They are at the end or along the course of the nerve cords, between which there may be few or many connecting commissures or a network of nerves.

In Rhynchocoela there appear for the first time ganglionated nerve cords, and the brain appears to be formed by the fusion of two pairs of ganglia. As summarized by Gibson (1972), a ganglionated dorsal nerve cord, such as is found in *Neuronemertea aurantiaca,* is probably unique among animals. The ganglia are "metamerically" arranged, may number 100, and are coordinated with the branchings of the lateral nerve cords.

Small ganglia, sometimes including a small brain, occur in Acanthocephala, Aschelminthes, and lophophorates.

The Mollusca show more diversity in gross features of the nervous system than any other phylum. In what are usually thought to be the primitive classes, there are nerve cords with ganglia and a brain. In the more advanced Gastropoda, the brain becomes more complex, but the cords seem much simpler, and each leads to a simple ganglion. In the sedentary Bivalvia, where there is no brain, the cords are even fewer and the number of ganglia reduced, generally not being paired. The Cephalopoda for the first time show the centralization and complexity required by an active animal; the CNS ganglia are nearly all concentrated in a mass around the oesophagus, and a foreshadowing of a ladder-type CNS may occur.

In Sipunculoidea, ganglia are not mentioned in any part of the nervous system, although there is a brain and a ventral nerve cord. The absence of ganglia seems to be correlated with the absence of nerve cell bodies (nuclei), but the presence of a brain that is not formed of fused ganglia is not explained.

In Echiuroidea there is mention of a small "cerebral ganglion" that does not show ganglionic swellings. Such swellings do not occur elsewhere in the adult system. In the larva there may be a paired row of ganglionic rudiments, segmentally arranged.

The basic plan of Annelida and Arthropoda is a ladder-like chain of paired segmental ganglia and a brain consisting of paired supra-oesophageal (or cerebral) ganglia either fused medially or with circumoesophageal commissures.

Ganglia are abundant in most Annelida, both along the cords and peripherally, but even when they are lacking peripherally, they may also be apparently nonexistent in the cords. Even in the brain this word is usually not used. The Arthropoda have paired ganglia in the central system, but these usually seem to be absent peripherally.

There are trends in several groups toward amalgamation of many ganglia into a large mass other than the brain. This amalgamation in the CNS has happened in Myzostomida (where the ventral cord is a single ganglionic mass many times as large as the brain), in Merostomata, Araneida, Solpugida, and Crustacea (both Branchiura and Decapoda), and in Insecta (at least in the thorax of some Diptera).

Terms relating to invertebrate ganglia include:

1. Axon tract — an area of synaptic connections between the dendrites and the axon terminals
2. Brain — any dorsal cephalic mass formed by fusion of ganglia
3. Connective — a longitudinal bundle of nerve fibers between adjacent ganglia of the CNS
4. Core — the fibrous inner zone of the invertebrate ganglion, containing most of the nerve endings, synaptic regions, and axons
5. Glia — same as Neuroglia
6. Neuroglia — accessory connective tissue cells in the nervous system
7. Neuropile — an area of tangled nerve fibers with synaptic connections
8. Rind — the outer region of the invertebrate ganglion, containing most of the cell bodies
9. Synaptic region — an area of many synaptic connections

2. Vertebrate Brain

The basic nature of the vertebrate brain is seldom described; no real distinction between these and invertebrate brains (or cerebral ganglia) is given. Although most books seem to assume that the vertebrate brain is different from those of invertebrates, some books admit that they are extremely complex ganglionic masses not fundamentally different from other ganglia; however, most vertebrate anatomy books cite the brain as unique, without stipulation of exactly how they differ from invertebrate ganglionic brains, but report that ganglia do occur inside the basal portions of the vertebrate brain.

In virtually all books, it is assumed that certain phyla are somehow involved in the ancestry of vertebrates. These are the phyla usually listed (because of requirements of chapter sequence) between the Arthropoda and the Vertebrata, namely, Chaetognatha, Pogonophora, Echinodermata, Pterobranchia, Enteropneusta, Tunicata, and Cephalochordata. It is fascinating that in an organ system as important as the nervous system there is in these groups almost no development toward, or anticipation of, the extreme development, cephalization, and complexity of the vertebrate brain. For example, in the Echinodermata the word brain is used only to deny its existence in any form. The Chaetognatha are at the level of the Rotifera, except that a large mid-ventral ganglion is larger than the simple brain. In the Hemichordata and Tunicata a brain is not even mentioned in most accounts, although a cerebral ganglion may be present. Even in the Cephalochordata no brain is visible, although the anterior end of the nerve cord may be considered a very simple brain. Nevertheless, the brains of vertebrates are known in great detail; they conform to a pattern clearly seen as an evolutionary sequence of the classes.

Terms relating to vertebrate brains are only sometimes distinct from those of invertebrates:

1. Glia — same as Neuroglia
2. Gray matter — areas in the CNS containing cell bodies, axon terminals, dendrites, and synapses
3. Neuroglia — same as for Invertebrates
4. Neuropile — same as for Invertebrates
5. White matter — areas in the CNS containing only myelinated nerve fibers

G. Nerve Cords

The longitudinal nerve cords in the various animal groups differ in several obvious ways:

1. Number — from one (Vertebrata) and two (Arthropoda) to at least eight (s.Turbellaria)
2. Position — mid-dorsal (Vertebrata) or mid-ventral (Arthropoda) or all peripheral (Turbellaria)
3. Centralization — varying from an integral part of the brain system (Vertebrata) or substantial isolation (Rotifera)
4. Relation of ganglia to ladder-type cords — serially and usually segmentally (s.Arthropoda); fused in masses along the cord, as in the thorax of some Arthropoda
5. Branched — the number and distribution of branches and commissures between them

Although the epidermal position of nerve cords in Platyhelminthes is considered primitive, and most later ones are beneath the epidermis, in Polychaeta many are epidermal, some are in the muscle layers, and in many others there is one free in the coelom. These arrangements often vary within a family or even a genus. Although two cords do sometimes occur in Annelida, it is more common for there to be only one, with little evidence of fusion. The more specialized worms tend to have only one. This is surprising when it is seen that the Onychophora have two widely separated cords, and most Arthropoda have at least clear evidence of two cords only partly fused. The simplest insects have a clear ladder-type system, but in advanced flying insects there is great condensation of the system into the head and also into the thorax, and the cords are fused anteriorly and largely absent posteriorly.

In Sipunculoidea the CNS consists of a definite brain and a ventral nerve cord with circumoesophageal connectives.

An unusually simple system is found in the Echiuroidea, where there is a single median ventral cord from which numerous nerves pass to the body wall. Anteriorly the cord divides to form a complete loop in the proboscis. There are no ganglionic swellings, and the lateral nerves often fuse dorsally, forming numerous rings about the digestive tract.

In Vertebrata is found the largest (proportionally) and the most complex longitudinal cord, the spinal cord. It carries impulses to and from the brain and also forms many reflex arcs in which stimuli produce reactions without intervention of the brain.

The cord is essentially ganglionic in nature, consisting of a central H-shaped mass of cell bodies of motor neurons and interneurons with large synaptic regions, these forming the gray matter. The rest of the cord is the surrounding white matter, consisting principally of axon fibers in tracts. This type of cord is practically an extension of the brain, functionally as well as structurally.

Descriptions of the structure of the cords in invertebrates are surprisingly few. In segmented animals the segmental pattern is clear in the ventral cord or pair of cords, with a pair of ganglia in each presumed segment and these joined longitudinally by connectives and transversely by one or two commissures. The ganglia are often regionally fused, either transversely or both transversely and longitudinally. The first ganglion of the cord is the suboesophageal ganglion. The longitudinal connectives contain many sensory and motor axons, as well as many interneurons. Nerve cells may occur along the connectives or be restricted to the ganglia.

H. Circum-Enteric Rings

A random viewing of diagrams of the CNS throughout the animal phyla could scarcely fail to show one unanticipated uniformity. In almost all groups, even the lowest, the CNS encircles the anterior part of the digestive tract, usually the oesophagus. If there is a brain, it is almost always above the oesophagus and encircles it to ganglia beneath. If it is a highly developed brain, the oesophagus will appear to pass through it. Even in Coelenterata and Echinodermata, where there is no brain, the nerves form a ring around the proctostome or mouth, respectively (Figure 22).

The exceptions to this are intriguing. In the Rhynchocoela the ring encircles the rhynchocoel, which opens terminally. In some species the digestive tract opens ventrally, clearly outside of the ring. In other species the mouth opening is into the rhynchocoel itself, from beneath, so that there is a common exterior opening; here also it appears that the nerve ring is far enough back to pass around only the rhynchocoel. It is interesting to note that in the embryology of these worms the rhynchocoel is formed by an invagination, similar to formation of an open blastopore, but it precedes the mouth (stomodael invagination). The significance of these peculiarities is not clear.

The obvious exception to the circumoesophageal ring is the Vertebrata, in which the dorsal nerve cord never surrounds the ventral digestive tract in such a manner.

IV. CHEMICAL CONTROL

A. Introduction

In animals, chemical control operates in at least four situations. It may operate within a single cell, where it is the expression of gene activity; between two adjacent cells, as in much neurohumoral secretion; between organs, as the classical endocrine gland and its target organ; and between individuals, as in the case of pheromones.

The first of these, the intracellular chemicals, are usually not dealt with in endocrinology books. Virtually no information is available to permit a comparative analysis of their nature or their distribution through the groups of animals.

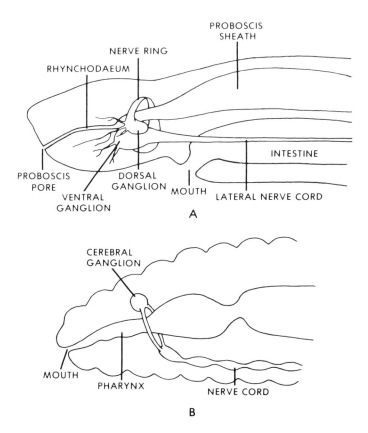

FIGURE 22.   Circumenteric nerve rings. (A) Rhynchocoel (nemertean); (B) earthworm.

The last, the interindividual chemicals or pheromones operate between individuals; they are briefly treated in the next section and in Chapter 22.

Until recent decades, the study of endocrinology in both vertebrates and invertebrates dealt almost exclusively with endocrine glands, their hormonal products, and their effects. The field of neuro-endocrinology is a relatively recent development that is now recognized as indistinguishable from the older field, although one is a cell diffusion phenomenon and the other is accomplished through the circulatory system.

B. Chemical Messengers

Endocrine cells and glands produce minute quantities of specific chemical substances which are carried in the blood or cell protoplasm to stimulate or inhibit specific effectors or to control certain aspects of metabolism and development. The secreted substances are the *hormones*, described as "chemical activators". Besides hormones there are two other kinds of activators in animals, the nerves (already described) and so-called mechanical activators.

1. Mechanical activation — for example, water currents in a sponge stimulating the osculum to remain open; earthworm segment contraction stimulating the segment behind to contract; vertebrate stomach distension stimulating secretion of enzymes
2. Hormonal activation (see below)
3. Nerve activation — impulse transmission from receptor to effector, receptor to another neuron, one neuron to another, or a neuron to an effector

Hormonal activation is accomplished by neurosecretion and endocrine activity. Both are processes that utilize so-called chemical messengers, which are similar in nature to the messengers between individuals (pheromones).

These messengers are more diverse than the usual list of hormones and neurohormones would indicate, as shown in a later list. General terms for the classes of these messengers include the following.

Neurohormones are the chemical messengers released by neurosecretory cells, most of which are associated with the CNS and carried by the blood. Two are well known in vertebrates as to chemistry and action: oxytocin and vasopressin.

Neurohumors are products of the neurons; they are called local hormones or diffusion hormones. They travel over the minute distance involved in crossing a synapse. Their actions are transient and highly localized. Examples are acetylcholine and norepinephrine.

Hormones were formerly defined as chemical agents synthesized by special ductless glands and carried by the bloodstream to other parts of the body where they evoke responses from specific target organs. The term is now sometimes used to include both the products of the ductless glands and the neurohormones.

Chalones are hormones that act on mitosis in certain tissues, as long-range inhibitors.

Ectohormones are chemical messengers acting outside the body and only on other individuals (see Pheromones).

Gamones are ectohormones produced by gametes and acting on the opposite sex.

Pheromones are hormone-like substances released from one individual to influence other individuals. Their role is in animal behavior, since they produce reactions in the behavior of whole individuals rather than in specific cells or organs of the producing individual.

Parahormones. The cells of all animals produce and release substances which change the chemistry of either its internal or its exterior environment. They are not hormones or neurohormones but can be grouped as parahormones (not to be confused with parathormones which are the hormones of the parathyroid gland). Example are carbon dioxide, urea, histamine, leukocyte attractants, and renin.

Phytohormones include growth and wound regulators in plants, but they are beyond the scope of this book.

Classification of chemical activators. — A revised scheme of chemical activators in animals was given by Jenkin (1970) and is abridged here:

1. Local Activators
   a. Intracellular messenger RNA
   b. Regional activators for chemodifferentiation
2. Diffusion activators
   a. Embryonic organizers
   b. Neurohumoral secretions at nerve endings
   c. Gamones (inter-sex "hormones")
   d. Ectohormones or pheromones
3. Hormones
   a. Neurosecretions
   b. Vascular hormones
   c. Chalones (growth inhibitors)

The present section deals with the vascular hormones (endocrinology) and the neurosecretions (neuroendocrinology), with their organs and mechanisms.

C. Endocrinology

1. Vertebrates vs. Invertebrates

For many years there appeared to be a great imbalance in the knowledge of animal endocrinology, because nearly all the detailed information applied to vertebrates, with the small remainder being all from arthropods. This imbalance seemed to grow rapidly, as most work was done with vertebrates, and yet the imbalance today seems to be decreasing.

It is seldom noted that this reversal of trend is due to the recent development of the field of neuro-endocrinology. The endocrine glands of classical endocrinology are virtually limited to the Vertebrata, but the secretion of neurohormones by neurons is apparently universal. Furthermore, these neurohormones seem to be more generally involved in the control of processes among some invertebrates than among vertebrates. Thus, the field of endocrinology has finally become truly comparative; i.e., there is coming to be comparable information from many groups. However, enough detail for tabulation of differences is still lacking.

2. Endocrine Glands

In the Vertebrata there are many glands that have been cited as endocrine. Their hormones are very briefly listed here:

1. Adenohypophysis or anterior pituitary (the "master" gland) (somatotrophin, thyrotrophin, corticotrophin, gonadotrophins such as follicle-stimulating hormone and luteinizing hormone, prolactin, intermedin or melanocyte-stimulating hormone, adenocorticotrophin, and corticosteroids such as glycocorticoids and mineralocorticoids)
2. Adrenal cortex (cortisone, aldosterone, corticosterone, deoxycorticosterone, progesterone)
3. Adrenal medulla (adrenalin or epinephrine, noradrenalin or norepinephrine)
4. Anterior pituitary (see Adenohypophysis)
5. Corpus luteum (see Ovary, below)
6. Hypophysis (see Adenohypophysis and Neurohypophysis)
7. Neurohypophysis (see under Neurosecretions, below)
8. Parathyroid gland (parathyroid hormone, parathormone)
9. Posterior pituitary (see under Neurosecretion, below)
10. Thymus gland (thymosin is recently found to enhance certain immunological abilities; it was earlier known to inhibit the effects of thyroxine)
11. Thyroid gland (thyroxine, calcitonin)

It is nowadays known that other organs may incidentally secrete hormone messengers. Among those cited are the lungs, the kidneys, the duodenum, the stomach, the placenta, the testis, and the ovary. The hormones include:

12. Duodenum (secretin, cholecystokinin, enterogastrone, enterocrinin)
13. Islets of Langerhans — in pancreas (insulin, glucagon)
14. Kidney — in some fishes and in mammals, there are tissues associated with the kidneys that produce renin which may be involved in endocrine activity
15. Ovary (ovarian follicles secrete estradiol while performing their other functions; later, the expended follicle secretes progesterone when it is called corpus luteum)
16. Placenta (progesterone, chorionic gonadotrophic hormone)
17. Stomach (gastrin, urogastrone)

To these vertebrate organs can be added two others that occure in the Tunicata but they may differ mainly in name: the endostyle seems to correspond to the thyroid gland; the subneural gland corresponds at least in part to the dual gland called hypophysis.

Although much work has been done on "endocrinology" of arthropods, most of it is now seen to relate to neurosecretory structures. Among the invertebrates true endocrine glands include these four:

1. Optic gland — hormones relating to sexual maturity (Cephalopoda)
2. Salivary glands (Cephalopoda)
3. Y-organ — molting hormones (Crustacea)
4. Androgenic gland — hormones relating to gonadal development and sex characteristics (Crustacea)
5. Prothoracic glands — ecdysone (Insecta)
6. Corpora allata — juvenile hormone (Insecta)
7. Ecdysial gland — molting hormones (Insecta)

3. Hormones

Hormones were once the only known "chemical messengers". They were defined as "specific chemical compounds synthesized in certain cells or tissues and exerting a specific action on other cells or tissues" or as "a substance elaborated by a ductless gland and carried by the blood stream to some other part of the body, which it excites".

Such a simple definition is unsatisfactory under the current understanding of the enlarged field of endocrine and neuro-endocrine substances. A hormone as now understood is one of the substances that produce an effect in a distant organ or in a neighboring cell, thus encompassing both hormones and neurohumors. Its function is to stimulate or inhibit some specific action or reaction. Hormones are principally proteins or lipoids. Most are steroids, although the juvenile hormone of insects seems to be of other lipoidal nature.

In the early days of invertebrate endocrinology, there were thought to be biochemical similarities between the hormones of different phyla, mostly Arthropoda and Vertebrata, which were the only ones known. Later workers "have failed to adduce convincing proof that hormones in different phyla are biochemically identical" (Lee and Knowles, 1965).

Several hormones are cited in these pages. No complete list can be produced because of the diversity of terminologies used. Such terms as follicular stimulating hormone (FSH) tell much about the hormone's activity but not of its chemical nature. These are not formally listed here. There are elaborate systems of descriptive terms that specify the function or the place of the effect, such as adrenocorticotropic and lactogenic. (Note that at one time all the -tropic terms were spelled -trophic, and all hormone names now beginning with e- were spelled oe-.)

a. Classification of Hormones

Hormones in the broad sense can be classified in several ways. They may be arranged by their distance from the target and the transfer method employed:

1. Local (diffusion activators): (a) intracellular (enzymes), (b) intercellular (embryonic organizers), (c) between nerve cells (neurohumors)
2. Distance (circulatory activators): (a) isolated cells (gastrin from a stomach cell), (b) neurosecretory cells (vasopressin), and (c) endocrine gland cells (insulin)

Hormones can be classified by their chemical nature:

1. Steroids (androgens, progesterone, cortisone, oestrogens)
2. Amino acids (thyroxine)
3. Polypeptides (pitressin)
4. Simple proteins (insulin)
5. Conjugated proteins (follicle stimulating hormone)

Hormones can be classified by the germ layer source, derived from these embryonic tissues: (a) ectodermal (juvenile hormone from corpora allata). (b) endodermal (insulin), and (c) mesodermal (cortisone).

They may be classified by the effect produced in the body:

1. Kinetic — acting on effectors (adrenalin)
2. Metabolic — controlling metabolic activities (insulin)
3. Morphogenetic — controlling cell division, growth, and differentiation (testosterone)

b. Hormone Functions

The kinetic hormones act upon effector cells or organs to produce repeatable reactions mainly concerned with feeding, digestion, and protective color change. Many of the relatively quick-acting kinetic hormones induce protective responses to the environment and maintain short-term changes in diurnal and tidal rhythms. Many of these are neurosecretory substances.

A sub-group of the kinetic are the hormones which stimulate the secretion of other hormones from endocrine glands. These are termed endocrinokinetic hormones by Jenkin (1962), from whom these descriptions are adapted; an example is the adrenocorticotrophin referred to as ACTH.

The metabolic hormones control the "internal milieu" in the tissue: while some tend to maintain a steady balance, others allow a relatively slow adaptation to environmental changes.

The morphogenetic hormones produce long-term changes that involve cell division, growth, and differentiation. Their effects can neither be reversed nor repeated, at least for a considerable time.

It is expected that hormones will be found in all animals. Some hormones are reasonably well known in Mollusca, Annelida, Arthropoda, as well as in Vertebrata, as cited under the organs, above.

These three principal types of hormones can be considered by functions:

Kinetic hormone functions

1. Control of muscles (Cephalopoda, Crustacea, Insecta, Vertebrata)
2. Control of pigmentary effectors (Cephalopoda, Crustacea, Insecta, Vertebrata)
3. Control of exocrine glands (Bivalvia, Gastropoda, Cephalopoda, Crustacea, Vertebrata)
4. Control of endocrine glands (Crustacea, Insecta, Vertebrata)
5. Control of reproduction (Crustacea, Insecta, Vertebrata)

Metabolic hormone functions (influencing metabolic rates)

6. Control of respiration (Crustacea, Insecta, Protochordata, Tunicata, Cephalochordata, Vertebrata)
7. Control of fat metabolism (Crustacea, Insecta, Vertebrata)
8. Control of carbohydrate metabolism (Crustacea, Insecta, Vertebrata)
9. Control of protein metabolism (Crustacea, Insecta, Vertebrata)

10. Control of electrolytes and water (?Arthropoda, Vertebrata)
11. Control of water balance (Crustacea, Insecta, Vertebrata)
12. Control of balance of calcium and phosphates (Crustacea, Insecta, Vertebrata)
13. Control of hibernation, diapause, etc. (Arthropoda, Vertebrata)

Morphogenetic hormone functions

14. Control of growth (Mollusca, Annelida, Arthropoda, Vertebrata)
15. Control of mitosis (Annelida, Arthropoda, Vertebrata)
16. Control of molting (Arthropoda, Vertebrata)
17. Control of metamorphosis (Annelida, Arthropoda, Vertebrata)

4. Effectors

The story of nervous and endocrine control is not complete without reference to the effectors, the organs that respond to the transmitted signals. These include all the organs of the body. One way to look at these is by the nature of the effect produced, in which they may be

1. Producers of mechanical action, especially the muscles
2. Producers of materials by secretion, such as glands
3. Producers of stimuli to produce effects in still other effectors, the neurons and endocrine glands

Whether the stimulus is by nerve or hormone, the stimulation itself seems always to be hormonal, as the activation of an effector by a nerve impulse is accomplished only by neuro-endocrine secretions which are also hormones.

D. Neurosecretions

Neuro-endocrinology is one of the fast growing fields of physiology. It is becoming clear that some of the endocrine functions recognized in the past are not related to glands but to secreting neurons. Thus, most endocrinology of arthropods, where much detailed work has been done, relates in reality to neurosecretions. These do not have a well-known distinctive class name. Neurosecretions are variously referred to under the terms hormones, neurohormones, neurohumors, and neurosecretions. There are reasonable distinctions among these that add greatly to understanding of these substances. Neurosecretions must include all messenger secretion of neurons. The messengers intended for action on neighboring neurons are called *neurohumors*. The messengers carried to more-or-less distant organs by the blood or other body fluids are called *neurohormones*; they are similar to vascular hormones in general.

Neurosecretions are known in all groups where there are neurons — from Coelenterata to Vertebrata. They are generally from cells in the ganglia (especially cerebral), the nerve cords, or the brain. They are recorded, for example, in *Hydra*, in Platyhelminthes (cerebral ganglia), in Rhynchocoela (brain), in Nematoda, Mollusca, and Sipunculoidea, in Annelida (cerebral ganglion), and in Arthropoda (in the CNS).

The neurosecretions are hormones very similar to the hormones produced by glands, but they are not usually identified by simple "hormone" names. Two exceptions which occur in the products of the hypothalamus are vasopressin and oxytocin. (These are released by and sometimes ascribed to the neurohypophysis or posterior pituitary.). Hormones in general are lipoidal (steroids) or proteinaceous (often being merely polypeptides or amines), but few books distinguish the nature of specific hormones in groups other than vertebrates, and few mention the chemical nature of the neurosecretions.

The function of neurosecretion in general is dual: to communicate with neurons (by neurohumors) and with distant organs (by neurohormones). The latter is well described by Turner and Bagnara (1971): "It is now generally agreed that most, if not all, nervous systems secrete neurohormones for the regulation of such processes as growth, reproduction, molting, water balance, pigmentation, and blood chemistry. Gland-like neurons are almost ubiquitous among the Metazoa and they occur with regularity in specific locations within the nervous system. They may be regarded as specializations that enable the nervous system to express itself in chemical terms over prolonged periods by utilizing both endocrine and non-endocrine targets. The discovery of such secretory neurons in organisms ranging in complexity from coelenterates to man has added a new dimension to endocrinology since many of the systemic adjustments to environmental factors are actually neuro-endocrine in nature."

E. The Message Systems by Phylum

To summarize the condition and extent of the three parts of the nervous and endocrine system (sense organs, nerves, and chemical messengers), it seems appropriate to bring these back together as a single functioning unit and to describe them briefly for each phylum. Although we have not seen this attempted before, the following may be considered a beginning.

Protozoa. No receptor organelles but some localized sites of irritability. No conducting or coordinating structures known; some conduction by plasma membrane. Neurosecretion impossible.

Porifera. No organs of sensation. No nerve cells. No neurosecretion possible.

Mesozoa. No control structures known.

Coelenterata. First ocelli, eyes, statocysts, and unicellular receptors. Neurons (without myelin sheath, synapses, or Nissl substance) and ganglion cells in an epidermal nerve net. Neurosecretory cells present. Nerves may be continuous throughout a colony.

Ctenophora. Subepidermal plexus; as in Coelenterata.

Platyhelminthes. Many receptors, unicellular and multicellular, including eyes, and statocysts. Nerves, subepidermal plexuses, CNS of 1 to 5 pairs of cords and a simple brain; peripheral system; circumoesophageal ring; ganglia; some giant fibers. Neurosecretion from cerebral ganglion and ventral cord.

Rhynchocoela. Many receptors, uni- or multicellular. Neurons; brain with paired cords, metamerically ganglionated; peripheral system; nerve ring around rhynchodaeum; nerve plexuses; giant nerve cells in brain. Neurosecretion at least in brain.

Acanthocephala. Very few receptors. Nerves paired, with ganglia; no real cords; no digestive tract and so no circumoesophageal ring. Neurosecretion unreported.

Rotifera. Numerous very small receptors. Nerves, simple brain, simple lateral cords with ganglia; eutelic. Neurosecretion unreported.

Gastrotricha. As in Rotifera.

Kinorhyncha. Receptors unreported. Nerves medullary; 4 cords with metameric ganglia; circumoral ring; nerves epidermal. Neurosecretion is unreported.

Nematoda. Variety of simple receptors, amphids, phasmids. Circum-enteric ring of ganglia, several longitudinal cords may be ganglionated; two sympathetic systems. Some neurosecretory cells.

Gordioidea. Few receptors. Ganglion around oesophagus; one cord; no peripheral plexus; giant nerve cells. Neurosecretion unreported.

Priapuloidea. No receptors clearly identified, "remarkably indifferent to chemical stimuli." System epidermal, circum-pharyngeal ring; ventral cord. Neurosecretion unreported.

Calyssozoa. Few receptors. Peripheral plexus (continuous in colony); subenteric ganglion but no ring; no cords. Neurosecretion unreported.

Bryozoa. Few receptor cells. Very simple; cerebral ganglion and circumoral ring; no cords; nerve net. Neurosecretion unreported.

Phoronida. Unicellular receptors only. Epidermal nerve net; dorsal ganglion and ring; giant fibers. Neurosecretion unreported.

Brachiopoda. Statocysts and simple receptors. Epidermal system; no cords; supra-oesophageal ganglion and ring. Neurosecretion unreported.

Mollusca. Receptors few and simple to many with some complex, including olfactory and proprioceptive; eyes in *Pecten* and Cephalopoda. Peripheral plexus; 2 pairs of cords and 2 rings in Monoplacophora; ganglia with connecting nerves; first identifiable nerves; giant axons; stellate ganglion and stomatogastric system in Cephalopoda. Hormones from salivary glands. Neurosecretion in major classes, at least.

Sipunculoidea. Many unicellular and a few simple multicellular receptors. Nerves without nerve cells; plexus beneath peritoneum; simple brain, ventral nerve cord, and rings. Neurosecretion assumed.

Echiuroidea. Unicellular receptors only. No brain; ventral nerve cord with "neural canal". Neurosecretion unreported.

Annelida. Simple receptors of several sorts, including free-ending nerve fibers. Nerves forming subepidermal plexus; ventral ladder-like cords with segmental ganglia; cerebral ganglion, circum-enteric ring; giant fibers. Neurosecretory control of reproduction, diapause, regeneration, color change, with neurohaemal organ.

Dinophiloidea. Little recorded but not inconsistent with Annelida.

Tardigrada. Sensory papillae. Four ganglia with two sets of connectives (ladder-like cords?), 2 circumoesophageal rings; no eutely of neurons. Neurosecretion unreported.

Myzostomida. Same level as Polychaeta but much simpler, with all abdominal ganglia fused into one mass; giant fibers. Receptors and neurosecretion unreported.

Pentastomida. Sensory papillae. Simple brain is sometimes a concentration of all ganglia around the mouth; sometimes ladder-like but cords and ganglia almost indistinguishable; fine structure as in Arthropoda. Neurosecretion unreported.

Onychophora. Sense organs simple papillae, especially on the mouthparts; eye with cup and lens. Circum-pharyngeal brain; ladder-like ventral pair of cords, the cord medullary and with simple ganglia; median dorsal nerve along heart; visceral system not well known. Neurosecretion not reported.

Arthropoda. Many unicellular and elaborate receptors, including compound eyes and wide variety of others, often numerous, sometimes clustered on appendages such as antennae; virtually all stimuli received in one or another species; especially proprioceptive in cuticle. Brain and suboesophageal ganglia forming ring; double ventral nerve cord usually fused into one, segmental ganglia; nerve plexuses in epidermis; stomatogastric system; all regional ganglia may be fused; giant nerve fibers. Several kinds of glandular endocrine organs; neurosecretory cells in CNS in most groups, control reproduction, pigmentation, cardio-acceleration, molting, yolk deposition in ova, metamorphosis.

Chaetognatha. Receptors are simple eyes and bristles, no statocyst. Two ganglia and circumoesophageal ring; basiepithelial plexus; no cords. Neurosecretion unreported.

Pogonophora. Sensory cells and a possible ciliated sense organ. Nerves entirely epidermal, a nerve net; indistinct brain with ring at base of tentacles (no digestive tract); longitudinal dorsal nerve trunk; giant nerve fibers. Endocrinology unreported.

Echinodermata. Sensory cells numerous; statocysts. Three networks at three levels; radial cords and nerve ring; primitive ganglion cells in epidermis. Neurosecretory cells but "no evidence of a truly endocrine organ".

Enteropneusta. Sensory cells only. Hollow collar cord; dorsal and ventral cords; giant neurons; circumoesophageal ring. Neurosecretion unreported.

Pterobranchia. Dorsal and ventral cords with nerve ring. Receptors and neurosecretion unreported.

Tunicata. Simple eyes, statocyst, sensory cells. Cerebral ganglion in mesenchyme; larva has "neural tube"; 5 nerves; a visceral plexus. Neurosecretion unreported.

Cephalochordata. Receptors a pigment spot and tactile cells and free nerve endings in skin; dorsal nerve cord but no obvious brain; no mixed nerves; somatic and visceral systems; giant cells and fibers. Neurosecretion unreported.

Vertebrata. Many receptors simple and complex, of general senses and special senses. Elaborate CNS with large brain; spinal cord with neural canal; autonomic system includes sympathetic and parasympathetic; neurons, interneurons, sensory ganglia, etc. A variety of endocrine glands and neurosecretory cells throughout the CNS.

REFERENCES

Bullock, T. H. and Horridge, G. A., *Structure and Function of Nervous Systems of Invertebrates,* 2 volumes. W. H. Freeman, San Francisco, 1965.

Case, J., *Sensory Mechanisms,* Macmillan, New York, 1966.

Ebling, J. and Highnam, K. C., *Chemical Communication,* St. Martin's Press, New York, 1969.

Gibson, R., *Nemerteans,* Hutchinson University Library, London, 1972.

Hall, P. F., *The Functions of the Endocrine Glands,* W. B. Saunders, Philadelphia, 1959.

Highnam, K. C. and Hill, L., *The Comparative Endocrinology of the Invertebrates,* American Elsevier, New York, 1969.

Imms, A. D., *A General Textbook of Entomology,* 8th ed., Methuen, London, 1951.

Jenkin, P. M., *Animal Hormones, Part I.,* Pergamon Press, London, 1962.

Jenkin, P. M., *Control of Growth and Metamorphosis:* Animal Hormones, Part II, Pergamon Press, New York. 1970.

Jennings, H. S., *Behavior of the Lower Organisms,* Indiana University Press, Bloomington, 1962.

Lee, J. and Knowles, F. G. W., *Animal Hormones,* Hutchinson University Library, London; Hillary House, New York, 1965.

Marshall, A. J., *Parker & Haswell, A Text-Book of Zoology,* Vol. 2, 7th ed., Macmillan, London, 1964.

Mill, P. J., Ed., *Structure and Function of Proprioceptors in the Invertebrates,* Chapman & Hall, London; John Wiley & Sons, New York, 1976.

Milne, L. J. and Milne, M., *The Biotic World and Man,* 3rd ed., Prentice-Hall, Englewood Cliffs, N.J., 1965.

Ochs, S., *Elements of Neurophysiology,* John Wiley & Sons, New York, 1965.

Prosser, C. L., Ed., *Comparative Animal Physiology,* 3rd ed., W. B. Saunders, Philadelphia, 1973.

Scharrer, E. and Scharrer, B., *Neuroendocrinology,* Columbia University Press, New York, 1963.

Tombes, A. S., *An Introduction to Invertebrate Endocrinology,* Academic Press, New York, 1970.

Turner, C. D. and Bagnara, J. T., *General Endocrinology,* 5th ed., W. B. Saunders, Philadelphia, 1971.

Wilson, J. A., *Principles of Animal Physiology,* Macmillan, New York, 1972.

Wolken, J. J., *Invertebrate Photoreceptors: A Comparative Analysis,* Academic Press, New York, 1971.

Chapter 18

INTEGUMENTS

TABLE OF CONTENTS

I.   Introduction...370

II.   Functions of Integument..370
      A.   The Functions in General..370
      B.   Primary Functions...370
            1.   Containment..370
            2.   Protection 371
            3.   Support..371
      C.   Secondary Functions...371

III. The Coverings of Protozoa...372

IV.   The Integuments of Invertebrates..372
      A.   Diversity 372
      B.   Integument Definitions...373
      C.   Histology of the Invertebrate Integument..............................374
            1.   Setae, Spines, Bristles...374
            2.   Setal Structures..376
            3.   Function of Setae 376
            4.   Setal and Nonsetal Terms...378

V.   The Skin of Vertebrates 378

VI.   Hard-parts of Animals 379
      A.   The Structures 379
      B.   Hard-part Substances...383

References 384

I. INTRODUCTION

The covering of the body of animals consists of a tissue or several tissue layers with their outer secreted materials and incorporated organs. In some cases there are body wall muscles and a peritoneum inside, so that the body is surrounded by a layered body wall that "contains" the organs and body fluids. This covering would be unique among tissues in many ways, and it is concluded here that it can best be treated as an organ system, defined earlier as a group of organs integrated into a functional whole for the accomplishment of a major group of body functions.

II. FUNCTIONS OF INTEGUMENT

A. The Functions in General

The principal function of integuments is containment. This helps to give shape to the body and to organs, provides for the maintenance of turgor inside, prevents the escape of tissue fluids and motile cells, and prevents the entrance of foreign materials.

As a second function, protection from the environment would be afforded by any integument, but some are especially designed to provide this. Even a thin epidermis has considerable strength and protects underlying tissues.

A third primary function is support, a function which it shares with internal skeletons. In the Arthropoda, the integument includes the exoskeleton, which is the chief support structure. Even a thin epidermis can aid in support if it forms a containment against internal pressure (turgor).

In this connection, a function is listed as primary if it is what the structure was designed to do. It appears that containment, protection, and support are primary functions of integument.

Secondary functions would be ones that may be performed incidentally, perhaps with special adaptations, but not interfering with the primary functions. These would include cooperation in the function of other organs, such as rhythmical movements of the integument to assist in movement of air in the tracheae of Insecta.

B. Primary Functions

1. Containment

This is a static function essential to all animals. In isolated animal cells, the cell membrane "contains" the cytoplasm, preventing its dispersal in the surrounding water. In multicellular animals, there is always an external enclosing tissue, often with its secreted cuticle, to confine the fluids and cells of the body.

The tissues and structures which will serve to contain the body of an animal include:

1. Cuticle — secreted by epidermis (Platyhelminthes, Acanthocephala, Nematoda, Rotifera, Gastrotricha, Gordioidea, Priapuloidea, Phoronida, Sipunculoidea, Echiuroidea, Myzostomida, Annelida, Pogonophora, Tunicata, and probably others
2. Epidermis — in all animals, so far as known (the term epithelium has sometimes been used for what is properly called epidermis; see descriptions later in this chapter of the condition in Trematoda and Cestoda)
3. Exoskeleton — a hardened cuticle (Arthropoda)
4. Perisarc — translucent layer secreted by epidermis of some Hydrozoa
5. Pneumatic layer — around some sponge gemmules
6. Shell — secreted by the epidermis (Brachiopoda, Mollusca)
7. Skin (see Section V, "The Skin of Vertebrates")

8. Tegument — the special form of epidermis in Trematoda and Cestoda
9. Tunic — a form of cuticle (Tunicata)
10. Zooecium — secreted by epidermis (Bryozoa)

The function of containment itself is one of those passive things, like "being transported", that cannot show any diversity in itself. The result of "transport" is always the same, to be at some new location, whatever the object used in the transport. The result of containment is to not spill outside, regardless of the nature of the containing structure or the contained materials.

Some containing tissues are much stronger than others, as exoskeletons of Arthropoda compared to the thin epidermis of sponges, for example. Some are perforated by apertures of various sorts, pores, duct openings, mouth and anus, etc. Some have surface features that produce color by light refraction, or texture, or contained pigments. The same layer which serves for containment may also serve other functions.

2. Protection

This function is served most directly by those integuments that are strengthened by secreted cuticle, exoskeleton, or shell. They may protect against:

1. Mechanical injury — such as puncture or mashing
2. Chemical injury — salt, acid, alkali, poisons, etc.
3. Radiation injury — such as by ultraviolet light
4. Heat — excess heat or heat loss
5. Infection — invasion by other organisms

The listed aspects of protection are not discussed further in this book.

3. Support

This is accomplished in several ways:

1. Maintenance of turgor
2. Formation of an exoskeleton
3. Secretion of a shell
4. Strengthening of the epidermis by ossicles or other hard deposits

Support is discussed in Chapter 20, "Miscellaneous Organ Functions".

C. Secondary Functions

The following are among the functions assisted by the integument:

1. Respiration — The selective passage of dissolved gases through the integument or special parts of it is a necessity in most respiratory systems, whether the organs are gills, lungs, tracheal tubes, respiratory trees, or the general body surface
2. Ingestion or feeding — In such animals as internal parasites, there sometimes is no digestive tract; food is digested either by the host or by secreted enzymes and must be absorbed as dissolved matter through permeable and often specialized integument
3. Excretion — When waste products of metabolism, such as salt and ammonia, pass out of the body through the integument, the process is usually less obvious than respiration because no special organs are involved; again they are dissolved in water and are selectively passed
4. Temperature control — The same selective passage permits water to be excreted

to cool the skin by evaporation; also regulation of chromatophores may control light penetration

5.   Protective coloration — Color may be used for display or camouflage
6.   Nutrition — Under the influence of incident light, the skin of mammals may manufacture vitamin D

In four of these secondary functions it is the selectivity of the integument that makes the activity possible. A particular substance is passed in or out, while the general environment is kept out and the body contents kept in.

The coverings of the Protozoa, the invertebrates, and the Vertebrata are similar in some functions, such as containment, but they are different both in structure and in terminology. They are here dealt with separately.

III. THE COVERINGS OF PROTOZOA

In Protozoa the cytoplasm is always surrounded by a unit membrane called the *plasma membrane* or *plasmalemma*. This covering is also called pellicle; it may be complex in structure as seen through the electron microscope; and it frequently produces organelles. The *pellicle* in simplest form is a cell membrane or plasmalemma, but it may include a shell, scales, a protein layer, cyst, lorica, or test, perhaps encrusted with inorganic substances (calcium carbonate or silica) or foreign bodies (sand or diatom frustules).

The scales may be of secreted silica and may form an entire layer over the surface. The cysts may be temporary or permanent and may occur in any developmental stage. They are common, especially in parasitic species, often involving an outer phosphoprotein layer and an inner cellulose layer, or an outer quinone-tanned protein layer and an inner lipo-protein layer.

Usually more or less separated from the envelope is the test, theca, capsule, shell, or lorica. These may be of cellulose, chitin, tectin, pseudochitin, protein, silica, calcium carbonate, or gelatin, which may serve to glue together extraneous debris (sand grains, diatom shells, sponge spicules, mica flakes, coccoliths, etc.).

IV. THE INTEGUMENTS OF INVERTEBRATES

A. Diversity

It has been stated that the integument or body covering in invertebrates consists of a single-layered epithelium plus materials secreted to the outer side of this epithelium. To this generalization there are several exceptions, among which the most obvious are some syncytial epithelia and some multilayered integuments.

The integument of invertebrates shows diversity in several ways. It is sometimes implied that all have a single-layered epidermis (although this layer is sometimes called hypodermis), but three apparent exceptions occur. The first of these is the Monoblastozoa, in which a single layer forms both body wall and digestive tract, so that there is no epidermis as such. In the Acanthocephala the epidermis is a thick syncytium that incorporates three fibrous layers, with the fibers apparently being noncellular protoplasmic strands. In the Chaetognatha, the epidermis is one-layered over much of the body but dorsally in front it becomes thicker and consists of large cells.

In the tapeworms, a normal epidermis has been thought to be lacking and was thus said to be functionally replaced by mesenchyme. It is now known that the Cestoda, like the Trematoda, do in fact have an epidermis, although one of unusual structure, in which the cells are columnar and basally syncytial. The nuclei are all near the bottom, where they were easily unnoticed, giving rise to the (erroneous) idea that the layer was actually a cuticle.

373

Thus, the histology of the epidermis varies considerably, but in most animal groups it secretes some sort of protective covering. These secreted coverings may be

1. Periderm or perisarc (Hydrozoa)
2. Cuticle of scleroprotein (Rotifera)
3. Cuticle of matricin and collagen (Nematoda)
4. Cuticle of protein and polysaccharides (Acanthocephala, Annelida, Pogonophora)
5. Cuticle of chitin (s.Mollusca, Pentastomida, Onychophora; see also exoskeleton and zooecium)
6. Cuticle of albuminoids (Tardigrada)
7. Cuticle of tunicin (Tunicata)
8. Cuticle of unknown but nonchitinous material (Gastrotricha, Kinorhyncha, Gordioidea, Priapuloidea, Calyssozoa, Phoronida, s.Mollusca, Sipunculoidea, Echiuroidea, Chaetognatha, Echinodermata, Cephalochordata)
9. Exoskeleton, chitinous and usually sclerotized (Arthropoda)
10. Zooecium, calcareous (s.Bryozoa)
11. Zooecium, chitinous (s.Bryozoa)
12. Shell, calcareous (s.Brachiopoda, s.Mollusca)
13. Shell, chitinous (s.Brachiopoda)

The exceptions, where no definite covering is secreted by the epidermis, include Porifera, Mesozoa, m.Coelenterata, Ctenophora, S.Platyhelminthes, Rhynchocoela, Myzostomida, s.Annelida, Echinodermata, Enteropneusta, and Pterobranchia.

B. Integument Definitions

The outer parts of invertebrates have been called by several names. Some of these can be made specific, and others usually are employed only in general ways:

1. Body covering — same as integument
2. Body wall — all layers from the outside inward to the body cavity
3. Coenoecium — a secreted encasement in Pterobranchia, of unknown composition (see also Zooecium)
4. Cuticle — a tough but not necessarily hard outer layer secreted by the outer layer of cells
5. Cutis — term sometimes used in Vertebrata for the combined epidermis and dermis; in Onychophora as a layer between the epidermis and the muscle layer
6. Cyst — the covering of transfer stages of many parasites (Trematoda, Cestoda)
7. Dermis — a little used term for the layer beneath the epidermis, in Acanthocephala, Annelida, and Holothurioidea
8. Epidermis — the outer layer of cells in the body covering, which may be the entire integument (as in Porifera) or may be underlain by other tissues or overlain by cuticle
9. Epithelioid membrane — the syncytial epidermis of sponges
10. Exoskeleton — chitinous skeletal elements forming the surface of an animal (i.e., not covered by any living tissue), as in Arthropoda; may be hardened into sclerites or impregnated with calcium carbonate
11. Hypodermis — sometimes used for an epidermis that secretes a cuticle
12. Integument — the covering of the animal body; in the invertebrates: that part of the body wall consisting of the epidermis, its basement membrane, and its secreted cuticle; in the vertebrates: the skin
13. Lorica — the thin cuticle in Rotifera

14. Mantle — the outer soft skin of Brachiopoda and Mollusca
15. Periderm — the chitinous tube of colonial Hydrozoa which protects and connects the hydranths and gonangia
16. Periostracum — horny shell covering in Mollusca
17. Perisarc — same as Periderm
18. Shells — secreted encasements; (a) eggshells in Platyhelminthes, Nematoda, Vertebrata, etc., of chitin or calcium carbonate; (b) in Brachiopoda and Mollusca, of calcium carbonate, silicon dioxide, or calcium phosphate
19. Tegument — sometimes used in Platyhelminthes for the integument, which is of unusual nature
20. Test — in Echinoidea, of calcium carbonate plates cemented together
21. Thecae — the calcium carbonate skeletons of Crinoidea
22. Tunic — a tough elastic outer layer usually of cellulose, in Tunicata
23. Zooecium — a case (gelatinous, chitinous, or calcareous) containing an individual animal or a colony, also called coenoecium (Bryozoa)

C. Histology of the Invertebrate Integument

As used in this chapter, the word integument is somewhat indefinite, being either the periderm in Hydrozoa or the complex exoskeleton of Arthropoda. It always includes an epidermis and often its secreted cuticle or exoskeleton. There is sometimes a second layer called dermis. One to three muscle layers may be intimately associated, and there may be a basement membrane either inside or outside of some of the muscles. There may be bristles or setae produced by the cells of the integument, and spines or stylets occur in a variety of forms and origins. Some of the simpler features of the integument are tabulated in Table 21.

1. Setae, Spines, Bristles

It would seem to be an easy matter to list the phyla in which the structures called setae occur. These include at least the Arthropoda and Annelida. In defining setae in the Arthropoda, they are said to be hair-like structures projecting from the body wall and each to be produced by a single cell. The apparent difference in the body wall of arthropods (exoskeleton) and annelids (cuticle) leaves some question of whether the setae on these are really identical.

When one also tries to add the movable "spines" of Chaetognatha, Mollusca, Brachiopoda, Bryozoa, and Platyhelminthes, and the "bristles" of Aschelminthes and Pogonophora, the question of basic similarity is beyond solution. It is even possible that some "immovable" spines or spicules may be comparable to setae in structure and origin.

In the Arthropoda distinction has sometimes been made between "cuticular appendages" (movable) and "cuticular processes" (immovable). These have also been cited as macrotrichia and microtrichia, but many quite large extensions are immovable and many setae are very small and movable. This distinction will serve to give us a definition of seta, in the broad sense, as an appendage of the cuticle, normally flexibly attached, and secreted by a single cell in the outer layers of the body wall.

In Insecta, at least, the flexibility of the seta is obtained by its own flexibility and also by ability to move on its base. The seta projects through the cuticle, appearing to rest in a socket. Its walls are continuous with the cuticle, which is thin at that point and recessed slightly. This thinness of the cuticle ("membranous ring") permits some movement.

There are at least 20 phyla in which structures like setae (spines, bristles) have been reported. The identity of these in structure and origin has usually not been elucidated. They are cited here with suggestion of what is reported, but the terms cannot be supposed to be distinctive.

Table 21
FEATURES OF THE INTEGUMENT

	Cuticle	Layers in epidermis, "hypodermis"	Dermis	Muscle layers	Spines, setae
Porifera	0	1	0	0	0
Mesozoa	0	0	0	0	0
Coelenterata	X/0	1,S	0	1/0	0
Ctenophora	0	1	0	Fibers	0
Turbellaria	0	1	0	3	0
Temnocephaloidea	X	1,S	0		0
Trematoda	X	1*	0	2/3	Spines
Cestoda	X	1*	0	Fibers	0
Acanthocephala	X	3,S	0*	2	Spines
Rhynchocoela	0	1	X	2—3	0
Rotifera	X	1,S	0	Bands	Bristles
Gastrotricha	X	1,S	0	Bands	Spines
Kinorhyncha	X	1,S	0	Bands	Bristles
Nematoda	X	1/0,S	0	1	Spicules
Gordioidea	X	1	0	1	0
Priapuloidea	X	1	0	2/1	0
Calyssozoa	X	1	0	1	Spines
Bryozoa	Zooecium	1	0	2/0	Spines
Phoronida	X	1	0	2	0
Brachiopoda	Shells	1	0	1	Bristles
Mollusca	Shells/X	1	0	(Various)	Bristles
Sipunculoidea	X	1	X	2/3	Spines
Echiuroidea	X	1	Cutis	3	Setae
Tardigrada	X	1	0	Bands	Bristles
Myzostomida	0			Bands	
Annelida	X	1	X/0	1/2/3	Spines
Dinophiloidea	X		0	1	
Pentastomoidea	X			X	
Onychophora	X	1	X	2/3	0
Arthropoda	Exoskeleton	1	0	Bundles	Setae, scales
Chaetognatha	X	1*	0	1	Spines
Pogonophora	X	1	0	2	0
Echinodermata	X/0	1	X	2/0	Spines/0
Enteropneusta	0	1	0	2	0
Pterobranchia	Coenoecium	1	0	1	0
Tunicata	Tunic	1	0	Bands/1	0
Cephalochordata	X	1	X	1	0
Vertebrata	0	1	X	Myomeres	0

Note: X, present in some form; O, absent; S, syncytial; *, of unusual nature; setae are produced by single cells, spines, and bristles usually by groups of cells (or as projections of the cuticle).

Platyhelminthes. Usually not cited under any term. Spines are reported in *Gyrocotyle* in the Cestodaria; it is not clear whether they are movable.

Acanthocephala. Small spines on the trunk; hooks on proboscis; both arise from the dermis, not the cuticle.

Rotifera. Sensory bristles of great length, "stiff hairs", "setose bristles", "skipping spines", sensory hairs.

Gastrotricha. Scales, spines, bristles; the spines are clearly not movable; the scales sometimes drawn to look like setae.

Kinorhyncha. Spines abundant, some movable by muscles.

Nematoda. Sensory bristles.

Gordioidea. Bristles that appear to be fixed spines. In *Nectonema* there are numerous natatory bristles, which must be movable.

Priapuloidea. Small spines are probably sensory; spines in and around the mouth.

Bryozoa. In drawings spines are shown (and labeled) on the zooecium.

Brachiopoda. Setae on the mantle edge, sometimes numerous and very long, each secreted by a single cell, movable; a seta sometimes with minute barbs or thorns; said to be chitinous.

Sipunculoidea. Body surface with scales, spines, thorns, and hooks; the spines and thorns generally hollow. It is said that each hook is secreted by a raised epidermal papilla covered by cuboidal epidermal cells. Some spines are continuous with cuticle but apparently movable.

Echiuroidea. "Anal setae" reported.

Tardigrada. Threads or thorns but no movable setae.

Myzostomida. Paired parapodia, each with a strong hooked seta; setae derived from setal sacs.

Annelida. Chaetae are movable setae. Chitinous or not.

Onychophora. Body surface with rings of papillae, each with a spine, sometimes associated with a sense organ.

Arthropoda. Chitinous exoskeleton has spines (immovable) and setae (movable). Sense organs may be tactile hairs; sensory hairs in statocyst. Scales are modified setae, others may be branched or plumose. Long setae on tarsi used for flotation. May contain poison.

Chaetognatha. Large grasping spines on each side of mouth; sensory bristles; large lateral tufts of bristles.

Pogonophora. Cutaneous bristles or teeth or thorns, not movable. Each epidermal platelet with a long bristle having a basal cell. Each bristle of metasoma formed inside a separate multicellular thin-walled sac; no one formative cell.

Echinodermata. The spines are part of the endoskeleton, movable but covered with epidermis.

Cephalochordata. Some sensory cells have hair-like structures.

2. Setal Structures

There are two ways in which setae, which are basically very simple organs, can be diverse. There are an astonishing variety of shapes and branchings of setae in different taxa, and setae can be integrated into groups that perform functions that are beyond the power of a single seta.

As shown in Figures 23 and 24, setae may be flattened into scales or spatulae, in endless shapes and surface sculpture; they may individually be long, slender, and flexible or short, thick, and rigid; they may be serrated or plumose; they may have a beaded shaft capped by a pear-shaped head; they may themselves be spiny; or they may be pointed and hollow to serve as weapons for transferring poison to anything touching them.

When set in close rows they can form combs. These are often used for cleaning other appendages. They may be used to form a sieve for straining out large particles of food.

They may stud a surface sparsely or densely or fringe any structure. They may occur on exoskeletal plates, in soft epidermis, or in sense organs.

3. Function of Setae

Setae serve a wide variety of functions:

1.   Cleaning — by combs of setae

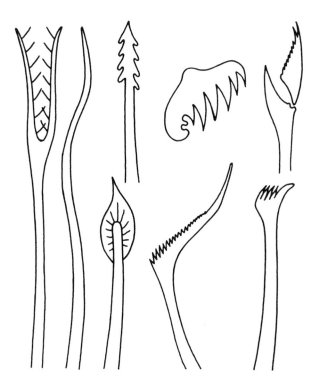

FIGURE 23.   Examples of setae from polychaete worms.

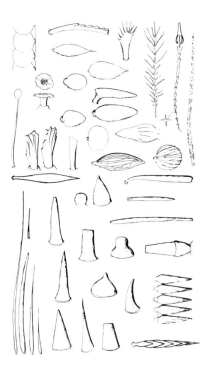

FIGURE 24.   Examples of setae from insects. (From Ferris, *Can. Entomol.*, 65, 1933.)

2. Transmission of poison — as in s.Lepidoptera
3. Sensing or tactile — on antennae
4. Ornamentation — in Crustacea and as scales in Lepidoptera
5. Locomotion — in Annelida
6. Respiratory movements
7. Reproduction
8. Support on water — by surface tension, as in aquatic Insecta
9. Excretion
10. Feeding — by straining food from the water, in m.Crustacea

4. Setal and Nonsetal Terms

Some of the terms employed in the Arthropoda and Annelida include:

1. Bristles — generally seta-like organs of multicellular origin
2. Macrotrichia — the movable processes, same as setae
3. Microtrichia — tiny immovable cuticular spines
4. Scoli — immovable processes or horns in some Insecta
5. Serrule — comb-like organs on chelicerae or pedipalpi of some Arachnida
6. Spines — in Insecta, immovable projections of cuticle
7. Spurs — large seta-like spines on tibiae of s.Insecta, but of multicellular origin
8. Uncinni — hooked setae of some Polychaeta

V. THE SKIN OF VERTEBRATES

The skin (or cutis) consists of epidermis (of ectodermal origin) and dermis (a mesodermal connective tissue). Both are said to be stratified, but the "layers" are not definite and would be more accurately termed zones. The *epidermis* consists of stratified squamous epithelium, and it gives rise to a variety of specialized structures ranging from feathers and hair to claws and glands.

The *dermis* (or *corium*) is also rather indefinitely subdivided into two layers. Beneath all of these is also a *stratum subcutaneum* of areolar tissue, which is usually closely associated with the fascia of the underlying muscles.

A *cuticle* is secreted by the epidermis only in cyclostomes. In fishes and aquatic amphibians, the epidermis is simple, but in higher forms it becomes thicker and indefinitely stratified. In terrestrial vertebrates the outer layer becomes cornified, the cells being filled with keratin. The surface cells die and are worn off or shed seasonally (as in snakes). In reptiles this cornified layer forms scales or scutes. In birds the scales have mostly evolved into feathers and in a few mammals scales persist, especially on the legs and tail and in the pangolin over most of the body.

Epidermal structures include scales, beaks, claws, nails, hoof, "true" horns (but not antlers), rhinoceros horns, feathers, hairs, and glands.

The dermis is a mass of fibrous connective tissue, with little diversity except in the bony fishes. There the dermis is full of bony scales or plates, forming a defensive armor. Among higher forms only turtles have such plates, although some elements of all skulls are of the same origin. Hair and feather follicles and glands usually project down into the dermis, where there are nerves and blood capillaries that are absent in the epidermis.

Functions of the vertebrate skin are numerous, besides the secretion of the corneous structures. Containment and protection are obvious in all; also defense against the invasion of microorganisms, warding off physical and chemical influences, regulating water absorption and loss, respiration, excretion, pigmentation, secretion, and temperature regulation.

VI. HARD-PARTS OF ANIMALS

A. The Structures

In many books with Vertebrate orientation, the bones, cartilages, associated structures such as teeth, nails, hooves, and antlers, and perhaps the skeletal muscles, are treated together as an organ system. The appropriateness of this is much reduced when one includes the entire animal kingdom. Because the exoskeleton of Arthropoda consists of epidermal structures that are indistinguishable from cuticles, they would not be called skeletons, and the various types of shells perform some support function, but do not classify well as skeletons. In other groups of animals there are other types of supporting mechanisms, often involving merely turgor or hydrostatic pressure.

It appears to be more realistic to treat the various skeletal structures in separate places. For uniformity with other books, vertebrate skeletons will be treated herein as a specialized organ system (Chapter 19). Arthropod exoskeletons are treated as epidermal structures or integument in the present chapter, and echinoderm endoskeleton will be treated as supporting structures in Chapter 20.

Many types of hard-parts are better known to paleontologists than to neontologists (students of animals that are not extinct), because they are often the only parts preserved in the rocks. Indeed, in several groups, they are the only parts known at all.

By structure, hard-parts may be classified as tests, spicules, thecae, loricas, tubes, chitinous exoskeletons, shells, dermal ossicles or plates, and scales, fin rays, carapaces, plastrons, beaks, feathers, hair, claws, nails, hooves, antlers, baleen, and horns. When viewed in terms of their tissue origins, a rather definite pattern appears.

Hard-parts may be secreted (1) on the outside of the body by the outer layer of tissue (epidermis), or by the surface layer of a protozoan cell. These include the tests of Foraminifera and other Protozoa, some of the coral of Coelenterata, the zooecia of Bryozoa, the shells of Mollusca and Brachiopoda, the exoskeletons of Arthropoda, and the dwelling tubes of Phoronida, Pogonophora, insect larvae, etc. The hard-parts may be secreted on the inside of the body, (2) by mesenchyme amoeboid cells (spicules in Porifera), (3) by the dermis or middle layer of the body wall — mesodermal in origin (dermal skeletons in Echinodermata and Vertebrata), and (4) by connective tissue — also mesodermal in origin (bones in Vertebrata).

Tests of unicellular animals are secreted by the surface layer of the cell protoplasm. They may extend into the cytoplasm or even into the nucleus, as happens in the Radiolaria. The tests may be extremely elaborate with spiraling chambers, radiating spines, and hollow lattice or lace-work structures of myriad shapes. (The so-called tests of Echinoidea are dermal plates cemented together.)

Spicules are produced in Porifera (by mesenchyme cells), in Alcyonarian corals (by mesogloeal cells), in Brachiopoda (by connective tissue), and in some Echinodermata (by dermal cells). These are all internal in origin, although sponge spicules may project to the outside.

Thecae or *calyces* may be either cup-shaped or conical. They may be a secretion of part of the animal body, or they may consist primarily of the main body wall itself, with or without hard-parts. Several other terms are applied to these parts in certain groups. The thecae of corals of the Hydrozoa and Anthozoa are ectodermal in origin; they may be calcareous or chitinous. The extinct Stromatoporoidea are also calcareous, and the extinct Graptozoa are chitinous. On the other hand, in the extinct Conularida the thecae are chitinophosphatic. In the Bryozoa a calcareous or chitinous zooecium is secreted by the epidermis. In pelmatozoan Echinodermata the theca is formed of dermal plates. In the Tunicata the tunic is composed of cellulose of mesodermal origin. A *lorica* is found in Ciliata, Flagellata, Suctoria, Rotifera, and larvae of Priapulida, but it represents merely the cuticle instead of a skeleton.

Table 22
PRINCIPAL CONSTITUENTS OF ANIMAL HARD-PARTS

	Calcareous	Siliceous	Phosphatic	Other inorganic	Organic	
					Also	Only
Protozoa						
Sarcodina	X 1	X 1	X 1	Al_2O_3, F_2O_3, $(Al,Fe)_2O_3$, MgO, CaO, P_2O_5, $SrSO_4$ [1]	X	
Flagellata						X
Ciliata						X
Porifera			X 2	$(Al,Fe)_2O_3$, MgO, CaO, P_2O_5, $CaSO_4$, SO_3 [2]		
Calcarea	X 3					
Demospongia						
Cyathospongia	X 4					X
Graptozoa						X
Conularida			X 4			X
Coelenterata						
Hydrozoa	X 2	X 4	X 1	$(Al,Fe)_2O_3$, MgO, CaO, SO_3, P_2O_5, $CaSO_4$ [1]		
Siphonophora						X
Stromatoporoidea	X 4					
Scyphozoa						X
Anthozoa	X 5	X 2	X 2	$CaSO_4$, $(Al,Fe)_2O_3$, MgO, CaO, SO_3, P_2O_5 [1]	X	
Platyhelminthes						X
Rhynchocoela						X
Acanthocephala						X
Aschelminthes						X
Calyssozoa						X
Bryozoa	X 4	X 2	X 5	$(Al,Fe)_2O_3$, P_3O_5, SO_3, CaO, $CaSO_4$ [1]	X	
Phoronida						X
Brachiopoda	X 1	X 2	X 1	CaF_2, $(Al,Fe)_2O_3$, MgO, CaO, SO_3, P_2O_5, SrO, $CaSO_4$, $FePO_4$ [1]	X	

Taxon				Notes				
Mollusca								
Monoplacophora	X 6					X		
Amphineura	X 2					X		
Solenogastres							Barium, fluorite	X
Gastropoda	X 5	X 2				X		
Bivalvia	X 7					X		
Scaphopoda	X 3							
Cephalopoda	X 2					X		
Sipunculoidea								X
Echiuroidea								X
Tardigrada								X
Myzostomida								
Annelida	X 4	X 4		$(Al,Fe)_2O_5$, P_2O_5, $CaSO_4$	1	X		X
Polychaeta			X 2	Sulphates, $CaSO_4$	2			X
Oligochaeta								X
Hirudinea								X
Pentastomida								X
Onychophora								X
Arthropoda								
Trilobita	X 8		X 9	$CaSO_4$	2	X		
Chelicerata	X 9		X 8			X		
Crustacea	X 9		X 9	$(Al,Fe)_2O_3$, P_2O_5, $CaSO_4$	1	X		
Arachnida								
Diplopoda	X 9		X 9			X		
Chilopoda								X
Insecta	X 9					X		
Chaetognatha								X
Pogonophora								X
Echinodermata	X 3,4	X 1	X 4	$(Al,Fe)_2O_3$, P_2O_5, MnO, $CaSO_4$ SO_3, $MnCO_3$, sulphates	2,5	X		
Enteropneusta								X
Pterobranchia								X
Tunicata								X
Cephalochordata								X
Conodontophorida			X					
Vertebrata	X 2		X 2	Strontium, barium	5	X		

Table 22 (continued)

PRINCIPAL CONSTITUENTS OF ANIMAL HARD-PARTS

1. Clarke, F. W. and Wheeler, W. C., The Inorganic Constituents of Marine Invertebrates, U.S. Geological Survey, Professional Paper No. 124, U.S. Geological Survey, Washington, D.C., 1922.

2. Nicol, J. A. C., *The Biology of Marine Animals*, 2nd ed., Sir Isaac Pitman & Sons, London, 1967.

3. Brown, C. H., *Structural Materials in Animals*, John Wiley & Sons, New York, 1975.

4. Nicol, D. and Eggert, D. A., Taxonomic summary of inorganic protective or supporting structures precipitated by animals and plants, *Trans. Ill. State Acad. Sci.*, 52(2), 95, 1965.

5. Prosser, C. L. and Brown, F. A., Jr., *Comparative Animal Physiology*, 2nd ed., W. B. Saunders, Philadelphia, 1961.

6. Hyman, L. H., *The Invertebrates*, Vol. 3, McGraw-Hill, New York, 1951.

7. Wilbur, K. M., Shell structure and mineralization in molluscs, in Sognnaes, R., Ed., *Calcification in Biological Systems*, No. 64, American Association for the Advancement of Science, Washington, D. C., 1960.

8. Moore, R. C., Lalicker, C. G., and Fischer, A. G., *Invertebrate Fossils*, McGraw-Hill, New York, 1952.

9. Richards, A. G., *The Integument of Arthropods*, University of Minnesota Press, Minneapolis, 1951.

Shells are properly only the secreted external hard-parts made by a mantle. They occur in Mollusca and Brachiopoda. They may be bivalved, spiraled, tubular, or in the form of a series of separate plates. In the Brachiopoda they are dorsal and ventral in position, whereas in the Mollusca they are lateral.

In the Brachiopoda the body wall consists of four basic layers: a one-layered epidermis, a layer of connective tissue, one or more muscle layers, and a peritoneum lining the coelom. The mantle lobes are extensions of this body wall, and they secrete the shells. The shells are either phosphatic or calcitic or both in alternating layers, covered externally by an organic *periostracum*. They consist of an outer and an inner layer.

In the Mollusca, the same structure appears, with the following exceptions: the epidermis is said to have a cuticle in most cases; there is no inner peritoneum because there is no evident coelom; the shells may be of aragonite, with two layers called *tegmentum* and *articulamentum*. There usually is a periostracum with up to four layers.

In both, the shell is secreted by the epidermis of the mantle, which is an extension of the body wall. The shells are usually covered by periostracum and consist of two layers of calcareous material.

A real chitinous *exoskeleton* occurs only in Arthropoda, where it is a thickening and hardening of the epidermal cuticle. It is divided into incompletely separated plates, and must be shed periodically to allow growth of the animal. It may be impregnated with calcium or magnesium carbonate or with tri-calcium phosphate.

Ossicles or plates secreted by the dermis and covered externally by epidermis are produced in all the Echinodermata. The plates may be free or may be united into a calyx or test.

Bones are found only in Vertebrata, where they are histologically related to cartilage. Both are of mesodermal origin. Bone consists of cells and the collagen/calcium phosphate secretions of these cells. Replacement of the hard-parts is continuous in bone, the cells resorbing and then re-forming the matrix.

Epidermal hard-parts are also universal in the Vertebrata. They include scales, "armor" plates, plastrons, teeth, hair, feathers, nails, claws, hooves, the outer keratinized sheath of many horns, and baleen (or whalebone).

Less obviously appropriate as skeletal objects but nevertheless hard-parts formed by action of the animals are the dwelling tubes of many groups. Phoronida may make a chitinous tube to which may adhere various debris. Or the tube may be made by cementing together fecal pellets. Many Polychaeta secrete tubes to hold back the surrounding sand. In Insecta and other Arthropoda these tubes are most likely to be spun or formed of silk fiber, perhaps with attached debris. The Pogonophora secrete a slender tube which fits closely to the body. The Pterobranchia live in aggregations of secreted tubes called coenoecia, of nonchitinous nature, but frequently with adherent foreign objects.

Among the unique hard-parts that occur in certain groups are the axial skeleton of some Anthozoa, the spiral brachidium of the lophophore of Brachiopoda, and the ossicles of the Aristotle's lantern in Echinoidea.

B. Hard-part Substances

The biochemical diversity of the hard portions of animals or their products is considerable. They include both organic and inorganic materials, as well as inclusions of both in a secreted matrix. The first include chitin, spongin, matricin, collagen, fibroin, tunicin, keratin, and other proteins or scleroproteins. The second include carbonates of calcium, magnesium, and strontium (all termed calcareous); oxide of silicon (siliceous); phosphates of calcium and iron (phosphatic); sulphates of barium and strontium; oxides of strontium, calcium, magnesium, and iron; and fluoride of calcium. The inclusions are fragments of soil, wood, etc., embedded in the organic secretions such as tubes.

The distribution of hard-part substances in the animal kingdom shows virtually no pattern. Each of the major substances occur in the Protozoa and in most of the large phyla. A few unique substances are found in just one group. There is usually a mixture of materials, such as calcium carbonate with magnesium carbonate, and the mixture may combine organic and inorganic substances, as chitin impregnated with calcium carbonate. Brown (1975) makes an incisive observation that "It is not possible to see any clear evolutionary trends in the type of structural material used or in the types of linkages employed."

Table 22 is a detailed list of the inorganic chemical substances found in the hard-parts of all animals. It is compiled from a variety of sources, as shown, and without standardization of citations. It is recognized that this is still a preliminary list. Only a few species in each class have been tested, and some tests have not been entirely trustworthy. There are also great differences in the proportions of the various materials in one type of hard-part. Especially is there diversity in the relative amounts of calcium carbonate and magnesium carbonate, and in the forms of calcium carbonate (calcite, aragonite, vaterite, and amorphous). For listing of organic components of hard-parts, see Chapter 8, under "Biochemicals."

REFERENCES

Barnes, R. D., *Invertebrate Zoology,* 1st ed., W. B. Saunders, Philadelphia, 1963.

Brown, C. H., *Structural Materials in Animals,* John Wiley & Sons, New York, 1975.

Clark, W. E. L., *The Tissues of the Body,* 6th ed., Oxford University Press, Oxford, 1971.

Clarke, F. W. and Wheeler, W. C., The Inorganic Constituents of Marine Invertebrates, U.S. Geological Survey, Professional Paper No. 124, U.S. Geological Survey, Washington, D.C., 1922.

Eaton, T. H., Jr., *Comparative Anatomy of the Vertebrates,* Harper & Brothers, New York, 1951.

Frey-Wyssling, A., *Submicroscopic Morphology of Protoplasm and its Derivatives,* 2nd ed., American Elsevier, New York, 1948.

Hyman, L. H., *The Invertebrates,* Vol. 3, McGraw-Hill, New York, 1951.

Imms, A. D., *A General Textbook of Entomology,* 8th ed., Methuen, London, 1951.

Ivanov, A. V., *The Pogonophora,* Consultants Bureau, New York, 1963.

Moore, R. C., Lalicker, C. G., and Fischer, A. G., *Invertebrate Fossils,* McGraw-Hill, New York, 1952.

Nicol, D. and Eggert, D. A., Taxonomic summary of inorganic protective or supporting structures precipitated by animals and plants, *Trans. Ill. State Acad. Sci.,* 58(2), 95, 1965.

Nicol, J. A. C., *The Biology of Marine Animals,* 2nd ed., Sir Isaac Pitman & Sons, London, 1967.

Prosser, C. L., Ed., *Comparative Animal Physiology,* 1st ed., W. B. Saunders, Philadelphia, 1950.

Prosser, C. L. and Brown, F. A., Jr., *Comparative Animal Physiology,* 2nd ed., W. B. Saunders, Philadelphia, 1961.

Richards, A. G., *The Integument of Arthropods,* University of Minnesota Press, Minneapolis, 1951.

Romer, A. S., *The Vertebrate Body,* 2nd ed., W. B. Saunders, Philadelphia, 1955.

Shrock, R. R. and Twenhofel, W. H., *Principles of Invertebrate Paleontology,* McGraw-Hill, New York, 1953.

Snodgrass, R. E., *Principles of Insect Morphology,* McGraw-Hill, New York, 1935.

Wilbur, K. M., Shell structure and mineralization in molluscs, in *Calcification in Biological Systems,* Sognnaes, R., Ed., No. 64, American Association for the Advancement of Science, Washington, D.C., 1960.

Chapter 19

UNIQUE ORGAN SYSTEMS

TABLE OF CONTENTS

I. Spongiocoel as a System 386

II. Demanian System of Nematodes 386

III. Tracheal System of Arthropods 387
    A.   The Nature of the System 387
    B.   Spiracles 388
    C.   Tracheae 388
        1.   The Tubes 388
        2.   Air Sacs 388
        3.   Tracheal Gills 388
        4.   Tracheoles 388
    D.   Diversity within the Tracheal System 389
    E.   Physiology of the Tracheal System 389

IV. Water-Vascular System of Echinoderms 389

V. Lateral Line System of Fishes 390

VI. Vertebrate Skeletal System 392
    A.   Bone Tissue 392
    B.   Classification of Skeletons 392
    C.   Individual Bones 393
    D.   Cartilage 393
    E.   Enamel and Dentine 394

References 395

I. SPONGIOCOEL AS A SYSTEM

Although sponges vary widely in shape and complexity, they are all built around a chamber or series of chambers into which the circulating water brings food and oxygen and carries out wastes. The cavity is a *spongiocoel* (commonly misspelled spongocoel). The entire life of the sponge is built around this system of chambers that carry the water that makes the life of the sponge possible. No such elaborate system, circulating water for respiratory and feeding purposes, exists in any other phylum.

The number and arrangement of chambers in the spongiocoel has been the source of a terminology of "canal types":

1. Asconoid — having one cavity unbranched, entry canals not flagellated, one exit canal (an ascon)
2. Syconoid — having one cavity but with many side chambers lined by flagellated cells, the entry canals numerous but not flagellated, one exit canal (a sycon)
3. Leuconoid — having multiple or branching chambers off the spongiocoel, lined by flagellated cells, numerous entry canals not flagellated, one or more exit canal (a leucon)
4. Rhagon — a developmental precursor of many of the leucons, with a large spongiocoel and flagellated side chambers

In all cases the incurrent canals open from the surface via pores called *ostia* (sing. *ostium*), often more numerous than the chambers. The excurrent canals, called *oscula* (sing. *osculum*), are always single in the ascons and in the sycons; they are often more than one but seldom numerous even in leucons.

The ostia are simply indentations of the outer surface, lined with a fine epidermis. Leading from each ostium is an incurrent canal, either short or long, also lined with epidermis but occasionally pierced by pores consisting of a single doughnut-shaped cell (*porocyte*) opening into an adjacent flagellated chamber. In all but the syconoid type, the flagellated chambers, which are branches of the exit canal, are completely lined with *choanocytes*. These are flagellated cells in which the flagellum is surrounded at its base by a transparent protoplasmic collar.

Water entering through the pores is passed over the collars by the stirring action of the flagella, and food particles are captured on the adhesive surface of the collar. Flow of water is apparently controlled by the slow constrictions of the porocytes and the osculum.

The function of the spongiocoel is to put water in contact with the tissues. This water brings food to the choanocytes and makes oxygen available to all the surrounding cells. It also brings in spermatozoa, to be captured by the choanocytes and passed on to the waiting ova.

II. DEMANIAN SYSTEM OF NEMATODES

Hardly to be classed as a mere organ is the system of tubes and other structures found in the females of one family of free-living marine Nematoda. The system may include a cell cluster in the wall of the intestine, a rosette of gland cells, some other glands, a duct along the uterus, and an external pore. It may be dual, with identical parts anterior and posterior to the ovary.

As described by Hyman (1951), "the system begins as a blind cell cluster in the dorsal wall of the midgut and runs posteriorly dorsal to the midgut as a thin-walled tube that gives off one or two connections into the adjacent uterus or uteri. These connections are encircled by a radiating cluster of gland cells termed the rosette. More posteriorly the tube forks and each fork, accompanied by a row of gland cells, the moniliform glands, opens to the exterior laterally shortly in front of the anus by a minute pore or set of pores.'' In some species there may be two uterine connections and even an opening into the vagina, or there may be fewer parts and connections.

The function of this system is not clearly understood. It is said to emit an adhesive fluid, which may play some role in reproduction. It is unlikely that so elaborate a group of organs could function only as a simple gland.

III. TRACHEAL SYSTEM OF ARTHROPODS

A. The Nature of the System

Nearly all animals have some method for obtaining molecular oxygen for their energy metabolism. This oxygen comes from either the surrounding air or the surrounding water. In most animals other than arthropods, the oxygen diffuses into the body through an epithelium either in a lung or on a gill, after which it must be transported to the cells by some means. In most arthropods the air itself is conducted to each cell by fine tubes called tracheae, and the oxygen is extracted at the cell surface.

Tracheal tubes occur only in the two related phyla, Arthropoda and Onychophora, but they are restricted therein to terrestrial species (sometimes secondarily living in water). In the Arthropoda they occur in the following classes: Arachnida (s.Araneida, m.Acarina, Phalangida, Solpugida, Chelonethida, Ricinulei), Chilopoda, Diplopoda, Symphyla, s.Pauropoda, and m.Insecta. They are also reported in the Crustacea (in the terrestrial Isopoda), where they are called pseudotracheae; these are merely lung cavities with short tubular branches.

In most arthropods the tracheae are organized into an elaborate system, which consist of spiracles, tracheae, and tracheoles. The segmentally arranged pairs of spiracles (the openings from the outside) usually each have a closing apparatus and an atrium or vestibule within. Elastic tubes (the tracheae) branch within their segment and unite with tracheae in adjacent segments (especially into longitudinal trunks). Sometimes tracheae are dilated into thin-walled vesicles or air sacs. Finally, each terminal tracheal branch ends among the body cells in minute and delicate canaliculi called tracheoles (often uniting into a capillary reticulum). Sometimes the tracheole actually penetrates into the cell. Most of these features may sometimes be lacking, or rarely all of them may be absent (see Apneustic, below).

The intimate association of these tubes with other organs is shown by these examples: in addition to actually penetrating the cells such as in some salivary glands, they may pass deeply into the ganglia of the CNS; they may enter between the fibers of muscles; and they are distributed over the organs of the digestive system, the reproductive organs, and even the Malpighian tubules.

In a slightly broader view of respiration, the tracheal systems of Insecta are described by these terms, which actually refer more to the spiracular openings:

1. Holopneustic — in which spiracles on the meso- and metathorax and eight abdominal segments are open and an elaborate system of trunks exists throughout the body
2. Hemipneustic — in which one or more pairs of spiracles are closed; subtypes of this include peripneustic with all open except on segments that do or will carry wings; amphipneustic with only the prothoracic and posterior abdominal spiracles open; and metapneustic with only the last pair of abdominal spiracles open
3. Apneustic — in which the spiracles are all either closed or entirely lacking, with the tracheae still either well-developed (operating with tracheal gills) or much reduced or absent (m.Collembola and s.Protura)

B. Spiracles

Spiracles may occur on any of the three thoracic segments and/or any of the nine abdominal segments. No adult insect has more than 11 pairs, although in some embryos the primordia of 12 pairs can be seen. Even 11 pairs is very rare in what are considered to be primitive groups. Two thoracic pairs and eight abdominal pairs is the prevalent number, but there may be one thoracic and six abdominal pairs, one or two thoracic and two abdominal pairs, just one or two thoracic and two abdominal pairs, or just one to three abdominal pairs alone. Other combinations also occur.

The spiracle is generally situated on a special plate of the exoskeleton, the peritreme, and the spiracle is assumed to also include the atrium and the closing apparatus. There seems to be no end to the diversity among spiracles, and the closing apparatuses vary from fixed combs that form a filter to plates movable by muscles and capable of forming a water-tight closure.

C. Tracheae

1. The Tubes

The tracheae are elastic tubes composed of three layers: a so-called basement membrane on the outside, a one-cell-thick epithelial layer (sometimes called ectotrachea), and an inner lining of chitin known as the intima (or endotrachea). The intima is continuous with the cuticle of the body wall of the insect and is cast off at each molt or ecdysis. On the inside the intima is finely ridged or thickened to form a spiral taenidium, which serves to keep the tube distended for the passage of air. These thickenings are usually spiral but interrupted at intervals; they sometimes form independent rings instead of spirals.

The arrangement of the tracheae is endlessly diverse, but they typically form trunks on each side connecting the spiracles, two dorsal trunks alongside the heart, two ventral trunks along the digestive tract and nerve cord, and many cross-connections between these trunks.

2. Air Sacs

The tracheae are sometimes dilated in various parts of the body into thin-walled vesicles or air sacs. They apparently are lined with intima but usually do not have the taenidia. They may be few and large as in worker bees or small and numerous as in some beetles. It was once thought that these air spaces lessened the specific gravity of the body by increasing the total volume. This is now seen as unlikely or negligible, and the sacs surely serve primarily as reservoirs for air (oxygen). They are well developed in most insects that spend much time in flight. Likewise, in several aquatic insects it is evident that the air sacs serve as storage depots for air. In one aquatic genus (*Chaoborus*) they serve as hydrostatic organs, their pressure being adapted to changes in ambient water pressure.

3. Tracheal Gills

There are in many aquatic insects gills that are filled with tracheae and tracheoles, rather than with blood. Oxygen diffuses from the surrounding water, so that the entire tracheal system is filled with molecular oxygen. Gaseous carbon dioxide is eliminated by the same mechanism.

4. Tracheoles

The terminal branches of the insect tracheal tubes are the tracheoles. These are delicate intracellular canaliculi, but closed at the extremity. They contain small amounts of fluid, which provides the moisture necessary for the diffusion of the oxygen through the tracheole membranes.

Although tracheal systems are reported in all classes of terrestrial arthropods and in Onychophora, it is seldom mentioned that in some of these groups tracheoles do not occur. This is apparently true of all except Insecta, although the details of tracheal endings are usually described only for insects. This difference would support the widely held theory that tracheae in the groups arose independently.

D. Diversity within the Tracheal System

Among the numerous diversities in the tracheal system of onychophorans and arthropods, one stands out: that tracheoles occur only in insects. In the others haemolymph must take over part of the transport, albeit for only very short distances.

Other differences seem to separate the insects from the others, including the nature of the spiracles, the extent of inter-connecting trunks, and other features. The diversity in many details is so great in the Insecta that the features of the other classes generally fall within this range. In the Insecta there may be no tracheae at all, simple tracheae may extend only in one segment; very elaborate ladder-like systems occur, and large expansions serve as air sacs. These do not seem to be constant in any one group but depend more on the manner of living of the species concerned. Aquatic insects of many orders have modifications such as permanently closed spiracles. In several orders species that fly continuously will have air sacs and highly developed trunk systems.

E. Physiology of the Tracheal System

Under this heading are sometimes listed the "respiratory movements" — rhythmical muscular movements of the body wall to move the air along the tracheae. These movements and diffusion are the only known mechanisms for movement of the oxygen, but how these movements affect the cylindrical and reinforced tubes is not clear, unless some of them are more elastic.

There is no question that oxygen reaches the cells principally through the tracheae and tracheoles, but the elimination of carbon dioxide is not merely the reverse of this. The carbon dioxide from the tissues diffuses in all directions and passes to the exterior partly through the integument and partly back into the tracheae. The proportions vary: in soft bodied insects the amount that leaves via the integument is large, and even in such hard bodied insects as beetles, much passes out through the intersegmental membranes.

Diffusion is the process that passes oxygen into the cells from the tracheoles, and where there are tracheal gills, diffusion brings oxygen in from the surrounding water. In case of very simple systems, or none, the oxygen passes from the tracheae into the haemolymph and then to the cells.

In certain larvae of Diptera that have only terminal abdominal spiracles, there is such a rich supply of tracheal branches to the hind part of the heart as to form a kind of lung.

IV. WATER-VASCULAR SYSTEM OF ECHINODERMS

In all Echinodermata, and peculiar to this phylum, is the water-vascular system, sometimes called the ambulacral system. The system is one of tubes in which hydrostatic pressure aids such functions as operation of the tube-feet or podia, but the functions of this system may include participation in locomotion, feeding, burrow-building, excretion, sensing, and respiration.

So much is still unknown about this system that it has been implied (Nichols, 1966) that little progress in its study has been made in 100 years. "Even today, almost every statement we make about the nature of the water-vascular system must be framed in similar uncertain terms and end with a question mark. For we still cannot state exactly the functional limits of the system, nor can we be at all certain of the role played by every part of it in the economy of the animal.''

The system basically consists of a ring canal around the oesophagus, a stone canal from this to the outer surface (usually dorsal), where it opens to the exterior through a pore or a sieve plate (madreporite), and a radial canal from the ring canal into each arm or along each ambulacral groove. In the ambulacra, the radial canals branch into many lateral canals, each of which connects to the ampulla of one tube-foot. The ampulla is a muscular reservoir that can contract to force water into the tube-foot, extending it.

The podium (tube-foot) itself is a tubular extension of the body wall, covered with epidermis and lined with peritoneum. It extends to the outside through pores between or through the skeletal plates. They are arranged in various patterns along the ambu-lacra and can be moved by muscles in the podial wall. The tip of the podium is often formed into a sucker, which can hold so tightly that the podium may break off before it lets go.

Other features of the system are a madreporic ampulla, to collect the ducts from the madreporite; a polian vesicle which may hang from the ring canal between each pair of radial canals, but there may be many or few; and Tiedemann's bodies on the ring canal which are thought to produce the amoebocytes in the canal fluid. The operation of this system is still much disputed, but tube-feet do sometimes help in locomotion and in food capturing and movement.

The frequent lack of assurance as to the function of parts of this system may be partly due to differences between groups, different emphasis on the several possible functions. It is supposed, for example, that the tube-feet (podia) were originally used only for food gathering, but in many recent echinoderms some of them serve also (or exclusively) a locomotory function. Although the stone canal may open to the exterior and admit seawater, in other cases it may open into the coelom.

There is almost endless diversity in the details of this system in the five Recent classes of echinoderms. The most obvious forms of this diversity are tabulated in Table 23.

V. LATERAL LINE SYSTEM OF FISHES

Recent books refer to an acoustico-lateralis system of sense organs that is found in all Craniata. It encompasses the lateral line system of fishes, the rostral canals of elas-mobranchs and aquatic Amphibia, and the labyrinth (inner ear) of all craniates. In most vertebrates these organs do not really form an organ system; the individual or-gans are united only by the nervous system. They are in part discussed in Chapter 17. The lateral line of fishes is such a complex of sensory organs with water channels and pores that it is usually treated as more than a series of sense organs. It is here described under its traditional name.

The *lateral line system* is described as consisting of canals and sense organs. The sense organs are neuromasts distributed in the skin, but particularly along a series of canals or grooves on the head and trunk. The canals may run nearly the length of the animal or form a complex pattern, but each has frequent pores to the surface. In both Chondrichthyes and Osteichthyes, some species may have the canals replaced with open grooves.

The nervous end-organs of this system consist of groups of sensory cells (neuro-masts) among the epithelial cells of the outer layer of the epidermis. Each has a pro-truding hair-process ensheathed in an elongated gelatinous cupula, waving freely in the surrounding water, and each is innervated by lateral line nerves. They thus respond to water movements, detecting both movement and very low frequency vibrations, and transmit their movement to the nerves. The placement of the sensory cells, in canals or

Table 23
WATER VASCULAR SYSTEM OF ECHINODERMS

	Tube-feet (podia)	Ring Canal	Stone canal	Madreporite or opening	Ampullae or podia	Polian vesicle	Tiedemann's bodies
Crinoidea	Mucus net food capture	Present	Many into coelom	None	None	None	None
Asteroidea	Feeding & locomotion	Present	One	Present	Yes	1 or more or none	5 pairs or 9 singles
Ophiuroidea	Mucus-producing	Present	One	To an ampulla	None	9 or more	None
Echinoidea	Mucus-producing	Present	One	Up to 5 or hydropore	Yes	5 "spongy bodies"?	None
Holothurioidea	Feeding & locomotion	Present	Usually 1 or many	Hydropore usually lost	Yes	1 to 50+	None

on the surface, enable the fish to detect currents, waves made by passing or approaching objects, the angle of such currents, the rate of movement, etc. Thus they are important orientation organs, as well as detectors of prey or enemies. It now seems unlikely that either hearing or temperature detection is involved. They occur in Pisces and aquatic larval Amphibia. In Amphibia the neuromasts occur without canals or grooves. Similar cells occur also in some invertebrate sense organs.

The so-called *acoustico-lateralis system* is one of those that consist of rather disparate elements, which is herein accorded less than system status. It includes the lateral line system (lateralis system), the rostral canals, and the labyrinth (inner ear). Although the latter is included as a sense organ in Chapter 17, the last two are briefly described here for those who wish to recognize the more inclusive system.

Occurring with the lateral line of elasmobranchs, a few teleosts, and aquatic Amphibia is a system of jelly-filled canals on the rostrum. They are called *ampullae of Lorenzini*. Some of the cells are innervated but specific functions seem to be uncertain.

The equilibration part of the inner ear of Vertebrata is better developed than the auditory part. This *membranous labyrinth* consists of a series of sacs and canals in the otic region on each side of the brain case. These form a closed system of cavities and tubes, lined by an epithelium and containing a fluid, the *endolymph*, not unlike the interstitial fluid. The sensory cells of the inner ear are comparable to the neuromasts of the rest of the lateral line system. Among the tubes are the *semicircular canals*. Altogether these structures register turning movements of the animals in all directions.

Labyrinths occur in all vertebrates but vary in many details from group to group. They are said to have four chief functions: maintenance and regulation of muscle tone, detection of angular acceleration, detection of gravity, and reception of sound.

Other sensory organs are found in the skin of fishes, but they are not nowadays considered to be part of the acoustico-lateralis system.

VI. VERTEBRATE SKELETAL SYSTEM

A. Bone Tissue

The supporting framework of most vertebrates consists principally of the tissues called bone and cartilage. In this they are distinguished from all other animals. This framework is a system in the sense that it consists of many organs — the individual bones, cartilages, and ligaments — and that besides support it serves the additional function as anchor for the muscles that operate the body. (Some aspects of this muscle/skeleton association are discussed in Chapter 20.)

One function of a bony skeleton is to support. This takes many forms and is accomplished in many ways. It is obviously incorrect to call the vertebrate skeleton an endoskeleton, without some reservation, because the part called the dermal skeleton may be external. The dermal skeleton can thus be like an arthropod exoskeleton in performing also functions of containment and protection.

B. Classification of Skeletons

The skeletons of vertebrates are usually described as consisting of two sorts called exoskeleton and endoskeleton according to whether the hardparts are in the skin or are in deeper tissues within the body. It must be remembered that this use of exoskeleton for deposits in the skin (either epidermal or dermal) is rather different from the exoskeleton of arthropods, which is actually a secreted cuticle almost always on the outside of the epidermis.

The epidermal hardparts, formed by cornification of epidermal cells and including scales, horns, hair, feathers, claws, nails, and hoofs, are dealt with under "Integument" (Chapter 18).

The dermal skeleton, formed by deposits in the dermis, includes scales, fin-rays, teeth, and bony armor. The endoskeleton includes the notochord and all bones or ossifications found interior to the skin of the body.

The skeletons of vertebrates are all much alike. The notochord is found in early development of all vertebrates. It persists into the adult in Cyclostomata and the more primitive Elasmobranchiata, Chondrostei, and Dipnoi. In all others it is replaced in the adult by part of the vertebral column.

The parts of the vertebrate skeleton are sometimes classified, as in Romer (1955):

Dermal skeleton
Endoskeleton
    Somatic skeleton
        Axial skeleton
        Appendicular skeleton
    Visceral skeleton

The number of bones in a vertebrate body is not great enough to require emphasis on such a scheme, and they are instead more likely to be dealt with in textbooks by the region of the body.

It should be noted that although the outer skeletal parts (bones) are usually cited as "dermal" and thus part of the skin, they are actually of mesenchymal origin.

C. Individual Bones

The more familiar bones are here listed. Each type occurs to some extent in all classes except where indicated otherwise.

1. Dermal skeleton — Plates, scales, scutes, denticles, teeth, antlers, carapaces, plastrons, part of skull and jaw
2. Axial skeleton — Skull, vertebrae, ribs, sternum (tetrapods only)
3. Appendicular skeleton
   a. Pectoral girdle — Clavicle, scapula
   b. Pelvic girdle — Ilium, ischium, pubis (together called the innominate bone)
   c. Appendages (all except Agnatha), including fins, flippers, legs, arms, wings; humerus, ulna, radius, carpals, metacarpals, phalanges; femur, fibula, tibia, tarsals, metatarsals, phalanges
4. Visceral skeleton — Gill skeleton (Pisces only), jaw elements (all except Agnatha), skull elements (all except Agnatha and Pisces)

Other hardparts occur on the surface of animal bodies, often in functioning connection with the skeleton, but these keratinized epidermal structures are not properly part of the skeleton.

Although *ligaments* form the attachment between bones, they are not themselves of bony nature. They are bundles of parallel connective tissue fibers and may be surrounded by a connective tissue sheath. Comparative data are not available.

D. Cartilage

Those internal skeletal structures which form the endoskeleton may be formed as cartilage in the embryo, but many of them are replaced by bone in the adult. Like all bone, cartilage arises from connective tissue. There are three possible developmental stages of the endoskeleton, as described by Hyman (1942): "mesenchyme, cartilage, and bone. The mesenchymal, also called membranous, stage is . . . the accumulation of mesenchyme in the skeletogenous regions. This is followed by the laying-down of cartilage in the mesenchyme, and this cartilage gradually takes on the shape of the parts of the definitive endoskeleton. In the lower vertebrates the endoskeleton may remain wholly or partly cartilaginous, and in that case the cartilage may be stiffened by the deposition in it of calcium salts. Such cartilage is said to be calcified. In most vertebrates, however, the cartilage is more or less replaced during development by bone, deposited by bone-forming cells. The skeleton is then said to be ossified. Bone produced in this manner by the replacement of pre-existing cartilage is known as cartilage bone.''

There are four principal types of cartilage, differing in the material interspersed in the matrix between the cells:

Hyaline cartilage. Flexible, rather elastic, with a translucent glass-like appearance, its matrix a complex protein with a network of collagenous connective tissue fibers in the intercellular substance, with rounded cartilaginous cells throughout. As on the opposed surfaces, of movable joints.

Elastic cartilage. Flexible, with many intercellular elastic fibers in addition to the collagenous fibers, opaque, and of a yellowish color. As in the external ear of mammals.

Fibrous cartilage (fibrocartilage). Little intercellular substance but large collagenous fibers parallel to each other, said to be essentially a densely arranged connective tissue. As in intervertebral discs.

Calcified cartilage. Hard, brittle, opaque; with a deposition of calcium salts in the matrix.

The above all occur widely in the phylum. One other type is found in larval lampreys. This is mucous cartilage, soft and diffuse, with branching cells.

Some invertebrates produce fibrous connective tissue. Ones that resemble cartilage are found in the radula of Gastropoda and the pen of Cephalopoda.

E. Enamel and Dentine

These are the major materials of vertebrate teeth. They differ from bone in structure and composition. Bone consists of fibrous connective tissue in lamellae, impregnated with calcium and magnesium salts (20%), and containing numerous branching bone cells. *Dentine* is usually harder than bone, with the secreting cells outside with long processes inward. It is the dentine of elephant tusks that is called ivory. *Enamel* is much harder, containing over 90% of the salts, which occur in long prisms, but with little other structure and no cells. Both bone and dentine are of mesenchymal origin, but enamel is of epidermal origin.

Teeth illustrate the contention that classification of bone is difficult. The teeth are unquestionably derivatives of dermal scales, so they are listed above as dermal skeleton. By moving into the oral cavity the teeth become functionally part of the digestive system and thus are listed also as part of the visceral skeleton. This mixture of embryonic origin and adult function as the basis of grouping is ineffective, but nothing better presents itself.

REFERENCES

Bremer, J. C. and Weatherford, H. L., *A Text-Book of Histology Upon an Embryological Basis,* Blakiston, Philadelphia, 1944.

Bourne, G. H., *The Biochemistry and Physiology of Bone,* Academic Press, New York, 1956.

Brown, C. H., *Structural Materials in Animals,* John Wiley & Sons, New York, and Sir Isaac Pitman, London, 1975.

Brown, M. E., *The Physiology of Fishes,* Vol. 2, Academic Press, New York, 1957.

Clark, W. E. L., *The Tissues of the Body,* 6th ed., Oxford University Press, Oxford, 1971.

Evans, F. G., Skeleton, vertebrate, in *Encyclopedia of the Biological Sciences,* Gray, P., Ed., Reinhold, New York, 1961.

Hyman, L. H., *Comparative Vertebrate Anatomy,* University of Chicago Press, Chicago, 1942.

Hyman, L. H., *The Invertebrates,* Vol. 3, McGraw-Hill, New York, 1951.

Imms, A. D., *A General Textbook of Entomology,* 8th ed., Methuen, London, 1951.

Jollie, M., *Chordate Morphology,* Reinhold, New York, 1962.

Marshall, A. J., *Parker & Haswell, A Text-Book of Zoology,* Vol. 2, 7th ed., Macmillan, London, 1964.

Nichols, D., *Echinoderms,* 2nd ed., Hutchinson University Library, London, 1966.

Romer, A. S., *The Vertebrate Body,* 2nd ed., W. B. Saunders, Philadelphia, 1955.

Chapter 20

MISCELLANEOUS ORGAN FUNCTIONS

TABLE OF CONTENTS

I.   Miscellaneous Organs and Organ Functions 398

II.   Body Spaces.. 399
        A.   Cavities as Organs 399
        B.   Embryonic Cavities... 399
                1.   Blastocoel.. 399
                2.   Archenteron... 400
        C.   Adult Body Cavities.. 400
                1.   Nature and Occurrence... 400
                2.   Pseudocoel 401
                3.   Coelom 401
                4.   Enterocoel.. 402
                5.   Schizocoel.. 402
                6.   Haemocoel 403
        E.   Function of Body Cavities 403

III.   Movement 403
        A.   Diversity of Movement 403
        B.   Brownian Movement.. 404
        C.   Diffusion... 404
        D.   Cyclosis 404
        E.   Amoeboid Movement (Pseudopodial Movement)........................ 405
        F.   Hydrostatic Movement 405
        G.   Ciliary and Flagellar Movement.. 406
        H.   Movement by Myonemes 406
        I.   Movement by Muscle Cell Contraction...................................... 406
                1.   Contractile Tissue.. 406
                2.   Muscles... 407
                3.   Muscle Innervation... 407
                4.   Muscle Striation.. 407
                5.   Phosphagens 409

IV.   Pumping Organs 410

V.   Supporting Structures... 411
        A.   Support in General 411
        B.   Turgor as a Support Mechanism 412
        C.   Skeletons and Miscellaneous Hardparts 412
        D.   Notochord 415
        E.   Terms for Supporting Rods 416

VI.   Organs of Defense... 416
        A.   Organs and Organelles.. 416
        B.   Trichocysts 416

C.   Nematocysts...417
D.   Ink Sacs 417
E.   Spitting Organs..418
F.   Poison Organs..418
G.   Pedicellariae...418
H.   Autotomy Plane..418
I.   Horns, Antlers, and Tusks 419

VII.   Secretory Organs...419
A.   The Organs 419
B.   The Secretions 420

VIII.   Storage Organs 420
A.   The Diversity...420
B.   Storage Sites 420
C.   Purpose of Storage 421
D.   Stored Materials...422
E.   Storage Behavior..422

IX.   Osmoregulation 422

References 423

I. MISCELLANEOUS ORGANS AND ORGAN FUNCTIONS

The following special organs are considered to be substantially independent of the six general systems described in preceding chapters:

1.   Body cavities
2.   Organs of movement
3.   Pumping organs
4.   Supporting structures, including notochord, but not the skeleton of vertebrates
5.   Organs of defense
6.   Secretory organs
7.   Storage organs

It must be noted that these classes of organs are not entirely exclusive, inasmuch as movement (of parts) cannot be clearly separated from locomotion and storage can be an activity of an organ, a tissue, or a cell, and also an activity of the whole animal. As nearly as possible distinctions are made as follows: treating such an event as representing a separate function or a complex activity of an individual; examining whether the function involves only a few or many organs, is largely independent of or dependent on brain control, or serves internally only a part of the organism or the organism as a whole.

It must be noted that many organs that are utilized in gross functions of the whole individual are not in the above list. They are dealt with in the following chapters on "Behavior" and include locomotion, grasping (for a variety of purposes), flotation, attachment, care of offspring (prenatal, before hatching, etc.), and feeding (grasping, sucking, masticating, etc.). It should be clear that although these are performed by organs, they are essentially activities of the whole individual.

II. BODY SPACES

A. Cavities as Organs

From the frequency with which the terms body cavity and tissue spaces are used in most textbooks, one might get the impression that animals are full of empty spaces. Even to speak of a body *cavity* in an animal can be misleading. There are no empty spaces — such a thing cannot exist in animals. Even the air sacs in fishes, birds, and some insects are full of air. Other cavities are always filled with organs and fluid, so that they too are not empty spaces at all. There are spaces between cells, tissues, and organs that are filled with some fluid; these are generally vesicles in that they are surrounded by an epithelium of some sort. Some are merely the large lumen of an organ. The contents of these spaces may be undiluted seawater, water charged with enzymes and food, intercellular or tissue fluid, pseudocoel fluid, coelomic fluid, or "blood".

Under some circumstances the body cavities of one animal may form a sort of system, as is the case with the haemocoel of arthropods, which is actually a major part of the circulatory system. Other cavities are very different, filled with blood, haemolymph, air, water, etc., and serving diverse purposes. It seems more realistic in animals in general to treat these cavities as organs rather than as systems.

As in so many other cases, the cavities of the body are referred to by numerous and sometimes ill-defined terms. These terms are also of several sorts, loose names for spaces of unknown nature and technical terms for specific cavities of known function and origin. The latter are usually called body cavities. It seems necessary to list them with explanations or definitions before they can be discussed systematically.

B. Embryonic Cavities

A few cavities appear in the early embryo, formed from intercellular spaces or by invagination of cell layers:

1. Archenteron — derived from an invagination into the blastula at the time of gastrulation; often the precursor of the digestive tract
2. Baer's cavity — same as blastocoel
3. Blastocoel — the cavity of a blastula (coeloblastula)
4. Gastrocoel — the cavity within the archenteron
5. Neocoel — body cavity formed by assembly of cells within a cavity (Remane, 1963)
6. Splanchnocoel — a specific coelomic cavity found within splanchnic mesoderm of an embryo

1. Blastocoel

In animals in which cleavage produces a hollow blastula (a coeloblastula) the cavity is a blastocoel. This is the earliest cavity in development in such animals, and remnants of it may persist into later stages (pseudocoel or haemocoel).

This type of blastula, and therefore this cavity, occurs in at least some members of these groups: Demospongia, s.Hydrozoa, Scyphozoa, Anthozoa, Gnathostomuloidea, Rhynchocoela, Gastrotricha, Nematoda, Gordioidea, Bryozoa, Phoronida, Brachiopoda, Amphineura, s.Gastropoda, s.Bivalvia, Scaphopoda, Echiuroidea, Archiannelida, s.Polychaeta, Oligochaeta, Hirudinea, Chaetognatha, Echinodermata, s.Pterobranchia, Enteropneusta, s.Ascidiacea, Cephalochordata, and Vertebrata.

Major groups in which no blastocoel occurs because a solid blastula is formed include: Hexactinellida, Siphonophora, Ctenophora, Platyhelminthes, Acanthocephala, Cephalopoda, and Arthropoda. For groups not in either list, information on the blastula type is not available.

The presence or absence of an identifiable blastocoel seems to have little effect on the type of gastrulation. For further treatment, see "Embryogenesis" in Chapter 5.

2. Archenteron

In those animals which produce a gastrula by emboly (invagination), the invaginated pouch is the archenteron. This occurs in at least the following groups: Porifera, s.Scyphozoa, s.Anthozoa, Rhynchocoela, Nematoda, Gordioidea, Calyssozoa, s.Gymnolaemata, Phoronida, Brachiopoda, s.Solenogastres, Amphineura, s.Gastropoda, s.Bivalvia, Scaphopoda, s.Echiuroidea, Archiannelida, s.Polychaeta, s.Oligochaeta, s.Onychophora (probable), Arachnida, s.Crustacea, Chaetognatha, Echinodermata, Pterobranchia, Enteropneusta, s.Ascidiacea, Cephalochordata.

It will be seen that there is only a rough correspondence between this list and the one of blastocoels. Invagination can take place into a solid stereogastrula as well as into a blastocoel.

C. Adult Body Cavities

1. Nature and Occurrence

As this word is usually used, the body cavities are the pseudocoel, the coelom, and the haemocoel of Arthropoda. To these customary ones, it seems appropriate in this book to add the spongiocoel, the gastrovascular cavity, and the rhynchocoel — all of quite different nature. The groups in which the first three occur are listed in later sections. The occurrence of the latter three are shown here, along with those in which there is no such cavity.

1. None — Mesozoa, Monoblastozoa, Cestoda, Cestodaria
2. Spongiocoel — Porifera
3. Gastrovascular cavity — Coelenterata, Ctenophora, Gnathostomuloidea, m.Platyhelminthes
4. Rhynchocoel — Rhynchocoela

In addition to these, it must be recorded that no actual body cavity is found in some of the groups that are listed as possessing them:

1. Mollusca — supposed to be coelomate but reported to be doubtfully present and, if present, of unknown manner of formation
2. Hirudinea — no cavity in adults, in which the organs are embedded in parenchyma, but there seem to be hints of coelomic pouches in the embryos
3. Pauropoda — supposed to have a haemocoel, but whatever cavity exists is filled with a large fat body
4. Ascidiacea — no coelomic cavity ever appears in the embryo

The terms that have been applied to body cavities include the following:

1. Abdominal cavity (see Peritoneal cavity)
2. Body cavity — any extensive space within the body
3. Cardiocoelom (see Pericardial cavity)
4. Coelom — a body cavity formed in the mesoderm and bounded by epithelium, in this position sometimes called mesothelium
5. Enterocoel — a coelom formed in mesodermal pouches from the archenteron
6. Gonocoel — (1) a coelomic cavity containing a gonad; (2) cavity of a gonad
7. Haemocoel — a blood-filled cavity derived from the blastocoel, in Onychophora and Arthropoda

8. Mesencoel — a coelom formed by re-arrangement of mesoderm cells
9. Pericardial cavity — chamber of the coelom that surrounds the heart, as in Mollusca and Vertebrata
10. Peritoneal cavity — the coelomic cavity posterior to the diaphragm (abdominal cavity), as in mammals
11. Perivisceral cavity — the abdominal coelom in Vertebrata
12. Pleural cavity — the coelomic cavity containing a lung as in mammals
13. Pseudocoel — body cavity derived from blastocoel and not completely lined with tissues of mesodermal origin
14. Schizocoel — a coelom derived from splitting of the mesoderm bands
15. Spongiocoel — the water channels of Porifera
16. Thoracic cavity (see Pleural cavity)

There are three principal types of body cavity in adult animals: the pseudocoel, the coelom, and the haemocoel. The distribution of these three, and of the two subtypes of coelom (schizocoel and enterocoel) is one of the basic characters used in the classification of animals. The distinctions seem clear-cut and important for this purpose, because they reflect different pathways in early embryology. Some peculiarities exist in the distribution of these cavities. The peculiarities are mostly well known but seem to be deliberately forgotten by classifiers, perhaps because they are embarrassing to the preconceived system. For example, see Priapuloidea, Brachiopoda, Tardigrada, and Vertebrata, in the following lists.

2. Pseudocoel

When the blastocoel persists into the adult stage, and no cavity appears in the mesoderm, this persistent cavity is called a pseudocoel. It is usually defined as not being completely lined with epithelium of mesodermal origin, but there is considerable diversity among the eight groups included.

The phyla (or classes) which are customarily classed as pseudocoelomate are these: Acanthocephala, Rotifera, Gastrotricha (some have three cavities, of which two seem to be coeloms), Kinorhyncha, Nematoda (thought by some to be enterocoelous), Gordioidea, Priapuloidea (unquestionably coelomate; Kaestner, 1967), and Calyssozoa.

Astonishingly, the Priapuloidea are usually described, even by some of those who accept this pseudocoelomate grouping, as having a coelom.

3. Coelom

The coelomic cavity is sometimes described as being separated from the body wall musculature by a peritoneal membrane of mesodermal origin, which also surrounds all enclosed organs, especially the digestive tract. There are some debatable cases, but it is clear that it must arise as a cavity in the embryonic mesoderm and that it must separate the body wall from the digestive tract. It may be formed as a split in the mesoderm (schizocoelous) or as pouches from the archenteron (enterocoelous). The former can also be formed by rearrangement of mesoderm cells (mesencoelous).

A coelom is found in most higher animals. There is no body cavity in the animals with a coelenteron or a gastrovascular cavity (GVC) and none in the Acanthocephala. The only groups in which the animals have an intestinal tract but not a coelom are the Rhynchocoela and the Aschelminthes. The former have no body cavity and the latter have a pseudocoel. However, there are exceptions of several sorts. The Priapuloidea are placed in the Aschelminthes but clearly have a coelom. Mollusca are always listed as coelomate, but the most careful writers admit that even the existence of a coelom in these animals is doubtful. From here on all groups are coelomate, with the following exceptions or difficulties:

1.   Dinophiloidea — apparently have no body cavity
2.   Hirudinea — coelom sometimes broken up or filled with cells
3.   Ascidiacea — coelom sometimes said to be entirely absent

It is possible that future work will clear up some of the inconsistencies noted in the foregoing and following lists. Until then this feature of the presence and nature of coeloms seems hardly usable in classification.

In several groups which apparently have a coelom, the manner of its origin is not known. They thus cannot be listed as schizocoelous or enterocoelous. These include Priapuloidea, Bryozoa, Phoronida, Myzostomida, Dinophiloidea, Archiannelida, Planctosphaeroidea, and perhaps Tunicata.

4. Enterocoel

The enterocoelous groups are usually listed as the following (difficulties are noted):

1.   Brachiopoda — in one of the two classes (Articulata) forms from one pair of pouches; the other class is schizocoelous
2.   Mollusca — coelom not obvious; source usually unknown but in some Gastropoda clearly neither schizocoelous nor enterocoelous; in Cephalopoda said to be a schizocoel
3.   Chaetognatha — from one pair of pouches
4.   Pogonophora — but clearly described as a schizocoel
5.   Echinodermata — from one pouch or one pair
6.   Enteropneusta — described as from one pouch or five
7.   Pterobranchia — (the number of pouches is not recorded)
8.   Tunicata — described as enterocoelous or as not enterocoelous; also recorded as none; said to form from one pair of pouches
9.   Cephalochordata — said to be from one pair or two pairs of pouches
10. Vertebrata — but always clearly described as a schizocoel

Some other groups, usually not listed among the enterocoelous groups include:

11. Tardigrada — clearly enterocoelous from 5 pairs of pouches
12. Pentastomida — clearly enterocoelous from 4 pairs of pouches

5. Schizocoel

The groups usually classified as schizocoelous are these (with difficulties noted):

1.   Bryozoa — said to be clearly not enterocoelous
2.   Phoronida — said to be clearly not enterocoelous
3.   Brachiopoda — the Inarticulata are said to be schizocoelous, but the Articulata are enterocoelous from one pair of pouches
4.   Mollusca — the coelom is not obvious, and its source is usually unknown; in some Gastropoda clearly neither schizocoelous nor enterocoelous; in Cephalopoda said to be a schizocoel
5.   Sipunculoidea
6.   Echiuroidea
7.   Tardigrada — the coelom is an enterocoel, from 5 pairs of pouches
8.   Myzostomida — the coelom is of undetermined nature but apparently not enterocoelous
9.   Annelida — the coelom may be absent in Hirudinea
10. Dinophiloidea — the coelom is of undetermined nature, if present

11. Pentastomida — the coelom is an enterocoel, from 4 pairs of pouches
12. Onychophora
13. Arthropoda — in at least one insect (*Musca*) it is said to be enterocoelous; Pauropoda are said to have neither coelom nor haemocoel

Other groups which seem to be schizocoelous include the following:

14. Priapuloidea — said to be neither enterocoelous nor pseudocoelous
15. Pogonophora — said to be definitely formed from one pouch, but pictured as forming from a single mass of mesoderm which later forms spaces; this seems to be schizocoely
16. Vertebrata — in spite of being always cited as having an enterocoel, in all groups the coelom forms by a clear-cut schizocoely, as always described for the chick embryo

6. Haemocoel

The only other major body cavity is the haemocoel of Onychophora and Arthropoda. Although this space is theoretically derived from the blastocoel as is the pseudocoel, it occurs only in animals with a coelom, although that cavity is greatly reduced. (Note that what is called "Haemocoel" in Mollusca is part of the coelom, called pericardial cavity.)

In Pentastomida the body cavity is said to be a haemocoel (Kaestner, 1968), but in this general account of segmented animals it is diagrammed as arising from four pairs of "pouches". If by pouches he means the usual pouches from the archenteron, the cavity would be an enterocoel. It is possible that the figures are intended to represent splits in the mesoderm; if so, this is a schizocoel which in part becomes a mixocoel (formed from several sources).

E. Function of Body Cavities

In general, body cavities such as coeloms seem to be included in the scheme of body structure to give the enclosed organs (viscera) liberty to move freely during their functional activity and to change more readily in size and shape during development.

In the Vertebrata, the coelom is partitioned by connective tissue into several cavities, including abdominal, pericardial, and two pleural, which serve to isolate some of the organs. Still other organs are not actually inside the cavity lined by the peritoneum but lie against its outside, pushing it inward. Sometimes these form hanging organs surrounded by the peritoneum, when they are said to be *retroperitoneal*.

In the Arthropoda, the haemocoel is functionally part of an open circulatory system. Such a system may have a pumping heart and a vessel extending into the head. The blood (haemolymph) leaves this dorsal vessel anteriorly and returns to the heart through the open haemocoel, bathing all the body organs on the way. It re-enters the elongate heart posteriorly through a pair of ostia in each segment.

III. MOVEMENT

A. Diversity of Movement

Movement occurs through the animate and inanimate worlds, and in animals it is familiar in two forms: the movement of organs and organelles and the translocation movement from place to place called locomotion. To these must be added the movements produced by physical forces: osmosis, streaming of air or water, gravity, and so on. The diversity of causes and results of movement make it difficult to isolate the translocation movements from the others. The following must be recognized:

1. Passive movement, being moved by exterior forces
    a. Materials, protoplasm, cells
    b. Individuals
2. Active movement
    a. Of protoplasm, organelles, cells, or organs, resulting in negligible translocation
    b. Of materials being moved about by action of organ or organelle: either outside of the individual animal or inside
    c. Of unattached cells (amoebocytes, gametes)
    d. Of unattached organs (urns, gametes, germ balls, ovarian balls)
3. Active movement resulting in translocation of the individual

Passive transport (1) is basically not produced by any action of the animal. It has the same result as locomotion: translocation to a new site, and it is briefly exemplified in Chapter 21 under "Locomotion". Item (3) is locomotion as usually understood. It is also discussed in Chapter 21 as an activity of animals. Although this leaves only (2) to be dealt with here, it does not remove all the problems. There is no sharp distinction between passive and active at the level of solutes, body fluids, and the surrounding medium. There is really no difference between the purposeful movement of some whole individuals and the purposeful movement of such detached cells (organs) as gametes.

The present section therefore deals with movement in ducts or body spaces, whether actively produced by the animal or resulting from physical forces, the movement of organelles and organs, and the contractions of cells and organs. It must be remembered that some forms of "movement", such as amoeboid movement, may simply change the relation of parts of the individual or may actually produce locomotion; similarly, ciliary movement may move part of the surrounding medium or may propel the individual.

Movement within the body is produced by a variety of forces. These are here discussed under the headings of Brownian movement, diffusion, cyclosis, amoeboid movement, hydrostatic movement, ciliary and flagellar movement, myonemes, and contractile cells. Morphogenetic movements are briefly cited in Chapters 5 and 11, on development and tissues, respectively.

B. Brownian Movement

The movement of very small particles in a liquid medium, due to their random bombardment by rapidly moving molecules of the medium, is called Brownian movement. It is not a biological phenomenon but a physical one caused by heat, a normal feature of colloidal suspensions. Any biological implications of this phenomenon are beyond the scope of this book.

C. Diffusion

In a solution, diffusion is movement of molecules from a region of comparatively high concentration to one of lower concentration. This is a physical process related to heat and occurs in all biological systems.

D. Cyclosis

Cyclosis is the flowing movement of protoplasm inside a cell. It is odd that this phenomenon, generally assumed to occur in many cells, is seldom referred to except in plants and Protozoa. In ciliates it moves the food vacuoles along what appear to be predetermined pathways.

Here again, there is no comparative data available on the diversity or distribution of this process among animals.

E. Amoeboid Movement (Pseudopodial Movement)

Movements of cells by means of changes in shape and by the streaming of cytoplasm to form pseudopodia are always described in Protozoa, where these may produce locomotion. Many cells move in body tissues, however, either passively or actively, and amoeboid movement is their principal form of locomotion.

As recounted in the chapter on cells, there are probably no animals without some sort of amoebocytes or wandering cells. These float in circulating fluids or actively force their way between the cells of other tissues. Although they are apparently ubiquitous, there is little information on how they differ from group to group. Various functions are ascribed to amoebocytes:

1. Spermatozoan transport — in Porifera
2. Spicule formation — in Porifera
3. Differentiation — into other types of cells as the need arises, especially in lower animals
4. Phagocytosis
5. Transport — of digestive enzymes
6. Transport — of wastes

Both general and specific terms have been used to specify these cells, including:

1. Alveolar phagocytes or dust cells — in lungs of Vertebrata
2. Amoebocyte — any cell capable of amoeboid movement
3. Archaeocyte — large wandering cell of Porifera
4. Basophil — a type of granulocyte with strong basophilic staining
5. Coelomocyte — an amoeboid cell in coelomic fluid
6. Eleocyte — cell derived from chloragogen tissue in Annelida
7. Eosinophil — a type of granulocyte with strong acidophilic staining
8. Granulocyte — a leukocyte with prominent cytoplasmic granules
9. Haemocytoblast — a form of leukocyte in lower vertebrates
10. Heterophil — same as neutrophil
11. Histiocyte — see macrophage
12. Kupffer cells — large phagocytes in liver of Vertebrata
13. Leukocyte — a white blood corpuscle in Vertebrata; including granulocytes, lymphocytes, and monocytes
14. Lymphocyte — a form of leukocyte in blood and lymph
15. Macrophage or histiocyte — a phagocytic cell in connective tissue spaces in Vertebrata
16. Monocyte — a form of leukocyte
17. Neutrophil — a type of granulocyte that stains lightly
18. Pseudocoelocyte — an amoeboid cell in the pseudocoel fluid
19. Steatocyte — a fat-destroying cell in some Insecta
20. Trephocyte — a coelomocyte that transports substances

F. Hydrostatic Movement

Hydrostatic pressure is a physical force originating in the pull of gravity or in any sort of pumping mechanism. The hydrostatic pressure produced by gravity is a static pressure that as often works against fluid flow as for it.

Although usually applied to liquids, the term hydrostatic will also cover all fluids and gases. The nature of the fluid under hydrostatic pressure in animals thus ranges from pure water through aqueous fluids like blood to air and molecular oxygen. Pressure from a pumping mechanism or from osmosis plays a part in many hydrostatic processes in animals, such as:

1. Flow of blood
2. Circulation of coelomic fluid
3. Eversion of probosces
4. Burrowing of worms and mollusks
5. Flow of water in the U-shaped tubes of *Chaetopterus* for feeding and respiration
6. Operation of leg segments in some Arthropoda
7. Movements of spine and palp in Arthropoda
8. Operation of tube-feet in Echinodermata
9. Erection of combs, peni, etc. in Vertebrata
10. Inflation of pouches, in Vertebrata
11. Movement of air in tracheae and lungs
12. Maintenance of organ or body shape by turgor

G. Ciliary and Flagellar Movement

There are several types of movement produced by cell processes of ciliary nature. These do not correspond to the usual distinction between cilia (short) and flagella (long). In the case of Protozoa, movement often produces locomotion of the organism. In the Metazoa there are a few small organisms (flatworms, larvae) in which locomotion by swimming or creeping is produced by cilia or flagella, but in most animals the ciliary movement propels fluids in ducts, passes materials along lining membranes, or sets up feeding currents in the surrounding water.

Cilia are hair-like cell organelles capable of bending forcibly in one direction, returning to their original position, and sometimes of reversing the direction of beat. Movement is now believed to be produced by bending of some of the internal fibrils (tubules), which itself seems to be produced by sliding movements of the fibrils over one another.

Flagella are similar in structure to cilia, although usually much longer, but their movement is more complicated and diverse. It is sometimes a corkscrew motion that pulls the cell forward, and sometimes a wave motion that pushes the cell. If the flagellum is covered with mastigonemes (threads), the effect of the corkscrew movement is reversed.

H. Movement by Myonemes

Myonemes are bundles of contractile fibrils in the cytoplasm of a few ciliate and gregarine Protozoa and in epidermal cells of some hydroid Coelenterata. They operate in much the same manner as simple muscle strands. Contraction is apparently initiated by a raised concentration of free calcium ions in the part of the cytoplasm in which the myonemes are located. In Protozoa they produce change of body shape or contraction of a stalk.

I. Movement by Muscle Cell Contraction
1. Contractile Tissue

Movement by muscle action is basically the result of shortening of the muscle cell or muscle fiber. It causes shortening of the body, withdrawal of extended organs, constriction of pores, peristalsis of intestines, distension of organs, propulsion of fluids in ducts, and others. These are not all distinct functions.

Contractile tissue exists in several forms. It occurs as isolated cells, as in the epitheliomuscular cells of Coelenterata; as separate strands, as in Rotifera; as whole muscles of many fibers, as in Vertebrata; as components of organs, such as the massive heart muscle or layers in the stomach wall; and as sheets of large extent, as in the body wall of animals from Platyhelminthes to Vertebrata.

Although muscle *cells* all serve the function of moving contraction, the muscle *or-*

gans serve the function of moving other parts of the body. The muscle movements are diverse, and the muscles themselves are structurally diverse. The term muscular system is sometimes used, but this exists with coordinated functions only in the muscles used in body movement and locomotion. In the Vertebrata, these muscles are part of the functioning skeletal system (Chapter 19). The other muscles of the body are treated here as special organs.

2. Muscles

The muscles of animals are diverse in a variety of ways: (1) the cells themselves are of several types, with some showing striations across the elongated cell; (2) they are innervated in at least two ways; (3) the contractile cells may act individually, or they may be joined in bundles that are the usual "muscles"; (4) the muscles may be discrete strands, or they may be arranged in layers; (5) the fibers of the body muscle layers run lengthwise (longitudinal muscles), around the body (circular), or diagonally; (6) these layers are combined in varying sequences in the body wall (see Table 14); and (7) the embryonic origin of muscles is diverse.

Many books classify muscles in three groups, called smooth, striated, and cardiac. This simple system obscures much diversity. As described by DuPraw (1968): "The gross appearance of muscle cells, as seen under the light microscope, is highly variable and includes cells that are conspicuously "striated" or cross-banded (but which vary widely in the details of banding), cells that show bands only during contraction, cells which show a diagonal or diamond-like pattern, cells which lack cross bands but have conspicuous longitudinal bands (sometimes in the form of coils or helices), and cells which appear to be entirely 'smooth' or without resolvable differentiations."

Although the distribution of these types is quite uniform among vertebrates, there is much diversity among invertebrates. To quote again from DuPraw: "in some molluscs the heart is striated while in others it is smooth; similarly, though Annelida, Onychophora, and Arthropoda have many structural features in common, most annelid and onychophoran muscles are smooth (including the locomotor muscles), while most arthropod muscles are striated (including the gut muscles). In scallops the adductor muscles contain two parts, one of which is striated and the other smooth."

3. Muscle Innervation

There are two methods of excitation of muscles. These are stimulation directly by nerves (neurons) and spread of excitation from cell to cell without involvement of nerves. The first of these is represented by any of three mechanisms. First, there may be a single synapse from a single neuron to a single muscle cell. Second, this single neuron may be multiterminal, providing synapses at more than one point on that muscle cell (at least as many as six can occur). Third, there may be innervation of one muscle cell by as many as five nerve fibers, each with a single terminal. These may be called (1) single innervation, (2) multiterminal innervation, and (3) polyneural innervation.

No clear indication of the distribution of these in the animal kingdom is available, but the first is presumably widespread; the second is cited in Crustacea and Insecta; and the third also in Crustacea and Insecta.

4. Muscle Striation

Muscle tissue is usually subdivided into three types: smooth muscle, striated muscle, and cardiac muscle, but it must be noted that both striated and cardiac muscle have cross-striations. However, there is a sharp difference between the so-called striated muscles of vertebrates and arthropods and other invertebrates in that the latter are in all other features similar to smooth muscle but with the striations added.

Table 24

OCCURRENCE OF MUSCLE STRIATION

	Smooth	Striated	Helical
Porifera	x	x	
Coelenterata	x	x	
Ctenophora	x		
Platyhelminthes	x	x	
Rhynchocoela	x		
Acanthocephala	?	?	
Rotifera	x	x	
Gastrotricha	x	x	
Kinorhyncha	x	x	
Priapuloidea	?	?	
Nematoda	x		
Gordioidea	x		
Calyssozoa	?	?	
Bryozoa	x	x	
Phoronida	x		
Brachiopoda	x		
Mollusca	x	x	x
Sipunculoidea	x		
Echiuroidea	x		
Annelida	x	x	x
Dinophiloidea	?	?	
Tardigrada	x		
Myzostomida	?	?	
Onychophora	x	x	
Pentastomida		x	
Arthropoda	x	x	
Chaetognatha		x	
Pogonophora	x	x	
Echinodermata	x	x	x
Pterobranchia	x	x	
Enteropneusta	x		
Tunicata	x	x	x
Cephalochordata	x	x	
Vertebrata	x	x	

It is usually not mentioned that in several groups the striations may be diverse, with some being described as helical or spiralled around the fiber. Striated muscle fibers have cross-banding, are unbranched, they are multinucleate (each derived from a syncytium of embryonic cells), the nuclei lie at the surface of the cells, and they are usually each innervated by one neuron. Smooth muscle fibers are not striated, have a single central nucleus, and are excited by spontaneous potentials spreading through the mass or by one neuron.

Cardiac muscle fibers are cross-striated and have periodic dark cross bands, intercalated discs, fibers branch and anastomose, the nuclei are central, and the fibers are excited by spontaneous potentials.

Although in Table 24 striated muscle is cited in many invertebrates as well as in vertebrates, there is a difference between those of lower invertebrates and those of arthropods and vertebrates, as reported by Beklemishev (1969): "We must point out that, when speaking of the striated structure of invertebrate muscle cells, we are thinking of the transverse striation of myofibrils as such and not of the striation of the cells as a whole. In the relative locations of contractile fibres, nuclei, and sarcoplasm, the transversely-striated muscle cells of different invertebrates usually resemble the smooth

Table 25

OCCURRENCE OF MUSCLE PHOSPHAGENS

	Phosphoarginine	Phosphocreatine	Other phosphagens
Protozoa	x		x
Porifera	x	x	x
Coelenterata	x	x	x
Ctenophora	x		
Platyhelminthes	x		
Rhynchocoela	x		
Mollusca	x	x	
Sipunculoidea	x	x	x[a]
Echiuroidea			x[a]
Annelida	x	x	x[a]
Arthropoda	x		
Echinodermata	x	x	
Crinoidea	x		
Asteroidea	x		
Ophiuroidea		x	
Echinoidea	x	x	
Holothurioidea	x		
Enteropneusta	x	x	
Tunicata	x	x	
Cephalochordata		x	
Vertebrata		x	

[a] In these three phyla there occur also the phosphagens listed as phosphoglycocyamine (s.Polychaeta), phosphohypotaurocyamine (s.Polychaeta), phospholombricine (all three phyla), phosphoopeline (s.Polychaeta), and phosphotaurocyamine (s.Polychaeta and s.Sipunculoidea).

muscle fibers of the same forms, and for the most part have nothing in common with the complex, polyenergid muscle fibres of arthropods and vertebrates.''

5. Phosphagens

The presence of two major phosphorus compounds in the muscle metabolism of animals has long been used to support the theory of the origin of vertebrates from echinoderms. Even today some physiology books say that all chordates and echinoderms utilize creatine phosphate whereas all other invertebrates utilize arginine phosphate. This is simply a case of continuing to copy an over-simplification after the facts have proved it to be wrong.

Phosphagens are guanidine phosphate compounds that are capable of storing energy. There are at least seven such compounds, of which only phosphoarginine and phosphocreatine are usually cited. These have recently been spelled phosphorylarginine and phosphorylcreatine and are also cited as arginine phosphate and creatine phosphate.

The reported occurrences of phosphagens in animals are shown in Table 25.

It is not easy to see evidence of phylogeny in this arrangement, just as it would be difficult to use such a character in a general classification of phyla. In the first edition of Prosser's *Comparative Animal Physiology* (1950), where a slightly less complete table is given, it is claimed that this distribution "supports the theory of the relation between this phylum (the echinoderms) and the chordates." In the second edition (1961), the same table is rearranged and simplified, omitting several occurrences mentioned in the text. This revised table is much more clearly in support of the echinoderm/chordate theory, but the conclusion has been reduced to this: "The presence of creatine in muscles of many polychaetes (not shown in the table) and of all chordates is an example of convergent evolution." In the third edition of that work (1973) the concluding statement is now: "The explanation of the extensive biochemical diversity of phosphagens of marine worms is unknown." We can only conclude that failure to recognize the diversity that exists can lead to unjustified conclusions.

IV. PUMPING ORGANS

All mechanisms called pumps move fluids from one place to another. In relation to the animal body, the purpose for which pumping is employed varies from the movement of a fluid from one place to another, to movement of water around the animal, and to locomotion of an individual by jet propulsion.

Examples of pumping and its purposes are cited here. There are similar devices in other phyla as well:

1. Protozoa — contraction of vacuoles, to discharge water
2. Porifera — slow contractions of parts of the body, to move water through the channels, aided by valves (porocytes and osculum)
3. Coelenterata — the contractions of the medusa bell in Hydrozoa and of the nectophores in Siphonophora, to produce locomotion by expelling water from the cavity
4. Rhynchocoela — muscular contraction of the blind rhynchocoel, to evert the very long proboscis
5. Mollusca — a chambered heart with muscular auricle, to maintain a partially open blood circulation
6. Cephalopoda — muscular constriction of the mantle, to eject water with sufficient force to produce rapid jet propulsion
7. Annelida — contractile vessels (hearts), to produce a pressure to move blood through the closed vessel system
8. Polychaeta — in tube-dwelling worms large fan-like parapodia may pump water through the tube (e.g., *Chaetopterus*)
9. Onychophora — muscular contractions of two storage glands to eject an adhesive material to entangle enemies
10. Onychophora — muscular dorsal heart tube, as in arthropods
11. Arthropoda — dorsal vessel or heart, aided by valves, to move haemolymph forward and eject it into the haemocoel
12. Crustacea — in some the maxillae are used as water scoops or bailers to drive water through the gill chamber
13. Insecta — a pharynx that sucks is expanded by muscles radiating to the head to suck in fluids, and then expels the imbibed fluids backward into the oesophagus by contraction of its own surrounding muscles
14. Insecta — in the fly *Phlebotomus*, "a piston-like chamber with a movable rod . . . is believed to regulate the seminal flow after the manner of a pump" (Imms, 1935)
15. Insecta — there are sac-like pulsatile organs in the legs of some Hemiptera that pump haemolymph independently of the heart
16. Insecta — a salivary pump, "the organ at the base of the stylet in piercing insects through which the products of the salivary gland are pushed into the victim" (Gray, 1967)
17. Pogonophora — a simple muscular heart with a complex closed circulatory system

18. Echinodermata — muscular contractions of the ampulla force water into the podium to produce its distension
19. Holothurioidea — pumping of water into and out of the muscular cloaca and rectal tree for respiration
20. Vertebrata — peristaltic muscle contractions, to force food along the intestine
21. Vertebrata — elaborate chambered heart to pump blood through a closed circulatory system

V. SUPPORTING STRUCTURES

1. Support in General

Because of our familiarity with vertebrates, the skeleton of bones seems to be an integrated system just as much as is the nervous system. In some other groups of animals there are a few instances of structures that seem to be comparable to bones and therefore could otherwise form part of a skeletal system, but in animals in general, there are no other instances of such special structures performing primarily the functions of support and muscle attachment. The so-called exoskeleton of arthropods is not structurally comparable to bones, because it is merely the hardening of the integument to the point where bones are unnecessary. Among its functions are included, however, those of support and muscle attachment. This apparent functional similarity is unrelated to their structure and location. It is therefore not reasonable to speak of all types of "skeletal systems" together as if they are comparable. Some of the various functions of the "skeletal" structures are discussed elsewhere.

Support mechanisms are sometimes referred to under the heading of "Supportive Tissue", where the nature of the material and cells is of most interest. Support may involve connective tissue (mesodermal in origin) or surface structures (epidermal). Some mechanisms like turgor may involve the entire organ or body. Support may be provided in these ways:

1. Turgor, the maintenance of cell and body shape by the pressure of the fluid contents; all soft-bodied animals
2. Hard spicules or ossicles in the body wall; in Porifera (in mesenchyme), in Anthozoa (in mesogloea), and in Holothurioidea (in mesenchyme)
3. A theca or calyx or zooecium of hard material to enclose the entire animal; in many Hydrozoa and Anthozoa, including coral made by mesogloea
4. Tunic of tunicin; in Tunicata
5. Shells secreted around the animal; in Brachiopoda, the shells of most mollusks may cover but do not really support the animal
6. Cylindrical tube, external, which encloses the animal and supports it; in Phoronida, s.Polychaeta, Pogonophora
7. Brachidium; in Brachiopoda, formed by epidermis of the mantle
8. Exoskeleton of hardened plates or rings; in Arthropoda (of sclerotized chitin)
9. Dermal plate; in Echinodermata
10. Test (endoskeleton); in Echinodermata, formed in the dermis (second layer of the body wall)
11. Cartilage and its relatives; in Cephalopoda and Vertebrata
12. Notochord; found only in Cephalochordata and Vertebrata (although similar tissues occur in Coelenterata, Mollusca, Arthropoda, Enteropneusta, Pterobranchia, and Tunicata, under various names)
13. Endoskeleton of bone; in Vertebrata (see Chapter 19)

Of these, the brachidium of Brachiopoda is treated under Hard-parts in Chapter 18. Vertebrate cartilage and bone are discussed in Chapter 19.

B. Turgor as a Support Mechanism

The maintenance of internal pressure or turgor is very important to many soft-bodied animals, especially to those like earthworms where locomotion is dependent upon constrictions of the body wall. In such animals there is not a single "space" distended by fluid but a separate space in each segment of the body, each using turgor to supplement the action of its body-wall muscles.

In the Rhynchocoela, turgor of the body is necessary for operation of the muscular pump that everts the proboscis. The pumping would not be effective if the soft body behind was not held rigid by turgor.

In Nematoda, where all movement is by alternate contraction of longitudinal muscles, turgor is essential to give something for the muscles to work against.

Turgor merges into hydrostatic pressure so that they can hardly be distinguished. Turgor is pressure in a closed space and is more likely to be maintained over long periods of time; it results in internal pressure that is hydrostatic in nature. If the system is open for flow, the hydrostatic pressure produces movement without building up a static turgor pressure.

C. Skeletons and Miscellaneous Hard-parts

Aside from vertebrate cartilage and bone dealt with in Chapter 19, the remaining support mechanisms are all "hard-parts" and mostly on or near the outside surface of the body. Such skeletal elements have one thing in common: they increase mechanical stability. These structures are described briefly here, but some of them are also described in the section on hardparts in Chapter 18 ("Integument").

Spicules. Porifera. Spicules are so well known in sponges that they are cited first. They are produced in the mesenchyme by amoebocytes (scleroblasts) but may project through the epidermis to the exterior. They are extremely varied in shape, but the shapes are specific to each species. The spicules may be few and fairly large or they may be small and very numerous. They are generally discrete, but they may be replaced by fibers of spongin that can form a dense network.

The spicules are either siliceous or calcareous. If the latter, they presumably each consist of a single calcite crystal, as it is the nature of calcite to form in this manner.

The gemmules of freshwater sponges may be amphidisks (dumbbell-shaped) which are specially produced by scleroblasts and placed radially in an outer layer. These are lost when the gemmule hatches.

Protozoa. It is not so well known that the skeleton of some Radiolaria may consist of separate spicules. These may be hollow rods or needles. They are siliceous (glassy) in composition. How these are formed projecting from a single cell seems to be little understood, except that the outer of the two layers of cytoplasm is capable of secreting the silica.

Coelenterata. In one group of Anthozoa, the Alcyonaria, the usual coral skeleton may consist of calcareous spicules. These are secreted by mesenchyme (mesogloea) cells; they may be fused together in various ways or cemented into groups. The spicules may be oval disks, spindles, rods, or needles, either smooth or warty or with longitudinal flanges.

Brachiopoda. In some brachiopods there are irregular calcareous bodies or spicules in the connective tissue of the mantle and lophophore. They are secreted by mesenchyme cells and may be very numerous. It is not clear whether these are of similar nature to certain long, thin fibers of calcite in the shells. The latter are each secreted by a single cell, and this presumably means that each consists of a single calcite crystal.

Holothurioidea. The dermis produces ossicles of many shapes, some of which are called spicules. The ossicles are generally of microscopic size and have also been called calcareous deposits. They are of endless shape and may be fenestrated, branched, wheel-like or dumbbell-shaped, or anchor-like. The ossicles are found in the general body wall, tentacles, podia, and the mesenteries. Larvae may have different types of ossicles than the adult of the same species. There is some question as to the chemical composition, but it is usually cited as calcite, sometimes replaced by iron phosphate.

Calyces. There is a great diversity in the terms used for the supporting structures that are roughly cup-shaped. The words commonly used are calyx, theca, zooecium, lorica, tunic, and hydrotheca. They occur in Protozoa, Coelenterata, Graptozoa, larvae of Priapulida, Bryozoa, Echinodermata, and Tunicata. It is not likely that in such a diverse list there should be much standardization of terms nor much similarity in the nature of the structures. They will be cited under the term that seems most appropriate in modern usage.

In Crinoidea, as in several of the extinct classes of Echinodermata, the endoskeleton forms a compact calyx and, usually, a stalk of superimposed disks called columnals. The cirri or arms are also supported by a series of cylindrical segments called cirrals. The calyx shows the pentagonal arrangement of the Echinodermata.

Loricas. In Protozoa, a lorica may surround the protozoan as a separate vase-like enclosure. In some it is chitinous and not clearly distinct from a test (see below). Loricas occur in Flagellata, Ciliata, and Suctoria.

In many Rotifera, the cuticle on the trunk is thickened and hardened into a lorica. This cuticle is secreted by the epidermis and is of scleroproteins, not chitin.

In the larvae of some Priapuloidea, a cuticular lorica is present, consisting of five somewhat separate longitudinal plates. It is lost by molting, as the larva becomes a juvenile.

Tunics. In Tunicata, a special mantle covers the body. It is composed of a cellulose called tunicin, found nowhere else among animals. It can be soft and delicate or tough and similar to cartilage.

Theca. In the Coelenterata, polyp members of both Hydrozoa and Anthozoa may form a cup-shaped theca, basically radial in appearance. In the former, it is called hydrotheca around a hydranth and gonotheca around a gonangium; these are both periderm secreted by the epidermis. Even a developing egg may be surrounded by a theca. In Anthozoa, the theca may be called a corallite; it may consist of two separate layers.

In the extinct Graptozoa, the tiny individuals of the colony are thecate. This theca is unique in being made of rings, each of which has overlapping ends forming an imbricated column up the theca.

Zooecia. The Bryozoa are often said to have a zooecium, which is a bilaterally arranged case broadly open above (filled by the polypide or living organism).

Shells. Like so many other words, shell has been used loosely for structures in many groups. Even the exoskeleton of a crab has been called a shell. If we disregard the "shells" of protozoans (tests), we can reasonably restrict "shell" to structures secreted by a mantle and composed of calcium carbonate or phosphate. These occur only in Brachiopoda and Mollusca.

In Brachiopoda, the shell may be of calcium phosphate and chitin (chitinophosphatic), as is usual in the class Inarticulata, or of calcium carbonate (calcitic), as in the Articulata. The shell always consists of two valves, dorsal and ventral, which may be different in size and shape.

In Mollusca, the shell is of calcium carbonate. It may be a single conical shell, a series of transverse plates, a spiral shell, or a pair of valves, one on each side.

Tubes. There are burrowing animals in most phyla. Animals in five of the phyla secrete external dwelling tubes, which serve as supporting structures. There is considerable diversity among these.

In Phoronida, a slender tube attached to the sea bottom is secreted by the epidermis. It is reported to be definitely chitinous.

In Polychaeta, dwelling tubes may be composed of various materials, such as sand grains or fern spores cemented together, or of a secreted organic material or of both. The secretions come from special ventral glands that lie in the coelom, each with a duct through the body wall. The tubes may be in the substratum, or encrusting various hard surfaces, or extending upward from the bottom. In Oligochaeta, the tunnels are produced by removal of the soil, and not enough is added to the walls to make a substantial tube.

In Insecta, some burrowing larvae line a short tube with silk, to make a chamber in which to pupate.

In Pogonophora, extremely long upright rubes are constructed, usually much longer than the worms — as much as 150 cm or nearly 5 ft. The tubes are elaborate, consisting of several layers, and often being variously annulated, even with each successive ring forming an encircling membranous cone. The material is a combination of chitin and a scleroprotein.

In Pterobranchia, the individual secreted tubes may form an aggregate called a coenoecium. It is not chitinous, but of otherwise unidentified material, secreted by epidermis in a glandular area of the cephalic shield.

Exoskeleton. The exoskeleton of Arthropoda is a sclerotized version of the chitinous cuticle. It is secreted by the so-called hypodermis (which is merely a cuticle-secreting epidermis). It consists of several layers and is made rigid by the incorporation of sclerotin, as the chitin does not by itself form more than a soft cuticle. The sclerotin is distributed to produce hard-plates (sclerites) separated by soft intersegmental membranes. A certain amount of growth is permitted by flexibility and expandibility of the membranes, but periodic shedding of the entire cuticle is required for further growth. The new exoskeleton forms beneath the old, with overlapping of plates and some temporary stretchability ensuring that the new skeleton will be larger than the old (at least during growth periods).

In many arthropods the chitinous cuticle is impregnated with minerals and said to be calcareous. The most common of these minerals is calcium carbonate, which may form as much as 95% of the cuticle and may occur in any of these three crystallographic forms: calcite, vaterite, and amorphous (thus excepting aragonite). Among the other elements that are usually present are silicon, aluminum, iron, magnesium, phosphorus, and sulphur.

Such calcareous exoskeletons occur in most Crustacea, many Diplopoda, and a few Insecta. (Example of the latter is the puparium of the fly *Rhagoletis cerasi*, where the calcium deposits come from the malpighian tubules at molting.)

This exoskeleton supports, contains, and protects, but it is also very important as the solid base to which muscles are attached. In this way it may function in locomotion, breathing, food handling, and other aspects of the life of the individual.

Endoskeleton of dermal plates. In all echinoderms there is an endoskeleton produced by the dermis and consisting of a calcite meshwork with large interstices. This endoskeleton may take the form of closely fitted plates forming a theca or test, or it may consist of small separate pieces called ossicles. Projecting spines and tubercles are also part of this endoskeleton; they are covered with epidermis.

In Crinoidea the endoskeleton forms a compact calyx (see above), which shows the typical pentagonal arrangement. In Ophiuroidea the superficial skeleton is of plates, the so-called shields, which are produced by the dermis but may be on the surface because of loss of the epidermis. A deeper skeleton is also present in the form of "vertebral ossicles" that form a support for the long arms. Such ossicles also form the five jaws of the Aristotle's lantern above the mouth.

In Asteroidea the endoskeleton consists of discrete calcareous ossicles that have the meshwork filled in with connective tissue. The dermal ossicles harden the body wall, and various sorts of projecting spines are covered with epidermis.

In Echinoidea the dermis produces an endoskeleton of closely fitted and cemented calcareous plates (forming a so-called test). There are 20 curved rows of these plates, forming 5 ambulacral grooves. The plates are unique in the phylum in being perforated for passage of the podia or tube-feet. In one family the plates overlap and the test is somewhat flexible. Spines, pedicellariae, and sphaeridia are covered by the epidermis.

In Holothurioidea the dermis produces the ossicle or spicules (see above).

Tests. The word test, referring to hard external parts of an animal, has no fixed meaning but is usually restricted to the groups Protozoa and Echinodermata. (The former is described below. The latter is described above.) In other groups such terms as shell, tunic, calyx, or zooecium are preferred.

Protozoa. The protective encasements of protozoans are variously termed pellicles, shells, tests, loricae, cyst walls, or cuticles. The word shell is most commonly used by protozoologists and in general textbooks, whereas in the large literature on fossil forms the word test is widespread. In some Flagellata, a gelatinous secretion incorporating foreign materials may be called a test. In Foraminifera the test may be siliceous, calcareous, or formed of various foreign objects (sand grains, sponge spicules) cemented by tectin (pseudochitin). The diversity of shape is very great, many of the tests have several chambers, some are spiralled. All these are secreted by the outer regions of the cytoplasm.

D. Notochord

One other possibly supporting structure needs to be recorded. The notochord is found in all vertebrates, at least in early development, but its distribution outside the phylum is colored by the common assumption that the ancestors of vertebrates must have had such a structure and that therefore homologs should be identifiable in the groups thought to occupy such a position.

In the embryonic development of higher vertebrates, a continuous unsegmented rod occupies the place later taken by the vertebral column. It persists throughout life only in Cyclostomata and in supposedly primitive members of the Elasmobranchii, Chondrostei, and Dipnoi, among the Pisces. The notochord forms from embryonic mesoderm or its precursors.

Basically a form of connective tissue, the tissue of the notochord differs greatly from that of cartilage or bone. The cells are thick-walled, their cytoplasm is homogeneous in appearance, and there is almost no intercellular material. The cells are also described as vacuolated, altogether surrounded by a laminated sheath secreted from within.

In Cephalochordata the cells are also vacuolated. The rod runs the whole length of the adult body and is universally called notochord.

In the Tunicata there is a "notochordal" structure only in the tadpole larva stage, a stage which is sometimes altogether lacking. The rod forms from certain cells of the archenteron, before mesoderm is formed. The structure of the rod and the nature of its tissue are neglected by most authors.

In Pterobranchia a structure resembling a notochord occurs. This structure is sometimes called a stomochord. It is a slender tube surrounded by about a dozen cells, running only from the buccal cavity into the proboscis.

In Enteropneusta, dorsally on the digestive tract, a long, narrow diverticulum extends as in the Pterobranchia only in the anterior part of the body. Histologically it is similar to the buccal tube. It is also called a stomochord.

Some textbooks now concede that the stomochord is not a notochord, but how then does one explain its location where a notochord would be expected, if one believes these two groups to be related to the Vertebrata?

E. Terms for Supportive Rods
1.   Notochord, a turgid rod of cells lying immediately beneath and parallel to the nerve cord in Cephalochordata and Vertebrata embryos
2.   Stomochord, a diverticulum of the buccal tube that projects into the protocoel of hemichordates
3.   Hypochord, a thin rod immediately below the notochord in some amphibian embryos
4.   Parachords, a pair of cartilages along the anterior end of the notochord in embryos of many Vertebrata
5.   Pygochord, in Enteropneusta, a structure is formed as a thickening of the gut wall or as a tube with an interrupted lumen opening at both ends into the gut; it lies in what may be called the caudal part of the body and extends back to the anus

Even beyond these structures, there have been suggestions of comparable organs elsewhere in the animal kingdom. In Turbellaria, Kaestner (1967) reports: "Especially interesting is the stiffness of the anterior end (of the body). It comes about by transformation of the cephalic intestinal branch, the cells of which form many vacuoles, become turgid, and obliterate the lumen. Sometimes the row of cells thus formed resembles early developmental stages of the notochord."

Jensen (1963) appears to support in detail the suggestion made in 1883 that the proboscis apparatus of the Rhynchocoela is homologous (and actually ancestral) to the notochord of vertebrates. Many details of the two are compared.

VI. ORGANS OF DEFENSE

A. Organs and Organelles
Defense is an activity that is frequently related to behavior of the whole individual rather than to activity of a single organ. There are, however, a number of organs whose principal function is defense, and they may react to stimuli without any recognition of the danger by the whole animal.

A list of the organs (and organelles) of defense would be long. In looking over such a list it would be evident that some of the listed organs have more than one function, with defense probably not the prime one. For example, defensive organs that are used also for food capture or feeding include trichocysts, nematocysts, spitting mucous glands, jaws or mandibles, beaks, fangs, and appendages armed with hands, claws, or talons. Although such organs with secondary defense functions are mostly omitted here, a few are of such great defensive importance that they will be described here.

In addition to organs there are two defensive structures in the Bryozoa, avicularia and vibracula, which are specialized individuals in the colony. They will be described under "Colonies" (Chapter 23). Organs for producing startling noises are cited under "Communication" in Chapter 22.

This leaves us with a manageable list of organs that are substantially defensive. With four additions from the structures cited above, they include trichocysts, nematocysts, ink sacs, spitting organs, poison spines, poison organs, pedicellariae, and abscission layers.

B. Trichocysts
Some of these are tiny vesicles that can "explode" to produce a thread with a ter-

minal dart (Ciliata and Dinoflagellata). Similar organelles may emit a toxin or mucus. The function of all of these is in question; defense is often assumed, but only food capture has been demonstrated. If defensive, they apparently fail when a *Paramecium* is attacked by a *Didinium*.

C. Nematocysts

The "stinging cells" commonly called nematocysts are diagnostic of the Coelenterata, although there have been reports of them in other phyla as well. In reality a nematocyst is an organelle produced by a cnidoblast cell. The cnidoblast or nematocyte lies in the epidermis, or rarely the gastrodermis, and its sole function is production of the "explosive" nematocyst organelles. The nematocyst is a capsule containing the mechanism. The term nematocyte denotes the cell containing the nematocyst, whereas the term cnidoblast is sometimes used for the cell during the period in which the mechanism is not yet mature.

The cnidoblast is derived from an interstitial cell; it moves into the epidermis (or rarely the gastrodermis) as it matures. The nematocyst develops as a capsule within the cnidoblast and is composed of a substance thought to be similar to chitin. Inside the capsule is a coiled tube (called a thread) which is attached at one end to the capsule wall. It discharges by eversion of the tube to the exterior. The tube may be open at the outer end (after eversion) or not.

At least 16 types of nematocysts are known, differing in the closure of the tube, its coiling, any ridges and spines on the tube (inside before eversion), and its visible division into a butt and a thread. In some, the tube is designed for penetration and anchoring of the prey, in others for emitting a toxic material, in still others for anchoring the animal.

The nematocyst is caused to discharge by appropriate stimulation of the cnidocil, a ciliary trigger projecting from the cell. The activation may be chemical or by touch. The stimulation is transmitted only to the capsule, which then expels the tube by releasing its pent up hydrostatic pressure.

The "sting" of an individual nematocyst of most species of coelenterate would not be perceptible to a human, because neither the dart nor the chemical penetrates the skin. If the nematocyst darts penetrate in sufficient numbers, one might experience both pain and more serious effects. On the minute animals of the plankton and nekton, the effect of one sting may be drastic, producing paralysis and leading to its capture.

The reports of nematocysts in other phyla are of three types. First, living nematocysts are saved from ingested hydras and utilized functionally by individuals in several phyla (see "Exploitation for Use of Transplanted Organelles" in Chapter 22). Second, in certain Ctenophora it is claimed that real native nematocysts do occur. This would be an unexpected development, as the phylum has regularly been distinguished from the Coelenterata because they did *not* possess nematocysts. Third, there are reports of nematocysts in Protozoa (s.Dinoflagellata). No matter how similar they are in appearance or function, the protozoan organelle is not formed in a specialized cell (cnidoblast) and would be better identified by a distinctive term.

D. Ink Sacs

In the region of the looped intestine, in such Cephalopoda as *Loligo* and *Sepia*, there is a large ink-producing gland with a reservoir and a duct opening into the rectum (in the mantle cavity). The gland secretes a brown or black fluid containing melanin pigment. The pigment is produced by oxidation of the amino acid tyrosin. It is stored in the reservoir and released when needed into the mantle cavity through the anus. Here it is mixed with seawater and is forcibly ejected through the funnel as a dense dark cloud, under cover of which the squid may escape from the threatening predator. It is also claimed that the ink, being an alkaloid, may itself be objectionable to predators, possibly by anaesthetizing the chemoreceptive senses.

E. Spitting Organs

More than one animal can emit substances from the mouth region to repel enemies or capture prey. The best example of defense by such a device is the Onychophora, which can eject from the tip of the oral papillae a slime that is effective in entangling would-be predators. The slime is a viscid albuminous fluid which soon hardens into threads in the air. It is not poisonous nor acrid but adheres to all objects except the onychophoran's own skin. It is produced in a pair of large slime glands lying in the haemocoel alongside the salivary glands. The ducts of these glands are long and dilated, to serve as reservoirs for the slime. The ducts open at the front end of the body and the slime can be ejected under considerable force, squirting three times the length of the body or more. Such animals as cobras may "spit" poison from a fang, but this would be under Poison Organs, below.

F. Poison Organs

Here are various spines, stings, and fangs that transmit poison from special glands. Spines that transmit poison are found in several groups: Polychaeta, Insecta, Echinodermata, and Pisces (at least). In some fishes the same function is served by certain specialized fin rays.

Among the polychaetes, for example, there are bundles of brittle setae, which contain a poison. The irritant is liberated when the setae are broken.

Among insects, some caterpillars of Lepidoptera possess so-called urticating hairs, which may have minute side spines, capable of tearing tender tissues, and which may also contain a poisonous secretion. Tubular setae are also known, filled with a poisonous secretion that is liberated upon fracture of the fragile setae.

In the Echinodermata, the echinoids particularly have spines which are part of the endoskeleton and therefore covered by the epidermis. In some cases, the spine is surrounded basally by a bluish poison bag composed of connective tissue and muscle fibers; the epidermis thus forms a poison sac that extends over the tip of the spine. Poison may be released when the spine is touched.

Poisonous devices other than spines are found in Arachnida, Insecta, Vertebrata, and others. They are tubular structures used to inject poison secreted by special glands. One need only mention the caudal stings of Insecta (Hymenoptera), the telson sting of scorpions, the cheliceral fang of spiders, and the specialized teeth (fangs) of some snakes. All of these are associated with poison glands, but there are probably no homologies between the various "stingers" or their glands. The poisons, of course, are diverse. Many animals secrete noxious materials, from the anal region (some insects, skunks, snakes) or from other parts of the body (some fishes, amphibians, lizards, turtles). For example, in the so-called horned toads, constriction of a blood vessel in the eye orbit forms a rupture through which blood is squirted at an attacker.

G. Pedicellariae

On the surface among the spines of Asteroidea and Echinoidea are curious structures called pedicellariae which often resemble a pair of pincers. They are part of the endoskeleton and may be variously modified from the pincer type and may have more than two projecting parts. Some of them snap shut on objects within their reach. They are thought to be defensive and to have also a surface cleansing function.

H. Autotomy Plane

Although autotomy is mentioned in many books, there appears to be no word in zoology to correspond with the botanical term abscission layer; yet in several animals there are regions at the base of appendages where the tissues permit breaking off of the appendage. Many books deal with the processes of autotomy and regeneration of the appendage; few deal with the nature of the tissue at the breaking point. Such a preformed breakage plane exists in some limbs of Crustacea and Insecta and in the tails of some lizards (Reptilia).

A very similar region of anticipated breakage is found in Polychaeta that undergo epitoky, although there is no protective function involved. The subsequent breakage is an act of autotomy, as cited in Chapter 21 on behavior).

Another unusual example of preformed zone of weakness is described by Hyman (1955) in the behavior of the Cuvierian tubules in some Holothurioidea. These blind tubules extend from the base of the respiratory tree into the coelom. In a threatened situation, these tubules are emitted from the anus, blind ends first, and entangle the intruder. "Reflection on the anatomy of the parts concerned will show that the tubules can emerge only through a rupture in the cloacal wall, and such rupture does in fact occur, probably at a preformed weak spot."

I. Horns, Antlers, and Tusks

Particularly among arthropods and vertebrates animals may have some sort of projecting "skeletal" parts that may be used for defense as well as for offense. In Arthropoda these are always outgrowths of the exoskeleton. They are described as spines in Chapter 18. In a few cases the "spine" may be very large, meriting the term horn. For example, a few beetles have very long horns on the head or pronotum; these may attain a length of three inches, or roughly as long as the body of the beetle.

Among the Vertebrata, horns are best exemplified in the Mammalia, where they are of several types: horns, antlers, fangs, and tusks, grading into mere spines. Horns also are of several types: in the rhinoceros a heavy horn is formed by fusion of many hairs; in some ruminants paired horns form from protrusions of the bones of the skull, and may be permanent or annual; in giraffes the horns are separate bones that fuse with the skull and are covered with hairy epidermis. In pronghorns the horns may be branched and shed annually. In cattle the paired bony processes are covered with a sheath of horny epidermal fibers. In deer the branched paired horns are bare bone (when mature) and are called antlers.

The tusks of elephants and sabre-tooths are very long teeth. The "tusk" of the narwhal is a single tooth developed into a long spear protruding from the head medially.

VII. SECRETORY ORGANS

A. The Organs

Secretion is the movement of material out of a cell. Although only cells secrete, when these cells form a tissue or organ, that structure is also said to be involved in the secretion. Secretory organs are called glands. The principal organ function is collection of the secretions from the component cells and direction of their delivery.

Glands may contain any number of cells, but they commonly consist of either many or only one. In higher animals they occur in great profusion and endless variety (104 are listed by Gray, 1967); and even in Coelenterata unicellular glands are numerous. Glands are usually classified by the function of the secretion. However, glands are sometimes described as *epicrine* (or *merocrine*), *apocrine*, or *holocrine*, even though these terms really apply to the cells only. Epicrine gland cells discharge through the cell membrane without damaging it. Apocrine cells discharge by rupture of the membrane and loss of some cytoplasm. Holocrine cells discharge by rupture resulting in destruction of the cell. (Merocrine is a term sometimes used in place of epicrine, but as the root mero- implies part or fragment, the term seems to be misplaced.)

The more familiar adjectives endocrine and exocrine have been applied to glands. They are intended to show the general place of discharge, endocrine into the blood-stream without a duct, exocrine through a duct into some other organ. This distinction has been somewhat blurred by the concepts of neuroendocrinology.

In some Oligochaeta and Hirudinea (together called the Clitellata), there is a region of 2 to 60 segments, called the clitellum, which has been cited as a reproductive organ. It may appear only at sexual maturity, and consists almost entirely of epidermis and glands, the latter secreting mucus, the wall of a cocoon around the egg mass, and albumin that surrounds the eggs. It can be regarded as a secretory organ, since that is its principal function.

There are a few secreting tissues that do not qualify as organs or parts of organs. For example, one is the chloragogen tissue, which envelops the digestive tract in all Annelida and fills the typhlosole of Oligochaeta. Another is an epidermis which se-cretes a cuticle or an exoskeleton.

There has been a distinction made in many books (especially with reference to ver-tebrates) between secretion of *useful products* and excretion of *wastes*. With these in separate chapters, one gets the impression that the two processes are unrelated, but in detailed descriptions of the activity of the excretory cells it is often evident that the process is actually one of secretion. Therefore in the list below such excretory products as seem clearly to be secretions of cells are included.

B. The Secretions

The purposes which the products of secretory organs may serve include at least the following: attaching (cement, byssus threads), attracting (scents, musk), cooling (sweat, water), digesting (enzymes), entangling (mucus, silk), excreting (sweat, honey-dew, amino acids, urea, uric acid, guanine, ammonia, inorganic salts), feeding (milk, mucus), insulating (fats and oils), lubricating (mucus), poisoning (toxins, saliva), pro-tecting (sepia, dyes, toxins, silk), regulating (hormones, water), supporting (spicules, cartilage, bone, spongin, collagen, nacre, cellulose, eggshells), and transporting (se-men).

VIII. STORAGE ORGANS

A. The Diversity

A variety of cells, organs, and structures are used to store materials of a wide variety, in a variety of places, and for a variety of purposes.

The processes by which substances can be stored in living beings are seldom treated together; each author is usually interested in the storage of a particular substance or class of substances only.

It is possible to store at least the following in cells, tissues, organs, or outside devices: food (both raw fresh food and digested nutrients), secretions, blood, inorganic chem-icals, organic compounds, water, and air or molecular oxygen, and even energy.

Among the substances often cited as not stored in living systems are proteins and amino acids, although several cases of temporary storage of protein are known (see below).

A few animals store material outside of the body. Besides humans, these would include earthworms, ants, birds, mammals, and probably others.

B. Storage Sites

Materials may be stored in the animal body in the following sites:

Cells. In Protozoa, a variety of metabolic materials are stored as granules, vacuoles, or crystals in the cytoplasm. These materials may be starch, glycogen, protein, and nucleic acid. In Metazoa, cells in the intestinal epithelium may store carbohydrates, fat, and even iron. Basal cells of the epidermis may store pigments. Much glycogen is stored in muscle. In many glands, even endocrine, the secretion may be stored as granules in the cytoplasm of the cells. Gastrodermal cells of *Hydra* may store protein, and the intestinal epithelium of starfish may do the same.

Tissues. Many cells store various materials, but the following tissues are multiple-cell storage sites:

1. Fat body — in Vertebrata and Insecta
2. Muscle tissues — glycogen
3. Epithelium — of the gut of Acarina and Insecta stores wastes; in Echinodermata it stores food as glycogen and fat
4. Connective tissue — may store chloride (salt)
5. Adipose tissue — stores "saturated natural fat"
6. Bone — stores phosphates, carbonates, and sulphates

Organs. There is much storage in organs, both in the cells of the organ and in its alveolar spaces. Examples include storage in the vertebrate liver (carbohydrates, lipoids, iron, water), in bone (calcium and magnesium salts), and in the spleen (red blood cells particularly); secretions include those from prostate and thyroid glands; other stored materials include air in the air sacs of some Insecta, ova or fertilized eggs in the ovarian system of many Insecta, and spermatozoa in special receptacles such as the spermathecae in Insecta.

In the ascidian *Perophora*, there are outgrowths from the stolons filled with mesenchymal cells and used to store substances to be used by neighboring buds. In some Cephalopoda, spermatophores are stored in a special reservoir off the mantle cavity (termed Needham's sac). In many animals a bladder stores excretory products until discharge.

Body cavities. In Acanthocephala the ovaries break up to form "ovarian balls" in the pseudocoel. Ova accumulate in the pseudocoel as well as in so-called "ligament sacs". In Echiuroidea the ova are in the coelom and accumulate in storage sacs on ciliated funnel tubes, that are probably modified nephridia. In Dinophiloidea the coelom functions as a uterus in storing eggs, and also as a spermatheca in storing spermatozoa in the female.

Of course, animals can also store such things as food outside of the body, in cavities or storage receptacles (see "Storage of Food" in Chapter 21).

C. Purpose of Storage

Materials can be stored for different purposes, such as:

1. As food, for later digestion
2. As nutrients (after digestion), for later use
3. As building materials, for later use or re-use
4. As accumulations of secretions, for later use
5. As accumulations of wastes, for later elimination
6. As accumulation of gametes, ova or spermatozoa, for mass liberation
7. As stores of spermatozoa in the female, for later use in fertilizing her ova
8. As isolation of foreign materials (such as insecticide poisons) to keep them from interfering with metabolism

D. Stored Materials

The following are among the materials that may be stored:

1. Food — both raw food and such nutrients as fats and carbohydrates as glycogen, starch (paramylum and leucosin)
2. Energy — as energy-rich bonds, especially in ATP
3. Water — for later metabolic use
4. Air or molecular oxygen — bladders, exterior bubbles, plastron, swim-bladder
5. Other inorganic chemicals — for later metabolic use (such as sodium chloride, calcium, magnesium, iron, lead, radium, carbonates, phosphates, sulphates)
6. Secretions — milk, yolk, saliva, hormones, wax, honey, silk
7. Wastes — excretions in bladders, nephrocytes, cuticle, fat body, calcareous corpuscles
8. Blood or blood cells
9. Reproductive products — spermatozoa, in male or in female; ova, in female
10. Sense impressions — in memory

E. Storage Behavior

Individual animals and also groups of animals store various materials outside of their bodies for later use. These activities are matters of behavior (see Part V).

IX. OSMOREGULATION

Virtually every aspect of an organism is normally under some sort of regulation. Most often cited are osmoregulation and ionic regulation. "Living systems at all levels not only react to changes in their environment (to re-establish equilibrium), but more, they control and regulate their reactions. Regulation of both structure and function is basic to the biological world." (Wilson, 1972). Within this framework there are two principal levels at which regulation can be discussed. These are the cellular and the organismic. The two are completely interdependent, but discussions usually are directed to one or the other.

Homoeostasis, the maintenance of normality in internal systems (metabolism), includes many processes working in an inconceivably complex interaction. Some of these processes have been suggested in our discussion of nerves and hormones, but an even larger portion are usually cited under such terms as osmotic and ionic regulation. The composition and volume of the body fluids, the production of secretions, and the maintenance of cellular contents are all subject to homoeostatic control.

One of the principal problems of animal life is described by Prosser (1973) as "to maintain inside the organism just the proper amount of water — not too much, not too little . . . Terrestrial animals must retain and use what water is available; freshwater animals must exclude water to prevent self-dilution; some marine and parasitic animals are in osmotic equilibrium with their medium, whereas others are more dilute than the medium and have the problem of taking in enough water while living in a plenitude of it" and, one might add, while excluding undesirable solutes.

In plants this regulation is primarily a function of individual cells. In animals there is a second level of regulation, by means of the circulatory and excretory systems, to provide for the operation of the organism as a whole.

Osmoregulation may be accomplished by any of the following mechanisms:

1. Limiting permeability to water
2. Limiting permeability to solutes, especially salts
3. Secretion (in or out) of salts against a gradient

4. Secretion (in or out) of water against a gradient
5. Storage of water or solute

In the writings on osmoregulation the only organs mentioned as performing this function are the excretory organs. Where individual cells are involved there may be contractile vacuoles. There is apparently much variation in the proportion of "excretion" devoted to osmoregulation as against nitrogenous waste removal, but these differences seem to be more related to the general habitat of the species than to its place in the classification of animals.

Osmosis, diffusion, and active transport are the chief processes involved in the maintenance of the equilibria. These act in mechanisms cited as excretion, resorption, ultrafiltration, and vacuole discharge. Experiments and measurements have been made of many animals, even many invertebrates, but the only comparative data are those related to excretory organs described in Chapter 16.

The second aspect of regulation is that of the concentration of inorganic ions. Seawater contains principally ions of chloride, sulphate, bicarbonate, calcium, magnesium, potassium, and sodium. Animals apparently tend to be similar in ion concentration to their medium, but there are many exceptions.

There is much analysis of the ion concentrations in different animals but little report of the mechanisms by which balance is maintained, nor of any differences between the phyla.

REFERENCES

Beklemishev, W. N., *Principles of Comparative Anatomy of Invertebrates*, (2 volumes), University of Chicago Press, Chicago, 1969.

Bremer, J. L. and Weatherford, H. L., *A Text-Book of Histology Arranged Upon an Embryological Basis*, Blakiston, Philadelphia, 1944.

DuPraw, E. J., *Cell and Molecular Biology*, Academic Press, New York, 1968.

Fry, W. G., Ed., *The Biology of Porifera*, Academic Press, New York, 1970.

Gray, P., *The Dictionary of the Biological Sciences*, Reinhold, New York, 1967.

Harrison, F. W. and Cowden, R. R., *Aspects of Sponge Biology*, Academic Press, New York, 1976.

Hyman, L. H., *The Invertebrates: Echinodermata: The Coelomate Bilateria*, McGraw-Hill, New York, 1955.

Imms, A. D., *A General Textbook of Entomology*, 3rd ed., Methuen, London, 1935.

Jensen, D. D., Hoplonemertines, myxinoids, and vertebrate origins, in *The Lower Metazoa*, Doughterty, E. C., Brown, Z. N., Hanson, E. D., and Hartman, W. D., Eds., University of California Press, Berkeley, 1963.

Kaestner, A., *Invertebrate Zoology*, Vol. 1 to 3, John Wiley & Sons, New York, 1967, 1968, 1970.

Kerkut, G. A., *Implications of Evolution*, Pergamon Press, Oxford, 1960.

Krogh, A., *Osmotic Regulation in Aquatic Animals*, Dover, New York, 1965.

Lockwood, A. P. M., *Animal Body Fluids and Their Regulation*, Harvard University Press, Cambridge, Mass., 1963.

Marshall, A. J., *Parker & Haswell, A Text-Book of Zoology*, Volume 2, 7th ed., Macmillan, London, 1964.

Potts, W. T. W. and Parry, G., *Osmotic and Ionic Regulation in Animals*, Pergamon Press, Oxford, 1963.

Prosser, C. L., *Comparative Animal Physiology*, 3rd ed., W. B. Saunders, Philadelphia, 1973.

Remane, A., The systematic position and phylogeny of the pseudocoelomates, in *The Lower Metazoa; Comparative Biology and Phylogeny*, Dougherty, E. C., Ed., University of California Press, Berkeley, 1963.

Richards, A. G., *The Integument of Arthropods*, University of Minnesota Press, Minneapolis, 1951.

Wilson, J. A., *Principles of Animal Physiology*, Macmillan, New York, 1972.

Part V
Behavior

"It has become obvious that greater attention has been paid to the behaviour and sensory physiology of insects than to the rest of the invertebrates . . . The mass of work still waiting to be done on invertebrates other than insects stands accentuated once again."

J. D. Carthy, 1958

Chapter 21

ACTIVITIES OF INDIVIDUALS

TABLE OF CONTENTS

I.   Introduction...428

II.   Response..429
        A.   Stimulus...429
        B.   Response Terms...430
        C.   Orientation 431

III.   Provision of Food 432
        A.   Food Capture...432
        B.   Provisioning...433
        C.   Entrapment and Tools...434
        D.   Storage of Food...434
        E.   Drinking 435

IV.   Prehension or Grasping 435

V.   Locomotion 436
        A.   Deliberate Movement 436
        B.   Methods of Locomotion 437
                1.   Aerial 437
                2.   Surface 437
                3.   Burrowing 437
                4.   Aquatic..438
                5.   Locomotion of Parasites...438
        C.   Migration 438
        D.   Prepared Transport 439

VI.   Protection 439
        A.   Direct Action 439
        B.   Evasion...439
        C.   Concealment 439
        D.   Control of Environment 440

VII.   Habitats...440
        A.   Diversity 440
        B.   Marine Habitats...441
        C.   Freshwater Habitats...441
        D.   Terrestrial Habitats..441
        E.   Parasitic Habitats...442
        F.   Distribution of Phyla 442
        G.   From Saltwater to Freshwater to Land 442

VIII.   Other Activities...443
        A.   Autotomy...443

    B.   Flotation 444
          1.   Flotation in Air 444
          2.   Floating on Water 444
          3.   Floating in Water 445
          4.   Flotation Mechanisms 445
    C.   Attachment 445
    D.   Bioluminescence 446
          1.   Light Production 446
          2.   Luminescent Organs 447
          3.   Occurrence of Luminescence 448
    E.   Thermogenesis 450

References 450

I. INTRODUCTION

Some books on animal behavior deal exclusively with senses, stimuli, and reactions to the stimuli. Others deal with the complex combinations of these as an animal performs its daily activities. These two approaches are roughly that of the two chapters in this Part, but both are usually called simply behavior. Thus, Simpson and Beck (1965) define behavior as "doing things", or as "externally directed activity".

In these two chapters a distinction was made on the basis of whether only the acting individual is involved or whether there is interaction between two. This is not a fundamental distinction and no formal terms are available for the two aspects. The interactions of Chapter 22 involve the same sort of activities as those described in Chapter 21, and both are behavior in anyone's definition.

So far, this book has dealt almost exclusively with parts of animals: cells, organs, and organ systems, and in a few cases with molecules. The so-called "organismal concept" warns us that each organism behaves as a unit, and much about that organism can be discovered only by studying it as a functioning whole. "Just as each animal species possesses its specific form which is different from that of all others, each species also is characterized by its own behavior" (Stern, 1938). This warns us that there is diversity in behavior — that animals are not all alike in the things they do as whole animals.

It is natural to think that related animals, those placed together in a group, will be alike in some aspects of behavior just as in structure. This assumption will often lead us into difficulties, as there are many cases in which "investigators, finding that one animal does a certain thing, take it for granted that all related species do the same thing. . . . We have observed numerous instances in which species of animals of the same genus are so closely related that microscopic inspection is necessary to distinguish between them, but in which the habits are completely different" (MacGinitie and MacGinitie, 1949).

This also means that although much diversity occurs it is at a level far below that at which diversity is tabulated in most of this book. Furthermore, the word behavior itself is used as a heading in this book with some trepidation. The modern field of animal behavior has become so highly specialized and attentive to certain experimental aspects of the responses of animals to stimuli that many of the day-to-day activities of whole organisms are slighted. It is principally these latter that will be included here.

Even within this framework, it may seen that scant space is given to this double field — the inherent activities of whole individuals or major parts of them *and* the activities that are loosely described as shared between two or more. The reason for this, as in other brief treatments in this book, is that although much is known about behavior of many animals, there is a great dearth of data that can be usefully compared between groups.

Therefore no attempt is made here to outline the entire field of the study of animal behavior. It will have to suffice to list the available data in those specific behavioral activities, such as locomotion and communication, in which it is found possible to tabulate differences between groups.

The reader will have noted that it has not been possible to make clear-cut distinctions between the subjects of some of the chapters and even of the parts of this book. This is particularly true of behavior, as it has seemed necessary and appropriate to deal with many aspects of behavior at the point where the structures are compared. As a result, at least the following specific aspects of behavior are dealt with elsewhere in this book, in the chapters indicated:

1. Asexual reproduction (Chapter 2)
2. Fusion of individuals and prereproductive behavior (Chapter 4)
3. Cleavage of zygote and apozygote and gastrulation (Chapter 5)
4. Emergence of larvae, torsion, epitoky, pupation, anamorphosis, strobilation, retrogression, inversion, metamorphosis (Chapter 6)
5. Molting, dormancy, regeneration (Chapter 7)
6. Behavior of cells (Chapter 10)
7. Behavior of organs (Chapters 12 through 20)
8. Behavior of colonies (Chapter 23)
9. Phagocytosis in Protozoa, feeding (Chapter 13)

The forms of animal behavior are exceedingly diverse, and they can be classified or categorized only with difficulty. The basic purposes of behavior are reasonably distinct; they are activities related to obtaining food, obtaining shelter and escaping from enemies, finding a mate and/or reproducing, and performing the physical and metabolic activities necessary to these. These are carried on in varying degrees in all life stages, but some stages and some individuals may not take part in some of these basic activities.

This chapter will show considerable overlap with Chapter 20, Miscellaneous Organ Functions. Although all behavior involves organs and their functions, it is sometimes possible to distinguish the direct function of an organ,' such as a gland, from an activity, such as attachment, that directly involves the whole animal. Even in the latter case, the activity is accomplished by organs, although it is serving the animal as a whole.

"Behavior" is herein dealt with as if it is a formal term with a definite meaning. It is in reality a word of such nontechnical origin that biology books and zoological dictionaries give no formal definition at all. It is apparently agreed that *behavior* is the sum of all the activities of an animal. It is also frequently noted that behavior results from the interactions of external and internal factors, of which the ones commonly referred to are called stimuli. The modern term for behavior in relation to environment is ethology.

II. RESPONSE

A. Stimulus

A stimulus is an influence that produces a change in part of the organism, frequently in a special organ called a sense receptor. The animal reacts to this change by action of such organs as muscles and glands.

The reaction is mediated to greater or lesser extent by the nervous and endocrine system. The reaction of the organ is a *response,* and the sum of the responses of the individual is behavior, but the term response is also used to signify the overall reaction of the individual to that stimulus. Thus, stimuli produce responses, the sum of which constitutes behavior.

Most of the response activities are discussed in sections of this book dealing with the relevant structures and their functions. There are, however, some general sorts of behavior that are involved with several of the basic activities and so need to be treated separately. They include at least feeding, orientation, locomotion, attachment, symbiosis and consortism, constructions, and habitats, as well as such aspects of social behavior as aggregations and societies, signalling, parasitic control, slavery, domestication, and parental care.

B. Response Terms

Two terms are used in referring to the responses of whole animals:

1. *Taxis* (pl.taxes) — a continuously oriented movement such as locomotion (applied to free-living animals)
2. *Tropism* — growth response (now generally restricted to plants and sessile animals

Taxes

1. Anemotaxis — movement in response to air currents
2. Chemotaxis — movement in response to a chemical stimulus
3. Galvanotaxis — movement in response to a direct electric current
4. Geotaxis — movement in response to the pull of gravity
5. Menotaxis — movement in response to a light stimulus, but at an angle to the source
6. Pharotaxis — navigational movements in response to landmarks, but thus requiring prior learning
7. Photo-horotaxis — movement in response to a sharp change from white to black in the background coloring
8. Phototaxis — movement in response to a light source (many Turbellaria respond negatively to light; many moths respond positively to a light source)
9. Rheotaxis — movement in response to a water current
10. Thermotaxis — movement in response to temperature differentials (one Turbellarian, *Crenobis alpina,* can distinguish water differing by as little as 3°C and chooses the cooler one)
11. Thigmotaxis — movement in response to a touch stimulus

Tropisms

1. Galvanotropism — a response to an electric current
2. Geotropism — a response in relation to gravity
3. Heliotropism — a response in relation to light from the sun
4. Phototropism — a response stimulated by light
5. Rheotropism — a response to flow of fluids
6. Thermotropism — a response to a heat source
7. Thigmotropism — response of part of an organism to a touch stimulus

The root -tropism, meaning a growth response, has been combined (especially in botany) into an endless number of compound terms, specifying not only the nature of the stimulus but the direction of reaction, the strength of the stimulus, or merely whether the response is positive or negative. The terms listed above are those most used in zoology, corresponding to the taxis terms.

Three other terms have been proposed as a system of classifying taxes: *telotaxis, klinotaxis,* and *tropotaxis.* These refer to use of two symmetrically placed receptors and experimental removal of one (see article on taxis by Carthy, in Gray's *Encyclopedia of the Biological Sciences*).

Although the responses intended here are of the whole organism rather than just one organ, they are still only the first level of what is collectively known as behavior. This is the sum of all the responses as they produce activities of the whole animal to accomplish some recognized purpose. These multiple activities are the ones whose diversities are briefly cited in the rest of this chapter.

C. Orientation

An animal orients itself by interpreting information received by sense organs. The orientation may be with respect to gravity, echoes of its own emissions, visual stimuli, other vibrational stimuli received, or chemicals in the medium. At a more specific level, these become more diverse. Individual invertebrates may orient themselves to water currents, to the edge of a rock or crevice, or along the stem axis of a seaweed. They may react to light, heat, pH, salinity, turbidity, water movement, and many others. Only a few examples of formal orientation can be described here.

Although all motile animals must orient themselves to a variety of stimuli, the literature on the subject is almost entirely on vertebrates. Here are found references to echolocation, sun-compass, lunar and star orientation, homing, the Coriolus force, and others. In most instances receptor organs are not known.

What they call a "sense of orientation" is described by MacGinitie and MacGinitie (1949) with respect to several responses: "A great many free-living animals of all groups show a definite response to water currents. This response is generally to head into the current. In most animals just what sense organs are concerned with making adjustments to current is not definitely known. In fishes the lateral line organs have been shown to function as perceptors of (water) current stimuli.

"Another response that is very common among marine animals is that of aligning themselves under the edge of a rock or with a crevice. This response is due to something more than the tactile sense, because animals will move sideways toward such edges or crevices before the sense of touch can come into play.

"Still another common response is exhibited by a great many animals that live among the seaweeds, that of orienting themselves along the main axis of the stem or frond of seaweed. Among animals that thus orient themselves are annelid worms, crustacea, gastropods, and fishes. When *Pentidotea resecata*, an isopod an inch or more in length . . . is taken from seaweed and placed crossways to it, the isopod immediately returns to a position parallel to the seaweed. It seems to have no particular choice as to whether it is heading up or down. If it is placed . . . at an angle of less than 90° it will turn toward the lesser angle. Certainly in the case of such an animal, the satisfactory result is obtained not through the sense of sight or response to gravity or through tactile stimulus, but through a sense that results in orientation parallel to the long axis of the seaweed. The other senses no doubt play a part, but the satisfaction derived from parallel orientation is something greater than that derived from a response to the stimuli received through any other known single sense organ."

III. PROVISION OF FOOD

A. Food Capture

Obtaining food is a procedure so different in different animals that the various methods seem to have nothing in common. Virtually all aspects of life can be involved in getting food, from locomotion, seeing or smelling, being born in the midst of the food, to growing one's own. There doesn't seem to be any simple way to describe the diversity that exists, except to single out some of the steps and tabulate the different means adopted.

Most animals cannot eat unless they first detect the food. This requires sense organs of some sort. These are described elsewhere, but quite a few animals have little use for food-detecting senses because during the feeding part of their life they live in the midst of the food and do not have to search for it. For example:

1.   In many plant-feeding insects the egg is laid in the tissues of the plant on which the newly hatched young is to feed.
2.   A parasite in an intestine lives in the midst of food that has been ingested by the host.

In many animals the adults feed the young directly by placing food in the mouth, so no detection is necessary on the part of the young animal (e.g., nestling birds are fed by the parents). Many other animals simply wait for food to come to them, with no direct detection and no direct action to overtake the food. For example:

1.   Detritus feeders — sit on the bottom of the sea and eat whatever falls upon them from above
2.   Ant-lions — build a trap and wait for their prey to fall in
3.   Clams — pump a current of water through the mantle cavity and select food from it.

Other animals burrow through the sand or soil, a slow form of locomotion, swallowing large quantities of the substrate, so that they can digest out of it whatever food is there and eliminate the remaining soil.

If animals are not fed and do not live directly in the food or where it will come to them, they must not only detect the food at a distance but take action to get to it and to take possession of it. This generally means locomotion, which may be running, flying, creeping, swimming, etc.

Some of these, and most other animals, have means to grasp food that they have reached or that has come to them and to manipulate it into their mouth. The mechanisms used for this ingestion may be

1.   Appendages — arms, legs, tentacles, proboscises, or jaws
2.   Special structures around the mouth — mouthparts or trophi
3.   Cilia — on exterior surfaces of small animals, whose food can be moved along ciliated surfaces
4.   Collars — of choanoflagellates
5.   Collar cells — in Porifera

Quite a few animals have no functioning mouth in this sense, taking their food directly into surface cells or by indirect means; for example:

Free-living animals

1. Protozoa by engulfing; using organelles such as choanocyte collars or pseudo-podia
2. Porifera by choanocytes in the water channels
3. Some Coelenterata in which there is little digestion in the GVC, with the food taken into cells directly
4. Colonial animals with the GVCs interconnected by tubes such as solenia (s.Hydrozoa, Anthozoa)
5. Nonfeeding colonial animals, specialized for other purposes, which are fed by their neighbors through interconnecting stomachs (s.avicularia of Bryozoa)
6. Most embryos, which receive nourishment from yolk previously stored in the egg
7. Placental animals, nourished from the blood of the parent through a placenta, as in Onychophora, Insecta (Dermaptera), and Mammalia

Parasitic animals

8. Those living in the ingested food of their host (Protozoa, tapeworms, Acantho-cephala)
9. Those living in other tissues (including blood) from which they can absorb food directly through the surface cells (Protozoa, Mesozoa, larval Trematoda and Gordioidea, male Echiuroidea)

If the food to be eaten is liquid it may have to be sucked in. This requires a muscular pump of some sort, usually called a pharynx. Feeding in this manner occurs all the way from protozoans to insects and to humans. Often a special tube is provided for this sucking function, as in the modified mouthparts of many Insecta.

Sometimes it is necessary, before liquid food can be sucked in, to puncture the prey in some manner; for example:

1. Teeth — as in vampire bats
2. Oral or buccal stylets (Nematoda, Tardigrada, Acarina)
3. Radulae — of some snails (Gastropoda)
4. Piercing mouthparts — of many Insecta (scale insects, mosquitoes, horseflies, aphids)

If the food is solid it may need to be torn to pieces or chewed, either in the oral cavity or outside; for example:

1. Chewing teeth, in mammals
2. Grinding by a mill formed by the gnathobases (the base of the legs), in horseshoe crabs
3. Grinding in a mastax, in Rotifera
4. Rasping by a radula, in s.Mollusca
5. Crushing or chewing by mandibles, in m.Insecta

The food is now in the digestive tract. The next activity is digestion. All further steps are treated in Chapter 13 under "Digestive Tract".

B. Provisioning

Provisioning is here taken to cover those instances in which animals store food in a "nest" or other place for later use by themselves or by their offspring. Besides humans, examples are well known in squirrels (nuts), ants (honey), and termites (grass and seeds). It is also represented by the "parasitic" wasps that supply paralyzed arthropods (often larvae or spiders) for their developing embryos. Other examples are cited under "Storage of Food", below.

Several forms of provisioning involve animals of two kinds. They include domestication and cultivation. These are cited briefly in Chapter 22.

C. Entrapment and Tools

Although it is sometimes said that only humans use tools in their activities, there are several forms of traps and lures that seem to be deliberately used for the fulfillment of a specific purpose. Although webs are perhaps better treated as constructions, in a later section, one may note the trapdoors and bolos of some spiders, the conical sand pits of ant-lions, and the lures used by some fish.

Because such traps and lures do partake of the nature of tools, we may mention some of the other tools used by animals. Sea otters use large stones to break the shells of the bivalves on which they feed; they carry these stones to the surface for this purpose.

Some arthropod appendages are used as tools. The coconut crab of the South Sea Islands is terrestrial: it is said that "Its food consists of coconut meat, which is obtained by hammering a hole in the 'eye' end of the coconut with its large chela (a drill) and extracting the meat from the inside through this hole by means of the smaller claw (a spoon)."

The radulae of gastropods are often used as tools, in much the same way as a file is used by humans.

The grains of sand in the statocysts of many animals are tools, turning a cavity into a delicate balancing instrument.

Even the fine hairs or darts fired by trichocysts of some Protozoa and by nematocysts of Coelenterata serve as tools. In use they are essentially lifeless objects.

An actual tool seems to be used by one spider. "In Australia there is a so-called 'Bolas spider' that secretes a short thread of silk at the end of which there is a sticky globule. This is whirled around and around by one of the legs and used to capture the spider's food" (Schechter, 1959).

D. Storage of Food

Storage of many things in the tissues or cavities of the body was tabulated in Chapter 20. Some animals also store materials outside of their body. *Homo sapiens*, of course, is the storer of virtually all things that exist on the earth, including other organisms, alive or dead, and energy in several forms. Aside from humans, food storage behavior is found in several animal groups. For example:

Food for the storer's use

1. Squirrels (nuts)
2. Shrikes (carcasses)
3. Woodpeckers (acorns)
4. Bees (honey)
5. Ants (converted food, seeds, etc.)
6. Termites (seeds, etc.)
7. Earthworms (dead leaves)
8. Spiders (immobilized prey)
9. Moles (living earthworms)
10. Shrews (living snails)

11.   Ants (partially digested food, in repletes)
12.   Parasitic insects (immobilized caterpillars or spiders)
13.   Ants and termites (leaf fragments or excrement, for cultured fungi)

Some ants store quantities of seeds. Germination is prevented by removing the radule. Deterioration is prevented by ventilation of the storage chambers or by occasionally bringing the seeds to the surface for drying in the sun. Among the ants that feed on fungi reared underground on cut leaves, the young queens store some fungal hyphae in a special pocket of the mouth, to start a new garden when a new colony is formed. Some other ants have a special pouch on the abdomen, into which food is placed by attendant workers, to be later drawn into the mouth and swallowed.

Earthworms often store leaf material in their holes. There it is enough to last them through inclement periods when they cannot forage.

In dealing with such storage behavior, it is not always clear that the "storage" is for more than a brief time, and it cannot always be specified who is to eat the stored food.

E. Drinking

An aspect of feeding that is often unmentioned is the intake of water for direct metabolic needs. In many animals enough or too much water enters with the food or as part of the food (such as blood), so that separate water intake is not required.

The only animals known to "drink" water as food are terrestrial ones: Arthropoda and higher Vertebrata. All others live in water (or aqueous fluid) and require no special intake of water, rather being often involved in processes of eliminating excess water.

"In many insect (eggs) . . . the absorption of water is the particular function of a specialized area of the shell and underlying embryonic tissues; these areas are sometimes called 'hydropyles'" (Davey, 1965).

IV. PREHENSION OR GRASPING

The structures used by animals to grasp objects (food, mates, enemies) are to some extent the same ones as used for burrowing, locomotion, and defense. They are found from the simplest animals to the most advanced:

1.   Pseudopodia (Protozoa)
2.   Trichocysts (Protozoa)
3.   Nematocysts (Coelenterata)
4.   Colloblasts (Ctenophora)
5.   Tentacles (Conularida, Dipleurozoa, Hydrozoa, Scyphozoa, Anthozoa, Ctenophora, Turbellaria, Temnocephaloidea, Trematoda, Rhynchocoela, Calyssozoa, Bryozoa, Phoronida, Brachiopoda, Hyolithelminthes, Monoplacophora, Gastropoda, Bivalvia, Cephalopoda, Sipunculoidea, Archiannelida, Polychaeta, Chaetognatha, Pogonophora, Holothurioidea, Pterobranchia, Ascidiacea)
6.   Captacula (Scaphopoda)
7.   Jaws (Oligochaeta, Arthropoda, Vertebrata)
8.   Proboscis, prehensile (Rhynchocoela, Sipunculoidea, Echiuroidea, Mammalia: Proboscidea)
9.   Jointed appendages (Arthropoda and Vertebrata)
10.   Podia (Echinodermata)
11.   Chelicerae (Merostomata, Pycnogonida, Arachnida)
12.   Spines, prehensile (Chaetognatha)

13. Tongues, prehensile (Amphibia, Reptilia, Mammalia)
14. Tails, prehensile (Mammalia)

V. LOCOMOTION

A. Deliberate Movement

Locomotion is movement, powered from within, from one place to another. The distance may be great or very small, the speed may be high or very low. Some forms of movement are difficult in practice to distinguish from locomotion, but deliberate action must be involved as well as change of location.

There are at least eight general forms of locomotion. These are amoeboid, swimming, burrowing, somersaulting, creeping/crawling, walking/running/jumping, looping, and flying. Some of these can be performed by a variety of organs or other means.

It is necessary to remember that animals may be able to produce locomotion in almost any developmental stage; the only one which usually cannot being the zygote. Developmental stages, or even adults, of many species do not make use of this form of behavior.

Other words are sometimes used to describe the locomotion of particular sorts of animals, but these can usually be referred to one or more of the above types. For example, climbing is usually either walking or crawling up a slope. In climbing a rope, a man is dragging his body and thus crawling up. The so-called euglenoid movement is partly amoeboid creeping and partly flagellar swimming.

The major forms of nonlocomotory movement in animals are discussed in Chapter 20. The emphasis there is on the mechanism producing the (active) movement:

1. Amoeboid movement
2. Ciliary movement
3. Flagellar movement
4. Myoneme contraction
5. Muscle contraction

Most such mechanisms of movement are capable in some circumstances of moving the entire animal, not just part of it, but individuals are not the only objects that can move themselves. Locomotion occurs at these five levels, with the mechanisms illustrated:

1. Cells — Protozoa and many isolated cells of Metazoa, by these organelles: cilia, ciliary membranelles, flagella, flagellar membranelles, undulating membranes, pseudopodia (which are the result not the cause of locomotion), tentacles
2. Organs — some detached organs, such as urns and gametes by means of cilia and flagella
3. Individuals — unicellular or multicellular, by organelles as in (1) above or by organs, such as: jointed legs in Arthropoda and Vertebrata, wings, jet-propulsion funnel, muscular foot, antennae for swimming as in some Crustacea, looping with suckers as holdfasts, tentacles, undulating bell, cilia for swimming or creeping, flagella, ctenidial cilia in Ctenophora, unjointed legs in Onychophora, fins for swimming in Vertebrata (in Chaetognatha and Cephalopoda the fins aid in steering but do not produce the motion), tube feet in Echinodermata for crawling by pulling the body along, and parapodia for swimming in Annelida
4. Colonies — of unicellular or multicellular animals, by organelles of the individual cells
5. Populations — through the locomotion of the individuals

All of these are independent units producing the movement and controlling it; the movement they produce is locomotion. It is more common to speak of the moving cells and organs as being motile, but there is no real distinction between motility and locomotion in respect to these isolated objects. Motility might not always indicate directed or purposeful movement, but for that matter even some locomotion seems to be largely random.

It is not easy to separate locomotion from simple movement, as there is an area of overlap. Furthermore, some animals move from one place to another at their own volition but without any activity that can be called locomotion. For example, a man may travel considerable distances on horseback, but the man produces no locomotion — he arranged for his transport by the horse (or by an automobile).

In the following paragraphs, the forms of locomotion are related to the medium or surface through or over which the movement is accomplished. Thus, a locomotion is surface if the animal is moving over the surface of the earth, whether the earth is at that point covered with air or with water. An "aquatic" insect creeping on the lake bottom is thus performing surface locomotion, not aquatic locomotion. The latter can only be done by swimming. The former is independent of the overlying material.

B. Methods of Locomotion

There are four principal sets of surroundings through which animals move. These are identified as aerial, surface, burrowing, and aquatic (freshwater and marine). In each of these there are various forms of propulsion.

1. Aerial

This is accomplished by only one method — *flying*. Four groups of animals have attained this most difficult form of locomotion: insects, reptiles, birds, and bats. There is little similarity among these except in having lightened bodies and the use of movable air foils (wings of different types). Other animals whose movement is sometimes erroneously assumed to be flying are the flying fish, which merely soar when in the air; spiders, which are passively carried by balloons; and flying squirrels, which are only planing, while falling.

2. Surface

This is represented by such terms as *walking* (with appendages), *creeping* (by body movements or by cilia or by amoeboid movements), and *somersaulting* (looping of the entire body). Walking would include running, jumping, climbing, and even dragging the body, if appendages are used. Walking is essentially restricted to animals with jointed appendages: Arthropoda and Vertebrata. Creeping in this sense is produced (1) by body movements, of snakes and worm-like invertebrates; (2) by an undulating surface, as in snails; (3) by cilia, aquatic but bottom-dwelling, by a few Protozoa, some minute ciliated Metazoa, and most free-living flatworms; and (4) by amoeboid movement, by some Protozoa.

3. Burrowing

This is movement through a solid material, either by compressing the material or by ingesting it. It is not entirely distinct from walking or creeping, because locomotory appendages may be used in the burrowing as well as in walking, and muscular waves of the surface may be used in creeping as well as in burrowing. *Burrowing* thus involves two activities intermixed, tunnelling and locomotion in the tunnel. It occurs in obvious form in many Mollusca, nearly all worm groups, Insecta (especially larvae), and many Vertebrata. All tube-dwelling animals are essentially burrowers, including Phoronida, some Polychaeta, and Pogonophora.

Burrowing is also the method of locomotion of many internal parasites, who move through the tissues of their host by this means.

4. Aquatic

This is usually labelled as *swimming*, regardless of the mechanisms employed. Swimming may be by jointed appendages (Arthropoda, Vertebrata); by undulatory body movements (s.Polychaeta, s.Hirudinea, s.Pisces, s.Reptilia); by ciliary or flagellar movement (Protozoa, Monoblastozoa, Ctenophora, Turbellaria, Rotifera, Gastrotricha, Dinophiloidea, larvae of Porifera and Coelenterata and of nearly all aquatic animals, and the spermatozoa of most animals); and by jet propulsion (medusae of Coelenterata, Cephalopoda, and something similar in Crustacea such as shrimps).

What we call ciliary movement is curiously diverse. True *cilia* are short and abundant, beating in one direction (sometimes reversible). The cilia may be united in bundles to form stronger *cirri* for creeping, or they may be in rows to form swimming *membranelles* with the cilia fused in sheets (both in Protozoa and Ctenophora). The *flagella* are long, generally occurring as one per cell, although in Protozoa two per cell may be more widespread and even more sometimes occur. Obviously, neither size nor number will provide a clear distinction between cilia and flagella.

A better distinction can be found in the mode of movement. Cilia apparently always move in one plane, with a backward directed stroke and a relaxed return. The flagellum, on the other hand, never beats in this manner but beats in some form of corkscrew or wave motion.

In a few Protozoa (e.g., *Trypanosoma*), the flagellum lies back over the animal to form an *undulating membrane* (for details of ciliary structure, see Chapter 10).

5. Locomotion of Parasites

It is sometimes forgotten that most parasites move about, at least at certain stages of their life history. Many internal parasites move through the tissues of their host, a movement that would usually be called burrowing. For example, many parasites gain entrance via the digestive tract, but at some stage they burrow through the wall of the intestine. Some enter one of the body fluids and thereafter move by swimming. Most protozoan parasites swim, as do the ciliated larvae of helminths, which are essentially aquatic at this stage. Even intestinal parasites are in a fluid medium, and some may be said to swim.

Ectoparasites generally move in the same manner as terrestrial animals, moving with appendages in a way that would be called crawling.

C. Migration

Some of the many phenomena called migration are listed by Newman and Lowery (1961) thus: "The exodus of whole faunas from one continent to another in prehistoric time and the daily passage of flocking birds to and from roosts; shifts of human population and rhythmic responses of marine invertebrates to tides; the suicidal cyclic outbreaks of lemmings and the equally suicidal emigrations of some insects; irregular southward influxes of boreal birds and sudden permanent range expansions, as that of the armadillo; the return of eels to the sea and of Pacific salmon in from the sea, to spawn at their birthplaces and die there. . . . A more stringent definition of migration (is) as a semiannual alternation between definite summer and winter homes. Animals of several classes show at least a semblance of such alternation: butterflies, moths, ladybugs, and dragonflies; various crustaceans and marine fish; toads and salamanders; bats, ungulates, seals, and whales; and, most clearly of all, a majority of nonsedentary birds."

Not clearly included in the above are the diurnal/nocturnal vertical migrations of many pelagic marine animals, which would seem to be necessarily related to the amount of light but which are in reality due to a complex of factors.

In spite of the mention (above) of insects and marine invertebrates, nearly all extensive discussions refer to vertebrates. Among these, matters of much discussion include the reasons for migration, the stimuli that determine choice of migration day and time, the navigational methods, and the clues used (among a variety of possible clues that exist).

"So it is certainly a mistake to look for *the* mechanism of orientation in any species. . . . To appreciate the actions of an animal in nature we must understand how various kinds of information interact in the fine adjustment of the orientation process" (Marler and Hamilton, 1966).

Migration is a notably diverse subject, both in its purposes and in the mechanisms of orientation. Comparative data are not available except perhaps for vertebrates, but even there the diversities of purposes and of mechanisms are usually not clearly sorted out.

D. Prepared Transport

On the fringes of locomotion, and also not clearly distinct from nonlocomotory movement, are the cases of active development of situations or devices for the purpose of obtaining passive transport. These may depend on physical features such as water currents, or on other organisms.

To obtain transport by air or water or blood currents, animals may develop floats or buoyancy, silk "balloons" (threads), foils for gliding, etc.; or they may place themselves where a physical event will move them, as rafting or a nematode that climbs onto a plant seed pod that is about to jactitate, throwing the nematode some distance.

To obtain transport on other organisms, an animal may develop hooks, claws, holdfasts, suckers, grasping proboscises or other appendages, or may enslave or domesticate the transporting animal.

A slightly different form of active "preparation" for a passive movement would be the attainment of swimming speed by a "flying fish" so that it can coast in the air above the water.

VI. PROTECTION

A. Direct Action

Some animals are protected from the elements, and even from their enemies, by passive existence in locations that happen to provide these protections. For example, internal parasites do not require individual protection from weather or from predators. Insects living in galls do not normally face either of these perils, but most animals require protection from a variety of dangers, and they must take direct action to avoid fatal circumstances. Among these actions are (1) evasion by locomotion, (2) concealment and camouflage, and (3) physical control of part of the environment.

B. Evasion

The active avoidance of enemies is by locomotion, whether running, swimming, flying, or burrowing. The organs utilized serve other purposes as well.

C. Concealment

Protection by concealment may be either active or passive. Many animals lurk in protective places and emerge only for necessary activities. For example, in small places a small animal is protected from a large predator, as well as from currents or storms. But the "small place" may be self-made, such as the cases of many aquatic insect larvae. Even shells may serve this function.

A major concealment that is passive or at least automatic is the assumption of shapes, textures, or coloration that either blend the animal with its surroundings or make it look like something else or warn of its presence. These are common among arthropods, where the individual may merge with background or be specially formed to look like part of it. These effects are entirely passive, in the sense that they were produced by evolution and are not under the control of the individual. Included among these are the situations called protective coloration, warning coloration, and mimicry.

Camouflage is the active adoption of means to make oneself look like something else. Aside from humans, it is practiced by some arthropods, such as the decorator crab, which attaches sponges, anemones, or algae to its carapace to hide or disguise it. In such cases there is exploitation of the second organism (see Chapter 22).

D. Control of Environment

Many animals exercise a modicum of control over their environment by their choice of habitat, but only a few are able to control even some of their surroundings by their own activity. Some of the constructions listed in a later section serve to control the environment in certain ways.

In a sense it is possible to think that gall-inhabiting animals have induced their host to produce tissues around them for their protection. Here would be the numerous gall insects (gall wasps and gall midges) and plant-parasitic nematodes. There is, however, no direct action by the individual to produce the gall, which is made by the host in response to mechanical or chemical stimuli resulting from the presence of the parasite.

It is sometimes implied that galls are produced also in animals, and it is true that in response to some parasites the host may form a sort of cyst around it. These do not seem to be the same as galls, which are always of characteristic form and do not primarily protect the host from the parasite.

The extreme example of the host modification occurs in ants parasitized by nematodes, where the condition is called mermithization. Instead of forming galls, the ant may be sharply altered in various ways: enlarged abdomen, decreased size of head and prothorax, atrophy of wings, and reduction of ovaries and fat body.

Direct control over physical aspects of the environment seems to have been achieved only in two classes: Insecta and Mammalia. In the former, both ants and termites build elaborate nests that require control of humidity and temperature, at least in some chambers. Termites, especially, may ventilate their nests with elaborate passageways; the air circulation serves for control of both humidity and temperature.

In the Mammalia, it appears that humans are the only species that deliberately controls the physical environment.

VII. HABITATS

A. Diversity

The place where an organism lives, or the general type of place in which all members of a species live, is its habitat; i.e., its natural environment. It is always a specific kind of environment, sometimes widespread, as the open sea, sometimes very limited, as the waters of a particular cave. In general the word habitat is used to specify the known distribution of the species, but in some cases the full distribution can only be guessed at. In these cases the "habitat" could include all the occupied areas, whether yet known or not.

When speaking of a small group of organisms, what is often called a local population, the habitat may be isolated and much restricted, a microhabitat. This might be a single plant, a dead animal, a fallen acorn, or the cavity of a certain jellyfish. The term thus has a wide range of coverage, and the terms used to describe the various kinds of habitats are legion.

The number and diversity of habitats is endless. Indeed, it is probable that each of the several million forms of life has a distinct habitat. It is possible, however, to group these helpfully, starting with the distinction between marine, freshwater, terrestrial, and parasitic. There is overlap, and a few organisms seem to live in more than one — either sequentially (the larva in one, the adult in another) or simultaneously (as a parasite in a marine animal).

B. Marine Habitats

"The habitats of marine animals may be divided roughly into five types: the open oceans, rocky shores, sandy beaches, estuaries, and ocean bottoms" (MacGinitie and MacGinitie, 1949). The open ocean and the shores are abruptly separated by wave action and depth, and rocky shores are clearly distinct from sandy beaches. Estuaries are places of mixing of freshwater and salt and of sand and silt; and the ocean bottoms merge at the edges with both sandy beaches and the mud of estuaries.

Likely to be forgotten in this five-part grouping are many rather distinct habitats, usually with no counterpart on land. These include coral reefs that may not be "shores" and may extend to considerable depths, providing a multitude of special habitats; regions of up-welling water, where the growth of algae and thus of other organisms is greatly favored; the lightless depths that have no extensive counterpart on land; and the large areas of low and variable salinity. It is these that contradict the common belief among biologists that the habitats of freshwater are more numerous and diverse than of the sea.

The groups of animals found in the marine habitats are listed here for comparison with the lists given later for freshwater, terrestrial, and parasitic habitats:

Marine exclusively: Ctenophora, Gnathostomuloidea, Kinorhyncha, Priapuloidea, Phoronida, Brachiopoda, Sipunculoidea, Echiuroidea, Myzostomida, Dinophiloidea, Chaetognatha, Pogonophora, Echinodermata, Pterobranchia, Enteropneusta, Planctosphaeroidea, Tunicata, Cephalochordata

Extinct marine: Receptaculitida, Cyathospongia, Graptozoa, Conularida, Hyolithelminthes, Cricoconarida, Coleolida, Calyptotomatida, Mathevioidea, Protonychophora, Stylophora, Homostelea, Homoiostelea, Cycloidea, Cyamoidea, Camptostromatoidea, Lepidocystioidea, Helicoplacoidea, Conodontophorida

Marine and others: Protozoa, Porifera, Coelenterata, Platyhelminthes, Rhynchocoela, Rotifera, Gastrotricha, Nematoda, Gordioidea, Calyssozoa, Bryozoa, Mollusca, Tardigrada, Annelida, Arthropoda, Vertebrata

C. Freshwater Habitats

Phyla that are exclusively in freshwater: (No phylum, but many species and even a few whole classes) Temnocephalida, Gordioidea with juveniles parasitic, and Phylactolaemata

Phyla that occur both in freshwater and other habitats: Protozoa, Porifera, Coelenterata, Platyhelminthes, Rhynchocoela, Rotifera, Gastrotricha, Nematoda, Gordioidea, Calyssozoa, Bryozoa, Mollusca, Tardigrada, Annelida, Arthropoda, Vertebrata

D. Terrestrial Habitats

The general types of terrestrial habitats are for animals that live on the surface (terricolous), those that burrow in the ground (fossorial), and those that spend much of their life in the air (aerial). There is much overlap or crossing-over between these. Among the burrowing forms are of course the ones which are more often called soil-inhabiting. Many of those that would be classified as "on the surface" actually never do touch the ground until they die, because they live on or in plants or other objects.

Phyla that are exclusively terrestrial: Onychophora
Phyla that occur both in terrestrial and other habitats: Platyhelminthes, Mollusca,
  Arthropoda, Vertebrata
Phyla that occur exclusively in soil: (None)
Phyla that occur both in soil and elsewhere: Rhynchocoela, Nematoda, Annelida,
  Arthropoda

E. Parasitic Habitats

Diverse in a different way than the habitats of the sea or of the land are those adopted by the very diverse animals that live in or on other animals. These are the parasites, whose habitats are as diverse as the organs of the hosts. As these animals are discussed in more detail in Chapter 22, this group of habitats will receive no further attention here.

Phyla that are exclusively parasitic: Mesozoa, Acanthocephala, Pentastomida
Phyla that include both parasites and others: Protozoa, Platyhelminthes, Nematoda,
  Gordioidea, Arthropoda

F. Distribution of Phyla

Out of 58 living and extinct phyla recognized in this book, the following have representatives living in the habitats as follows (exceptional occurrences are not listed):

53 have marine representatives
37 are exclusively marine (of which 19 are extinct)
16 have freshwater representatives
 0 are exclusively freshwater
 5 have terrestrial representatives
 1 is exclusively terrestrial
 5 have soil-dwelling representatives
 0 are exclusively soil-dwelling
 1 has terrestrial saline representatives exclusively
 8 have parasitic representatives (more than exceptionally)
 3 are exclusively parasitic

G. From Saltwater to Freshwater to Land

It is usually understood that the evolutionary passage of any kind of animal between major habitats is a very drastic thing. Thus, the change from a freshwater habitat to a marine or a terrestrial one, or vice versa, is not easily accomplished. Nevertheless it is interesting to note how many times this has happened, as evidenced by existence of species of a group in two or three of these environments. In these examples the direction of passage is not shown. (The following symbols are used: F = freshwater, M = marine, P = parasitic, T = terrestrial but including interstitial forms in water films.)

Protozoa	M---F---(T)---P
Porifera	M---F
Coelenterata	M---F
Platyhelminthes	M---F---T---P
Rhynchocoela	M---F
Rotifera	M---F
Gastrotricha	M---F
Nematoda	M---F---T---P
Calyssozoa	M---F

Bryozoa	M---F
Mollusca	M---F---T
Annelida	M---F---T
Arthropoda	M---F---T---(M)
Tardigrada	M---F
Pisces	M---F---(T)
Amphibia	M---T
Reptilia	T---(F)---(M)
Mammalia	T---(F)---(M)

The changes to other habitats shown in parenthesis represent animals not adapted for respiration in that new environment.

VIII. OTHER ACTIVITIES

A. Autotomy

Autotomy is self-mutilation, usually the removal of some appendage, body part, or group of organs. It can be very simple, involving little more than scratching the skin, or it can be an extremely drastic action involving nearly all internal organs and requiring many weeks of rebuilding.

The process is closely associated with regeneration, which is the restorative reaction, that prevents the mutilation from being fatal, or at least crippling (which in nature is usually the same thing).

In some Crustacea there is "a highly developed ability to drop an injured appendage" (Waterman, 1960). Although there are several ways in which a limb may be severed, the word autotomy is often used to cover them all. Some writers now recognize three ways in which an arthropod may discard a limb: (1) autotomy (in strict sense) is severance at a preformed breakage plane by means of a reflex; (2) autospasy is separation at a preformed plane when the appendage is pulled by an outside agent; and (3) autotilly is the severance at a preformed plane with the assistance of that individual's own mouthparts, claws, or legs.

The processes of autotomy (defined in the broad sense) include:

Amputation, removal of (damaged) appendages by direct action of the individual

1. Legs — in Crustacea, mostly after mutilation in fighting
2. Wings — in termites, cast off after the nuptial flight, when they are no longer needed; the action is voluntary and occurs at a predetermined breaking point
3. Wing part — in hemipterous Insecta, where the membranous portion is broken off by direct use of the legs; apparently deliberately to expose the abdomen for mating
4. Siphons — in certain burrowing clams
5. Scales — of some annelid worms
6. Tail — in lizards, usually when held by an enemy, and breaking at a predetermined point

Fragmentation

7. Arms — many echinoderms can regenerate broken-off arms; there is direct evidence that the breaking is often self-induced
8. Trunk segments — some Annelida break off posterior trunk segments when disturbed; this also occurs in Rhynchocoela
9. Proboscis — in Rhynchocoela

10. Calyx — from colonial Calyssozoa, leaving stolons to regenerate new individuals
11. Tentacular crown — in Phoronida
12. Body fragments — in Holothurioidea

Evisceration (autoevisceration)

13. Viscera — in Holothurioidea especially, in which some external stimuli prompt the animal to cast out all the viscera through the mouth, leaving the metabolic organs all to be replaced by regeneration before feeding or breathing or excretion can be resumed

Disassociation

14. Cells — the extreme form of regeneration is the restitution that can be accomplished in some sponges and simple coelenterates after the cells have been completely dissociated and left in a heterogeneous pile (this can also occur in nature; see Chapter 11)

Although many other animals have good regenerative powers and can replace parts that have been cut off, it is usually clear that self-mutilation did not occur (see also section on regeneration in Chapter 7).

B. Flotation

This concept (and that of attachment, to be discussed later) are related to locomotion (and its absence) and to the physical feature called buoyancy. Flotation is a means of obtaining support or transport without locomotory organs. This subject might have been included in a chapter on control mechanisms, as control of buoyancy is usually the basic feature involved.

Some animals are designed to float or to be suspended in water, and they have structures or activities to maintain the desired position. These are the flotation devices. Others will stay on the bottom because they are either heavier than water or have means of attaching themselves to the substrate. Those that are to live at an intermediate position must adjust their buoyancy to exactly match that of the desired level.

The same situation really applies in air, but it turns out to be somewhat simpler. There is effectively no upper surface, and most control of elevation is by locomotion rather than control of buoyancy directly. Weight can sometimes be controlled, but "attachment" is not a useful concept as no animal is in danger of floating off the earth because of being lighter than air.

1. Flotation in Air

This seems to have been attained only a few times among animals. Aside from man's use of balloons filled with gases that are lighter than air (hot air, hydrogen, helium), this seems to have been achieved only once in the animal kingdom by spiders. Young spiders can spin out fine threads of silk so long that the lift of rising air currents can carry the spiderling for long distances with no further expenditure of energy. (The same result is obtained by spores of microorganisms and plants, which are light enough to be carried long distances by moving air.) This type of buoyancy is in part the result of wind resistance; it would fail if there were no movement of the air.

2. Floating on Water

This can be partly active or wholly inactive. The former is a form of swimming. The latter is due to differential specific gravity of the object and the liquid. So long as the object is lighter than the fluid, it will float. It does not float on up into the air because the air is lower in specific gravity than the object.

Very few individual animals float *on* water (i.e., at the surface). Some marine siphonophore colonies do so (see below) and egg masses of such freshwater animals as insects may do so. One type of statoblast in Bryozoa floats and is called a floatoblast. These all can float because they trap enough gas to keep their total specific gravity below that of the water.

3. Floating in Water

Very many animals, both marine and freshwater, float *in* the water; i.e., below the surface but above the bottom. They have adjusted their buoyancy to equal that of the water level in which they live, and some of them can change their buoyancy in order to rise or sink to other levels. Nearly all plankton animals are of this sort, except that many of them also swim. In fact, true floating with no locomotion may be rare below the surface.

Floating is sometimes related to viscosity of the water. Ocean water is more viscous than fresh, and cold water is more viscous than warm. Many floating organisms have projecting feathery or hair-like structures which retard sinking during periods when buoyancy temporarily falls too low and sinking might be fatal.

4. Flotation Mechanisms

It does not seem possible to usefully tabulate the devices concerned with flotation. Some examples will give an idea of the range of such mechanisms.

Siphonophora. Although some siphonophores can swim by means of nectophores and weak jet propulsion, most also have gas-filled pneumatophores which serve as floats to sustain the entire colony near the surface of the ocean.

Gastropoda. The oceanic snail *Janthina* forms an elaborate float from which it can hang upside down from the surface. The float has "cells" filled with secreted gas.

Cephalopoda. Empty chambers in the spiral shells of *Nautilus* are filled with secreted gas. The shells thus serve as floats.

Polychaeta. A swimming animal such as *Tomopteris*, flattened and with broad parapodia, can quickly sink to a lower level by rolling into a ball, thereby reducing the surface resistance.

Insecta. In the aquatic larva of *Chaoborus* the main longitudinal tracheal trunks are strongly dilated into two pairs of sacs, which are filled with oxygen. This larva can vary the size of the sacs and adapt very rapidly to changes of pressure, as well as adjust its depth by changing the specific gravity.

Pisces. The swim-bladder of fishes is well known. Among its functions is keeping the fish at the same specific gravity as the surrounding water. Adjustments are made by secreting or dissolving the contained gas.

C. Attachment

Many animals live all or part of their lives firmly attached to some substrate, and many others can attach themselves temporarily. At least four major means are employed in a variety of ways, either by sedentary animals or by parasites.

Cell organelles

1. Stalks (s.Protozoa)
2. Polar filaments — to intestinal wall of host (s.Protozoa)
3. Trichocysts (Ciliata)

Body structures (regions)

4. Scolex — with hooks and suckers (Cestoda)
5. Spiny proboscis (Acanthocephala)
6. Pseudoscolex (Cestoda: s.Cyclophyllidea)

Glands

7. Adhesive-secreting (Gastrotricha)
8. Cement-secreting (Crustacea: barnacles)
9. Silk-secreting (Arachnida)
10. Tube-secreting (Phoronida)
11. Secretion of byssus thread (Bivalvia)

Organs other than glands

12. Suckers (Trematoda, Cestoda, hagfish)
13. Hooks (Cestoda, Pentastomoidea, s.Crinoidea)
14. Antennae (Cirripedia)
15. "Foot" (Rotifera)
16. Spicules or spongin (Porifera)
17. Stolons (s.Hydrozoa)
18. Pedicle (Brachiopoda)
19. Mouthparts (s.Insecta)
20. Root-like organ (Brachiopoda, Crinoidea)

In many of these it is only the adult that is attached, with the larval stage (and even the embryo) being motile, but in different animals examples of all stages can be found that are attached. For example, the eggs of many insects are attached by the mother to a substrate, often the food for the hatched larva. The second larval stage of some Scyphozoa is attached while undergoing strobilation. The adults of all Bryozoa are attached, usually in a dense colony.

There is a curious dual use for the term *sessile* (from the Latin sessilis, *to sit,* the same root that gives us sedentary). Sessile animals are those that "sit" and do not move about, thus being set off from the motile animals, but the word sessile is also used in Protozoa to make a distinction between animals with stalks and those without — stalked vs. sessile. In the latter usage the "sessile" ones "sit directly" on the substrate without being attached by a stalk.

D. Bioluminescence
1. Light Production

The production of light by organisms is called luminescence, bioluminescence, and photogenesis. *Luminescence* covers a wide variety of light-producing physical and chemical reactions, from friction and oxidation to radioactivity. No one would misunderstand the word in connection with organisms, but the prefix bio- has been used to give notice that it is due to an oxidative chemical reaction that occurs only in living tissues.

This light-producing reaction has always seemed to involve a substance called luciferin and an enzyme called luciferase. Because these latter are not specific chemicals but classes of chemicals, various animals have slightly different forms of this reaction system. Other systems for light production have also been isolated. In at least some coelenterates, the process appears to consist merely of the mixing of a special protein with calcium. Tabulation of such systems and their occurrence does not seem possible, but it cannot be assumed that luciferin/luciferase is universal.

The term *photogenesis* is appropriate for animal light production, but its adjective form, photogenic, has been rendered objectionable by its use in the entirely inappropriate popular meaning of being suitable for photographing.

The term *phosphorescence* is sometimes used for light production by organisms. Although clear distinction is not usually made even in dictionaries, phosphorescence usually includes, or is restricted to, the emission of light following irradiation.

Animals such as cats have been described as having luminous eyes. It is believed that all such cases have been conclusively shown to be due to reflection of light. However, in some invertebrates the light-producing organ may have a lens and take on some appearance of an eye.

Humans can use light for signalling, even though they cannot produce light chemically in their own bodies. It is natural to assume that the numerous animals that can produce light do so deliberately and for some purpose. Two purposes are suggested for light production: illumination of surroundings and signalling to other organisms. Although it is tempting to assume that all luminescence is designed to serve one of these purposes, there is in fact almost never any scientific evidence that either function is actually important to the organism.

A possible third function is identification, by means of the light pattern, in the same manner as color patterns serve for recognition. Here we would list such insects as fireflies, in which the light and its flashing pattern do serve for recognition by others of the species.

Clear-cut examples of any of these are rare. It is intriguing to note that in some animals none of these functions can be served by luminescence. Examples are given by MacGinitie and MacGinitie (1949): "Some of our most brilliantly luminescent animals, e.g. the worm *Chaetopterus* or the clam *Pholas,* live in burrows, and, in the case of *Pholas,* not only is the animal within a burrow but the light is within the shell. So far as we know, neither animal has any sense organ that would detect or could use its own light; and no warmth is derived from it. In fact, since luminescence is the result of a physiological process and such processes require energy, when an animal luminesces it expends energy from which it derives no apparent benefit."

Much luminescence in the sea is caused by luminescent bacteria, which may also be in or on an animal. These are sometimes "cultivated" in special organs or on special surfaces and are thus not entirely accidental.

2. Luminescent Organs

The production of light may be in special organs, in the cytoplasm in general, or outside of the body by reaction between extruded enzymes and luciferin. In bacteria it seems to be general in the cell, and luminescent bacteria are the cause of "luminescence" in some animals, in which the bacteria are symbionts. Here the light is usually emitted continuously, but in dinoflagellates it is in brief flashes. (The bacterial light can also be made intermittent by movement of a shutter.)

In Metazoa the light may arise in special cells, called *photocytes,* usually in specific sites on the body. Or there may be special organs called *photophores.* These may be similar to eyes in structure, having a cornea, a lens, and a retina-like cup of photocytes backed by a reflective layer.

Light may be produced inside certain cells, in the body cells in general, or in secretions of cells. In either case the reaction may or may not involve luciferin. The cells may be in organized groups, organs, or they may occur singly. Many animals may use two methods, and of course, symbiotic bacteria are the source of light in some, though not in as many as once believed. The following occur:

1.   Light from symbiont bacteria (s.Cephalopoda, s.Crustacea, s.Pisces)

2. Light from ingested food in transparent animals (s.Crustacea)
3. Light from protoplasm in general (?s.Protozoa, s.Hydrozoa)
4. Light from photocytes singly (s.Anthozoa, Rhynchocoela)
5. Light from photogenic organs containing photocytes
    (dinoflagellates, s.Crustacea, Diplopoda, Insecta: fireflies, s.Pisces)
6. Light from secretion of glands, usually called slime (s.Anthozoa, s.Bivalvia,
    s.Polychaeta, s.Crustacea, Enteropneusta, s.Pisces)

3. Occurrence of Luminescence

Luminescence has been reported in some species of the following 25 groups. (If this luminescence is believed to be in some cases due to bacteria, it is so annotated.)

1. Protozoa: Flagellata and Sarcodina
2. Porifera: Calcispongia, Sclerospongia
3. Coelenterata: All classes
4. Ctenophora
5. Rhynchocoela
6. Bryozoa: Gymnolaemata
7. Mollusca: Gastropoda, Bivalvia, Cephalopoda (s.bacterial)
8. Annelida: Polychaeta, Oligochaeta
9. Arthropoda: Pycnogonida, Crustacea, Chilopoda, Diplopoda, Insecta
10. Echinodermata: Ophiuroidea
11. Enteropneusta
12. Tunicata: Thaliacea, Larvacea
13. Vertebrata: Pisces (s.bacterial)

Some transparent Crustacea are illuminated by phosphorescent food ingested. Developmental stages may be luminescent: eggs of ctenophores, pluteus larvae of ophiuroids, trochophore larvae of polychaetes, and nauplii of crustaceans.

The following are examples of luminescence in the different phyla:

PROTOZOA. Only in Sarcodina and Flagellata. Sarcodina: Radiolaria apparently emit light only from symbiotic bacteria and dinoflagellates. Flagellata: Such dinoflagellates as *Gonyaulax* and *Noctiluca* are the source of most of the brilliant luminescent displays in the sea; the light is produced by reactions in the cytoplasm; it may be either constant or flashing.

PORIFERA. Occurs only in Calcarea, as in genus *Grantia;* source and mechanism not known.

COELENTERATA. Hydrozoa: Many species, including *Obelia, Oceania,* etc.; produced by granules in the cells of hydranth, stalk, or tentacular bulbs; as blue flashes. In *Aequoria* and *Halistauria* a mechanism is present that involves only the mixing of a special protein with calcium. (It is reported by Hyman (1940) that many of the Siphonophora are luminescent.) Scyphozoa: A few, especially *Pelagia noctiluca,* in which the light comes from scattered spots and streaks. Anthozoa: Many Pennatulacea emit a slime from mucus gland cells of the epidermis, with the slime containing luminous granules and spherules and the animals sometimes responding with flashes. Recent work confirms Harvey's (1920) belief that this light is produced by a process different from that of mollusks and arthropods.

CTENOPHORA. In most species, especially *Mnemiopsis leidyi,* light either continuously or in flashes, by outer cells of the coelenteric canals beneath the comb rows.

RHYNCHOCOELA. One species, the Japanese *Emplectonema kandai,* can luminesce, either as local flashes or over most of the body. The light is produced in epidermal gland cells and does not involve luciferin.

BRYOZOA. Reported several times among Gymnolaemata, but all the early records are doubted by later workers. In *Acanthodesia serrata* light is given off from special areas of gland cells.

MOLLUSCA. Gastropoda: The pelagic *Phyllirhoe bucephala* has luminous spots all over the body, each being a gland cell or cluster; luminescence occurs in several nudibranchs and in a New Zealand freshwater limpet *(Latia neritoides)*. Bivalvia: The clam *Pholas dactylus* is luminescent with simple epithelial organs that release secretions into the inhalent siphon. Cephalopoda: Many species luminesce, often with ectodermal pockets filled with luminescent bacteria; others have their own special organs, which may involve a lens and a reflector, or there may be a luminous secretion. The squid *Histioteuthis bonelleii* has "dozens of large complicated light organs on the mouth, funnel, head, and arms and enormous terminal light organs on the three upper arm pairs . . . probably under nervous control" (Kaestner, 1967).

ANNELIDA. Polychaeta: Several produce a luminescent slime from gland cells on body and tentacles; in at least some the reaction is by the luciferin/luciferase reaction. Oligochaeta: Luminescence has been reported and is believed to be due to a luminous slime exuded from the anus or the prostomium. It is specifically reported in *Diplocardia*, a genus of earthworms from New Zealand.

ARTHROPODA. Crustacea: The euphausiid *Meganyctiphanes norvegica* has a photophore with a lens and a retina-like cup of photocytes, backed by a reflective material; in *Cypridina* a photogenic gland secretes both luciferin and luciferase, which react when released into seawater. Chilopoda: Such species as *Scolioplanes crassipes* and *Geophilus carpophagus* have so-called repugnatorial glands which also secrete a luminous material visible inside the cells (neither bacterial symbionts nor air from tracheae is involved). Diplopoda: *Luminodermus sequoiae* is continuously luminescent over the entire integument. (Another species, or the same under a different name, *Amplocheir sequoia*, is also reported). Insecta: Light production is known in the orders Collembola, Ephemeroptera, Coleoptera, Diptera, and Lepidoptera. The larvae of *Bolitophila luminosa*, a mycetophilid fly from New Zealand, emits light (luminous materials?) from the malpighian tubules, which "may be seen streaming out of the (cage) ventilators at a distance of several feet" (Imms, 1951). Some other insects (Ephemeroptera, Diptera, Lepidoptera) are thought to harbor luminescent bacteria. The best known luminescence occurs in the fireflies (beetles of the families Lampyridae and Phengodidae), but the brightest by far is in the elaterids related to *Pyrophorus noctilucus*, which have two large organs on the edge of the pronotum, visible from above and from below, with yellow light, and a single organ at the base of the abdomen beneath, with reddish light. In this species even the eggs and larvae are luminous, the larva having a row of luminous spots along each side. The so-called "glow-worms" include the *Pyrophorus* larvae but also the larvae and larviform females of fireflies.

ECHINODERMATA. Luminescence occurs only in several species of Ophiuroidea, including *Amphipholis sinuatus*, where it emanates from the spines on the arms and is apparently produced by gland cells.

ENTEROPNEUSTA. Only in Ptychoderidae such as *Glossobalanus minutus* is there luminescence, where the green light comes from a slime secreted over much of the body.

TUNICATA. Thaliacea: In the colonial *Pyrosoma spinosum*, two groups of cells in the region of each mouth apparently emit slime that may cover the colony and be stimulated to luminesce. "Moseley states that he traced his name on the surface of a large specimen with his finger, and describes how 'in a few seconds his name came out in letters of fire' " (Sedgwick, 1909). Ascidiacea: The only record seems actually to refer to *Pyrosoma* (see above). Larvacea: Luminescence is reported in *Oikopleura*.

VERTEBRATA. Pisces: In *Cyclothone microdon* there is a large organ under the epidermis with lens, pigment cup, and reflector. In other species such organs may be few or many over the body; in still others there may be symbiotic bacteria. Luminescence occurs also in the selachian *Spinax niger,* in the teleosts *Myctophum* (lantern fish), *Stomias,* and in many bathypelagic forms.

Two specialized fish organs are described by Hardy (1956): " . . . tropical East Indian fish cultivate their luminous bacteria on special areas of the surface and so make their photophores by symbiosis: they give nourishment to the bacteria in exchange for light . . . . *Photoblepharon* has a fold of black pigmented skin, like an eyelid, which it can draw across the (bacterially) lightened area as a blind to cut off the light. In another fish, *Anomalops,* a similar bacterial photophore is made like a little culture-plate on the back of a hinged shutter . . . ."

E. Thermogenesis

It would be useful in comparative physiology to list the animals in which heat is deliberately produced, the mechanisms used, and the purposes for which the heat is needed. Only hints of these matters occur in most groups, although in birds and mammals one finds some reference to production of heat for maintenance of body temperature.

At least some muscle contraction produces heat, but this seems to be merely a by-product of the muscle inefficiency. (Less than 25% of the energy liberated performs work and the rest becomes heat.) This heat may be useful in some way, but except for shivering it is not produced *for the purpose* of heating the body.

Nearly all references to heat in animals are concerned with control of temperature (especially reduction of heat loss), heat as a by-product of muscle action, and tolerance of environmental heat — usually in vertebrates only.

REFERENCES

Andrew W., *Textbook of Comparative Histology,* Oxford University Press, New York, 1959.

Brown, M. E., *The Physiology of Fishes,* Vol. 1 and 2, Academic Press, New York, 1957.

Carthy, J. D., *An Introduction to the Behaviour of Invertebrates,* George Allen & Unwin, London and Hafner Publishing, New York, 1958.

Carthy, J. D., Taxis, in *Encyclopedia of the Biological Sciences,* Gray, P., Ed., Reinhold Books, New York, 1961.

Davey, K. G., *Reproduction in the Insects,* Oliver & Boyd, Edinburgh, 1965.

Hardy, A. C., *The Open Sea; the World of Plankton,* Collins, London, 1956.

Harvey, E. N., *The Nature of Animal Light,* J. B. Lippincott, Philadelphia, 1920.

Harvey, E. N., *Bioluminescence,* Academic Press, New York, 1952.

Haxo, F. T. and Sweeney, B. M., Bioluminescence, in *The Encyclopedia of the Biological Sciences,* Gray, P., Ed., Reinhold, New York, 1961.

Hedgpeth, J., *Ricketts and Calvin, Between Pacific Tides,* 4th ed., Stanford University Press, Stanford, 1968.

Hyman, L. H., *The Invertebrates,* Vol. 1, McGraw-Hill, New York, 1940.

Imms, A. D., *A General Textbook of Entomology,* 8th ed., Methuen, London, 1951.

Jennings, H. S., *Behavior of the Lower Organisms,* Indiana University Press, Bloomington, 1962.

Johnson, F. H. and Shimomura, O., The Chemistry of Luminescence in Coelenterates, in *Chemical Zoology,* Vol. 2, Florkin, M. and Scheer, B. T., Eds., Academic Press, New York, 1968.

Kaestner, A., *Invertebrate Zoology,* Vol. 1, Interscience, New York, 1967.

MacGinitie, G. E. and MacGinitie, N., *Natural History of Marine Animals,* McGraw-Hill, New York, 1949.

Marler, P. and Hamilton, W. J., III, *Mechanisms of Animal Behavior*, John Wiley & Sons, New York, 1966.

Newman, R. J. and Lowery, G. H., Jr.,Migration, in *Encyclopedia of the Biological Sciences*, Gray, P., Ed., Reinhold, New York, 1961.

Nicol, J. A. C., *The Biology of Marine Animals*, 2nd ed., Sir Isaac Pitman, London; John Wiley, New York, 1967.

Schechter, V., *Invertebrate Zoology*, Prentice-Hall, Englewood Cliffs, N.J., 1959.

Sedgwick, A., *A Student's Text-Book of Zoology*, Vol. 3, Swan Sonnenschein, London, 1909.

Simpson, G. G. and Beck, W. S., *Life; An Introduction to Biology*, Harcourt, Brace & World, New York, 1965.

Stern, C., Biology, in *An Orientation in Science*, Watkeys, C. W., Ed., McGraw-Hill, New York 1938, chap. 7.

Waterman, T. H., *The Physiology of Crustacea*, Vol. 1, Academic Press, New York, 1960.

Chapter 22

INTERACTIONS OF ANIMALS

TABLE OF CONTENTS

I.   Introduction... 454

II. Communication 454

III. Symbiosis 456
     A. Definitions... 456
     B. Cooperation.. 459
     C. Competition.. 459
         1. The Term 459
         2. Competition for Territory 459
         3. Competition for Food 459
         4. Competition for Shelter 459
         5. Competition for Mates 459
     D. Exploitation.. 460
         1. Purpose 460
         2. Exploitation for Food 460
             a.   The Methods 460
             b.   Cultivation 461
             c.   Predation 462
             d.   Micropredation... 463
             e.   Plant-Feeding 463
             f.   Parasitism 464
             g.   Ectoparasitism... 466
             h.   Endoparasitism.. 467
             i.   Cleptobiosis or Food Stealing............................ 468
             j.   Gleaning 468
         3. Exploitation for Shelter 469
         4. Exploitation for Use of Labor 469
             a.   Outline 469
             b.   Domestication 470
             c.   Slavery... 471
             d.   Social Parasitism... 471
         5. Exploitation for Camouflage 471
         6. Exploitation for Transport 471
         7. Exploitation for Use of Body Parts and Products 472
         8. Exploitation for Use of Transplanted Organelles 472
         9. Exploitation for Man's Purposes 473
         10. Exploitation for Care of Nonfeeding Individuals............... 473
         11. Exploitation for Care of Offspring.............................. 473
     E. Other Concepts... 477
         1. Commensalism 477
         2. Mutualism 478
         3. Host.. 478

F.   Parasitology 479
       1.   Usages 479
       2.   Parasite Life Cycles 479

IV.   Reproductive Behavior 480

References 481

I. INTRODUCTION

Activities involved in the interaction between two animals, whether of the same species or of widely different ones, are diverse but seldom listed. Only certain obvious ones are dealt with here: communication (by use of sounds, light, or chemicals), competition (for necessities of life), exploitation (for securing benefits from the other), and reproductive behavior (briefly, as it relates to bisexual reproduction).

A term sometimes used for some interactive activity is *social behavior.* This is usually restricted to the few animals that produce societies, almost exclusively vertebrates and insects. This level of interaction is only briefly mentioned herein, under such headings as cooperation and exploitation.

It has been found that other aspects of behavior are not recorded in such a way as to be readily compared from group to group.

II. COMMUNICATION

Information can be transferred within or between animals by a variety of mechanisms. Such transfer within an organism is primarily by nerve impulses and hormones; these are dealt with in Chapter 17. Between individuals, communication can be by means that are chemical, vibratory, or visual, in the broad sense of each word. Such communication is accomplished by organs that produce the signal in one animal and ones that receive the signal in another.

Information can be transferred from one individual to another without any purpose, essentially by accident, but to be included here as communication the sending of the information must be intended to accomplish some result, even if the organism is not capable of human rationalization. The most obvious purposes, aside from those of humans, are to attract some and to warn others to stay away. These may include:

1.   To attract possible mates
2.   To hold together a family group or herd
3.   To call others to a food source
4.   To identify an individual and its territory
5.   To warn others of danger
6.   To frighten intruders

It must be emphasized that most of the activities listed here as communication may not be so in other circumstances. Luminescence produces communication *only* if the luminescing individual is purposefully attracting or warning some other individual and does produce the desired reaction by it (at least theoretically). There is a fine line difficult to specify between a continuous luminescense that may possibly serve as a recognition sign and the flashing of fireflies in which the frequency and color of flash transmit not only the identity of the sender but its location, with the intent of attracting a mate or warning a predator.

Many animals produce characteristic odors as part of their normal life. These may serve as means of identification, but there is no deliberate communication with other animals. Some animals, however, produce specific odors at certain times with the apparent purpose of influencing other animals. These may include sex attractants or general repellants. Here again, emission of the potentially communicative signal may or may not be a deliberate communication.

Some examples of deliberate signals can be cited to show the diversity:

1. Vocalization by larynx (Amphibia, Reptilia, Aves, Mammalia)
2. Appendage waving (s.Crustacea)
3. Thumping on ground (s.Crustacea, s.Insecta, s.Mammalia)
4. Stridulating (s.Crustacea, s.Insecta)
5. Visual display (s.Reptilia, s.Aves, s.Mammalia)
6. Odor secretion (s.Insecta, s.Mammalia)
7. Snapping (s.Crustacea, s.Aves)
8. Vibration of appendages (s.Crustacea, s.Insecta)
9. Tapping the other individual (s.Crustacea, s.Insecta)
10. Vibration of tympanic membrane (s.Insecta)
11. Light emission (s.Insecta)

Diversity appears also in the organs designed to produce the signals:

Sound-producing organs

1. Vocal cords (s.Vertebrata)
2. Roughened areas on movable parts — for stridulation (s.Arthropoda)
3. Tympana — vibrated by muscles (especially s.Insecta)
4. Jaws and claws — for snapping sounds (s.Crustacea)
5. Rattles (s.Vertebrata)
6. Nasal passages — for snorting (s.Vertebrata)
7. Mouth passages — for whistling, hissing (s.Vertebrata)
8. Glands — to secrete explosive fluid (s.Insecta)
9. Appendages — used as hammers (s.Crustacea)

Chemical-producing organs

10. Exocrine glands — sweat glands, scent glands
11. Miscellaneous tissues and organs — repugnatorial glands

Color-producing organs, as in warning coloration

12. Chromatophores

Light-producing organs, controlled luminescense

13. Photophores

To complete the communication there must also be reception of the signal by the second individual. This is accomplished by a sense organ, as described in Chapter 17.

III. SYMBIOSIS

A. Definitions

"Organisms living in any given area, whether large or small, are associated together in what are known as biotic communities" (Odum, 1953). These organisms are associated in space and time, but nothing is said about the nature of the association. In the community there will be much interaction between individuals of different kinds, and also between individuals of the same kind. These associations or interactions between individuals, are diverse, not only in physical relations but also in behavioral purposes and in the effect on the two participants.

It is customary to arrange these by the physical relations, whether one lives in or on the other, whether the relation is brief or extended, and whether it is loose or close. The behavioral purpose seems to be thought to be of less importance even than whether the relationship is injurious or not to one or both.

For the purposes of the present book, emphasizing the diversity of purpose seems to have several advantages. It helps one to avoid the highly confusing differences in the definition of terms; it seems to help emphasize the multiplicity of relationships (so often hidden by the use of only three or four headings); and it helps to show the excessive diversity in these interactions when all animals are considered. Hyman (1951) lists 19 distinct forms of "parasitic" interaction in Nematoda alone.

Associations between organisms are of several sorts. These may be accidental or purposeful; among the former are found only those that were unavoidable: adjacent individuals in a colony, sessile animals that had no control of where they settled, juxtaposition of the two by a third agency. These form part of the life of those individuals, but they are not considered further here.

Purposeful associations (interactions) may be for cooperation (mutual benefit), for competition for physical needs, or for exploitation. These three are the principal subject matter of this chapter, under the three headings of Cooperation, Competition, and Exploitation.

Nearly all discussions and definitions of terms for the various sorts of animal interactions (predation, symbiosis, parasitism) specify or assume that the term is restricted to the interaction between two individuals of distinct species, often individuals of widely different groups. Yet within a species there may be found most of the same interrelationships. For example:

Individuals of 2 species	Both of 1 species
Predation	Cannibalism
Endoparasitism	Parasitic males
Phoresy	Domestication (part)
Dulosis	Slavery
Organ Transplant	Implantation of organ

There seems to be no biological reason to study these in separate places, as they are all examples of interactions between two animals. In order to emphasize the similarities and avoid use of arbitrary distinctions of closeness of relationship, these conditions will be herein discussed in pairs (between individuals of two species and between individuals of one species).

Symbiosis can thus be defined as the condition of two organisms of different species living together in close association. This is essentially the definition of both zoological dictionaries (Pennak, 1964 and Gray, 1967).

Nearly all the terms applied to these interactions are now so confused by diverse usage that they can no longer be used for transmitting facts or ideas accurately. These include symbiosis, commensalism, mutualism, and even parasitism. They will be avoided when possible or used in restricted sense.

It is also obvious that most discussions and most terms apply only where both organisms are animals, but the same interrelationships apply between animal and plant (and even between two plants).

Consortism. This is interaction of some sort between individuals. When individuals of one kind consort or interact with each other in groups larger than a family (parents and offspring) the groups are called *aggregations*. If the groups involve individuals of two or more such aggregations, the situation is called *association*. Thus, consortism includes both aggregation and association — all meaningful interaction between individuals. These terms are not universally used in these meanings, but they are adopted herein.

Many animals tend to live in groups. The reason for this is not always obvious, but it may be for protection, cooperation, or reproduction. Only one form of such aggregation is described in this book: colonies, in Chapter 23. This aggregation involves physical union between the individuals and comes close to being a family group rather than an aggregation because the members are all the asexual offspring of one individual and their descendants.

Association of species may be beneficial to individuals of both, or beneficial to one and harmful to the other. Only in very exceptional cases would it be harmful to both, as when a parasite prematurely kills the host and therefore itself dies for lack of food.

The relationships between different species of organisms are sometimes said to be, in the words of a recent book title, *Partners, Guests, and Parasites.* More technically these are sometimes called mutualism, exploitation (which includes both guests and parasites, as well as many others), and competition.

It is easy to keep competition separate from exploitation; in *competition* there is no direct use of the other organism for benefit, but merely getting space, food, or shelter before the other can take it. In *exploitation* one directly obtains some benefit (food, shelter, transport, etc.) from the other at the latter's expense.

On the other hand, mutualism is hard to define or to exemplify. Many books cite instances, from the birds that clean ectoparasites from large mammals (with obvious benefit to both) to the tending of aphids by ants. Apparently, if one takes the viewpoint of one of these "partners", the relationship is exploitation, and the other "partner" would also be exploited. One is left to wonder if mutual exploitation is really any different biologically from ordinary one-way exploitation.

Cases of mutualism are described in which survival of each species is dependent on the continued association with the other, but in the lives of every animal there are many factors essential to its continued existence. In mutualism, it merely happens that each member of the twosome finds the other to be essential to it in some way. The relationship is often the result of evolution of one or both partners, but as behavior it is still exploitation of each by the other.

Thus, in general discussions of the relation between individuals of two species, there is no place for the words cooperation, mutualism, partners, or guests. These words can still be used in some discussions of natural history, but even here there are apt to be anthropomorphic overtones that are unscientific.

Under this interpretation there are just two general aspects to be dealt with in describing the nature of the interaction between two species, competition and exploitation. It must not be forgotten here that these interactions are always between *individuals* of these two species. (It is not really an exception that sometimes two or more individuals cooperate on one side; they merely choose for the moment not to compete with each other but only with the individual of the other species.)

Table 26
THE FORMS OF ANIMAL INTERACTIONS

	Purpose	Damage	Terms or descriptions
1	For food	Slight to fatal	Parasitism, predation, micropredation, bloodsucking, scavenging, stealing
2	For use of "labor"	Moderate	Slavery, domestication, dulosis, digestion, care of young
3	For transport	Slight to moderate	Phoresy
4	For shelter	Slight	
5	For camouflage	Slight or none	
6	For use of construction/product	Slight or none	Domestication
7	For use of transplanted organs	Moderate to fatal	Predation
8	For man's purposes (esthetics, sport, experimentation, commerce, sacrifice, medicine)	Moderate to fatal	Domestication, predation

The usual terms			Descriptive words	
A	Symbiosis	1 (part), 2 (part), 4	I Cooperation	A (part), E, I (part)
B	Commensalism	1 (part), 2 (part), 4	II Competition	C, D, F, G, I, J
C	Parasitism	1 (part), 2 (part)	III Exploitation	A (part), B, C, D, F, G, H, I, J
D	Predation	1 (part), 7, 8		
E	Mutualism	1/2, 1/4		
F	Micropredation	1 (part)		
G	Parasitoidism	1 (part)		
H	Phoresy	2 (part), 3		
I	Domestication	1, 2, 3, 6, 8		
J	Slavery/dulosis	2, 6, 8		

All interactions between two animals of different species would seem to be either accidental or purposeful. Upon closer examination, however, it appears that all are purposeful at least to the extent that there is competition for a space to occupy. It is often further indicated that these contacts or associations (interactions) are for cooperation, competition, or exploitation. Again a closer look reveals that cooperation (at least aside from humans) is actually mutual exploitation.

Competition is for shelter, food, and territory. There may be physical struggle between the individuals, but there is not necessarily any physical damage. This is a matter of actively isolating itself from others.

Exploitation is more complicated. Animals are exploited for food, shelter, use of labor, camouflage, transport, use of constructions, use of transplanted organs, and such human purposes as experimentation, sacrifice, sport, etc.

In exploitation for food there are two groups: those in which the action is normally fatal to the prey, and those in which the prey is not normally killed. The first includes predation, whether by carnivores or by plankton feeders, and micropredation, in which a small predator developing inside the prey, gradually consumes it. Micropredation is sometimes called parasitoidism, but the latter term is less expressive of the final result.

If not fatal, the relationship may be ectoparasitism, endoparasitism, or commensalism.

Association for other forms of exploitation are exemplified in Table 26.

It should be noted that there is no place in this scheme for the term parasitism. Micropredators have usually been included with both ecto- and endoparasites, and commensals as well as animals living in a single confined space are often also called parasites, or at least dealt with under the general heading of parasitism.

B. Cooperation

There can be no question that cooperation for mutual benefit occurs between some members of most kinds of animals. Care of the young is the most obvious example, but swarming or herding is also common. Cooperation between individuals of two kinds is sometimes cited, but it is very doubtful if apparent cooperation is ever more than each acting for its own benefit in circumstances in which there is no need for direct competition. This latter is often called *mutualism,* variously defined, but it is here treated as mutual exploitation, under "Exploitation".

In effect, then, this subject encompasses only interactions between two individuals of the same species. Here there may be two aspects, cooperation to benefit the species (as in bisexual reproduction) and cooperation in forming a larger unit such as a colony or a society, where the activities of the higher unit to some extent replace those of the individuals. The forms of cooperation are

1.   Bisexual reproduction (most species in most phyla)
2.   Societies (Insecta and Mammalia, although some simple approaches to this occur in animals that deliberately cluster, and in other communal Vertebrata)
3.   Colonies, with interdependence through division of labor among the individuals (Coelenterata and Bryozoa, especially)

C. Competition

1. The Term

True competition, as distinct from exploitation, does not necessarily involve "living together", because the result of the competition will be that one effectively withdraws from the association. Competition seems to be effectively restricted to struggles for territory, food, shelter, and mates. It can be either interspecific or intraspecific.

2. Competition for Territory

Two animals cannot occupy exactly the same place at the same time, so there may be competition for the space. An internal parasite is not an exception to this because it occupies space, however small, that the host would otherwise use. From this minute amount of competition, there extends a range up to the territoriality of an individual that seeks to drive out of a region all species that could compete.

3. Competition for Food

Most animals compete for food with others of the same species as well as with individuals of other species. Two lions may fight over a kill, and the winner may still have to fight off jackals to finish his meal. Any animal that obtains food and stores it, will find other animals, of the same or very different kind, trying to steal that food. A squirrel stores nuts, but insects may have laid eggs on the nuts so that their new larvae can feed, thereby consuming the squirrel's food.

4. Competition for Shelter

Competition for shelter is the third type which may involve individuals of the same or of different species. For example, birds will fight over possession of a nesting site, either with others of their species or with another species; and primitive men would kill a bear in order to get possession of its cave only to risk being driven out by other men.

5. Competition for Mates

Competition for a mate occurs in all bisexual animals, but not normally between species. It may take the form of male courtship displays or of fighting with other males.

D. Exploitation
1. Purpose
One animal may exploit another of a different species for any of the following purposes, which should be taken with very broad meanings, as described in the succeeding sections:

1. Food
2. Shelter and protection
3. Use of labor
4. Camouflage
5. Transport
6. Use of body parts or products
7. Use of transplanted organs
8. Man's purposes

Most of these exploitations can also be found among individuals of the same species, plus these others:

9. For care of non-feeding individuals in a colony
10. For care of offspring

Exploitation may be for several of the purposes at once. The many "guests" in the nests of social insects are examples, where they obtain shelter, food, and transport from their hosts. An interesting sidelight on the relation between ants or termites and their many "guests" is that the latter commonly develop *physogastry*. This is swelling of the entire abdomen often with curling upward, which is supposed to arise from their being overfed by the solicitous hosts, resulting in hypertrophy of the ventral fat body.

An even better example of multiple purpose for exploitation is *domestication* by humans. The purpose of domestication may be stated as assuring the availability of the "prey" whenever the human wishes to utilize it for food, labor, transport, experimentation, etc. (This subject is herein discussed under "Exploitation for Use of Labor".)

Note that herein the word "exploitation" refers only to use by one individual of another individual, for the purpose indicated, not utilization or exploitation of a general food source.

2. Exploitation for Food
a. The Methods
Under this term are included the materials to satisfy all metabolic needs of the exploiter. Some exploiters normally kill the prey, others do not individually do so. Among the killing behaviors are those known as predation and micropredation. Among the nonkilling behaviors are those known as ectoparasitism and endoparasitism.

In the discussion that follows, attention will be centered on the interspecies relationships. Similar interactions between members of one species will be cited for comparison.

One organism may exploit another for nutriment in any of the following ways (interspecific/intraspecific):

1. By killing it from the outside and eating all or part of it or feeding it to its own dependents (predation, micropredation, plankton-feeding, filter feeding, domestication/cannibalism)

2. By killing it from the inside and consuming all of it (micropredation, parasitoid-ism/no term)*
3. By eating part of it from the outside without serious damage to it (ectoparasitism, plant-feeding/no term)
4. By living inside it and consuming insignificant parts of it, or part of its food, or part of its by-products (endoparasitism/placentation)
5. By stealing part of its food, from the outside (cleptobiosis/no term)
6. By eating food fragments dropped by the other (gleaning/gleaning)
7. By eating secretions on the outside (domestication/trophallaxis, brooding)

b. Cultivation

Cultivation sometimes means "tilling the soil", and man is the only animal which does that directly, but several animals deliberately grow or culture or protect other organisms to exploit them. They cultivate (raise or foster the growth of) the other organisms for their own benefit.

The "gardening" of plants for food is little more common among animals than the use of domestic animals. Among the best known are the cultivation of fungi upon the decaying leaves of certain plants in underground nests. This is done by the leaf-cutting ants, which carefully tend the fungi for eventual food. An example of similar nature is cited in an earlier chapter (13) of a moth that utilizes as food the conidia of a fungus harbored in its digestive tract.

Organisms are cultivated for various purposes, with varying amounts of care and of intent. For example:

For food

1. For direct consumption of the organism: by humans (many animals and plants), ants, and moths (fungi)
2. For consumption of exudates or secretions: by termites (various insect symbionts), ants (aphids, butterfly larvae), ants (various insect symbionts), humans (certain mammals for milk), and humans (bees for honey)

For dead body parts (other than meat)

3. By humans (wool, fur, hair, leather, feathers)

For labor

4. For draft by humans (horses, oxen, elephants, dogs)
5. For transport, by humans (directly by dogs, horses, mules, cattle, reindeer, camels, porpoises, etc., and humans (carrying of small objects: carrier pigeons)
6. For hunting, by humans (dogs, pelicans, cormorants, falcons)

There are at least two instances (besides many examples by humans) in which individuals of a species are reared in protective custody by another species, without the permanent control of slavery. For example: (1) Certain ants tend aphids from the egg stage, in the ant nest, then place the nymphs on a food plant, and defend them from enemies. (In return the ants receive desirable secretions from the aphids). (2) Certain ants keep larvae of lycaenid butterflies in their underground nests, bringing them up to feed on ant-selected plants and protected from enemies; the pupae are also pro-

---

* In three cases the expression "no term" is used to suggest that, although some activity of the sort can occur between individuals of a species, there is no explicit term to designate that activity.

tected. At least the first of these is an example of *trophobiosis*, as association in which one species obtains secreted food from another in return for tending and protecting it (see also "Domestication").

The exploited animal is fed and protected so far as necessary to maintain it, and it may be bred in captivity. As outlined here, cultivation is even broader than domestication, which it includes. Mere dependence on some other organism would not qualify as cultivation, unless one of the organisms actively fosters the life of the other. Thus, termite dependence on intestinal Protozoa for digestion of their food is accidental in the sense that the termite takes no deliberate action to cultivate the protozoans. Again, the attachment of anemones to the shell of a snail does not qualify, as nothing is done to cultivate the anemone, even if the snail does incidentally benefit from the arrangement.

On the other hand, as reported by the MacGinities (1949): "One crab of the California coast, *Podochela hemphilli*, uses rather delicate seaweed . . . to cover its back and legs . . . If allowed to become hungry, this little crab makes use of the garden on its back for food, being at least a partial vegetarian." They also warn that "masking crabs show no intelligent use of the masking instinct". Perhaps the "garden" is not intentionally provided and is eaten only in a final extremity.

c. Predation

Predation is the practice of catching and killing another animal (the prey) for food. Not always included in such a definition are two additional ideas. First, the catching must be active, and second, the predator must be larger (or stronger) than the prey. A third idea is usually not considered: whether the "predator" intends to consume the prey or intends to feed it to others.

The question of activity arises when one considers the case of a sessile animal that consumes whatever falls upon its surface. It is doubtful if this is ever completely passive, as nearly all sessile animals have tentacles or other devices to capture food that comes near.

The question of the size of the predator arises because there are thousands of animals smaller than their prey who eat them from the inside over a period of time. These are distinguishable as *micropredators*.

The question of who is to eat the prey cannot be clearly answered because it may be (1) the predator, (2) another individual of the same predatory species, (3) an individual of another predatory species, or (4) combinations of these. For example, a steer is butchered by a person, who sells the meat to a customer, who feeds it to a pet dog. In this situation, only the butcher fulfills the above definition exactly. However, in such higher animals as these humans, the "predator" can be thought of as a system that includes the "eater" (the dog) and his agents (the butcher and the customer). In social insects this system may include several individuals: the one who kills the prey, the one who carries it to the storehouse, and the one who feeds it to the young, with the latter being the real although inactive predator. In this viewpoint, the true predator is the individual that consumes the prey.

It is not customary to include under predation the eating of minute animals in the plankton (zooplankton), perhaps because the prey are minute in size and extremely numerous. There is, however, nothing in the above definition of predation to exclude this plankton feeding.

The word predation has some other confusing features. If we define it as the relationship between species A and species B, with A killing and eating B, we make it seem that B is essential to A, whereas in fact A may actually feed on any available species from B to Z. Predators vary from seeking out and eating individuals of one species to feeding on almost anything that comes along. This makes it inappropriate to define the term in reference to a single prey species.

In most discussions of predation, there is emphasis on the long-range effects on the prey population. This legitimate approach reveals a diversity among animals that should be of interest in a comparative analysis such as used here. However, it appears that nearly all large groups contain examples of many sorts of predatory relationships, and tabulation at the class level shows most feeding methods occurring in most groups. An attempt will be made here to show and exemplify the diversity of the interactions but not to discuss their population aspects or the adaptations that permit their successful competition.

In a recent major biology textbook (Keeton, 1980), it is recognized that feeding on animals and feeding on plants is not basically different. That book therefore defines predation as "the feeding of free-living organisms on other organisms", thus including plant-feeding as a form of predation. Even here, the nature of the food would give rise to the terms carnivore and herbivore. (The term herbivorous is commonly used for vertebrates, whereas phytophagous is more widespread for plant feeding by other animals.)

This mixing of plant feeding with animal feeding under the term predation would not be acceptable in entomology, where carnivorous and phytophagous are widely distinguished. The two concepts are herein kept separate because not only is the food different, but also the manner of its "capture".

d. Micropredation

An animal may kill and eat another animal without being large or strong enough to challenge it directly, or even to find it. Many of the insects that are loosely called parasitic do actually kill and eat their "hosts" and are thus true predators. Because of their small size, relative to the hosts, they can usefully be called micropredators.

The term *parasitoid* has been applied to these small predators, but the term has also been restricted to insects that live for a time as internal parasites and only later consume the hosts. Thus, these in a sense represent an intermediate between predation and endoparasitism, or at least a combination of the two.

Among these micropredators are "egg parasites" that develop from eggs laid in or near the egg of the "host" previously deposited. Thus the mother of the micropredator determines what her offspring will eat and in effect transports it to the place. Such well-known wasps as spider wasps are sometimes treated as predators, but the mother merely captures spiders (or in other species caterpillars) to provision her nest. She then lays one or more egg on the surface of the host or inside of it, and the larva, being inside or burrowing in, feeds on and thus eventually kills the prey (host). These are micropredators, but they are sometimes called either parasites, endoparasites, or parasitoids.

e. Plant-Feeding

Animals feed on plants in several ways. Some plants are destroyed by the animal, and some are not, but this is not usually made the basis of a distinction between plant feeders and plant parasites. Most multicellular plants are used as animal food only by consumption of fragments. Insects, for example, feed on leaves, buds, shoots, branches, bark, wood, roots, and flowers. They also feed on plant products, such as fruit, seeds, nectar, and sap. Microscopic phytoplankton is the object of "predation" in the same way as zooplankton: the organisms are eaten in large quantities.

Many terms have been used to describe these plant-feeding habits or the feeding animals. For example:

1. Algophagous — alga-feeding
2. Anthophilous — living on or frequenting flowers

3.   Gall makers (Nematoda, Insecta)
4.   Leaf-miners — feeding on interior tissues of leaves
5.   Phytophagous — plant feeding
6.   Seed feeders (Insecta, Aves)
7.   Wood-borers — in cambium, etc. (Insecta)
8.   Xylophilous — wood-boring or eating

Such terms as browsing, foraging, and grazing specify the animal's activities rather than the nature of the plant food utilized.

f. Parasitism

Many animals of diverse groups each live in close association with another animal, deriving essential nutrients therefrom. Among these are the ones called parasites. In many cases there are no problems associated with this terminology, but borderline cases and special situations are legion.

There is diversity in definition of the term parasitism, especially between biology texts, books on parasitism and symbiosis, and textbooks of parasitology. Among the many situations that make difficult the definition, and therefore the accurate employment, of the words parasite and parasitism are these: (1) the diversity of animal associations is very great and is not clearly divisible into a classification. The factors of this diversity include: (a) location in the body, (b) stage of parasite's life cycle, (c) stage of host's life cycle, (d) duration of parasitic phase, (e) material utilized (tissues, blood, digested food, secretions, wastes), (f) adaptation of the parasite, (g) effect on the host, and (h) responses of the host; (2) formal definitions are diverse; none is dominant among all books on the subject; (3) examples cited often do not fit the accompanying definition; (4) emphasis is often in the clinical aspects of parasitology, where interest in the biology of parasitism is subordinated.

One of the best of the definitions of parasite is given in Dogiel (1966), which is a book on parasitism. "Parasites are those animals which use other living animals as their environment and source of food, at the same time relinquishing to their hosts, partly or completely, the task of regulating their relationships with the external environment."

Even here, Dogiel finds it necessary to add that the host and parasite must be of different kinds. By this he excludes "the intrauterine development of the foetus", as in mammals. (It seems clear that under this viewpoint there would be excluded also the cases in other phyla of animals where placental arrangements occur.) He exemplifies as a parasite the glochidium of a clam when it is on the gill of a fish but not when it is in the gill of its mother.

This raises the question of biological justification for Dogiel's exclusion of "parasitism" between members of one species. Parasitologists will surely continue to exclude these developmental situations from parasitism, but it is well to note that they duplicate most aspects of the parasitism of separate species.

The elements usually involved in parasitism include the following:

1.   Intimacy of association
2.   Length of association
3.   "Recognized" as a foreign object
4.   Recognition of host
5.   Harmful to host (pathogenicity)
6.   Dependency of parasite on host (physiological or metabolic)
7.   Interaction of life cycles
8.   Site of interaction

A definition of parasitism should take into account most of these factors, but the appropriateness of each to the diverse forms of parasitism will vary. For this purpose, one might define *parasitism as the way of life of two individuals of different species living in extended close association, with interaction of the life cycles and harm done to one (the host) by the other (the parasite)*. The "harm" ranges from negligible loss of nutrients or tissues to substantial interference with the physiology of the host or its development.

Mechanical action on organs or tissues

1. Organ distention and impairment
2. Irritation to organs or tissues by attachment, locomotion, or feeding

Interference with host's metabolism

3. Robbing the host of part of its food
4. Secreting anticoagulants
5. Inhibition of host's enzymes
6. Starvation of the gonads
7. Production of toxic excretory products
8. Production of haemolytic substances
9. Irritating secretions by ectoparasites

Facilitation of other infections or diseases

10. Through surface wounds by ectoparasites
11. Appendicitis by whipworm
12. Intestinal injuries admitting pathogenic bacteria
13. By migrating larvae as carriers of disease
14. General lowering of resistance

Usually more than one of these influences occurs in a given case of parasitism. The extreme case of parasitic effect is direct control by the parasite over certain actions of the host. One of these is already mentioned as exploitation, including domestication, always involving two kinds, and slavery, involving either one kind or two. Here the control is by physical domination.

In other cases social hormones are the means of colony-wide control, as in some ant colonies. In grooming the queen and each other, the ants imbibe chemical substances that result in actions beneficial to the colony rather than to the individual. The workers are thus induced to tend the young and perform the many other chores of the colony. Indeed, the feeding of the young, under the influence of these social hormones, actually controls their development, producing various castes as required. The passing of food in this way, or rather control of actions by such feeding is called *trophallaxis*. The direct control of activities and the control of caste development are two forms of this chemical influence.

And third, a parasite may interfere with action of the control system in the host, thereby affecting its behavior. For example:

1. Control of ant by fluke cercaria in suboesophageal ganglion
2. Control of amphipod by cystacanth of acanthocephalan
3. Control of fish by fluke metacercaria in eye lens
4. Control of grasshopper habitat selection by a juvenile horsehair worm
5. Castration of the host, as in hermit crabs by a parasitic barnacle
6. Control of development and sex determination, in crabs by a parasitic barnacle

A few special terms applied to parasitism may be exemplified:

1. Coelozoic — living in a body cavity
2. Cytozoic — living inside a cell
3. Ectoparasitism — infestation by external parasite (see discussion below)
4. Endoparasitism — infestation by internal parasite (see section below)
5. Epiparasitism — same as ectoparasitism
6. Facultative parasitism — "the parasitic life of those animals that normally lead an independent existence but on settling accidentally on or in a suitable host immediately change to parasitism" (Dogiel, 1966) (s.Hirudinea, s.Insecta)
7. Haemoparasitism — living in the host's blood
8. Histozoic — living in tissues rather than body spaces
9. Hyperparasite — an animal whose host happens to be itself a parasite
10. Imaginal parasitism — with the parasite being adult (imago of Insecta)
11. Myiasis — any infestation by dipterous (fly) larvae in vertebrates (particularly mammals) and Insecta: (a) cutaneous (warble flies), (b) in cranial cavities (sheep botflies), (c) in digestive canal (horse botflies) (many other species merely pass through), and (d) in haemocoel, feeding on blood and fat body (the fly *Thrixion* in other insects)
12. Obligate parasitism — typical parasitism, in which the life cycle includes parasitism as an indispensable phase
13. Protelean parasitism — with the parasite being a larva
14. Pseudoparasitism — survival (like a parasite) of an animal not normally parasitic in that host (larvae of houseflies, blowflies, etc.)
15. Symparasitism — presence of competing parasites of two or more species in one host
16. Xenoparasitism — infection of an abnormal host through a wound

Parasites are universally distinguished as ectoparasites and endoparasites, depending on where they live — on or in the host. However, difficulties in making this distinction are referred to below, and there are animals that are clearly both. For example, the ichneumon fly *Hemiteles biannulatus* is ectoparasitic on a caddis fly larva and then changes to endoparasitic in the same individual by penetrating into the haemocoel.

g. Ectoparasitism

Ectoparasites are animals that live on or in the surface of other animals of different kind, obtaining most of their nutritional needs from tissues or products of the host. There is great diversity in the food, the method of its attainment, the motility of the parasite, the part or parts of the life history spent on the host, the amount of damage done to the host, and so on. Ectoparasites occur in the following classes, at least:

1. Ciliata — a few, on various aquatic hosts
2. Suctoria — a few, others by attachment only (see also Endoparasitism)
3. Turbellaria — a few, which may be commensals
4. Trematoda: Monogenea — mostly on fishes
5. Rotifera — some, attached by the mastax
6. Gastropoda — a few on bivalves, polychaetes, echinoderms
7. Bivalvia — glochidium larvae on fishes
8. Polychaeta — a few on crustaceans and fishes
9. Hirudinea — some on fishes
10. Myzostomida — a few, in body wall of echinoderms
11. Pentastomida (see Endoparasitism)

12. Pycnogonida — a few on polyps
13. Crustacea — a few that feed on emitted blood or tissue fluid
14. Arachnida: Acarina — many, in great variety of relationship with terrestrial vertebrates
15. Insecta — including all Anoplura, Mallophaga, Siphonaptera
16. Agnatha — some adults on other fish

Just what is meant by being ectoparasitic is not always clear. Some ectoparasites are half buried in the skin tissues; some are fully buried but just under the surface. Lung mites are sometimes treated as ectoparasites, as are gill parasites, whereas they are at other times treated as endoparasites. One of the best definitions of *ectoparasitic* (Dogiel, 1966) is "inhabiting the external surfaces of the hosts, their skin or gills".

h. Endoparasitism

In spite of the great diversity of organisms involved, endoparasitism is the easiest form to identify, presumably because their location inside the body is obvious; furthermore, it always involves striking adaptations for this special habitat. As used here, an *endoparasite* is an animal that lives at least part of its life inside an animal of a different species and obtains its nourishment therefrom.

Endoparasites are of three types with regard to their life history: (1) they may spend their entire life as parasites, (2) they may spend only the larval stage as parasites, with the adult free-living, and (3) they may be free-living as larvae but parasitic as adults. In the latter two cases, the species is not parasitic but only the stage — adult or larva. Thus, even though the free-living stage may feed in normal manner, no endoparasite obtains its nourishment from any source other than its host or the host's food.

More commonly noted in parasitology books is the distinction based on the number of hosts that are successively parasitized by the successive stages of the parasite during its life history. There may be one, two, or more hosts in the sequence, depending on the species of parasite and its life history. These do correlate to some extent with the previous types (spending all or only part of their life as parasites). The following are the possibilities:

1. One host, parasitized only by a larva (horsehair worms, botflies)
2. One host, parasitized only by an adult (hookworms)
3. One host, parasitized continuously by both larva and adult (mites)
4. Two hosts, one each for a larva and the adult *(Taenia)*
5. Three hosts, two for larvae and one for adult *(Opisthorchis, Dibothriocephalus)*
6. Four hosts, successively, three for larvae and one for adult (the trematode *Alaria*)

Without being concerned about exceptional occurrences of which the interpretation may differ, one finds ten classes of animals that consist entirely or almost entirely of endoparasites; these are Sporozoa, Rhombozoa and Orthonectida in the Mesozoa, Trematoda, Cestoda, Cestodaria, Acanthocephala, Gordioidea, Nectonematoidea, and Pentastomida. There are six others that include considerable numbers of endoparasites, including Sarcodina, Flagellata, Ciliata, Nematoda, Crustacea, and Insecta.

In many other groups there are a few exceptional parasitic species. But those among which endoparasites are entirely unknown include Porifera, Gnathostomuloidea, Gastrotricha, Kinorhyncha, Priapuloidea, Calyssozoa, Bryozoa, Phoronida, Brachiopoda, Mollusca except for Gastropoda and Bivalvia, Sipunculoidea, Echiuroidea, Tardigrada, Dinophiloidea, Onychophora, Myriapoda, Chaetognatha, Pogonophora, Echinodermata, and all the "chordate" groups.

Distribution of Endoparasites Among the Body Tissues

In digestive tract

Sarcodina	Cestoda	Nematoda
Sporozoa	Cestodaria	Bivalvia
Ciliata	Acanthocephala	Myzostomida
Trematoda	Rotifera	Insecta

In (external) passages (reached through the tissues)

Ciliata	Polychaeta	Crustacea
Mesozoa	Oligochaeta	Arachnida: Acarina
Nematoda	Pentastomida	Insecta

In other tissues and organs

Flagellata	Trematoda	Gastropoda
Sarcodina	Cestoda (larvae)	Polychaeta
Sporozoa	Cestodaria	Myzostomida
Ciliata	Rotifera	Pentastomida
Suctoria	Acanthocephala	Crustacea
Mesozoa	Nematoda	Arachnida: Acarina
Hydrozoa	Gordioidea	Insecta
Turbellaria		

i. Cleptobiosis or Food Stealing

Many animals live always in close association with another and derive their food from it without being truly parasitic. One group of these feed on food stolen from that gathered by the other, often taking it practically out of the mouths of the "hosts". For example, in the tube of a burrowing echiuroid worm may be found individuals of the polychaete worm *Harmothoe adventor,* which "seizes some of the mucus-bag by which its host carries out filter feeding" (Nicol, 1967). These cleptobionts seem to be on the borderline between independent living and parasitism.

Other examples are found among vertebrates, such as the fish-stealing birds and the jackals, when they take food that would otherwise benefit the "host". In a sense, some wasps (Chrysididae) steal the food (an anaesthetized larva gathered by and intended for the embryo of another wasp), by laying a fast-developing egg alongside the egg of the latter to consume the anaesthetized larva before the slow-maturing egg can develop enough to feed on it. A more complex example is the hermit crab accompanied in its shell by a *Nereis* worm, which it thus transports and protects; the worm actually seizes food from the jaws of the crab.

j. Gleaning

When the food eaten by one animal is part of that rejected, or left over, or dropped by another, the situation is slightly different from the food-stealing mentioned above. In cleptobiosis, a small amount of actual damage occurs through the loss of the stolen food. In gleaning, the food is not really stolen because it has already been lost to the "host" by its own volition or its own clumsiness. The gleaner is thus merely a scavenger.

Gleaning also, in this sense, is carried on by the jackals. There is usually no direct tie between the scavenger and the "host"; the former is on the lookout for such sources of food and does not care who furnishes them. Other examples are the pilot fish and the remora (which is also a phoretic and may even be considered as ectoparasitic).

3. Exploitation for Shelter

Many animals obtain shelter by making use of the body or the constructions of other animals or even of plants. There may be substantial or slight damage to the "host" or none at all. The variety of the relationships between two animals with regard to shelter can be exemplified thus:

1. Use of empty snail shell
2. Use of cloaca of holothurian
3. Living among the nematocysts of sea anemones
4. Hiding next to a larger animal to discourage predators
5. Residence in the tube of a polychaete worm
6. Living as "guests" in the nest of ants or termites (inquilinism by beetles)
7. Living in the abode provided by the parents
8. Aggregation to present a stronger defense (herding of ungulates)
9. Attachment of one organism to another for support only (epizoism)

Shelter is often only one of the benefits derived by the association of two organisms, and some of the terms applied to "sheltering" involve plants as well as animals:

1. Epizoism (and epiphytism) — the habit of growing upon or suspended from another animal (or plant) without otherwise harming the "host" or benefitting therefrom
2. Gall-formation — production by a plant of special tissues or structures in response to presence of an insect egg or a nematode
3. Herding — the aggregation of many individuals of a species for such benefit as protection
4. Inquilinism — the residence of individuals of one species within the "nest" of another species (usually of ants or termites); such "guests" may be symphiles, synoeketes, or synechthrans
5. Mermithization — parasitization of an ant by a nematode of the genus *Mermis*, causing pathological body form changes in the ant
6. Parabiosis — habitual intermingling of two or more species, such as mixed herds of ungulates
7. Symphiles — welcome guests that make some return to their hosts
8. Synechthrans — scavengers or predators tolerated or unsuccessfully challenged in the nest
9. Synoeketes — indifferently tolerated guests

4. Exploitation for Use of Labor
a. Outline

Several species of animal obtain the benefits of the activity of other individuals. Some of these are listed elsewhere in this section:

1. Enslavement of other species (or other individuals of the same species) to use them as domestic servants (dulosis among ants, slavery)
2. Domestication (horses, dogs, cattle, swine, sheep, goats, chickens)
3. Taming (elephants, reindeer)
4. Cultivation (by leaf-cutting ants)
5. Ingestion of microorganisms for their digestion of cellulose (termites)
6. Use of foster parents to rear young (cuckoos, humans)

One set of ideas and corresponding terms cuts across this classification by purpose. These are dealt with in the following section.

b. Domestication

Only one animal species exploits other species of animals by the extreme form of life domination called domestication. Under this term are included exploitations for food, for use of labor, for transport, and many others — even for benefit of humans esthetically and through companionship. Most of these exploitations are cited in paragraphs below, and domestication is here dealt with as if only labor was involved.

In a book on diversity of animals, domestication would seem to be a sterile subject, since it is "well known" that only humans domesticate other animals. The accuracy of this assumption may be questioned, because there is no appreciable difference between domestication and the process of interspecies slavery among ants termed *dulosis.* Furthermore, slavery among humans is not basically different, even though it involves only humans.

Domestication is defined in dictionaries as being made part of the household, tamed, and examples are well known. As shown below, this definition is too general, omitting the most important feature which is control by the domesticator of the reproduction of the animal dominated. In more technical terms a domestic animal "is one that has been bred in captivity for purposes of economic profit to a human community that maintains complete mastery over its breeding, organization of territory, and food supply: (Clutton-Brock, 1981, quoted further below).

Thus a distinction is made between domestic animals and those tamed animals which will not produce a continuing population under the care of the humans. This distinction has been called *domestic* and *domesticated.* In the book cited, those are called man-made animals and exploited captives respectively.

Man-made animals (domestic) are those "that have been molded by man for his personal satisfaction and gain . . . (when) the livelihood and breeding of the animals is entirely under human control . . . " The list is not long. It includes:

1. Dogs — of all breeds (from wolves)
2. Horses — from "wild horses" and Przewalski horses
3. Donkeys — from wild asses
4. Mules — from hybrids of donkey with horse
5. Sheep — from the mouflon
6. Goats — from the bezoar
7. Cattle — from the aurochs; including zebu
8. Pigs — from wild boar

In order to be domestic in this sense, an animal must live in populations that through direct selection by man "have certain inherent morphological, physiological, or behavioural characteristics by which they differ from their ancestral stocks."

Man's domestication and selective alteration of organisms is not confined to animals. As pointed out by Jones (1967), the giant grasses (cereals) are not only of immense importance to humans, who are heavily dependent on them for food, but the cereals cannot now seed themselves but must be planted, protected, and carefully nourished by man; without man they would become extinct.

Exploited captives (domesticated). When the "individuals . . . have been made more tractable or tame but whose breeding does not involve intentional selection" they are called domesticated. There is not always a clear distinction.

Almost any individual mammal can be tamed, if the process is started at an early age, but the following species are domesticated only in this sense of taming, without giving up their freedom of breeding. "The reason that there has been little human interference with the breeding of these exploited captives is because it is their perfect adaptation to a harsh environment that is of the greatest benefit to man" and therefore he does not need to tamper with it. Such animals are cats, elephants, camels, llamas, reindeer, and the cattle of Asia (mithan or gaur, bali cattle or banteng, yak, and water buffalo).

Thus, the principal difference between the domestic and the domesticated ones, as defined by Clutton-Brock, is that the former are populations maintained by man but the latter are individuals that have been more or less tamed.

Cats are listed here because the vast majority of household cats are free to breed without intervention of humans, and many of them live partially wild lives. They actually exploit the humans, rather than the other way around.

A number of small mammals are not included in either of these lists. They include rabbits, mice, rats, foxes, ferrets, Guinea pigs, dormice, hamsters, chinchillas, muskrats, coypus (nutria), minks, etc. They are reared and exploited by humans, may be subjected to selective breeding, and therefore may be considered as belonging in either one or both lists.

These lists include only mammals. Many other vertebrates seem to warrant inclusion, such as fowls, cage birds, aquarium fishes, and terrarium reptiles and amphibians. However, most of these will not fit neatly into the domestic/domesticated scheme. For example, turkeys and chickens are usually man-made; waterfowl may be mixtures.

c. Slavery

It is not usually noted that enslavement of humans by other humans is biologically the same as domestication. The slaves are exploited captives, which just happen to be members of the same species. Certain ants enslave other species of ants and exploit them, making captured individuals, not reared populations; this "slavery" among ants is termed dulosis, above.

d. Social Parasitism

This is exemplified by the case of the cuckoo, which lays its eggs in the nest of a bird of some other kind. The "host" bird supposedly does not recognize the foreign egg as such and so proceeds to hatch and feed the nestling, thus saving the cuckoo much travail.

Much the same thing occurs in some insects, though not referred to by this term. Some wasps build a nest and provision it with a paralyzed insect such as a caterpillar. By laying an egg upon it, they have provided the larva that hatches from that egg with a supply of food. However, a "parasitic wasp" of different kind may lay its egg in the food supply even before it is enclosed, and its larva will hatch sooner and eat the stored food and probably the other larva too. The second wasp has exploited the first wasp to hunt down and transport the food, as well as to make the cell where all are protected.

There can be an approach here to cleptobiosis, above; and there is close similarity to enslavement of another species.

5. Exploitation for Camouflage

Camouflage is obtained both by accident and by deliberate action. For example, hermit crabs deliberately place sea anemones on the stolen snail shells they inhabit, thus helping to hide the crab; hydroids growing on an oyster illustrate the accidental condition, neither animal having taken any action to achieve the attachment.

6. Exploitation for Transport

Many animals are carried about by other animals. This carrying may be passive: their need is to be on the animal rather than to be transported elsewhere. Or it may be active: the attachment is deliberate, to attain transport to a desired place by domestication of the animal, such as a horse (by a human) or by attachment to a flying insect (by some other insect). The appropriate term for this, although seldom applied to horseback riding, is *phoresy,* with the "rider" called a *phoretic.*

Phoresy has been reported in at least ten classes of animals, but most of these are only accidental attachments. The following obtain transport on other animals by deliberate action of the transported individual:

1. Nematoda — juveniles on insects
2. Arachnida: Acarina — mites on insects
3. Insecta — flies on dung beetles
4. Mammalia — humans ride on horses, camels, elephants, cattle, dogs

However, the term phoresy (or phoresis) is another of those that are in danger of losing their true meanings because of loose usage by some writers. The phore- root, from the Greek phoreus, means that which is carried; it is related to phero, to carry. The word is sometimes defined as an association involving only passive transport, but the examples are of species that deliberately use other animals to get to a desired place. There is a clear distinction here, and it is usually possible to recognize when one animal is using the locomotion of another to get to a desired place. If one includes in the definition all animals that attach themselves to others for any reason, the assemblage of forms with diverse reasons for being on another animal becomes meaningless. Accidental attachment even to a dead shell could not be excluded. Among the latter are the many marine animals that normally live attached to other animals, even ones that move about. For example, the ciliate *Vorticella* often attaches itself to shells, but this is accidental and there is no advantage of transport to a predetermined place.

The word *endophoresis* has been used for a vorticellid protozoan attached to the gill filaments of a mussel. Of course, no transport is involved.

Two other associations bear some resemblance to phoresy. In some cases the substrate animal is responsible for the association. Here the "rider" is exploited for camouflage or even for food; these are cited under "Exploitation for Shelter" above. In some Insecta, the mother deliberately lays an egg in a "host" individual (such as a caterpillar) so that the hatched larvae may feed on or in that prey individual. The intent is on the part of the parent not of the rider.

The term phoresy should thus be restricted to the situations in which the smaller animal deliberately uses the larger animal to reach a desired place (situations for which the slang expression hitch-hiking would not be inappropriate). The animals that are merely incidentally attached to some other animals could then be called squatters.

7. Exploitation for Use of Body Parts and Products

Other than as food: fur, feathers, leather, bone, ivory, hair, shells, pearls, dried insect bodies; by humans only.

8. Exploitation for Use of Transplanted Organelles

Nematocysts are found in the epidermis of a few Turbellaria. They originate from ingested coelenterates. When freed by the digestion of the soft parts of the jellyfish, the nematocysts are phagocytized by the gastrodermis and passed into the mesenchyme, where they are engulfed by mesenchyme cells. They are carried to the epidermis by these amoeboid cells and can then be employed against prey, being discharged when sufficiently stimulated.

The turbellarian eats the hydras only when in need of more nematocysts, because it prefers other food. It is reported that some flatworms will reject hydras if the worm is already supplied with nematocysts and will regurgitate other food to make room for hydras when more nematocysts are needed.

Such use of "transplanted" nematocysts occurs in at least four phyla: Ctenophora, Platyhelminthes, Rhynchocoela, and Mollusca (Gastropoda).

9. Exploitation for Man's Purposes

The purposes included here are such as esthetics (decoration), experimentation, sport, commerce, religious sacrifice, and medicine. (Man's purposes, of course also include food, shelter, labor, transport, and probably others.) They are not cited further here.

10. Exploitation for Care of Nonfeeding Individuals

In some colonies a neighboring individual provides the food directly into the digestive tract (but see also under no. 11). Colony members may be fed entirely from neighboring individuals (gonangia in Hydrozoa, avicularia and vibracula in Bryozoa).

11. Exploitation for Care of Offspring

In virtually all animals there is some parental care of offspring, at least in the form of a supply of nutrients (yolk) in the ovum. In such a case the offspring is passively exploiting the parent for nourishment.

Many animals liberate their gametes before fertilization and never see their own offspring. Among the rest, there are a variety of means for providing for the protection and needs of the young until they can fend for themselves. Mammals are thought of as unique in care of the foetus through a placenta and the young by provision of milk, but neither of these are really unique in the animal kingdom as a whole. Such care of the offspring takes at least the following forms:

1. Supplying the ovum with nutrients (yolk) in advance
2. Keeping the developing embryo inside the mother, for protection
    A. Viviparity in which embryos are nourished by a placenta, in Mammalia, Onychophora, a few Insecta (with a so-called trophic membrane or trophamnion around the embryo); similar arrangements are found in some Porifera ("nutritive trophic membrane"), some Phylactolaemata; a few Arachnida; some Thaliacea, and possibly in some other forms merely listed as brooding or viviparous (placental viviparity)
    B. Viviparity involving retention of the egg and possibly the ensuing larva in the uterus (ovoviviparity, larviparity)
    C. Brooding, protection of the hatched larva, usually in a special organ
3. Providing an external site for protection of the embryo or larva
4. Providing food for the larva by provisioning or by placing the egg on the right food organism
5. Feeding the young, by suckling, regurgitation, bringing food, trophallaxis, etc.
6. Carrying the young about, for protection

Even among those animals which release their gametes into the surrounding water for chance fertilization, the mother has already stocked the ovum, and thus the zygote and embryo, with food in the form of yolk. This is always sufficient to last the new individual until some other form of food is available to it. These include most Coelenterata, Ctenophora, Brachiopoda, many Mollusca, Sipunculoidea, most Echiuroidea, most marine Annelida, some Echinodermata, some Pterobranchia, Enteropneusta, some Tunicata, Cephalochordata, and a few Vertebrata.

Aside from these aquatic forms, all animals must provide for the nutrition of their offspring, and the mechanisms employed are quite diverse. They may be roughly grouped as yolk (as above), viviparity, placentation or brooding of the embryo, and direct feeding and care of juveniles. Yolk is discussed in Chapter 13, with some indication of which groups depend on this nutrition source.

Among animals that produce zygotes (or apozygotes) inside the female, there is maternal care at least until the egg or embryo or foetus or larva is liberated. As this series implies, there is great diversity in the developmental stage which is first released: from an ovum and a spermatozoon to a larva that has already entered the pupal or resting stage (almost adult). But even this is not all the diversity, because some ova, zygotes, or embryos, upon birth, are deposited in exterior brood pouches, where they may be protected and nourished until development is nearly complete.

Formal tabulation of these processes among the groups of animals has not been feasible. Examples of the diversity are given below, with definitions in the following list of terms.

In many Suctoria, such as *Tokophrya lemnarum,* a ciliated larva is "budded" internally and then released into a brood pouch formed by invagination of the cell surface, from which it is later released. Any such form of parental care among Protozoa appears to be extremely rare.

In the Hydrozoa, both hydroids and medusae may have gonophores or brood chambers, in which the eggs develop to a planula larva or later stage.

In those Turbellaria that produce composite eggs (see Chapter 5), an egg or a few eggs are placed in a capsule in which there are many yolk cells, perhaps as many as several thousand, to provide nourishment.

In Trematoda eggs may be laid before development begins, or the eggs may remain in the uterus until they contain fully developed larvae. In one family the larva may even hatch in the uterus, a process called ovoviviparity.

In parthenogenetic Rotifera the females may be ovoviviparous. These may lack an oviduct, in which case the young are liberated through a rupture in the body wall.

Many Nematoda are oviparous but there is ovoviviparity in *Trichinella* and such groups as filarial worms. It is said that some parasitic nematodes can occur in two forms, oviparous and ovoviviparous, a condition that has been termed *dimorphobiosis.*

In Bryozoa there are many forms of brooding: in the coelom, between the two cuticles, or in an external pouch called an ovicell or ooecium.

In some freshwater Bivalvia, one pair of gills may be used as a marsupium to brood embryos and early larval stages. In some species these embryos actually attach to the wall and draw nourishment from it; this has been cited as a simple form of placentation.

In Polychaeta, the members of the genus *Polynoe* have overlapping scales on the upper surface, under which the young can develop.

In Hirudinea, "brood care often involves the attachment of each of several dozens of embryos to the ventral body wall of the parent by a curious ectodermal ball-and-socket joint and the parent may hold the embryos under her body for many weeks, passing a current of water over them by gentle dorso-ventral undulations" (Mann, 1961).

In Onychophora most species are viviparous, with part of the uterine wall forming a placenta with a trophoblast around the embryo.

Several groups of Crustacea provide care for their young. This varies from transport in masses attached to the appendages, with parental care limited to "aeration", to retention within a brood pouch, and to living in the empty test of a tunicate provided and guarded by the mother. The brood pouch may be called a marsupium.

In Insecta, there are a variety of modes of parental care, as would be expected. In many, the eggs develop in a protective case or ootheca formed by the mother. In some Dermaptera, eggs are cared for "in the soil in a group, and the female rests over them very much like a hen and her chickens'' (Imms, 1951), and drives away predators. Some wasps build an earthen cell, stored with food, and seal the egg into this chamber. Dung and carrion beetles deposit their eggs on buried masses of food, for consumption by the larva after hatching. Viviparity is widespread but never common, occurring in Orthoptera, Dermaptera, Homoptera, Ephemeroptera, Coleoptera, Lepidoptera, and Diptera, at least. Ovoviviparity is also widespread but never common in any group. It is said to occur in thrips, some roaches, some scale insects, in various flies, etc. The terms *larviparity* and *pupiparity* are used to denote the stage of the insect when it is finally deposited outside.

Although most Echinodermata are oviparous, viviparity is reported in some Ophiuroidea. Brooding is said to be very diverse in the phylum. There are a variety of brood chambers, marsupia, incubatory sacs, stomach pouches, the oral cavity, or bursae; or the eggs may even be brooded in the coelom.

In Tunicata (Thaliacea), eggs may be attached to the atrial wall, from which they obtain nutrients by a diffusion placenta.

In the Vertebrata, parental care takes its most elaborate and diverse forms. In general, the diversity includes all the forms listed for other animals, and more besides. Among the fishes there is viviparity, with either ovarian gestation, follicular gestation, or uterine gestation. There may be yolk-sac placentae with an umbilical cord, or a uterine glandular area that secretes a uterine milk that can be aspirated into the oral region of the embryo through the spiracles. There may be as many as 70,000 villi lining the uterus, termed *trophonemata*. In ovarian gestation elaborate extensions of the ovarian wall may grow into the gill cavities and mouth of the embryo to transfer food. Special ribbon-like extensions of the anal region of the embryo, called *trophotaeniae*, become closely associated with the folds of the wall of the ovary. Or vascular extensions of soft tissue between the rays of the vertical fins perform this transfer. ''As proof of the efficiency of this arrangement it may be mentioned that male *Cymatogaster* sometimes remain in the ovary until sexually mature'' (Hoar, 1957, quoting Turner).

In Amphibia, eggs may be deposited externally in pits on the dorsal surface, where they are nourished by their own yolk sac but where gaseous exchange takes place between the maternal tissues and the expanded leaf-like tail of the developing larva. This is termed *pseudoplacentation*. In some salamanders there may be ovoviviparity, with intrauterine cannibalism. Oral absorption of *uterine milk* may provide the nutrition for larvae hatched in the oviduct. Some frogs and toads construct nests or shelters for development of laid eggs. Eggs may be carried on the body of either parent or in pockets of the surface; they may be transferred to the immense vocal sacs on the ventral surface.

In the Reptilia, some lizards and some snakes are ovoviviparous and some viviparous. In the latter there may be yolk-sacs or a chorio-allantoic placenta. There may be incubating chambers in the oviducts, where a special blood supply is provided.

Apparently all birds are oviparous, so embryonic care is limited to provision of yolk in the egg. Parental care is nearly universal in the form of nests, feeding, and a rudimentary training of the fledglings.

In the Mammalia, viviparity is nearly universal, except for the egg-laying monotremes. Yolk is absent in eggs of the placentals. The fertilized egg is implanted in the uterine wall, where an elaborate placenta is formed for each. In marsupials there is a placenta, but the young are very early passed to the outside to be nurtured in a pouch or marsupium. Here they are nourished by milk from mammary glands, as in all higher forms. Much care of young by the parents occurs among mammals.

List of terms. The following are some of the terms that refer to care of the young by the parents:

1. Brood pouch or chamber — any cavity provided for the protection of eggs, embryos, or larvae
2. Brooding — protection of a group of eggs, embryos, or larvae, usually by a parent
3. Bursal brooding — retention of eggs in a pouch (bursa) of the body wall (Ophiuroidea)
4. Dimorphobiosis — occurrence of free-living ovoviviparous worms in species normally parasitic and oviparous
5. Gestation — the development from fertilization to birth in viviparous animals: (a) follicular, in the ovarian follicles of some Pisces; (b) ovarian, in the ovary but released from the follicle, in some Pisces; and (c) uterine, in the uterine wall of some Mammalia
6. Gonophore — the blastostyle of Hydrozoa, when used for brooding (this word is also used to refer to a portion of the body set aside, usually detached, to carry the gonads)
7. Incubation — the protection of the young by maintaining suitable temperature
8. Larviparity — viviparity that results in birth of a larva (s.Insecta)
9. Marsupium — an external pouch for brooding one or more eggs, embryos, or larvae
10. Milk — a nutritious emulsion secreted from mammary or other glands for nourishment of offspring
11. Ooecium — same as ovicell
12. Ootheca — protective capsule around one or several eggs (Insecta)
13. Ovicell — an external brood chamber (Bryozoa)
14. Oviparity — the condition in which eggs hatch outside of the mother's body
15. Oviparous — laying eggs that hatch outside of the body of the mother
16. Ovoviviparity — the condition in which living young hatch from the eggs inside the mother just before birth and are therefore not nourished by her
17. Ovoviviparous — giving birth to young through ovoviviparity
18. Placenta — an organ formed by close association of tissues of mother and offspring for transfer of nutrients, oxygen, and wastes; see also pseudoplacenta, trophoblast, trophamnion, etc.; includes: (a) chorio-allantoic placenta, formed of the chorionic and allantoic membranes of the embryo (s.Mammalia), (b) diffusion placenta, one formed from follicle and oviduct cells of the parent and ectoderm cells of the embryo (Thaliacea), and (c) yolk-sac placenta, one formed by an external yolk sac in intimate contact with the uterine wall (Pisces, s.Mammalia)
19. Placentation — the provision of nourishment to embryo or foetus through a placenta
20. Pseudoplacenta — placenta-like nutritive arrangement (s.Insecta; but here called a placenta)
21. Pupiparity — condition in which a larva is retained inside the mother until it has pupated (s.Insecta)
22. Semiplacenta — One in which the chorionic villi are closely associated with, but not fused with, the uterine lining (s.Mammalia)
23. Trophic membrane — one that supplies nutrients to the embryo (see Trophamnion)
24. Trophamnion — a nutritional envelope of some insect eggs
25. Trophoblast — the outer coat of the implantation stage of the early embryo of placental mammals; see also Onychophora
26. Trophonemata — villi on the surface of the uterus, involved in nutrient transfer to the embryo, in some viviparous fishes

27. Trophotaeniae — ribbon-like extensions of the anal region of the larva to form a placenta with folds of the maternal ovarian epithelium, in some viviparous fishes
28. Uterine milk — a nourishing secretion of the uterine mucosa, in a few sharks, amphibians, snakes, and lizards
29. Viviparity — the condition in which young develop inside the body of the mother and are nourished by her tissues: (a) exgenito-viviparity, with the larva nourished in the haemocoel (s.Insecta); and (2) intussuctio-viviparity, with the larva nourished in the uterus (s.Insecta); but the term would also apply to Mammalia
30. Viviparous — giving birth to young through viviparity
31. Yolk — the intracellular food reserve of an ovum, zygote, or embryo; sometimes contained in nurse cells
32. Yolk-sac — reservoir for nutrients for developing oviparous embryos of birds and most fishes and reptiles

It should be noted that the terms viviparity and ovoviviparity do not form a contrasting pair. All animals that "lay" eggs are said to be oviparous; all that produce living young are said to be viviparous. Among the latter some can be seen to harbor the young inside eggs retained in the mother, hatching just before birth; these are called ovoviviparous. In reality, ovoviviparity is a form of oviparity, in which the hatching of the egg occurs before or during the egg-laying. The important feature is not the condition at birth (egg or young) but whether the young have been nourished by the mother before birth. Thus, oviparity and ovoviviparity involve no maternal nutrition after fertilization, whereas in viviparity the developing embryo is directly nourished by the mother.

E. Other Concepts
1. Commensalism
Another term, frequently used for some form of exploitation, has had an unfortunate history. Commensalism means "eating together" and was originally applied in this correct sense: living in association with an individual of another species for the purpose of obtaining food. This food could be stolen, gleaned, or consist of material rejected by the "host". In recent years, that meaning has been both enlarged and restricted to designate associations in which the "commensal" benefits in any way, but the "host" is not clearly damaged.

Most recent books that use this term are in agreement on its definition. This should make it easy to apply the word in practice. Unexpectedly, it turns out that nearly all examples given in these books, although actually fitting the definition, do not have much to do with symbiosis. In the oft-cited pilot fish, for example, there is no interrelationship between the individuals. The pilot fish has merely found a niche that it likes and exploits it, in the same manner that another species uses a hole in a coral reef as its niche. It is no more symbiosis than is predation or the scavenging of a jackal. The relationship is not necessary to either animal, nor is it host-specific.

Nevertheless, parasitologists often treat it along with parasitism. And among organisms of medical interest to man, there are some whose damage to the host is virtually nil but which benefit from it themselves. These are generally internal symbionts, ones which happen to feed on materials of no essential use to the host. They are like endoparasites except for this lack of damage. Actually there are all possible variants, from no damage to severe damage and death.

It is clear that the diversity of animal interrelationships cannot be covered by the usual series of terms: symbiosis, parasitism, commensalism, and mutualism. Symbiosis is so general as to include the other three; parasitism is used to cover real endoparasites but also temporary ectoparasites, phoretics, and accidentals; commensalism is used for two very different sorts of relationships; and mutualism does not really occur at all, as all examples are merely mutual exploitation. No better system of terms is available, but the diversity was exemplified as in Table 26.

Terms that seem to apply to commensalism rather than to parasitism or any other form of symbiosis include these:

1. Ectocommensal — living on the outside of another animal to obtain food without injury to the animal
2. Endocommensal — living on the inside of another animal to obtain food without injury to the animal
3. Endozoic — living within another animal
4. Epizoic — living on the exterior surface of another animal
5. Myrmecophily — living by association with ants
6. Synoeketes — indifferently tolerated guests in any nests
7. Trophobiosis — symbiosis in which there is an exchange of food

2. Mutualism

This is often defined as an extended association that is beneficial to both individuals. If individual A makes use of products or facilities of species B, A is exploiting B. If at the same time species B makes use of products or facilities of species A, it is also exploiting. This is mutual exploitation. The term mutualism is thus useful where it is desired to indicate that each animal exploits the other. Because the duration and closeness of the association vary, and the amount of benefit derived by each one varies greatly, and may be necessary to either or to both, the term does not connote much about the relationship.

In some cases of mutualism one of the individuals could live alone, not absolutely requiring anything from the other, even though accepting the benefit when offered. In other cases neither species can exist without the other. There is sometimes implication that one deliberately benefits the other in order to obtain the benefits. No case has been found that would justify this view.

3. Host

The word host is one of the terms related to parasitism that is used in a variety of ways, but it usually does not thereby become confusing. It can be informally defined as the animal which is exploited, in all forms of symbiosis. The host is not even distinguishable from prey, except that in general one survives the exploitation and the other does not.

This word is apparently not considered a technical term, as it is seldom defined or indexed. In the case of hosts of parasites, there are some descriptive terms in use:

1. Definitive host — the host in which the parasite reaches adult stage, or becomes sexually mature
2. Final host — same as definitive host
3. Intercalary host — one which is entered passively and in which no development occurs
4. Intermediate host — the host that is parasitized by an immature stage of the parasite, which later moves to another host for further development; there may be one, two, or even three intermediate hosts in one life cycle, leading finally to the definitive host
5. Paratenic host — sometimes defined as "an intermediate or transport host" but in parasitology restricted to a host in which there is no development (i.e., transport host)

6.   Provisional host — same as intermediate host
7.   Reservoir host — an animal other than a human that is normally infected with a parasite which can also infect humans
8.   Transport host — a host in which no development takes place while waiting to infect a definitive host (see paratenic host)

It is an odd thing that many books describe a host as an animal that "harbors" parasites. The verb to harbor is here transitive and implies activity to provide a safe haven for another. No parasites are harbored in this sense, but some symbionts are welcomed and may be provided for. However, any parasite may be said to harbor *in its host*.

Hosts occur in every group of animals. Presumably, every individual of every species is host to some symbionts (especially parasites) during most of its life.

F. Parasitology

1. Usages

Parasitology is literally the study of parasites and parasitism. Although this definition would usually be acceptable to anyone, it is in fact not the definition by which the word is used. There are many books on "parasitology", usually using that word in the title. There are many other books that use the word "parasitism" in the title, and there is usually a sharp distinction between the two.

For parasitology, many books deal largely with the medical and veterinary aspects of parasitic animals. Parasitologists are generally associated with the practive of medicine, and their international societies are associated with public health organizations. In these books there may be more than just clinical parasitology, but interest is primarily in the life of those parasites that directly or indirectly affect humans.

Under *parasitism,* and even more under symbiosis, a more biological approach is usually taken. Here parasites (or symbionts) are studied without exclusive regard to clinical aspects of any particular species. In books on either of these subjects, a broad view of symbiotic relationships will lead to understanding of the immense diversity that exists, and the present chapter is designed to give that broader view.

2. Parasite Life Cycles

There are a few interests of parasitologists that have not so far been discussed herein. In describing the life cycles of parasites, much emphasis is sometimes placed on adaptation of the parasite cycle to that of its host. When the life span of the host may vary from a few days (Protozoa and Rotifera) to many years (Mammalia), it is obvious that the cycles of the parasites must be different and that they must be such as to fit that parasite to live in that host or series of hosts. The requirements of parasitic life are sometimes strict, but so are the requirements of many other animal lives. So there is no sharp distinction here.

Parasites are described as requiring a high biotic potential because of the vicissitudes of their life. However, it is true of many other animals also that continuation of the species requires production of multitudinous gametes and also extra reproduction by asexual means.

Many parasites live in environments that seem unusual and harsh to the observer. The hosts impose physical and chemical factors that restrict the parasite throughout its life cycle, but free-living animals may also live in harsh environments (hot springs, petroleum or saline pools, for example) and it does not seem that the factors are necessarily different in kind, rigor, or number.

Much is made of the mechanisms (adaptations) that may have produced a parasitic relationship. It is supposed that parasitism arose independently in each group, that ectoparasitism may or may not have led to endoparasitism, or that the same may hold for other forms of symbiosis. In any case one must ask how this differs from the adaptation of other animals to their special environments (plural because most of them also live in several different conditions, as embryo, larva, and adult).

It seems necessary to conclude that, neither in biotic potential, nor in harshness of environment, nor in adaptation to special situations, do parasites fall beyond the already wide range of free-living organisms.

The term *hyperparasitism* has been used for the occurrence of parasites within (or upon) other parasites. Some books treat this as a special adaptation, worthy of a special section; or these parasites-upon-parasites are called secondary. It is quite certain that most parasites are themselves parasitized routinely. For example, many parasitic Crustacea (Isopoda or Cirripedia) are parasitized by other ectoparasitic Crustacea of the same or other groups. Microsporidia of several species live in the cells of certain flukes and tapeworms, which themselves live in the intestine of some vertebrates.

Many hyperparasites are cited among insects. For example, one moth caterpillar is known to have 23 parasites (6 flies and 17 wasps). These 23 in turn have at least 13 parasites (called secondary but primary to the 23 hosts), and the 13 themselves have several parasites (called tertiary but actually primary to their 13 hosts). It must be noted, however, that many insects called parasitic are actually predaceous, so such an example as this may not involve real hyperparasitism.

A *hyperparasite* is simply a parasite of an animal which itself happens to be a parasite. There is nothing unusual about the hyperparasite; it is just another parasite that must live in a suitable host. One does not hear of hyperpredators, and yet many feed on other predators and must take advantage of the life of that prey.

IV. REPRODUCTIVE BEHAVIOR

Reproduction is usually thought of as a cooperative process involving two individuals, as in all bisexual reproduction. There are thousands of species in which "sexual reproduction" is merely unisexual; parthenogenetic. Much reproduction is even asexual. Reproductive behavior is treated under social behavior merely to reflect the common view of bisexual reproduction.

Behavior is nowadays often described as a highly specialized subject using the most refined techniques and synthesizing data from a wide variety of fields, both observational and experimental. Behavior also covers many simple reactions of an organism, some of which can be described in reasonably simple terms. Even these comparatively simple behaviors show great diversity, as we have seen in the sections on animal feeding, locomotion, and excretion. This book deals mostly with gross features, rather than with molecular and cellular ones, and, at the general level of the whole individual, the behavior is not such an esoteric subject.

Some behaviorists treat reproduction as the most important subject in behavior. This is presumably because virtually all behavior contributes to reproduction in some way. The chapters on reproduction have already touched on such behavior as gamete liberation, spermatozoan transfer, budding, and fragmentation. More generally, the behavior related to reproduction would include also courtship, territoriality, home building, oviposition or birth, brooding of eggs, and care of the young. The first three of these are largely restricted to vertebrates, although there are occasional examples among invertebrates.

For example, there are courtships and mating dances in some Arachnida and in some flies. There is building of homes in some Crustacea and some Tunicata. There is even a sort of territoriality in many parasites, in which one gives off some influence that prevents others from becoming established there. The birth of living young that have been nourished inside the mother occurs in Onychophora (where there is an actual placenta) and in some of the brooding species in many marine groups.

REFERENCES

Blackwelder, R. E. and Dyer, W. G., Animal Interactions. *Transactions of the Illinois State Academy of Science*, 72(3), 1, 1980.

Caullery, M., *Parasitism and Symbiosis*, Sidgwick & Jackson, London, 1952.

Chandler, A. C. and Read, C. P., *Introduction to Parasitology*, 10th ed., John Wiley & Sons, New York, 1961.

Cheng, T. C., *The biology of Animal Parasites*, W. B. Saunders, Philadelphia, 1964.

Clutton-Brock, J., *Domesticated Animals from Early Times*, University of Texas, Austin, 1981.

Dogiel, V. A., *General Parasitology*, revised, Academic Press, New York, 1966.

Gray, P., *The Dictionary of the Biological Sciences*, Reinhold, New York, 1967.

Hoar, W. S., The gonads and reproduction, in *The Physiology of Fishes*, Brown, M. E., Ed., Vol. 1, *Metabolism*, Academic Press, New York, 1957, chap. 7.

Hyman, L. H., *The Invertebrates*, Vol. 3, McGraw-Hill, New York, 1951.

Jones, A. W., *Introduction to Parasitology*, Addison-Wesley, Reading, Pa., 1967.

Keeton, W. T., *Biological Science*, 3rd ed., W. W. Norton, New York, 1980.

MacGinitie, G. E. and MacGinitie, N., *Natural History of Marine Animals*, McGraw-Hill, New York, 1949.

Mann, K. H., *Leeches (Hirudinea); Their Structure, Physiology, Ecology and Embryology*, Pergamon Press, Oxford, 1961.

Nicol, J. A. C., *The Biology of Marine Animals*, 2nd ed., Sir Isaac Pitman & Son, London, 1967.

Odum, E. P., *Fundamentals of Ecology*, W. B. Saunders, Philadelphia, 1953.

Pennak, R. W., *Collegiate Dictionary of Zoology*, Ronald Press, New York, 1964.

Schmidt, G. D. and Roberts, L. S., *Foundations of Parasitology*, C. V. Mosby, St. Louis, 1977.

Simon, H., *Partners, Guests, and Parasites; Coexistence in Nature*, Viking Press, New York, 1970.

Part VI
Coloniality

"A prerequisite for this analysis is an understanding of the term 'colony'. We define it as a group of individuals, structurally bound together in varying degrees of skeletal and physiological integration, all genetically linked by descent from a single founding individual. 'Colony', then, includes a range of structures grading from those in which all polyps are completely individualized with independent functions and no soft-part connections, to those in which soft parts, skeleton, and functions are communal."

A. G. Coates and W. A. Oliver, Jr., 1973

Chapter 23

COLONIES

TABLE OF CONTENTS

I.   Coloniality 486
      A.   Orientation 486
      B.   Colonies 486
      C.   Noncolonies 487

II.   Colonies by Group 490

III. Motility of Colonies 492

IV.   Colony Terms 492

V.   Reproduction of Colonies 494
      A.   Sexual Reproduction 494
      B.   Asexual Reproduction 495
            1.   Budding 495
            2.   Division 495

References 495

I. COLONIALITY

A. Orientation

The headings in this book make it appear that the nature and life of animals can be clearly separated under a number of subject titles. This is a notably false appearance. Many subjects have had to be mentioned in several places, and some have had to be placed in arbitrary positions. So it is with individuality and coloniality, which affect our account of diversity in several ways.

The various ways in which organisms exist in groups of many individuals are suggestd in Chapter 22 under "Consortism". Here we exclude the flocks of birds and hives of bees that are sometimes loosely called colonies, because they do not really come under the term coloniality. The present discussion includes only the colonies that are physically interconnected groups of organisms produced by asexual reproduction with incomplete separation. The components always retain some individuality, but the colony also achieves individuality of a higher order, sometimes potentially of endless extension, sometimes as clearly delimited as ordinary single individuals.

One seldom finds clear-cut definitions of either individual or colony, any more than of cell, organ, or process. This is because an organism which is always highly integrated can show more or less individuality, and a colony which may show more or less individuality may also show more or less integration. This varying amount of distinctness of individuals was one of the first diversities encountered in this volume; it arises again as one of the last. In spite of the existence of animals that cannot clearly be called either colonial or noncolonial for certain, one can make a definition that will cover the most frequently seen situations: *coloniality is the tendency of animals to form clonal aggregations of individuals in physical contact.*

B. Colonies

A colony in zoology is a variously defined group of individuals of one species. The only factor common to all the definitions is that more than one individual is involved. It is customary to deal with animals as if they were always distinct individuals (see "Individuality" in Chapter 1). A variety of exceptions to this general situation are easily overlooked. There are at least 18 classes of animals in which "individuals", formed asexually, remain attached to each other in some form of colony. The type of interconnection, the duration of it, the form of the colony, its mobility, and the extent of its integration, all vary considerably.

To be classed as a colony rather than as an aggregation, the individuals composing the colony must be derived from one original individual. Most of them will retain physical contact and will usually remain in protoplasmic connection, forming a permanent colony of a fairly uniform shape and structure. This definition would eliminate such temporary "colonies" as those formed by strobilation in the scyphistoma of Scyphozoa, the transverse fission of Turbellaria and Polychaeta, and the lateral buds or attached larvae of other Polychaeta. It also eliminates the temporary strobilation in both Ciliata and Mastigophora and the syzygy of some Sporozoa.

A colony is a group of individuals produced asexually from one progenitor and remaining in physical and frequently protoplasmic contact.

The true colonies so defined are found only in sessile organisms, although the colonies themselves may be free-floating or locomotory. (Both of the latter are found in the Hydrozoa, the Graptozoa, and the Tunicata.) In each case the colony may arise from stolons or the individuals may be budded directly from earlier individuals.

Sessile colonies occur in the stalked Ciliata and Suctoria, where connection is through the stalk. Colonies connected by the horizontal extensions called stolons are produced in some of the Hydrozoa, Graptozoa, Endoprocta, Bryozoa, Pterobranchia, and Tunicata. Colonies produced by budding or division of individuals and not clearly stolonate are found in some of the Stromatoporoidea, Anthozoa, Bryozoa, and Tunicata.

Motile colonies, including pelagic ones, are produced by stolons in Graptozoa and Tunicata, but some of the latter seem to bud without stolons. Some members of two classes of Protozoa produce colonies by division of the cell; these are the Mastigophora (e.g., *Volvox*) and the Sarcodina (some Radiolaria). Siphonophora in the Hydrozoa produce polymorphic floating colonies by budding.

C. Noncolonies

Several animals form aggregations built up of separate individuals rather than connected progeny of one. These are not colonies, but they might be taken for such. They include some of the tube-dwelling Phoronida, the Polychaeta, and the Pogonophora, which may occur in tangled masses of tubes; the Brachiopoda and Mollusca, which may grow attached to each other's shells; and the Cirripedia (barnacles), which may grow in dense clusters. Some Sarcodina form gregaloid "colonies", in which individuals become attached to one another by means of pseudopodia in an irregular form. In the Gregarinida two individuals may come together in a front-to-rear manner called syzygy. There is also an unusual association in the Polychaeta, when side branches remain attached and form an arborescent mass.

Strobilation produces "colonies" in some groups with a comparatively permanent status. In the Radiolarian *Collozoum*, the Ciliata, and some Dinoflagellata, a chain is produced by successive cell divisions, but this is not strobilation, which requires that new individuals be produced at one point in the chain, not at the ends. In Scyphozoa a strobilus forms a temporary chain by strobilation. In rhabdocoel Turbellaria a temporary chain may be produced, and in certain Polychaeta a temporary chain may be produced by successive division of the body in what seems to be strobilation. (Only in Cestoda is strobilation the source of an entire chain which lasts to maturity, each proglottid dropping off when it is mature and when it reaches the end of the chain.) However, these proglottids are not individuals; they are detached organs to carry the gonads until gametes are released.

In some discussions of coloniality there is extensive reference to viviparity, and viviparous animals are listed as colonial. Nothing seems to be gained by treating this reproductive/behavioral condition as related to coloniality.

Thus, the terms individual and colony do not form an exclusive system into which all animals can be fitted. At least the following associations occur in this system:

1. Completely separate individuals
2. Aggregations of separate individuals that have become attached to each other: (a) by their tubes (Phoronida, Polychaeta, Pogonophora), (b) by their shells (Brachiopoda, Mollusca, Crustacea: Cirripedia), (c) by cell wall as gregaloidy (Sarcodina) or as syzygy (Sporozoa), or (d) by body wall and internal tissues (panorpa larvae of Trematoda, s.larvae of Polychaeta)
3. Temporary connection of several arising from one: (a) by strobilation (Ciliata, Flagellata, Scyphozoa, Cestoda), (b) by incomplete transverse fission (s.Ciliata, Turbellaria, Polychaeta), or (c) by incomplete lateral budding (Hydrozoa, Polychaeta)
4. Incomplete separation of dividing cells, the colony form indefinite (Flagellata)
5. Incomplete separation of dividing cells, with great uniformity and individuality to the colony (Sarcodina: Radiolaria, Flagellata, Ciliata): (a) floating colonies (Siphonophora Graptozoa, s.Tunicata), or (b) motile colonies (s.Bryozoa, s.Tunicata)

6. Colonies of multicellular individuals, the colony form indefinite (s.Hydrozoa, s.Anthozoa, Bryozoa, S.Tunicata)
7. Multiple structures with great individuality and composed either of individuals or of organs (as variously interpreted (Siphonophora)
8. Compound structures composed of individuals sharing certain organs (Tunicata)
9. Siamese twins, partially separated pairs (Mammalia)
10. Plasmodia, masses of protoplasm with many nuclei but with no cell membranes (Sarcodina: Mycetozoa)

Number 1 represents undoubted individuals. Numbers 4 to 6 are undoubted colonies. Numbers 7 and 8 are usually called colonies but can be argued to be super-individuals. In number 9 the twins are not a colony but merely an incomplete separation in polyembryony. Number 3 includes a few colonies called catenoid, such as *Radiophrya* in the Ciliata. Number 10 represents fusion masses rather than colonies; these groups are endlessly argued as colonies or not (what the ''not'' represents usually being unspecified).

These diverse situations do not form a sequence, although there are some intermediates. The individual/colony distinction is incapable of dealing with the diversity, and it is necessary to invent additional terms or use descriptive modifiers.

Syzygy is usually described as the front-to-rear attachment of two individuals, found only in the gregarine Protozoa. This definition fails to tell much about this unusual process and its purpose or function. A detailed, although somewhat technical account is given in Sleigh (1973), where it is shown that the two individuals are gamonts, that they become enclosed in a cyst wherein each gamont undergoes multiple fission to produce many gametes. The gametes may be either isogametes, so that the gamonts have no evident sex, or they may be anisogametes so that the gamonts can be recognized as male and female. Fertilization takes place inside the cyst, after which each zygote becomes a spore that will develop into a few sporozoites. After infecting new hosts, these sporozoites will develop into the original form (trophozoites) that will become gamonts in the next cycle of syzygy.

Two other situations are sometimes mentioned with respect to coloniality. The first is hermaphroditism, in which one individual has the reproductive organs of both male and female, being in fact a dual animal so far as sex is concerned. The second is viviparity, the bearing of living young, in which two individuals are temporarily connected (in the cases of placentation). Each of these could be worked into the foregoing list (both in no. 3), but they seem a little farfetched for even a ''complete'' tabulation of multiple structures. The occurrence of both are listed in part II of this book.

With respect to the great diversity of cellular and colonial structures, the following situations exist among animals (see Figure 25):

1. Individual cells (Protozoa)
2. Indefinite colonies of cells (Ciliata)
3. Individualized colonies of cells (*Volvox*)
4. Plasmodia (Sarcodina: Myxomycetes)
5. Multicellular individuals (Metazoa)
6. Indefinite colonies of multicellular individuals (Bryozoa)
7. Individualized colonies of multicellular individuals (*Physalia*)
8. Chains of fragments that can never become separate individuals (Cestoda)
9. Chains of fragments that can become separate individuals (Scyphozoa)
10. Compound structures consisting of many incomplete individuals sharing some organs (Ascidiacea)

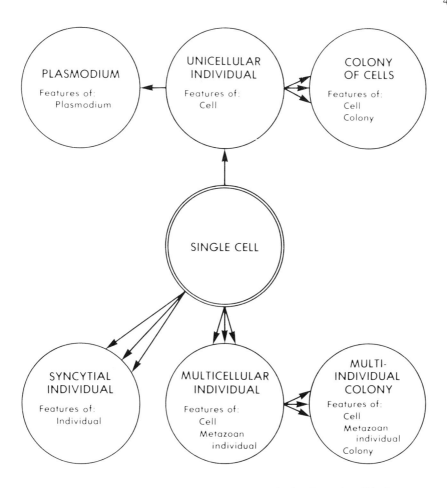

FIGURE 25. Relationships of cells, individuals, and colonies. From the cell in the center, individuals of three types may be seen to be derived. Two of these can subsequently become colonies.

The factors that must be considered in determining coloniality include these:

1. Multiplicity of individuals (at least presumed)
2. Clonality. They must be of one species only, which is assured by the necessity that they are all derived asexually from a single individual (either still present or replaced) and thus form a clone
3. Continuity. There must be structural continuity between individuals, and there must be or at some time have been protoplasmic continuity also
4. Dependence. There must be some independence among the "individuals", to establish that they are such; and some interdependence, to show a degree of colonial integration
5. Permanence. They must not be merely a temporary phase in development
6. Normalcy. They must be a normal feature of the life cycle, not merely the result of a developmental accident

These colonies grade off into temporary attachments, such as monodisk strobilation in Scyphozoa (see under "Asexual Reproduction" in Chapter 2) and into compound individuals in Tunicata, where interdependence is so great as to involve substantial common organs. They will also be confused with plasmodia (in Myxomycetes) as well as with clusters of separate individuals that grow together after a separate existence (such as barnacles).

Even beyond these, there are problems with the sponges, which show only some of the required factors of coloniality. Furthermore, two genera of pelagic siphonophores, which are highly integrated, have been listed as colonial but now appear merely as unusually large and specialized medusae (*Velella* and *Porpita*).

Thus there are many forms of colonies and of noncolonies. They occur very widely among animals.

II. COLONIES BY GROUP

These aggregations are described briefly in the various phyla with examples cited.

PROTOZOA

Flagellata. Linear: such forms as *Ceratium* and *Haplozoon* may form chains of several individuals, by the daughters remaining attached lengthwise; there is some polymorphism. Arboroid: as in *Dinobryon*, the daughter cells remain attached in a treeform. Discoid: as in *Gonium*, the cells form a roughly circular mass in one plane. Spheroid: as in *Volvox*, with or without protoplasmic connections; both somatic and reproductive individuals.

Sarcodina. Heliozoa, chains formed, by incomplete fission, as in *Rhaphidiophrys*.

Ciliata. Chains, as in *Radiophrya*, by transverse fission. Arboroid: as in *Carchesium* and *Zoothamnion*. Massive: as in *Ophrydium*.

Suctoria. Arboroid, as in *Dendrosoma*, where the macronucleus extends as a branched axis throughout the colony; many micronuclei.

Sporozoa. The multicellular "spores" in many species have been called colonies.

PORIFERA

Clear-cut colonies do not seem to exist among living species, but multiple structures are common and have been interpreted as being composed of many individuals. Some fossils, such as *Titusvillia*, appear to consist of budded individuals in linear succession to form branching colonies.

†GRAPTOLITOIDEA

The extinct graptolites were all minute and colonial. This extinct group produced both sessile and floating colonies. The individuals were arranged in rows on one or both sides of the branches, with colonies dendritic, frondose, or radiating.

COELENTERATA

Hydrozoa. The varieties of colony-like assemblages is almost endless. Frequently the "colony" is merely a stage in the division into several zooids. *Caspionema* forms double individuals, base to base. In *Gastroblasta,* formation of many proctostomes leaves a circular body with only a suggestion of individuals, which may later become separate by fission. Other colonies may be arboroid or stolonate in many varieties. Multiple budding may produce temporary "colonies" in either polyp form *(Lafoea)* or medusa *(Hybocodon).* (Siphonophora and Stromatoporoidea are cited separately.) Massive colonies of interconnected tubes occur, as in *Millepora*.

†Stromatoporoidea. An extinct group of animals forming colonies, massive irregular, laminar, or tubular dendroid. The colonies were presumably formed by budding and there seem to have been protoplasmic connections between individuals.

Siphonophora. These are all polymorphic pelagic colonies, consisting of specialized polypoid and medusoid individuals of several sorts. Two major types occur: Medusoid colonies are composed of as many as seven forms of individuals, as in *Physalia;* linear colonies such as in *Muggiaea* and *Agalma* may also consist of as many as seven forms of individuals. (Such forms as *Velella* and *Porpita* have been described as highly integrated colonies but are probably merely large medusae. If so, they show the great similarity between organs and specialized individuals.)

Scyphozoa. In such forms as *Chrysaora* and *Aurelia*, the scyphistoma stage strobilates like a stack of saucers, appearing like a linear colony. The connection is always temporary, and thus does not form a colony.

Anthozoa. Corals exist in a wide variety of colony forms. Some phaceloid colonies, tubular or dendritic, such as *Syringopora*, have connection between individuals, others do not. Discoidal colonies, such as *Renilla* and *Fungia*, may have a distinctive colony shape. Cateniform or *"chain-colonies"* occur in *Cystihalysites*, where the tubes are united into sheets. Encrusting forms are numerous, and there are many terms to describe the arrangement of the polyps. Many dendritic forms occur, such as *Pennatula*, *Ctenocella*, *Acanella*, and *Gorgonia*.

PLATYHELMINTHES

Turbellaria. Some rhabdocoels, such as *Stenostomum*, undergo transverse fission to form chains which are temporary and therefore not colonies.

Trematoda. Two sorts of very odd multiple individuals occur. In *Gyrodactylus*, an embryo may exist with a second embryo already formed inside, with a third inside the second, and even a fourth already inside the third. These are apparently formed successively from a single germ ball, carried along inside each generation of embryos. In *Diplozoon*, a diporpa larva may exist that is dual in nearly all respects; it is formed, however, by the fusion of two larvae in an X-shape. Neither of these are colonies.

Cestoda. Here also there are at least two types of multiple individuals. First, in most tapeworms, such as *Taenia*, the body produces a long chain of proglottids by strobilation; this has been held to produce a chain of individuals, asexually produced; it is now certain that these are not individuals but detached organs — gonophores, structures to carry the gonads just until gametes are liberated and then to die. Second, such larval stages as hydatid cysts in *Echinococcus*, produce internal buds resulting in a sac of several embryos; it is of course merely a temporary stage in the life cycle and therefore not a colony.

ROTIFERA

Monogononta. The pelagic *Conochilus* forms radiating masses said to be colonies. Similar but attached aggregates are formed in stalked forms such as *Lacinularia*. These aggregations are of stalked individuals attached to the parent at the base, but they are attached only by gelatinous threads with no organic connection. These eutelic animals were obviously not budded but arose from eggs laid in the jelly around the foot. What appears to be a clear-cut colony thus turns out to be an association of separate individuals.

CALYSSOZOA

The endoprocts frequently form stolonate colonies, by budding, as in *Pedicellina*, or somewhat dendritic, as in *Urnatella*.

BRYOZOA

In both classes (Gymnolaemata and Phylactolaemata) budding produces colonies in all species, with a wide variety of forms: encrusting *(Pectinatella)*, arborescent *(Cothurniella)*, frondose *(Flustra)*, stolonous *(Aetea)*, or free-living discoidal *(Cristatella)* in which the colony is capable of creeping as a unit. None of these are pelagic.

PHORONIDA

These tube-dwellers often grow in dense masses, usually thought to arise from individually settling zygotes. In at least some cases there is fragmentation (architomy) of a worm inside the tube with each half regenerating, a septum forming between them, and the lower one opening a new aperture to one side; each continuing to extend its own tube. These two are thus a clone and together qualify as a colony. The masses therefore may be aggregations of separate individuals, or true colonies, or both.

MOLLUSCA

Gastropoda. In *Crepidula,* it is noted by Urbanek (1973) that hormones passed by "skin-to-skin contact" are similar to pheromones in insects, and he claims that this integration of separate individuals produces "pseudocolonies". As in the insects these are interactions of individuals and not colonies at all.

ECHIUROIDEA

In *Bonellia,* the same effect of hormones is described as in Gastropoda (above), again resulting merely in "pseudocolonies".

ANNELIDA

Polychaeta. *Syllis ramosa* is exceptional in giving rise by lateral branching (budding) to a much-branched but permanent colony. Others such as *Autolycus* form chains of individuals, usually as a temporary step before separation of each.

Hirudinea. A "colonial" leech is reported as a fossil under the name *Lecathylus.* Pictures show this animal with no sign of coloniality of any sort.

ARTHROPODA

Crustacea. Barnacles often live in dense aggregations, but they each arise from a separate zygote and merely become cemented together by their shell-like carapaces.

Insecta. Social insects are often cited as forming colonies; they are better described as forming societies. They occur in the order Hymenoptera, Isoptera, and Embioptera, with less obvious examples in Lepidoptera and Coleoptera.

PTEROBRANCHIA

In *Cephalodiscus,* the individuals arise by budding but do not remain connected by protoplasm; a secreted coenoecium surrounds the mass. This colony consists of upright tubes in an erratic dendritic form.

In *Rhabdopleura,* the colony is recumbent and stolonate and the individuals are in contact, especially by the so-called black stolon.

TUNICATA

Ascidiacea. There are stolonate colonies, as in *Clavellina,* and also compound structures, such as *Botryllus,* where many budded individuals are enclosed in a common tunic and may share certain organs.

Thaliacea. As in Ascidiacea, such forms as *Pyrosoma* share organs to form a compound "individual".

III. MOTILITY OF COLONIES

It is natural to think of colonies as being attached to objects, often encrusting them or forming reefs. On the other hand, the swimming colonies of *Volvox* are well known, and also the floating ones of the siphonophores.

Floating colonies occur in Coelenterata, Graptozoa, and Tunicata, in each of which the colony itself achieves much individuality and has a specific form.

Swimming colonies are well known in Protozoa, where they may move by flagella, as in *Cyclonexis* and *Volvox.* In the siphonophores some locomotion is produced by the nectophores or swimming bells, as in *Muggiaea,* in much the same manner as a medusa moves. The compound tunicate *Pyrosoma* swims by a form of jet propulsion.

One true colony creeps over the surface. The bryozoan *Cristatella* is a colony with a flattened oval shape; it can move along and around the branches of submerged objects. It has a high level of individuality.

IV. COLONY TERMS

There are a number of terms relating to structure and development of colonies and noncolonies:

1. Arboroid — branched, arborescent, dendritic
2. Catenoid (linear) — in the form of a chain
3. Dendritic — (see arboroid)
4. Discoid — flat and rounded
5. Frondose — leaf-like
6. Gregaloid — in tandem
7. Monopodial — with growth zone at the terminal hydranth
8. Phaceloid — like a bundle of filaments
9. Sacciform — in the form of a pouch or sack
10. Spheroid — round, as a ball
11. Sympodial — with the terminal hydranths alternating

Parts of the colony

12. Coenobium — a protozoan colony having a constant shape as well as arrangement and number of cells
13. Coppinia — a fruiting stolon of some siphonophores
14. Corbula — colonial organ, fruiting stolon formed by union of many individuals (s.Hydrozoa)
15. Corm (cormus) — an isolated group of individuals in a colony (used in Hydrozoa)
16. Cormidium — group of interacting individuals of several types; part of a colony; in some Siphonophora
17. Ersaea — a eudoxid without sexual medusoids
18. Eudoxid (eudoxome, eudoxia) — a cormidium which has broken loose from the colony to live separately
19. Heterozooid — zooid lacking sexual reproductive function
20. Hydrocaulus — branched upright portion of the hydrozoan colony; a stalk
21. Medusoid — a medusa-like member of a siphonophore colony
22. Nectosome — part of the stolon bearing the swimming bells
23. Ovicell — a modified zooecium that serves as a brood pouch; in Bryozoa
24. Polypoid — a polyp-like member of a siphonophore colony
25. Pseudocolony — individuals "united" only by pheromones
26. Siphonosome — part of the stolon bearing the cormidia
27. Solenia — gastrodermal tubes connecting adjacent polyps in certain Coelenterata
28. Stolons — a cylindrical structure connecting certain individuals in some colonies
29. Strobila — the chain of proglottids in a tapeworm; or the scyphistomal constrictions like a pile of saucers in a scyphozoan larva
30. Zoarium — a colony of animals, especially of bryozoans
31. Zooecium — the case containing a zooid
32. Zooid — any individual in a colony

Polymorphic forms within the colony

33. Autozooid — fully-formed feeding polyp
34. Avicularium — a specialized zooid shaped like a bird's head, in Bryozoa
35. Blastostyle — a gonozooid
36. Bract — a leaf-like protective zooid in a siphonophore
37. Cystozooid — polyp individual with small pore in place of a mouth; possibly excretory

38. Dactylozooid — elongated hydranth without a mouth but with many tentacles
39. Gastrozooid — a hydranth with an oral manubrium and four short tentacles; a feeding polyp
40. Gonozooid — a polyp specialized for reproducton, in siphonophores
41. Kenozooids — zooids without feeding or reproductive structures; probably supportive or connective
42. Machopolyp (machozooid) — protective or capturing polyp in hydrozoans; with reduced or absent coelenteron
43. Nannozooecium — a dwarf zooid
44. Nannozooids (nanozooids) — small zooids of unknown function, in Bryozoa
45. Nectophore — medusa-like locomotory individual in siphonophores; same as swimming bell
46. Nematophore (nematocalyx) — minute thread-like dactylozooid; phagocytic
47. Nematozooid — a zooid bearing nematocysts, for defense in a hydrozoan colony
48. Palpon — a tactile zooid in some siphonophores
49. Phorozooid — nurse zooid in tunicates, bearing the gonozooids
50. Pneumatophore — the air sac of a siphonophore
51. Siphonozooids — small polyps of some hydrozoan colonies; tentacles and septae reduced or absent; functions in pumping water
52. Swimming bell — medusa-like locomotory individual of a siphonophore; same as nectophore
53. Tentaculozooid — a polyp in a hydrozoan colony; merely a single long tentacle
54. Tentilla — tentacle-bearing zooid of a siphonophore
55. Vibraculum — bryozoan zooid like a whip-like filament, sweeping the surface free of debris

Colony development

56. Ancestrula — the first-formed individual of a bryozoan colony
57. Astogeny — the postlarval development of a colony
58. Blastozooid — an individual resulting from asexual reproduction
59. Calyconula — a siphonophore larva with a swimming bell and a tentacle
60. Cormogeny — ontogenesis of a colony
61. Cyathozooid — primary or stem zooid in some tunicate colonies
62. Oozooid — a zooid that has arisen directly from an egg (an ancestrula)
63. Siculozooid — an oozooid, which later becomes the sicula or basal individual of the colony
64. Siphonula — a ciliated larva of some siphonophores
65. Syzygy — end-to-end attachment of gregarine Protozoa

V. REPRODUCTION OF COLONIES

A. Sexual Reproduction

Although colonies seldom reproduce by bisexual reproduction, in the flagellate genus *Volvox* there may be production of gametes by the individual cells. Some gametes fuse in karyogamy, but some larger gametes develop parthenogenetically. The former give rise to zygotes and the latter to apozygotes. Both will eventually undergo many cell divisions to form daughter colonies.

Some colonies of Calyssozoa consist of male and female individuals and some consist only of individuals of one sex. In at least some, the ova are fertilized to form a zygote that will start a new colony.

In Pterobranchia such as *Cephalodiscus,* the colony may consist of members all of one sex, or it may consist of individuals of both sexes.

B. Asexual Reproduction

1. Budding

In *Volvox* it is sometimes implied that the daughter colonies are formed inside the sphere by budding. In more detailed treatments it is clear that the daughter colonies arise by fission of a zooid free inside the colony. Thus, these undoubted colonies do produce daughter colonies, but inasmuch as each colony is a clone, the fertilization is clonal, producing less genetic diversity than in cross-breeding animals (See "Fertilization" in Chapter 3).

No other reports of colony budding have been found.

2. Division

Some form of colony division or fragmentation occurs in two classes of Protozoa and in four other phyla.

Sarcodina. In some Radiolaria, the colony constricts to produce two daughter colonies.

Flagellata. Such colonies as *Chrysomonadina* may split into two parts. In others the division may be so unequal that only one cell detaches, to divide into a new colony.

Porifera. In some sponges any detached piece is capable of growing into a complete sponge, although the process is very slow.

Hydrozoa. As Hyman (1940) described: "Branches and portions of colonies containing coenosarc may be constricted off and develop into new colonies."

Siphonophora. In many Calycophora, sections called cormidia break loose and presumably grow into new colonies.

Bryozoa. In Kume and Dan (1968) it is reported that in some (unnamed) species there is repeated division of the fan-shaped colony. Vorontsova and Liosner (1960) also describe new colony formation by "detachment of parts of the old colony", but neither the species nor the class is identified.

Tunicata. Whether the compound ascidian tunicates are colonies or not is a moot question. In *Amaroecium*, however, separation of several blastozooids seems to be related to colony fission.

REFERENCES

Beklemishev, W. N., *Principles of Comparative Anatomy of Invertebrates,* Vol. 1, *Promorphology,* University of Chicago Press, Chicago, 1969.

Boardman, R. S., Cheetham, A. H., and Oliver, W. A., Jr., *Animal Colonies; Development and Function through Time,* Dowden, Hutchinson & Ross, Stroudsburg, 1973.

Coates, A. G. and Oliver, W. A., Jr., Coloniality in Zoantharian corals, in *Animal Colonies,* Boardman, R. S., Cheetham, A. H., and Oliver, W. A., Jr., Eds., Dowden, Hutchinson & Ross, Stroudsburg, 1973.

Hyman, L. H., *The Invertebrates,* Vol. 1, 3, 5, McGraw-Hill, New York, 1940, 1951, 1959.

Kudo, R. R., *Protozoology,* 5th ed., Charles C Thomas, Springfield, Ill., 1966.

Kume, M. and Dan, K., *Invertebrate Embryology,* NOLIT, Belgrade, 1968.

Mackie, G. O., Siphonophores, bud colonies, and superorganisms, in *The Lower Metazoa,* Dougherty, E. C., Ed., University of California Press, Berkeley, 1963.

Sleigh, M. A., *The Biology of Protozoa,* American Elsevier, New York, 1973.

Urbanek, A., Organization and evolution of Graptolite colonies, in *Animal Colonies,* Boardman, R. S., Cheetham, A. H., and Oliver, W. A., Jr., Eds., Dowden, Hutchinson & Ross, Stroudsburg, 1973.

Vorontsova, M. A. and Liosner, L. D., *Asexual Propagation and Regeneration,* Pergamon Press, London, 1960.

Part VII
End of Existence

"Death, the permanent cessation of the vital functions in the bodies of animals and plants, the end of life or act of dying.

"Neither senescence nor natural death is a necessary inevitable consequence or attribute of life. Natural death is biologically a relatively new thing, which made its appearance only after living organisms had advanced a long way on the path of evolution."

Raymond Pearl, 1929

Chapter 24

DEATH

TABLE OF CONTENTS

I.   End of Existence 498
    A.   Perspective 498
    B.   Fragmentation 498
    C.   Death 498
    D.   Fusion 499
    E.   Change of Genome 499

References 499

I. END OF EXISTENCE

A. Perspective

It could be argued that the end of the existence of an individual is a subject comparable in significance to the beginning of that existence. In reality the beginning of life for an organism is a complex of processes and preparatory activities, showing great diversity, whereas the death of an organism is usually sudden, not preceded by any preparations, and in general merely the cessation of the life processes.

This does not mean that there is no diversity in the termination of the life of individuals. At least the following terminations occur:

Cessation of vital processes

1. Natural death — internal failure of an essential organ (principally in humans and domestic animals)
2. Predation — being consumed by other animals (nearly all animals)
3. Suicide — deliberate action of the individual with intent to terminate its own life (humans)

Separation of the individual into two or more, none of which can be identified with the original individual

4. Binary fission (Protozoa)
5. Multiple fission (Protozoa)
6. Division — longitudinal or transverse (Coelenterata)
7. Fragmentation (Rhynchocoela, Annelida)
8. Polyembryony (Cestoda, s.Insecta, Mammalia)

Fusion with another individual permanently, so that they both lose their identity

9. Fusion — Zygotes (s.Anthozoa), embryos (s.Turbellaria), larvae (s.Porifera, diporpa of Trematoda), adults (hologamy in s.Sarcodinia, s.Flagellata), and buds, pyloric budding (s.Ascidiacea)

Change of genome

10. Conjugation — interchange of pronuclei (s.Protozoa)

B. Fragmentation

The end of the life of an individual through breaking into two or more new individuals has been discussed at length as a reproductive process in Chapter 2. Although the original individuality is lost, the living substance is preserved by forming the new individuals. Thus, there is no death of an organism but only realignment of its living substance in the formation of new individualities.

C. Death

The cessation of vital processes may be due to senescence, to accidental damage, or to deliberate action of that individual or some other animal. In nature, few animals except humans survive predation and accident long enough to die "a natural death", but all will eventually do so if exterior causes do not intervene. The nature of senescence if largely unknown, even in humans, but it requires failure of only one vital activity to bring on collapse of the entire metabolic system.

Accidental death is basically similar to senescence in that accidental interruption of even one vital process will result in failure of the entire system. Thus, an earthworm stepped on will die if any vital organ is disrupted, even though much of the body may be undamaged. (By "vital" is meant necessary to continued existence.) Multitudes of small animals die merely by being trod on by larger animals (or their machines).

Predation is undoubtedly the principal cause of death among animals, if only because uncountable numbers of plankton animals are consumed by other aquatic and marine ones. So far as the individual prey is concerned, this is also accidental. The term predation does not specify the identity or even the nature of the predator. One form that has received a name is cannibalism, in which the prey is consumed by another member of its own species. The word is commonly used with reference to humans alone, but many animals eat their own kind indiscriminately along with other prey. For example, most plankton feeders liberate their gametes or zygotes into the water, and these and the subsequent larvae may be part of the plankton that is filtered and consumed.

As in this example, it must be assumed that cannibalism is an exceptional process, because if it was general the species would become extinct.

It cannot be assumed that cannibalism is deliberate only in humans. Such insects as ants deliberately kill and consume maimed or superannuated individuals to conserve available food.

A curious use of the word cannibalism has crept into careless speech. For this the definition would be eating humans. Under this man-oriented usage, any man-eating predator (tiger, shark, wolf) would be a cannibal. This is simply predation that seems unusually important to the humans who might be the prey.

A comparatively few animals die by their own action. Humans can commit suicide, but there seem to be no certain cases of this in other animals. The lemmings that are drowned in the sea were not seeking death but following some internal drive that ended in drowning. Some animals make preparations for death, but they do not themselves produce fatal metabolic failure.

D. Fusion

When two living individuals merge their substance into one, there have been two terminations as well as the start of a new individual. Fusion of individuals of some sort occurs in Protozoa (hologamy), Porifera (certain larvae), Coelenterata (zygotes, adults, colonies), and Trematoda (two larvae to form a diporpa.) These are listed in more detail in the section on fusion in Chapter 4.

E. Change of Genome

An animal is assumed to be what its complement of genes produces. There seem to be no internal mechanisms that alter that genome during the life of the individual, although of course control of the genome varies during development and with outside influences. But if new genes are incorporated into an individual at some point in its life, the original genetic identity is destroyed, and the individual has in effect ended one life and assumed another.

Such a genome change occurs only in Protozoa. It may be by conjugation, endomixis, autogamy, or hemimixis. The processes are discussed in Chapter 4 under "Para-Reproductive Processes".

REFERENCES

Blackwelder, R. E. and Shepherd, B. A., The Diversity of Animal Reproduction, CRC Press, Boca Raton, Fla., 1981.
Pearl, R., The Biology of Death, J. B. Lippincott, Philadelphia, 1922.
Pearl, R., Death, in Encyclopaedia Britannica, 14th ed., Vol. 7, Encyclopaedia Britannica, New York, 1929.

Part VIII
Classification

"Classification, as a process, is a fundamental necessity in human life. Indeed, we can see that this ability to classify is necessary to the ability to communicate. Nouns and adjectives, our chief classifiers of the world about us, are an absolute necessity for the exchange of information."

B. H. Burma, 1954

"The classification of animals is still very much a field in which discovery and revision are continuing, even after two hundred years of study. The importance of classification in biology increases every year, because the experimental and practical fields find increasing need for accurate identification of animals and for understanding of comparative relationships."

R. E. Blackwelder, 1963

Chapter 25

THE CLASSIFICATION OF ANIMALS

TABLE OF CONTENTS

I.   The Nature of Classification 504

II.   The Groups of the Animal Kingdom 507
     A.   The Parameters 507
     B.   The Groups 508

References 517

I. THE NATURE OF CLASSIFICATION

Classification is a device in logic whereby a multitude of things are made manageable by being grouped; this converts the multiplicity to a usable order. In the case of animals, classification is what produces that order, and it also helps us to understand how their diversity develops.

There cannot really be any question that there has been successive change among animals through time. The animals living today are not the same as those that lived in earlier times (as shown by the fossil record). This successive change is evolution, and it may be the only aspect of evolution that can be said to be demonstrated beyond doubt. It is known that some genetic and selective mechanisms could produce some change, but it is not certain that they have done so or which specific changes were caused. It is known that in a few groups, such as the Vertebrata, there is enough comparative information to make reasonable a belief that one can see evidence of the path of evolution among the subgroups, but in most of the animal phyla such evidence is questionable, absent, or directly contradictory.

Most published classifications are deliberately simplified in one or more ways. That elementary textbooks should use such simplified classifications is not surprising, because of space limitations and to enable comprehension by beginning students, but it is astonishing that evolutionary conclusions have often been based on such simplified and misleading classifications.

The textbook writers are working under great pressures to keep down the length of their book. They are not specialists in classification. They may warn their readers that the arrangement of animals into a classification is not a settled matter, but they seldom do justice to the existing diversity of animals because they do not make clear the exceptions and oddities — the endless diversity that has been discovered but often left buried in the older literature.

The simplifications that have been employed by writers of such textbooks are of several sorts: first, only living animals are included, with rarely a reference to such extinct subgroups as the Trilobita and the Ostracodermi. One false impression given by this is that few groups have become extinct; nothing could be farther from the truth. Another false impression is that extinct groups are simply relatives of well-known groups; the fact is that there are thousands of fossils that cannot be placed in modern groups, and there are small groups like the Cricoconarida and Helicoplacoidea that cannot with assurance be related to any known phyla.

Second, it is assumed that there are so-called important groups and unimportant ones, and it follows that the latter need not be mentioned at all; no one will know the difference. This simple but fallacious reasoning results in omission from most books of some of the most important diversities among animals.

Third, certain numerically minor groups, that somehow must not be omitted, are appended to major groups, whether or not they meet the stated features of those groups. Thus, the Calyssozoa (Endoprocta) are appended to the Bryozoa, which in reality they scarcely resemble in phylum characteristics. It is hereby implied that small groups are automatically unimportant ones that can be omitted or submerged into larger groups. In reality, what is known of possible mechanisms of evolution and extinction of animals should lead one to expect to find, at any given point in evolutionary time, groups of a wide range of size, some large and some small. It cannot be expected that small but distinct groups can be reasonably united (as in Aschelminthes) or incorporated into larger ones (as in Chordata).

Fourth, in some cases a group has been commonly included inside another group, leading later authors to assume that it is covered therein. In this manner *Dinophilus* is usually lost inside the Annelida (or even in the Archiannelida), with which it actually has almost nothing in common, and its distinctive features are therefore not even recorded.

Fifth, the desire to have chapters of equal length, even where the groups vary from 1 species to 800,000, has led to clustering of groups that have little in common. For example, at the end of Arthropoda may be clustered the Merostomata and Pycnogonida (which are chelicerates), the Trilobita (which stand alone), the four groups of myriapods (which are mandibulates), the Onchyophora (which is usually accepted as a separate phylum), and the Pentastomida and Tardigrada (whose basic features place them far from the Arthropoda, and from each other). This assemblage cannot be defined in any way more specific than to say that they are all Metazoa.

One thing is often forgotten in discussing the differences between classifications: there is almost never any real difference of opinion as to what groups do exist. Every classifier in the last 100 years recognizes that there is a group that is usually called Tardigrada. The most common argument is whether this groups is a subphylum of Arthropoda or a class of it or a separate phylum in its own right. Those who regard it as a separate phylum differ as to whether it should be placed near the Arthropoda or near the Rotifera.

The *groups* are in effect objective — they exist, and there is agreement on that. The *placing of the groups* is highly subjective; there is controversy either about the category or level to which they are assigned or about the placing of them among the other groups at that level.

For example, the Protozoa that employ pseudopodia comprise a clear-cut group of protozoans. This group is considered by Hyman (1940) to be a class (Rhizopoda), by Copeland (1956) to be a phylum (Protoplasta), and by Honigberg (1964) to be a superclass (Sarcodina). There has never been any way to determine which of these rankings is correct. The classifier must try to make the different parts of his scheme consistent, to use the same grade of evidence to support each part. And this can only be done by a serious effort to base the decisions on all available evidence, not merely on the features usually cited and not merely on the specialist's greater knowledge of one of the groups.

When one adds to this problem of ranking the fact that many groups have several names, often differently selected by different classifiers, it appears that there is great difference between classifications. In reality there seldom is. For example, one may compare three published classifications of Protozoa in Table 27.

At first glance there is little similarity between these three classifications, but if some of the unfamiliar names are replaced by better-known synonyms and the nominal levels of the taxa are not indicated, these three schemes appear as in Table 28.

There are still differences between these three, but in reality they are slight:

1. Assignment to categories, with use of 2, 3 or 5 levels
2. Choice of names (synonyms)
3. Placement of controversial groups (Opalinida, Suctoria)
4. Possible subdivision of Sporozoa into three: Piroplasmea (to go into Sarcodina), Sporozoa in strict sense, and Cnidospora

All of the groups in Honigberg are represented also in Hyman, where they would show up as lower levels (subclass or order). Although the Honigberg classification was put forth as an authoritative scheme, by the Society of Protozoologists, it has not received wide acceptance.

It appears now that there is still question about the placement of Opalinida and Suctoria, although the two groups are recognizable; the breaking up of the Sporozoa is

Table 27
THREE CLASSIFICATIONS OF PROTOZOA

Hyman (1940)	Copeland (1956)	Honigberg (1964)
Phylum Protozoa	Phylum Phaeophyta	Phylum Protozoa
SP.Plasmodroma	Cl.Heterokonta	SP.Sarcomastigophora
Cl.Flagellata	Phylum Pyrrhophyta	SpC.Mastigophora
Cl.Rhizopoda	Cl.Mastigophora	Cl.Phytomastigophorea
Cl.Sporozoa	Phylum Protoplasta	Cl.Zoomastigophorea
SC.Telosporidia	Cl.Zoomastigoda	SpC.Opalinata
SC.Cnidosporidia	Cl.Mycetozoa	SpC.Sarcodina
SC.Sarcosporidia	Cl.Rhizopoda	Cl.Rhizopoda
SC.Haplosporidia	Cl.Heliozoa	SC.Lobosia
SP.Ciliophora	Cl.Sarcodina	SC.Filosia
Cl.Ciliata	Phylum Fungilli	SC.Granuloreticulosia
SC.Protociliata	Cl.Sporozoa	SC.Mycetozoia
SC.Euciliata	Cl.Neosporidia	SC.Labyrinthulia
Cl.Suctoria	Phylum Ciliophora	Cl.Piroplasmea
	Cl.Infusoria	Cl.Actinopodia
	Cl.Tentaculifera	SC.Radiolaria
		SC.Acantharia
		SC.Heliozoia
		SC.Proteomyxidia
		Sp.Sporozoa
		Cl.Telosporea
		SC.Gregarinia
		SC.Coccidia
		Cl.Toxoplasmea
		Cl.Haplosporea
		SP.Cnidospora
		Cl.Myxosporidea
		Cl.Microsporidea
		SP.Ciliophora
		Cl.Ciliatea
		SC.Holotrichia
		SC.Peritrichia
		SC.Suctoria
		Spirotrichia

Table 28
THE THREE CLASSIFICATIONS SIMPLIFIED

Hyman (1940)	Copeland (1956)	Honigberg (1964)
Protozoa	Mychota (part)	Protozoa
Plasmodroma	Phaeophyta	Sarcomastigophora
Mastigophora	Mastigophora (pt.)	Mastigophora
		Opalinida
	Protoplasta	
Sarcodina	Sarcodina	Sarcodina
		(+Sporozoa pt.)
Sporozoa	Sporozoa	Sporozoa (pt.)
		Sporozoa (pt.)
Ciliophora	Ciliophora	Ciliophora
Ciliata	Ciliata	Ciliata
(Opalinida)	(Opalinida)	(+Suctoria)
Suctoria	Suctoria	

justified, but it was so recognized even by Hyman (at the subclass level). It is hard to see how greater unanimity could be achieved in these classifications, although for some purposes it may be more helpful to use a simpler scheme (more like that of Hyman) and for other purposes a more complex scheme (such as that of Honigberg).

Much the same situation obtains in all classifications of animals at the phylum and class levels. There is no question of the groups, but how they are to be combined into higher groups or subdivided into lower ones is debated. Of course, the many names and synonyms further confuse the picture.

What may be called "classification by specialists" exaggerates these problems. As suggested above, a classification must be consistent between its different parts. There must be as much correspondence as possible between the groups cited as phyla, or among the groups cited as orders. If a large classification is made by merely combining the schemes of the specialists in each subgroup, the result is likely to be inconsistent. It is also likely to be unnecessarily complex. These faults seriously detract from the usefulness and acceptability of the classification. Furthermore, arbitrary selection of unfamiliar names can militate against acceptance of a scheme by specialists and student alike.

Of the three schemes, Hyman's classification alone shows neither of these problems. The unusual arrangements are discussed, and choice of names explained. Both of the other classification partake of both the faults cited.

The list given in the present chapter is not strictly a classification because assignment to categories (levels such as phylum and class) is not considered as important as identifying and describing the groups (taxa at the phylum and class levels). Groupings unacceptable to us as taxa are included for the reader's convenience. It largely accepts the classification of Blackwelder (1963).

II. THE GROUPS OF THE ANIMAL KINGDOM

A. The Parameters

As suggested above, the purposes for which classifications are presented in different books are diverse. To be appropriate in the present book a classification of animals must do one thing: permit the display of the diversity which exists. All forms of simplification tend to obscure the extent of that diversity. The goal must here be to display the true picture of the groupings of animals, even if this causes some inconvenience. (This is not to say that in other circumstances, where the requirements are different, there can be no abbreviation, but it should always be stated how this is done and to what extent. For example, it is of no advantage in a beginning textbook to try to list all the extinct groups, but the fact that there are many of these should be made clear.)

The chief aim of the present book is to correct these three common misconceptions: (1) that all animals are much alike, (2) that well-known features really do occur in all members of a group, and (3) that there are only a small number (12 to 20) of basic forms. The data that refute these beliefs are tabulated throughout this book; they consist of the numerous exceptions, the almost random distribution of some basic features, and the number of groups whose placement is controversial.

Another "fact" implied in many books is that there are 19 (or 27, or 16, or 33) phyla of animals, even counting some extinct ones. The truth is that if one can separate Protozoa from Porifera, Coelenterata from Ctenophora, and Annelida from Arthropoda and from Onychophora, as almost all classifiers do, then one cannot logically place together the groups that differ as much as these do; for example, Coelenterata and Conularida, Rotifera and Nematoda, or the classes of Echinodermata and eight of the fossil groups that have been lumped with them.

At least hundreds of fossils have been described that are so unique that no one presumes to place them in any group. Aside from these, however, there are at least 19 extinct "classes" that can be clearly distinguished from known living animals, but cannot with certainty be placed in a phylum with any of them. (These are mostly "relatives" of Coelenterata, Mollusca, and Echinodermata.)

As a result it is necessary to understand that there are surely as many as 60 groups so distinct that a zoologist must recognize each of them as a phylum if he uses that term for any. At the level of class, these phyla can be logically subdivided into at least 125 classes, readily distinguishable and each reasonably homogeneous in the present state of knowledge.

The following list includes all groups referred to in the text or tables as well as all other groups that should be considered for recognition at the phylum and class levels. The level or category of the groups is not important here and is not directly shown, but in general CAPITALS indicate phyla, italicized words indicate classes. Boldface Roman type indicates groups used for convenience only. Names in parentheses are approximate synonyms. The dagger (†) indicates extinct groups.

B. The Groups

PROTOZOA. Individuals consisting of a single cell, although some are colonial, multinucleate, or plasmodial.

> (Classification of this phylum is still in a state of flux. In some recent books the Protozoa are removed from the Kingdom Animalia and placed in a separate kingdom usually called the Protista. General textbooks often use a simple 4- or 5-class arrangement, and some much more elaborate systems have been proposed. It is here necessary to use an intermediate scheme in order to record the diversity assembled.)

Sarcodina (Rhizopoda). With pseudopodia as the major means of locomotion and food intake; rarely also with flagella.

Flagellata (Mastigophora). With one to many flagella as locomotor organelles throughout life or intermittently or in young stages.

Opalinida (Protociliata). Endocommensals of lower Vertebrata, ciliated over the cell in oblique rows; no cytostome; nutrition by absorption of fluids; two or many nuclei of one kind; no conjugation.

> (A group long recognized as aberrant among the Ciliata but usually listed as an order of them. If they are not Ciliata, they must be given separate class status, because they do not fit even as well in any other class.)

Ciliata. With cilia as locomotory and food-catching organelles; with two kinds of nuclei; conjugation.

> (This group at one time included the Opalinida. It nowadays often includes the Suctoria, with the combined group called Ciliophora.)

Suctoria. Cilia present only in young stages; adults without mouth; with tentacles; mostly sessile, stalked.

> (These are usually separated as a subgroup of Ciliata, (or of the Ciliophora). They feed by a unique and little understood process of sucking body contents from the prey. Listed here as a group of still-undetermined rank and position.)

Sporozoa. Endoparasitic, transmitted by simple spores usually produced by multiple fission.

> (This class has for long contained at least the following six groups: Gregarinida, Coccidia, Haemosporidia, Haplosporidia, Sarcosporidia, and Cnidosporidia. The isolation of Cnidosporidia, with their polar capsules and filaments, leaves the other groups in a state of controversy. The sources of data listed in the present book usually do not identify the subgroups of Sporozoa, so it is retained in the old inclusive sense, without prejudice to any modern ideas of its proper subdivision.)

Cnidosporidia. Endoparasitic, with spores containing polar capsules containing a spirally coiled thread that can be discharged for anchoring.

(Includes Myxosporidia and Microsporidia.)

†CHITINOZOA. Usually symmetrical (radial) microfossils with a test probably of pseudochitin, usually bottle-shaped open at the top; sometimes in chains.

(As only the test is known, it is uncertain whether these organisms were protozoans or metazoans)

Metazoa. Adult individuals composed of many cells in tissues.

(A taxon of convenience, more often divided into Parazoa, Mesozoa, and Eumetazoa or into Invertebrata and Vertebrata. Herein it includes all animals except Protozoa.)

MESOZOA (Moruloidea). Cellular endoparasites; an outer cell layer or syncytium enclosing one or more reproductive cells; no cavities; eutelic.

Rhombozoa (Dicyemida). In nephridia of Cephalopoda; primary nematogen is vermiform and ciliated; not minute.

Orthonectida. In spaces of Turbellaria, Rhynchocoela, Bivalvia, Annelida, and Ophiuroidea; a multinucleate plasmodium that reproduces by fragmentation into agametes; sexual forms are minute and ciliated.

MONOBLASTOZOA. A tube enclosed by a single layer of cells, ciliated inside and out; possibly with unicellular ciliated larvae.

(A single species *(Salinella salve)* seen only once — in 1897 — and recently supposed to be a hoax. It is, however, a reasonable animal not out of line with the Mesozoa and some simple planula larvae. Failure to rediscover it — in salt beds in Argentina — is insufficient reason to declare it nonexistent.)

PLACOZOA. Minute planula-like animals of roughly circular shape; dorsal and ventral epithelia separated by a few cells in an intermediate layer; "ova" produced but spermatozoa not known.

(*Trichoplax adhaerens* has been placed in the Mesozoa or thought to be merely a larva of some unidentified hydrozoan. Not enough is known to permit any such assignment.)

PORIFERA (Parazoa). Metazoa with tissues from germ layers not embryologically corresponding to ectoderm, endoderm, and mesoderm. With large water channels lined with flagellated collar cells (choanocytes).

Calcarea. Skeleton of separate calcareous spicules; produces gemmules; all marine.

Hexactinellida (Hyalospongia). Skeleton of siliceous spicules, sometimes united; epidermis as a trabecular net; gemmules may be formed; all marine.

Demospongia. Skeleton of siliceous spicules or horny fibers or both; produces gemmules and reduction bodies; marine or freshwater.

†Sclerospongia. Basal calcareous skeleton of aragonite spicules overlain by siliceous spicules and spongin fibers, marine.

†RECEPTACULITIDA. Extinct; globular or discoidal skeletons of ossicles (plates) of calcite without perforations; may have had an apical opening; apparently never attached; skeletons different from any sponges.

†CYATHOSPONGIA. Extinct; the shape is that of an inverted cone; with one or two walls around a central cavity, the walls perforated; the cone open at the top, calcareous; rarely colonial; catenulate, massive or dendroid.

(Until recently divided into three classes: Monocyatha, Archaeocyatha, and Anthocyatha; recent changes give two classes: Regulares and Irregulares.)

Eumetazoa. The Metazoa exclusive of the Mesozoa and Porifera.

†GRAPTOZOA. Minute, colonial, marine; cup-shaped but without symmetry; a secreted calyx of chitin in imbricating plates.

(This extinct group has been placed in the Hydrozoa and in the Hemichordata. This extreme discrepancy emphasizes its peculiarities. It does not show clearly the basic features of either group and cannot be logically maintained in either on the basis of assured facts. Its true nature can be elucidated only by keeping it separate until comparative studies demonstrate the relationships of several coelenterate-like groups and several "hemichordate" groups.)

†CONULARIDA. Marine, moderate-sized, with a four-sided chitinophosphatic calyx; probably with tentacles.

(This extinct group is almost always cited as an early form of Scyphozoa. Aside from the fact that it cannot be proven to have any of the basic coelenterate features, its quadriradiate skeleton of chitinophosphatic nature is completely unique among the possible coelenterates.)

†DIPLEUROZOA. Flattened, bell-shaped, elliptical, thus bilateral; ridged in radiating pattern on each side; margin with lappets, each with a tentacle.

†STROMATOPOROIDEA. Marine colonies with calcareous skeleton; surface usually with single or branched cylindrical extensions; marine.

Radiata. The supposedly radially symmetrical Coelenterata and (usually) Ctenophora.
    (Few of them are clearly radial and most Ctenophora are clearly bilateral — sometimes erroneously called biradial.)

COELENTERATA (Cnidaria). Marine or freshwater; tentaculate with more or less radial symmetry; may have chitinous periderm; a large interior coelenteron with proctostome; solitary or colonial; flagella inside and out; with nematocysts.

†Protomedusae. Radially lobulate; stomach with radial canals, oral arms but no tentacles; marine.

Hydrozoa. Marine or freshwater; with no skeleton or a calcareous calyx or chitinous periderm; solitary or colonial; polyps or polyps and medusae; without gastral filaments or septae; symmetry various.

Milleporina. Massive colonies with calcareous skeletons; usually with tentacles; with simple medusae or attached gonophores; marine.
    (This and the following group are usually placed in the Hydrozoa, even in the Hydroida, but their massive colonies seem to make this inappropriate.)

Stylasterina. Branching colonies; with interconnecting canals; polymorphic; marine.
    (See note under Milleporina, above.)

Siphonophora. Marine, colonial, swimming or floating; no skeleton; polymorphic member individuals; "organs" are specialized individuals.
    (These colonial forms are coelenterate in basic structure but the exclusively colonial nature is not linked by intermediates to Hydrozoa or Scyphozoa (but note recent removal of *Velella* and *Porpita* to Hydrozoa. Their unique features seem to demand separate treatment at the present time.)

Scyphozoa. Marine; medusae except for polyp larvae; no skeleton; clearly quadriradiate; coelenteron with gastric filaments. (Conularida are not included.)

Anthozoa. Polyps only; hexamerous, octomerous, or mixed with bilaterality; coelenteron with septa.

CTENOPHORA. (Acnidaria). More or less spherical and quadri- or octoradiate but usually internally bilateral; with colloblasts but no nematocysts; with or without tentacles; no skeleton; eight comb rows.

Tentaculata. With two tentacles; sometimes very long (wide); comb rows may be present only in larva; mouth small.

Nuda. Without tentacles; bell-shaped with wide mouth; some coelenteric canals have numerous side branches.

Bilateria. The Eumetazoa that are not "radially symmetrical"; first occurrences of eutely.

GNATHOSTOMULOIDEA. Members of the marine interstitial fauna; with flagella but no internal cilia; no skeleton or body cavity; a GVC; no excretory, circulatory, or respiratory organs; without cuticle; not eutelic.

PLATYHELMINTHES. Flattened worms with little cephalization, no body cavity, anus, circulatory, or respiratory systems; flame-bulb excretion; not eutelic, although certain organs may show cell constancy.

Nemertodermatida. Marine; external cilia only; no excretory organs; no digestive cavity; hermaphroditic; no oviducts; circular and longitudinal muscle layers.

Xenoturbellida. Marine; external cilia only; no excretory organs; sac-like GVC; mouth serves as gonopore; no localized gonads.

Turbellaria. Marine, freshwater, or terrestrial; cilia inside and out; GVC may be branched; body wall muscles circular, diagonal, and longitudinal; flame-cell excretion.

Temnocephaloidea. Ectocommensals in fresh water; no cilia or few; 2 to 12 tentacles; posterior adhesive disks.

(This group has had many resting places in the Platyhelminthes but is now usually placed as an order in Turbellaria. They would be the only members of that class with tentacles, with an ordinary cuticle, or that are all ectocommensal.)

Trematoda. Endoparasitic except for ectoparasitic Monogenea; external cilia only on larva; peculiar "cuticle" is actually an unusual epidermis; GVC usually branched; flame cells; body wall muscles in three layers but variable.

Cestoda (Eucestoda). Endoparasitic; usually strobilated and with a holdfast; cilia internal except on the larvae; peculiar "cuticle" is actually an unusual epidermis; no GVC; flame cells; body wall muscles in two layers; with well-developed parenchymal musculature forming a cylindrical separation between inner and outer body regions; larvae diverse.

Cestodaria. Endoparasitic; not strobilated; no GVC; flame cells; larva a lycophore.

(A small group of "tapeworms" that do not form proglottids. They are distinguished by arrangement of holdfasts, by the lack of ciliation on the larva, and by its 10 hooks.)

RHYNCHOCOELA (Nemertinea). Acoelomate, complete intestinal tract; closed circulatory system present; flame-cell excretion; eversible proboscis or rhynchodaeum dorsal to digestive tract; not eutelic.

(Two groups, Enopla and Anopla, are here considered to be unnecessary groupings of the four orders, not distinguishable at the class level.)

Pseudocoelomata. Metazoa with body cavity a pseudocoel, derived from blastocoel.

(A group of phyla supposedly including the phyla having a pseudocoel: Acanthocephala, Aschelminthes [6 phyla], and Endoprocta. Two of the groups [Priapuloidea and Endoprocta] clearly have a coelom, so the group can include only Acanthocephala and the rest of the "Aschelminthes" and is not recognized formally here.)

ACANTHOCEPHALA. Endoparasitic; with pseudocoel and retractable proboscis; no digestive tract; flame cells in some; eutelic.

Aschelminthes. A convenience taxon sometimes used as a phylum to include the next five phyla, which are then treated as subphyla or classes.

ROTIFERA. Marine, freshwater, terrestrial, or parasitic; microscopic; ciliary corona; pharynx with mastax; one pair of flame cells; eutelic.

(Subdivision into three classes and five orders may be justifiable, but that decision is not required by our treatment.)

GASTROTRICHA. Marine or freshwater; microscopic; no corona; with cilia, spines, scales; two or more adhesive tubes, with or without flame cells; pharynx as in Nematoda; eutelic.

(Two classes, Macrodasyoidea and Chaetonotoidea, are not referred to in this book.)

KINORHYNCHA (Echinodera). Marine; microscopic; no cilia; superficially "segmented"; mouth spiny and invaginable; one pair of solenocytes; eutelic.

NEMATODA. Marine, freshwater, terrestrial, or parasitic; no cilia, flame cells, or bristles; cylindrical; longitudinal muscles only; triradiate pharynx; eutelic.

GORDIOIDEA (Nematomorpha). Very long cylindrical; parasitic as juveniles; no pharynx; digestive tract often degenerate; eutelic.

> *Gordioidea.* Fresh-water, with parasitic stage in insects or myriapods; cuticle without natatory bristles; much mesenchyme in pseudocoel.

> *Nectonematoidea.* Marine; parasitic stage in Crustacea; 2 rows of natatory bristles; pseudocoel large.

CALYSSOZOA (Endoprocta, Entoprocta, Kamptozoa). Marine or rarely freshwater; solitary or colonial, stalked; with pseudocoel, circlet of ciliated tentacles, flame bulbs; looped digestive tract with anus inside tentacle ring; not eutelic.

> (At one time placed in the Bryozoa, this group was then properly called Endoprocta. When completely separated from the Bryozoa, it seems inappropriate to use the class name Endoprocta for the phylum, because the phylum Bryozoa is not usually called Ectoprocta.)

Coelomata. General term for Metazoa with a coelom, either schizocoel or enterocoel.

PRIAPULOIDEA. Marine; moderately large; introvertible proboscis; solenocytes; with coelom; not eutelic.

> (This small group cannot be placed in the Aschelminthes, because of its coelom. The absence of details of early development leave this group without clear relationships.)

Lophophorata. General term for the three following phyla; with lophophore; digestive tract recurved; larvae interpreted as trochophores; coelom confused, usually not enterocoelous; not eutelic.

BRYOZOA (Ectoprocta). Marine or freshwater; in sessile colonies; with a lophophore but anus outside; recurved digestive tract; no excretory or circulatory system; coelom of questionable origin but not enterocoelous.

> *Phylactolaemata.* Lophophore horsehoe-shaped; muscle layers in body wall; coeloms continuous between zooids; monomorphic; all in fresh water.

> *Gymnolaemata.* Lophophore circular; no body wall muscles; no coelomic connections between zooids; polymorphic; almost all marine.

PHORONIDA. Marine tubicolous coelomates with lophophore; digestive tract recurved; closed circulatory system with erythrocytes; nephridia; coelom not enterocoelous.

BRACHIOPODA. Marine; coelomate with dorsal and ventral shell valves; attached by a stalk; a paired lophophore; open circulatory system; nephridia.

> *Inarticulata.* Valves not hinged; no internal skeleton in lophophore; anus present; enterocoelous.

> *Articulata.* Valves with hinge; lophophore with two internal (spiral) skeletons; anus absent; schizocoelous.

†HYOLITHELMINTHES. Small conical shells; shell laminated, of calcium orthophosphate; operculate.

> (This and the next three groups, plus Mathevioidea, have been listed by paleontologists as groups, usually classes, of Mollusca. They cannot be clearly associated with mollusks because of complete ignorance of all but the shells. The fact that these are similar to shells of Mollusca is inconclusive, as there are similar hardparts in other animals. Furthermore, calcium orthophosphate apparently does not occur in the Mollusca.)

†CRICOCONARIDA. Small, marine, paleozoic shells; ringed cones, shell of calcium carbonate; aperture only at large end; walls laminate; usually radially symmetrical.

(See note under Hyolithelminthes, above.)

†COLEOLIDA. Elongate-conical shells of small size; thick wall is laminated; no opercula or septa; paleozoic.

(See note under Hyolithelminthes, above.)

†CALYPTOTOMATIDA. Paleozoic, small, crudely conical shells of calcium carbonate; open only at large end which is operculate; partly chambered; sometimes with curved lateral rods.

(See note under Hyolithelminthes, above.)

MOLLUSCA. Marine, freshwater, or terrestrial; free-living; never colonial; questionably coelomate; unsegmented; with open circulatory system with one or more hearts; usually with a mantle, a muscular foot, a shell, a kidney, and gills; often with a radula in the pharynx.

> No clear-cut features distinguish this phylum, but the animals usually have a mantle, (often with a shell), a muscular foot, gills, an open circulatory system (with hearts), kidneys, and a radula in the pharynx.

Monoplacophora. Untorted, univalve shell; with some serially repeated organs; paired kidneys; marine.

> (It is sometimes claimed that these animals are segmented, the only such in the phylum. Inasmuch as segmentation is defined as serial compartmentation of the coelom, the presence of which has not been established in these animals, it seems premature to assume that the serial repetition of some organs indicates segmentation.)

Amphineura (Polyplacophora). Untorted, flattened, head indistinct; eight shell plates; with foot, gills, radula, coiled intestine, and kidney; marine

Solenogastres (Aplacophora). Untorted, vermiform without head or shell, with mantle and foot questionable; with kidney, radula, and calcareous spicules; with or without gill; straight digestive tract; marine.

> (Usually said to be unsegmented, but serial repetition shows up at least in the shell plates, the nervous system, and the numerous gills.)

Gastropoda. Torted and sometimes detorted; usually with spiral shell; with tentacles, eyes, radula, gill, and kidney; marine, freshwater, or terrestrial.

Bivalvia (Pelecypoda, Lemellibranchiata). With bivalved shell, valves left and right; intestine coiled; with kidney, and gills; no nerve cords; marine or freshwater.

Scaphopoda. With long conical shell open at both ends; digestive tract J-shaped, with radula; no gills. marine.

Cephalopoda. Spiral shell or remnants or none; digestive tract J-shaped, with jaws but no radula; with gills, closed circulatory system, and well developed eyes; marine.

†MATHEVIOIDEA (Matheva). Extinct; thick-walled short conical shells with two cavities; calcium carbonate; always with shells of two sizes, possibly front and rear.

> (See note under Hyolithelminthes, above. The original genus was *Mathevia*, from which the group name Matheva was coined. This is an unacceptable word, because the root of the source name is Mathevi-. The phylum name should be distinctive and is here altered.)

SIPUNCULOIDEA. Marine; large worm-like; digestive tract J-shaped; with nephridia; no circulatory or respiratory organs; no segmentation, molting, or colonies.

ECHIUROIDEA. Marine; worm-like (males vestigial); digestive tract coiled; with nephridia; no respiratory or circulatory organs, segmentation, molting or colonies.

Echiurida. With proboscis, setae, and paired nephridia; circular muscle layer outside.

Saccosomatida (Sactosomatida). Without proboscis or setae; circular muscle layer inside; with single nephridium.

TARDIGRADA. Minute, aquatic, cylindrical, bilateral; digestive tract straight or with diverticula; excretory organs as pouches off rectum or none; no respiratory or circulatory organs; five pairs of coelomic pouches; eutelic.

> (This is one of the most anomalous groups of animals. Most features would place it in the Aschelminthes, but the clearly enterocoelic coelom removes it far from these as well as from all segmented animals, which are schizocoelous.)

MYZOSTOMIDA. Minute, ciliated symbionts of echinoderms; marine; flattened circular, bilateral; digestive tract with diverticula; two nephridia; no circulatory or respiratory systems; coelom formation obscure.

DINOPHILOIDEA. Minute, marine, ciliated; epidermal nervous system; flame cells in some; coelom obscure; digestive tract complete or lacking; no circulatory or respiratory system; circular muscle only.

> (Usually placed in the Annelida, either in the Polychaeta or in the Archiannelida. They differ greatly from these in the protonephridia, a single layer of muscle in the body wall (circular), and in the absence of a trochophore larva.)

ANNELIDA. Minute to large; freshwater, marine, or terrestrial; segmented; digestive tract straight; with nephridia, or rarely solenocytes; respiration by gills or epidermis; coelom a schizocoel.

> *Archiannelida*. Marine or freshwater; ciliated; closed blood system, nervous system epidermal; longitudinal muscles only; at least sometimes with trochophore larva.

> *Polychaeta*. Marine, freshwater, or terrestrial; not ciliated externally; with nephridia or solenocytes and a closed blood system; gills in some; parapodia with setae; larvae trophophores.

> *Oligochaeta*. Terrestrial, freshwater, or marine; with nephridia and a closed blood system; without parapodia or gills; few setae or exterior cilia; no larvae.

> *Hirudinea*. Freshwater, terrestrial, or marine; no external cilia or parapodia; setae rare; with nephridia and a closed blood system or none; gills in some; no larvae.

PENTASTOMIDA (Linguatulida, Pentastomoidea). Parasitic; doubtfully segmented; coelom enterocoelous from four pairs of pouches; with a haemocoel and two pairs of anterior hooks; no excretory or respiratory organs; no cilia or setae.

†PROTONYCHOPHORA. Extinct; marine; segmented externally; with possible unjointed legs; two "pro-antennae".

> (The similarity of this marine animal to the terrestrial Onychophora, usually cited in palentology books is superficial. The gap of nearly 600 million years makes the association almost ridiculous, when it is remembered that Onychophora are among the least likely animals to have moved from the sea to the land.)

ONYCHOPHORA. Terrestrial; with two "pro-antennae", with chitinous cuticle, nephridia, and tracheae without tracheoles; no cilia but setae present; haemocoel but coelom questionable.

ARTHROPODA. Terrestrial, fresh-water, or marine; segmented with a sclerotized exoskeleton; no ordinary cilia; with jointed appendages; body cavity a haemocoel, circulation sometimes in blood vessels, or absent; coelom a schizocoel.

> †*Trilobitomorpha*. A subphylum that includes the Trilobitoidea and the Trilobita.

> †*Trilobitoidea*. Marine; trilobite-like arthropods not divided by longitudinal grooves into three "lobes".

>> (Although listed as a single class, this extinct group consists of fossils that would surely be placed in several classes if there were more species known. They are all of Cambrian age.)

> †*Trilobita*. Marine, divided by longitudinal grooves into three "lobes", with large head shield.

> *Chelicerata*. A subphylum that includes Merostomata, Pycnogonida, and Arachnida.

Merostomata. Marine or rarely fresh-water; digestive tract J-shaped; coxal gland excretion; with book gills, chelicerae, and chelae.

Pycnogonida. Marine; digestive tract straight but with diverticula into the legs; no excretory or respiratory organs; with chelicerae but no chelae.

Arachnida. Terrestrial or fresh-water; digestive tract variable and may be incomplete; with coxal glands, malpighian tubules, book lungs or tracheae, chelicerae, and chelae.

Mandibulata. A subphylum that includes Crustacea, Myriapoda, and Insecta, which all have mandibles.

Crustacea. Marine, fresh-water, terrestrial, or parasitic; usually with cephalothorax and abdomen; two pairs of antennae, one biramous; digestive tract straight, coiled or absent; open circulatory system but sometimes with blood vessels to the gills; with coxal glands, gills, jaws, and chelae.

Myriapoda. A convenience taxon to include the four classes with more than eight legs: Chilopoda, Diplopoda, Symphyla, and Pauropoda.

Chilopoda. Terrestrial; digestive tract straight; head and trunk; one pair of legs per segment; one pair of simple antennae; with malpighian tubules, tracheae, and jaws; no chelae or chelicerae.

Diplopoda. Terrestrial; digestive tract straight; head and trunk, two pairs of legs per apparent segment; antennae simple, with malpighian tubules, tracheae, and jaws; no chelae.

Symphyla. Terrestrial; digestive tract straight; head and trunk, 1 pair of legs on each of 12 segments; antennae simple; with malpighian tubules, tracheae, and jaws; no chelae.

Pauropoda. Terrestrial; digestive tract straight; head scarcely distinct from trunk, one pair of legs on each of nine segments; antennae biramous; with malpighian tubules and jaws; without circulatory or respiratory organs; no chelae.

Insecta. Terrestrial or freshwater; three pairs of legs on thorax; with wings or without; head, thorax, and abdomen; antennae not biramous; digestive tract straight or coiled or diverticulate; with malpighian tubules, tracheae, and jaws; no chelae or chelicerae.

CHAETOGNATHA. Marine; fusiform with lateral and tail fins; no appendages except prehensile spines on head; complete digestive tract; no excretory, circulatory, or respiratory organs; cilia external and internal.

POGONOPHORA. Marine; elongate tube-dwelling worms; no digestive tract or respiratory organs; with tentacles, nephridia, and closed blood system.

†HOMALOZOA (Carpoidea). An extinct group of three types of asymmetrical animals that show little similarity.

(See note under Echinodermata.)

†*Stylophora.* Marine; asymmetrical; an oval theca with a unique jointed brachial process; surface of large plates of calcite.

†*Homostelea.* Marine; asymmetrical; a discoidal theca of large and small plates of calcite; with a pedunculate appendage or stele.

†*Homoiostelea.* Marine; asymmetrical; a shapeless but lobed theca of large and small calcite plates; with a long stele and a flexible arm.

†CYCLOIDEA. Marine; thimble-shaped of five plates, with two planes of symmetry; skeleton of calcite plates

†CYAMOIDEA. Marine; half-lens-shaped, elliptical in apical view; two planes of symmetry; skeleton of calcite plates

†CAMPTOSTROMATOIDEA. Marine; medusiform, with radial symmetry; skeleton of calcite plates.

†LEPIDOCYSTIOIDEA. Marine; conical, possibly with radial symmetry; skeleton of calcite plates.

†HELICOPLACOIDEA. Marine; spirally arranged; skeleton of calcite plates.

ECHINODERMATA. Marine; pentaradiate after larval bilaterality; digestive tract complete or incomplete; no certain excretory or circulatory organs; no segmentation and usually no cephalization; water vascular system with podia (tube feet) arranged in ambulacral rows, passing through the skeletal plates by means of pores; spines usually; coelom an enterocoel.

> (Of the 13 extinct classes usually placed in this phylum, we reject those that are not basically pentaradiate. These are connected to the Echinodermata by only one distinctive feature: their skeletal plates each consist of one calcite crystal, a feature not uncommon in other animals. With all these groups included, the phylum cannot be effectively defined; without them the pentaradiate arrangement serves clearly.)

†Edrioasteroidea. Shape discoidal; without stalk or arms; theca flexible; pores for podia.

†Cyclocystoidea. Discoidal and apparently pentaradiate; ambulacra as branching grooves.

†Ophiocystoidea. Discoidal shape; pentamerous theca with five ambulacra; podia and giant podia.

†Eocrinoidea. Attached and subglobular; with stem and five arms, sometimes branched; imperforate thecal plates.

†Paracrinoidea. Attached and thecate; with stem and arms; thecal plates perforated.

†Cystoidea. Stemmed or stemless with globular test; plates may be asymmetrical, with thecal pores.

†Blastoidea. Stemmed and thecate, strongly pentamerous; with hydrospire, brachioles, and thecal pores.

Crinoidea. Bud-shaped, extinct species usually stalked, living species usually free-living; with pinnules or not, on movable arms, usually branched; theca rigid.

Somasteroidea. Five short arms; ambulacral pores but no grooves; skeleton of spicules and ossicles.

Asteroidea. Flattened, pentagonal, with five (or more) inflexible arms, each with ambulacral groove; skeleton of separate ossicles; with pedicellariae and podia.

Ophiuroidea. Flattened with small disk and five long flexible arms, sometimes branched; no ambulacral grooves; with pedicellariae and podia.

Echinoidea. Spheroidal, discoidal, or cordiform; movable spines; test of calcareous plates, perforated for podia but without grooves along the ambulacra.

Holothurioidea. Elongated with secondary bilaterality over the pentamery; skeleton of spicules; podia present or absent but without ambulacral grooves; with tentacles around the mouth.

Hemichordata. General term for the three following groups. Solitary or colonial; with enterocoelous coelom and epidermal nervous system; without nephridia or gill slits; tentacles in some; tornaria larva in some.

PTEROBRANCHIA. Marine; colonial or solitary; body in three regions; possible "stomochord"; arms with tentacles; coelom an enterocoel.

ENTEROPNEUSTA. Marine, worm-like and burrowing; colonial or solitary; "stomochord" present; body in three regions; coelom an enterocoel.

PLANCTOSPHAEROIDEA. Transparent, spherical; apparently larval digestive tract L-shaped; with ciliary band and coelom.

Chordata. General term for the Tunicata, Cephalochordata, Vertebrata; sometimes also the Hemichordata.

Protochordata (Prochordata). Older grouping of Tunicata and Cephalochordata, sometimes also with the Enteropneusta.

TUNICATA (Urochordata). Marine, sessile or pelagic, vase-shaped, usually with test of tunicin; "notochord" in larva only; coelom indefinite.

Ascidiacea. Solitary or compound; usually sessile; sometimes with calcareous spicules.

Thaliacea. Solitary or compound; free-swimming; with transparent test.

Larvacea (Appendicularia). Transparent, free-swimming; larviform; gelatinous test frequently discarded and replaced; pharynx with two stigmata.

CEPHALOCHORDATA (Acrania). Marine, swims and burrows in sand; no head or brain; fish-like shape; solenocytes; reversing blood flow; a notochord as the principal supporting structure; coelom an enterocoel.

†CONODONTOPHORIDA. Tooth- and jaw-like microfossils of calcium phosphate.

(This group is supposed to be vertebrate because the fossils are phosphatic as are vertebrate teeth, but, of course, phosphatic hardparts are common throughout the animal kingdom. The animals thought to have borne these structures are supposed to have other similarities to Vertebrata, but there is much doubt of the assignment. There is also no direct evidence to transfer them to any other position.)

VERTEBRATA (Craniata). Skull present, usually with jaws and paired limbs; gill slits but no atrium; coelom a schizocoel; notochord usually only in embryo, being replaced by the vertebral column.

Pisces. General term for all fish-like vertebrates. Used here for convenience to cover the next four classes.

Agnatha. Freshwater or marine; skeleton cartilaginous but rarely with bony elements, no jaws or paired fins; notochord persistent.

†*Placodermi.* With skeleton and heavy armor plates of bone; with hyoid gill slits; notochord probably persistent.

Chondrichthyes. Marine or freshwater; skeleton of cartilage, persistent notochord, two-chambered heart; gill slits, jaws, and spiral valve in intestine.

Osteichthyes. Marine or freshwater; with bony skeleton; notochord sometimes persistent; with two-chambered heart, gill slits and jaws.

Amphibia. Freshwater, terrestrial, or amphibious; with bony skeleton, three-chambered heart, gills or lungs or gill-slits, jaws, and two pairs of limbs.

Reptilia. Freshwater, terrestrial, or marine; with bony skeleton, four-chambered heart, lungs or cloacal respiration, and two pairs of limbs.

Aves. Terrestrial or aerial; with bony skeleton and feathers, four-chambered heart, lungs, syrinx, and two pairs of limbs including two wings.

Mammalia. Terrestrial but may be secondarily aquatic; with body skeleton and hair, four-chambered heart, lungs, larynx with vocal cords, and two pairs of limbs.

REFERENCES

Barrington, E. J. W., *The Biology of Hemichordata and Protochordata*, Oliver & Boyd, Edinburgh; W. H. Freeman, San Francisco, 1965.

Binyon, J., *Physiology of Echinoderms*, Pergamon Press, Oxford, 1972.

Bird, A. F., *The Structure of Nematodes*, Academic Press, New York, 1971.

Blackwelder, R. E., *Classification of the Animal Kingdom*, Southern Illinois University Press, Carbondale, Ill., 1963.

Blackwelder, R. E., *Taxonomy; A Text and Reference Book*, John Wiley & Sons, New York, 1973.

Boolootian, R. A., Ed., *Physiology of Echinodermata*, Interscience, New York, 1966.

Breder, C. M., Jr. and Rosen, D. E., *Modes of Reproduction in Fishes,* Natural History Press, Garden City, N.J., 1966.

Brown, M. E., *The Physiology of Fishes,* 2 volumes, Academic Press, New York, 1959.

Copeland, H. F., *Classification of the Animal Kingdom,* Pacific Books, Palo Alto, Calif., 1956.

Croll, N. A. and Matthews, B. E., *Biology of Nematodes,* John Wiley & Sons, New York, 1977.

Dales, R. P., *Annelids,* 2nd ed., Hutchinson University Library, London, 1967.

Davey, K. G., Reproduction in the Insects, Oliver & Boyd, Edinburgh, 1965.

Edwards, C. A. and Lofty, J. R., *Biology of Earthworms,* 2nd ed., Chapman & Hall, London; John Wiley & Sons, New York, 1977.

Farmer, J. N., *The Protozoa; Introduction to Protozoology,* C. V. Mosby, St. Louis, 1980.

Gibson, R., *Nemerteans,* Hutchinson University Library, London, 1972.

Gordon, M. S. et al., *Animal Function; Principles and Adaptations,* Macmillan, New York, 1968.

Green, J., *A Biology of Crustacea,* H. F. & G. Witherby, London, 1961.

Grell, K. G., *Protozoology,* Springer-Verlag, Berlin, 1973.

Hagan, H. R., *Embryology of the Viviparous Insects,* Ronald Press, New York, 1951.

Honigberg, B. M., A revised classification of the phylum Protozoa, *J. Protozool.,* 11, 7, 1964.

Hyman, L. H., *The Invertebrates,* Vol. 1, McGraw-Hill, New York, 1940.

Imms, A. D., *A General Textbook of Entomology,* 8th ed., Methuen, London, 1951.

Ivanov, A. V., *Pogonophora,* Academic Press, London; Consultants Bureau, New York, 1963.

Kudo, R. R., *Protozoology,* 5th ed., Charles C Thomas, Springfield, Ill., 1966.

Larwood, G. P., *Living and Fossil Bryozoa; Recent Advances in Research,* Academic Press, London, 1973.

Laverack, M. S., *The Physiology of Earthworms,* Pergamon Press, London; Macmillan, New York, 1963.

Lee, D. H. K., *The Physiology of Tissues and Organs,* Charles C Thomas, Springfield, Ill., 1950.

Lee, D. L., *The Physiology of Nematodes,* Oliver & Boyd, Edinburgh and W. H. Freeman, San Francisco, 1965.

Lenhoff, H. M. and Loomis, W. F., *The Biology of Hydra and of Some Other Coelenterates,* University of Miami Press, Coral Gables, Fla., 1961.

Mann, K. H., *Leeches (Hirudinea); Their Structure, Physiology, Ecology and Embryology,* Pergamon Press, Oxford, 1961.

Marshall, A. J., *Parker & Haswell, A Text-Book of Zoology,* Vol. 2, 7th ed., Macmillan, London, 1964.

Mill, P. J., Ed., *Physiology of Annelids,* Academic Press, New York, 1978.

Nichols, D., *Echinoderms,* Hutchinson, London and Hillary House, New York, 1962.

Parker, T. J. and Haswell, W. A., *A Text-Book of Zoology,* Vol. 2, 7th ed., Macmillan, London, 1964.

Patt, D. L. and Patt, G. R., *Comparative Vertebrate Histology,* Harper & Row, New York, 1969.

Pearse, A. S., *Zoological Names; A List of Phyla, Classes, and Orders,* American Association for the Advancement of Science, Durham, N.C., 1949.

Rice, M. E. and Todorovic, M., *Proceedings of the International Symposium on the Biology of the Sipuncula and Echiura,* Vol. 1 and 2, Institute for Biological Research and Smithsonian Institution, Kotor, 1970.

Riser, N. W. and Morse, M. P., *Biology of The Turbellaria,* McGraw-Hill, New York, 1974.

Romer, A. S., *The Vertebrate Body,* 4th ed., W. B. Saunders, Philadelphia, 1970.

Rudwick, M. J. S., *Living and Fossil Brachiopods,* Hutchinson University Library, London, 1970.

Runham, N. W. and Hunter, P. J., *Terrestrial Slugs,* Hutchinson University Library, London, 1970.

Ryland, J. S., *Bryozoans,* Hutchinson University Library, London, 1970.

Sadleir, R. M. F. S., *The Reproduction of Vertebrates,* Academic Press, New York, 1973.

Schmitt, W. L., *Crustaceans,* University of Michigan Press, Ann Arbor, 1966.

Sleigh, M., *The Biology of Protozoa,* American Elsevier, New York, 1973.

Smyth, J. D., *The Physiology of Trematodes,* W. H. Freeman, San Francisco and Oliver & Boyd, Edinburgh, 1966.

Smyth, J. D., *The Physiology of Cestodes;* Oliver & Boyd, Edinburgh and W. H. Freeman, San Francisco, 1969.

van Tienhoven, A., *Reproductive Physiology of Vertebrates,* W. B. Saunders, Philadelphia, 1968.

Wardle, R. A. and McLeod, J. A., *The Zoology of Tapeworms,* University of Minnesota Press, Minneapolis, 1952.

Waterman, T. H., Ed., *The Physiology of Crustacea,* Vol. 1 and 2, Academic Press, New York, 1960, 1961.

Index

INDEX

A

Abscission point, 43
Absorption, 286
Acanella, 491
Acanthella larva, 146
Acanthocephala, 511
  asexual processes, 20
  blastopore fate, 130
  blood pigments, 324
  body openings, 256
  body wall muscle layers, 242
  chitin, 189
  cilia, 220
  circulatory systems, 302
  egg coverings, 71
  excretory devices, 337
  flagella, 220
  hard part constituents, 380
  integument features, 375
  message systems, 366
  morphological features, 196—197
  muscle striation, 408
  reproduction, 28, 90, 97
  respiration, 312, 325
  setae, 375
  spermatozoa ducts, 254, 255
  tissue products, 246
  zygote covering, 120
Acanthocystis, 37
Acanthodesia serrata, 449
Acanthor larva, 146
Acanthosoma larva, 146
Acarina, 153—154, 271, 282
  ectoparasitism, 467
  excretory mechanisms, 339
  exploitation for transport, 472
  storage sites, 421
  tracheae, 319, 387
Acineta, 36
Acoela, 151, 243, 278
Acoustico-lateralis system, 390, 392
Actinomere, 198
Actinophrys, 24, 85
Actinotrocha larva, 146
Actinula, 37, 146
Activation, 53, 59—60, 82, 84, 112
Active transport, 273
Activities of individuals, see also Individuals, 427—451
Adelphophagia, 290
Adenocorticotrophin, 362
Adenohypophysis, 362
Adhesive sac, 129, 132
Adipose tissue, 421
Adrenal cortex, 362
Adrenalin, 362
Adrenal medulla, 362

Adults, see also specific topics, 48, 94, 112, 155, 160—161, 181—423
  biochemicals, 188—191
  body cavities, 400—403
  cells, 213—233
  circulatory systems, 293—305
  difficulties of, 161
  digestive system, 265—291
  division, 39
  endocrine system, 341—368
  excretion, 327—340
  integuments, 369—384
  metabolism, 191—192
  miscellaneous organ functions, 397—423
  morphology, 193—212
  nervous system, 341—368
  organs and organ systems, 247—263
  physiology vs. anatomy, 186—187
  respiration, 307—326
  strobilation, 42
  structure vs. function, 183—192
  tissues, 238—246
  unique organ systems, 385—395
Aepyornis titan, 119
Aequoria, 448
Aerial phyla, 441
Aeropyles, 312
Aestivation, 173
Aetea, 491
Afferent vessels, 300
Agalma, 490
Agamete, 11, 22, 29—30, 34, 38, 47, 64, 95, 162
Agamogenesis, 32—33
Agamogony, 20, 28, 34—35, 90—92, 113
Agamont, 51
Ageniaspis fuscicollis, 25
Aggregations, 430, 457, 486—490
Aging, 177—178
Agnatha, 393
Air, storage, 422
Airborne chemicals, 347
Air-breathing, 311—312
Air capillaries, 320
Alaria, 467
Alcohol, 284
Alcyonaria, 379, 412
Aldosterone, 362
Alecithal, 289
Algae, 272, 440, 441
Algophagous, 463
Alima larva, 146
Alimentary openings, 253
Alimentation, 286
Alimentation system, see also Digestive system, 257—258
Allantois, 71
Allogamy, 49
Allometry, 208—209

Allozygote, 121
Alternation of generations, 36, 43, 51, 95, 164, 165
Alveoli, 318, 320
Amaroecium, 495
Amblypygi, 310
Ambystomidae, 107
Ameiosis, 29
Ameiotic parthenogenesis, 28
Ametabolous, 150
Amitosis, 227
Ammocoetes larva, 146
Ammonia, 340
Ammonotelic animals, 340
Amnion, 71
Amoeba, 33, 236
Amoebocyte, 57, 116, 224, 226, 258, 334, 405
    movement of, 250, 405, 436
Amoebula larva, 146
Amphibia, 78
Amphibians, 318, 332, 418, 471, 477
Amphiblastula, 126, 146
Amphigastrula, 146
Amphigenesis, 48
Amphigony, 46, 49
Amphilina foliacea, 152
Amphimixis, 29, 31—32, 48
Amphioxus, 211
Amphipholis
    sinuatus, 449
    squamata, 154
Amphipnous, 311, 318
Amphipod, 465
Amphipoda, 153, 320
Amphitoky, 83
Amplocheir sequoia, 449
Ampulla, 411
Ampullacea, 347
Ampullae of Lorenzini, 392
Amputation, 443
Amylase, 284
Anabiosis, 135, 144, 173
Anabolism, 191
Anaerobes, 309, 320
Anal pores, 276, 278
Anal sacs, 283
Anamorphosis, 152, 156, 205
Anatomy vs. physiology, 186—187
Anaxonic, 198
Ancestrula, 65, 494
Androdioecious, 99
Androecism, 100
Androgenesis, 83, 103
Androgenic gland, 363
Andromonoecious, 99
Anemones, 440, 462
Anemotaxis, 430
Anisogametes, 49, 58, 66
Anisogamonty, 55, 105—106
Anisogamy, 49
Anisotropy, ova, 69
Annelida, 514

asexual processes, 20
blastopore fate, 130
blood pigments, 324
body openings, 256
body wall muscle layers, 242
chitin, 189
cilia, 220
circulatory systems, 298, 302—303
colonies, 492
excretory devices, 338
flagella, 220
hard part constituents, 381
integument features, 375
luminescence, 449
message systems, 367
molting, 168
morphological features, 196—197
muscle phosphagens, 409
muscle striation, 408
pumping organs, 410
regeneration, 175—176
reproduction, 28, 91, 97
respiration, 313, 325
setae, 376
spermatozoa ducts, 254, 255
tissue products, 246
Anomalops, 450
Anoplophyra, 205
Anoplura, 467
Antennae, 349
Antennary gland, 334
Antennules, 349
Anterior pituitary, 362
Anthogenesis, 83
Anthophilous, 463
Anthozoa, 189
Anthraquinone, 323
Anticoagulant, 284
Antimeres, 198
Antlers, 419
Ant-lions, 432, 434
Ants, see also specific types, 268, 272, 457
    casts, 208
    control of, 465
    cultivation of food, 461
    digestion, 287
    enslavement, 469, 471
    exploitation for shelter, 469
    food storage, 434—435
    guests, 268
    host modification, 440
    myrmecophily, 478
    parasitism, 465
    protective custody, 461
    provisioning of food, 433
    storage organs, 420
Anus, 253, 275, 283
Aphids, 89, 433, 457, 461
Aphis, 25
Apocrine glands, 419
Apodeme tension receptors, 350

Apomixis, 31—32
Apozygote, 31, 60, 68, 71—72, 84—85, 112, 118—122
Appendicularis larva, 146
Appendicular skeleton, 393
Apterygota, 153
Aquarium fish, 471
Aquatic Hemimetabola, 153
Aquatic Insects, 378
Arachnida, 78
Araneida, 319, 357, 387
Arboroid colony, 493
Archaeocytes, 230, 405
Archenteron, 127, 137, 290, 399—400
Archigastrula, 127
Archihiston, 177
Archimedes, 211
Architomy, 20—21, 29, 39—40
Aristotle's lantern, 253, 281, 383, 415
Armadillo, 87
Arrhenogeny, 83
Arrhenotoky, 83
Arteries, 303
Arthromere, 204
Arthropoda, 514—515
  asexual processes, 20
  blastopore fate, 130
  blood pigments, 324
  body openings, 256
  body wall muscle layers, 242
  chitin, 189
  cilia, 219—220
  circulatory systems, 302—303
  colonies, 492
  excretory devices, 338
  flagella, 220
  hard part constituents, 381
  integument features, 375
  luminescence, 449
  message systems, 367
  molting, 168
  morphological features, 196—197
  muscle phosphagens, 409
  muscle striation, 408
  pumping organs, 410
  regeneration, 176
  reproduction, 28, 91, 97
  respiration, 313, 325
  setae, 376
  spermatozoa ducts, 254, 255
  tissue products, 246
Arthropodin, 189
Articulamentum, 383
Articulata, 402
Ascaris, 59, 119
Aschelminthes, 380, 511
Ascons, 386
Asexual reproduction, see also specific topics, 18—21, 27—28, 32—44, 61, 84, 87, 89, 93, 113, 495
Asphyxy, 173

Asplanchna, 25
Assembled bodies, 29
Asses, 470
Astacus, 218
Asteroidea, 391
Asthenobiosis, 173
Astogeny, 494
Asymmetrical, 198
Athrocytes, 231, 334
Atoms, structure, 188
Atrocha larva, 146
Attachment, 430, 445—446
Atubaria, 154
Auditory organs, 348
Aulophora, 153
Aurelia, 24, 491
Auricularia larva, 146
Aurochs, 470
Autoevisceration, 444
Autogamy, 22, 31, 35, 55, 59, 105—106, 499
Auto-intoxication, 173
Autolycus, 492
Automixis, 31, 49, 54, 96, 104—106
Autospasy, 443
Autothecae, 207
Autotilly, 443
Autotomy, 11, 40, 43, 177, 443—444
Autotomy plane, 418—419
Autozooid, 493
Avicularia, 65, 207, 473, 493
Axes, 196, 199—200
Axial organ, 304
Axial skeleton, 393
Axoblasts, 34, 222
Axon, 353

B

Bacteria, 222, 447—448
Baer's cavity, 399
Balance organs, 349
Balanoglossus clavigerus, 154
Baleen, 280, 383
Bali cattle, 471
Balloons, 439
Banteng, 471
Barnacles, 446, 487, 490
Basic Bisexual Reproduction (BBR), 28, 48—49, 87—89
Basiconica, 347
Basophil, 405
Bathypelagic fish, 450
Batillipes, 205
Bats, 267, 437
Beaks, 378
Bear, 459
Bee moth, 268
Bees, 208, 351, 434, 461
Beetles, see also specific types, 208, 268, 419, 469
Behavior, see also specific topics, 22, 425—518

animals' interactions, 453—481
classification of animals, 503—518
colonies, 485—495
death, 497—499
individuals' activities, 427—451
reproductive, 480
Bezoar, 470
Bilateria, 510
Bile, 284
Binary fission, 9, 22, 38
Biochemical diversity, 4
Biochemicals, 188—191
Bioluminescence, 446—450
Biota, 188
Bipinnaria, 145, 146
Birds, 68, 282, 378, 457
competition for shelter, 459
flying, 437
nephron kidneys, 332
oviparous, 475
storage organs, 420
yolk sac, 477
Birth, 140
Bisexuality, 26—27, 46—49
Bisexual reproduction, see also specific topics, 19,
23—24, 27, 45—80
basic, 48—49
bisexuality, 46—49
gametophores, 76—79
gonophores, 76—77
reproductive system, see also Reproductive system, 60—76
sexual reproductive processes, 49—60
Bithecae, 207
Blastema, 177
Blastocoel, 127, 136, 399—400
Blastocyst, 136
Blastoderm, 125—126, 133, 136, 237
Blastodisc, 136
Blastokinesis, 135
Blastomeres, 29, 60, 103, 119—120, 122, 125,
136, 232
Blastopore 129—132, 135
Blastostyle, 476, 493
Blastozooid, 494
Blastula, 112, 122, 125—126, 136—137
Blepharisma undulans, 167
Blood, 239, 241, 294, 304, 322, 422
Blood cells, 422
Blood circulation, 301—304
Blood gill, 315, 320
Blood lacunar system, 297
Blood pigments, 323—324
Bloodsucking, 271
Bloodsucking Insecta, 267
Blood vessels, 259, 294, 297—299, 301—303
Blowflies, 268, 466
Body arrangement, 200—210
Body cavities, 296, 421
Body covering, 373
Body forms, 23

Body openings, see also specific types, 253, 276—277
Body spaces, 259, 399—403
Body wall, 373
Bolas spider, 434
Bolitophila luminosa, 449
Bombardier beetles, 288
Bone, 224, 239, 383, 393, 421, 472
Bonellia, 103, 289, 492
Bony armor, 393
Bony fish, 317
Book gills, 310, 320
Book lungs, 311, 317, 319—320
Botflies, 466, 467
Bothrioplana, 71
Botryllus, 492
Botryoidal tissues, 334
Bougainvillea multitentaculata, 79
Bowman's capsule, 332
Brachidium, 383, 411
Brachiolaria larva, 146
Brachiopoda, 512
asexual processes, 20
blastopore fate, 130
blood pigments, 324
body openings, 256
body wall muscle layers, 242
chitin, 189
cilia, 220
circulatory systems, 302—303
excretory devices, 337
flagella, 220
hard part constituents, 380
integument features, 375
message systems, 367
morphological features, 196—197
muscle striation, 408
reproduction, 28, 90, 97
respiration, 313, 325
spermatozoa ducts, 254, 255
tissue products, 246
Bract, 493
Brain, 356—358
Branchiae, 320
Branchial basket, 282
Branchiura, 357
Breakage plane, 443
Bristles, 246, 374—376, 378
Bromatophores, 268—269
Bronchi, 318
Bronchioles, 318, 320
Bronchus, 320
Brood chamber, 120
Brooding, 141, 287, 461, 473, 476
Brood pouch, 75, 476
Brown body, 332, 334
Brown funnels, 334
Brownian movement, 404
Browsing, 464
Bryozoa, 512
asexual processes, 20

blastopore fate, 130
blood pigments, 324
body openings, 256
body wall muscle layers, 242
chitin, 189
cilia, 220
circulatory systems, 302
colonies, 491
excretory devices, 337
flagella, 220
hard part constituents, 380
integument features, 375
luminescence, 449
message systems, 367
morphological features, 196—197
muscle striation, 408
regeneration, 175
reproduction, 28, 90, 97
respiration, 313, 325
setae, 376
spermatozoa ducts, 254, 255
tissue products, 246
Bubble statocysts, 349
Buccal cavity, 280—281
Buccal chamber, 280
Buccal stylets, 433
Bud, 9—10, 19, 22—23, 29—30, 36, 42, 94, 113, 251
    detached, 252
    fusion, 106
Budding, 11, 20—21, 23, 34, 36—37, 43, 113
    colonies, 495
    double, 37
    endogenous, 36
    exogenous, 36
    multiple, 37
    pyloric, 36, 103
    secondary, 40
    stolonization, 37
Bugula, 25, 95, 152
Buoyancy, 439
Burrowing, 436—438
Bursa, 132, 320, 334
Bursa copulatrix, 75
Bursal slits, 253
Butterfly, 156, 461

C

Caddis fly larvae, 146, 466
Cage birds, 471
Calcareous shell, 373
Calcitonin, 362
Callyspongia diffusa, 243
Calyces, 411, 413
Calyconula, 494
Calycophora, 495
Calyptotomatida, 513
Calyssozoa, 512
    asexual processes, 20

blastopore fate, 130
blood pigments, 324
body openings, 256
body wall muscle layers, 242
chitin, 189
cilia, 220
circulatory systems, 302
colonies, 491
excretory devices, 337
flagella, 220
hard part constituents, 380
integument features, 375
message systems, 366
morphological features, 196—197
muscle striation, 408
reproduction, 28, 90, 97
respiration, 312, 325
spermatozoa ducts, 254, 255
tissue products, 246
Camels, 461, 471, 472
Camouflage, 440, 471
Campaniform sensilla, 350
Camptostromatoidea, 515
Canals, see specific types
Cannibalism, 271, 456, 460
Capillaries, 222, 299, 302
Capitellidae, 285
CAP organs, 350
Captacula, 435
Capulus hungaricus, 152
Carapus acus, 154
Carbon dioxide, 295, 308
Carchesium, 490
Cardiocoelom, 400
Carion beetles, 475
Carnivorous, 271
Carrier pigeons, 461
Cartilage, 239, 393—394, 411
Caspionema, 490
Castes, 207—209
Catabolism, 191
Catenoid colony, 493
Catenulida, 249
Caterpillar, 146, 156, 471
Cats, 447, 471
Cattle, 419, 461, 469—472
Caudal filaments, 310, 320
Cavitation, 128
    gastrulation by, see Gastrulation
Cavities, see specific types
Cell as a unit, 8
Cell body, 353
Cell membrane, 70
Cells, 250
    adults, 213—233
    aggregation, 236
    blastomeres, 232
    chloride, 231
    cilia, 217—221
    components, 217
    division, 38, 226—228

duct, 231
dust, 405
epitheliomuscular, 230, 406
flagella, 217—221
flagellated epithelia, 230
flame, 330, 335
functions, 224—229
gametes, 232
glandulomuscular, 230
inclusions, 221—222
Kuppfer, 225, 405
locomotion, 436
migration, 117, 296—297
mormyomast, 351
motility, 228—229
muscle, 406
nematocysts, 223
nerve, 353
nucleus, 221
oddities, 223—224
organelles, 217
origins, 216
outer coverings, 223
packet-gland, 231
phagocytosis, 224—225
protoplasm, 214—215
protozoan cell functions, 229
rhabdite gland, 230
rheoreceptive, 231
secretions, 222, 224
setae, 222
shape, 216—217
skeletons, 223
spicules, 222, 224—225
spindle, 231
storage, 421
structure, 188, 216—223
theory, 215—216
transplanted, 253
transport between, 295
transport by, 226, 259
trichocysts, 223
tubular, 231
types, 229—232
unique, 230—232
universality of types of, 232
wandering, 134
zygotes, 232
Cellularity, 7—9
Cellulose, 189
Centralized nervous systems, 352
Central nervous system, 352
Centrolecithal, 289
Cephalization, 196, 201
Cephalochordata, 517
 asexual processes, 21
 blastopore fate, 131
 blood pigments, 324
 body openings, 256
 body wall muscle layers, 243
 cilia, 220

circulation, 298, 302—303
excretory devices, 338
flagella, 220
hard part constituents, 381
integument features, 375
message systems, 368
morphological features, 196—197
muscle phosphagens, 409
muscle striation, 408
reproduction, 28, 92, 97
respiration, 314, 325
setae, 376
spermatozoa ducts, 254, 255
tissue products, 246
Cephalodiscus, 100, 154, 492, 494
Cephalopoda, 71, 77, 120, 410
Cephalothrix, 152
Cephalotrocha larva, 146
Cerata, 287, 310, 316, 320
Ceratium, 490
Cercaria larva, 146
Cerci, 348
Cerebratulus, 152
Cestoda, 375
Chaetognatha, 515
 asexual processes, 21
 blastopore fate, 130
 blood pigments, 324
 body openings, 256
 body wall muscle layers, 242
 chitin, 189
 cilia, 220
 circulatory systems, 302
 excretory devices, 338
 flagella, 220
 hard part constituents, 381
 integument features, 375
 message systems, 367
 morphological features, 196—197
 muscle striation, 408
 reproduction, 28, 91, 97
 respiration, 313, 325
 setae, 376
 spermatophores, 78
 spermatozoa ducts, 254, 255
 tissue products, 246
Chaetopterus, 406, 410, 447
Chain-colonies, 491
Chaining, 209
Chains of individuals, 41, 201—202
Chalones, 361
Chaoborus, 388, 445
Chelicerae, 435
Chelonethida, 319, 387
Chemical activators, 360, 361
Chemical bonds, 4
Chemical control, 359—368
Chemical messengers, 360—361, 363—365
Chemoreception, 346, 347
Chemosynthesis, 271
Chemotaxis, 430

Chickens, 469, 471, 475
Chilopoda, 78
Chinchillas, 471
Chitin, 189, 245, 383
Chitinous shell, 373
Chitinozoa, 509
Chlamydomonas perty, 65
Chloragogen tissue, 239, 241, 243, 334—335, 420
Chlorocruorin, 323—324
Chlorogogen cells, 232
Chlorogogue cells, 232
Choanocyte, 57, 116, 218, 230, 386
Choanoflagellates, 432
Cholecystokinin, 362
Chondrichthyes, 279
Chondrostei, 393, 415
Chordamesoderm, 237
Chordata, 516
Chordotonal organ, 348, 350
Chorion, 70—71, 120
Chromatin, 51
Chromatophores, 455
Chromosomal determination, 103
Chromosomes, 49, 51
Chrysaora, 491
Chrysididae, 468
Chrysomonadina, 495
Cilia, 217—221, 438
Ciliary movement, 406
Ciliata, molting, 167
Ciliated funnels, 333
Ciliated urns, 333, 336
Ciliospores, 34
Cimex, 268
Circulation, 295—300
  blood, see Blood circulation
Circulatory system, see also Circulation, 257—260
  adults, 293—305
  blood circulation, see also Blood circulation,
    301—304
Circum-enteric rings, 359
Circumoesophageal ring, 359
Cirri, 218—219, 438
Cirripedea, 120, 146, 269, 446, 480, 487
Cisterna chyli, 300
Cladocera, 156, 173, 208
Clams, 200, 432, 443, 447, 449, 464
Clariallabes petriola, 154
Classification of animals, 503—518
  categories, 505
  groups of the animal kingdom, 507—517
  nature of, 504—507
  objectivity, 505
  protozoa, 506
  subjectivity, 505
  synonyms, 505
Clavellina, 492
Claws, 378, 383, 392
Cleavage, 112—113, 122—126, 135—136, 139
Cleavage spindle, 200
Cleft, see also Gill slit, 320

Cleptobiosis, 461, 468
Climatic polymorphism, 206
Climbing, 437
Cloaca, 283
Clonal fertilization, see Fertilization
Clones, 32—34, 55
Clothes moths, 268
Clymenella, 153
Cnidoblast cell, 417
Cnidocils, 217, 417
Cnidocysts, 261
Cnidocytes, 230
Cnidospora, 505
Cobras, 418
Coccidae, 275
Coccoliths, 372
Cockroaches, 272
Coconut crab, 434
Cocoon, 70, 120
Coelenterata, 510
  asexual processes, 20
  blastopore fate, 30
  blood pigments, 324
  body openings, 256
  body wall muscle layers, 242
  cilia, 220
  circulatory systems, 302
  colonies, 490—491
  excretory devices, 337
  flagella, 220
  hard part constituents, 380
  integument features, 375
  luminescence, 448
  message systems, 366
  morphological features, 196—197
  muscle phosphagens, 409
  muscle striation, 408
  pumping organs, 140
  regeneration, 175
  reproduction, 28, 90, 97
  respiration, 312, 325
  spermatozoa ducts, 254, 255
  tissue products, 246
Coelenteron, 274, 276—277
Coeloblastula, 126, 133
Coelogastrula, 127
Coelom, 64, 137, 225, 304, 400—402'
Coelomata, 512
Coelomocytes, 225—226, 335, 405
Coelomoducts, 56, 335
Coelozoic, 466
Coenobium, 493
Coenoblast, 237
Coenoecium, 373, 383
Coenurus bladders, 37
Coenurus larva, 146
Cognettia
  glandulosa, 83
  sphagnetorum, 33
Coiling, 289
Cold, 343

Coleolida, 513
Coleoptera, 449, 475, 492
Collagen, 190, 383
Collar cells, 57, 116
Collembola, 210, 310, 319, 339, 387, 449
Colloblast, 211, 230, 435
Collozoum, 487
Colon, 283
Coloniality, 486—490
Colonial polymorphism, 207
Colonies, 11—12, 95, 485—495
    aggregation distinguished, 486
    coloniality, 486—490
    cooperation, 459
    development, 494
    forms, 493
    groups described, 490—492
    individuals vs., 11—12
    locomotion, 436
    motility, 492
    parts of, 493
    polymorphic forms within, 493—494
    reproduction, 494—495
    structure, 188
Color phases, 208
Combs, 376
Commensalism, 477—478
Commissure, 354
Communication, 454—455
Communities, structure, 188
Competition, 457—459
Concealment, 439—440
Conchiolin, 190
Conducting devices, 351
Cone shells, 284
Conjugants, 105, 106
Conjugation, 19, 27, 55—56, 96, 104—106, 498—499
Connective, 354
Connective tissue, 421
Conochilus, 491
Conodontophorida, 381, 517
Consortism, 430, 457
Constructions, 430
Containment, 370—371
Contractile tissue, 406—407
Contractile vacuoles, 410
Contractile vessels, 410
Control system, 257, 262—263
Conularida, 189, 380, 510
Cooperation, 458—459
Copepoda, 153, 173, 207, 268, 285
Coppinia, 493
Copromonas subtilis, 72
Coprophagous, 271
Coprophagy, 272
Copulation, 53—54, 56, 57
Copulatory area, 58
Coracidium larva, 146
Coral, 200, 246, 281, 379, 411, 491
Corallite, 413

Corbula, 493
Cordyli, 349
Corema, 347
Coremata, 347
Coriolus force, 431
Corium, 378
Corm, 204, 493
Cormidium, 493
Cormogeny, 494
Cormorants, 461
Cornification, 392
Corona, 218
Corpora allata, 363
Corpus luteum, 362
Corticosteroids, 362
Corticosterone, 362
Corticotrophin, 362
Cortisone, 362
Corysterium, 76
Coscinasterias, 40
Cothurniella, 491
Coxal gills, 310, 320
Coxal glands, 331, 335
Coypus, 471
Crabs, see also specific types, 462, 465
Craniates, 390
Crawling, 436
Crayfish, 153, 212
Creeping, 436—437
Crenobis alpina, 430
Crepidula, 492
Cribiform organ, 320
Crickets, 272
Cricoconarida, 513
Crinoidea, 391
Cristatella, 491—492
Crocodiles, 318
Crop, 282
Cross-breeding, 55
Cross-fertilization, 49, 54, 59, 90—92, 102
Crossing-over, 33, 51
Crustacea, 78, 410
Cryptomitosis, 227
Crystalline style, 283
Ctenes, 218
Ctenidium, 320
Ctenocella, 491
Ctenodrilus, 33, 65
Ctenophora, 510
    asexual processes, 20
    blastopore fate, 130
    blood pigments, 324
    body openings, 256
    body wall muscle layers, 242
    cilia, 220
    circulatory systems, 302
    excretory devices, 337
    flagella, 220
    integument features, 375
    luminescence, 448
    message systems, 366

morphological features, 196—197
muscle phosphagens, 409
muscle striation, 408
reproduction, 28, 90, 97
respiration, 312, 325
spermatozoa ducts, 254, 255
tissue products, 246
Cuckoos, 469, 471
Cultivation of food, 461—462, 469
Cunina, 35, 53
  proboscidea, 123
Cupula, 390
Cuticle, 373, 375, 378
Cutis, 373
Cuttlefish, 252
Cuvierian tubules, 419
Cyamoidea, 515
Cyanopsin, 346
Cyathospongia, 380, 509
Cyathozooid, 494
Cycle
  defined, 85—86
  reproductive, see Reproductive cycles
Cycloidea, 515
Cyclomorphosis, 206, 208—209
Cyclonexis, 492
Cyclosis, 258, 295, 404
Cyclostomata, 393, 415
Cyclostomes, 378
Cyclothone microdon, 450
Cyclotrichium meunieri, 269
Cydippid larva, 146
Cymatogaster, 475
Cyphonautes larva, 146
Cypridina, 449
Cypris larva, 146
Cyst, 373
Cystacanth, 465
Cysticercius, 37, 146
Cystihalysites, 491
Cystozooid, 493
Cytochrome, 323
Cytogamy, 31, 55, 105—106
Cytozoic, 466

D

Dactylozoites, 36, 39
Dactylozooids, 207, 277, 494
Daphnia, 346
Daphniarubin, 323
Dasypus novemcinctus, 25
Daughter cells, 51
Death, 112, 115, 497—499
Death-feigning, 173
Decapoda, 147, 153, 156, 317, 357
Decorator crab, 440
Dedifferentiation, 112, 144, 171, 173
Deer, 419
Defense, 295

Defense organs, 416—419
Definitive host, 478
Delamination, 113, 128, 133
Demanian system, 76, 386—387
Dendrite, 353
Dendritic colony, 493
Dendrosoma, 490
Dentine, 394
Deoxycorticosterone, 362
Dermal branchiae, 310, 320
Dermal plates, 411, 414—415
Dermal skeleton, 393
Dermaptera, 433, 475
Dermis, 373, 375, 378
Desiccation, 173
Desmoscolecida, 283
Desmoscolex, 205
Desor's larva, 146
Determination, 138—139
Detorsion, 199
Detritus feeders, 432
Detritus-filtering, 272
Deuterostomatous, 131, 137
Deuterostome, 129
Deuterotoky, 83
Deutoplasm, 75
Development
  arrested, 173
  direct, 144, 151
  epimorphic, 156
  indirect, 144, 151
  individuals, see Development of individual
  site of, 139—140
Development of individuals, see also specific topics,
    109—179
  cycles of, 114—115
  defined, 112
  diversity in, 113—114
  embryology, 111—142
  larva to adult, 143—158
  life cycles, 159—179
  reproduction distinct from, 23—26
  unity in, 113
Developmental cycle, 115
Developmental polymorphism, 206—208
Developmental stages, 112—113
Diapause, 173
Diapedesis, 229
Diatoms, 212, 372
Dibothriocephalus, 467
Dibranchiata, 205
Dichogamy, 101—102
Dichromism, 209
Dicoryne, 77
Didelphys, 68
Didinium, 417
Diecdysis, 169
Differentiation, 112—113, 133
Diffusion, 273, 404
Digamety, 103
Digenea, 278

Digestion, 266, 268—269, 286, 288
Digestive system, 257—258
   adults, 265—291
   coelenteron, 276—277
   functions, 273—291
   gastrovascular cavity, 277—278
   intestinal tract, 278—284
   protozoan nourishment, 273—274
   structures, 273—291
   unusual features, 284—286
   utilization of food, 266—267
Digestive tract, see also Intestinal tract, 266
   embryonic origin, 290—291
   food and feeding, see also Food, 267—273
   metazoan, 274—275
   openings into, 275—276
Dimegaly, 68
Dimorphism, 209
Dimorphobiosis, 474, 476
Dinobryon, 490
Dinoflagellata, 261
   chains, 487
   luminescence, 447—448
   metamerism, 205
   nematocysts, 223
   outer coverings of cells, 222
   photogenic, 448
   trichocysts, 223, 417
Dinophiloidea, 514
   asexual processes, 20
   blood pigments, 324
   body openings, 256
   body wall muscle layers, 242
   cilia, 220
   circulatory systems, 302
   flagella, 220
   integument features, 375
   message systems, 367
   morphological features, 196—197
   muscle striation, 408
   reproduction, 28, 91, 97
   respiration, 313, 325
   spermatozoa ducts, 254, 255
Dinophilus, 98, 504
Dioecious, 100
Dioecious organs, 61
Dioecism, 54, 100
Dioecy, 100
Diphygenesis, 208—209
Diplauxis hatti, 218
Dipleurozoa, 510
Dipleurula larva, 146
Diploblastic, 117
Diplocardia, 449
Diplogaster, 98
Diploidy, 29, 47, 85
Diplozoon, 151, 491
Dipnoi, 317, 393, 415
Diptera, 146, 208, 357, 389, 449, 475
Disassociation, 444
Discoblastula, 126, 128, 133, 135

Discogastrula, 127
Discoid colony, 493
Discorbis, 218
Dispermy, 56
Dispersal, 148
Dissymmetry, 198
Distaplia, 24
Diurnation, 173
Diversity, see also specific topics, 4
   levels of, 93—96
   reproduction, 47
Division, 19, 22, 28, 39—41, 90—92, 498
   cells, 226—228
   colonies, 495
DNA, 191, 226, 228
Dodecaceria canulleryi, 40, 43
Dog, 461, 462, 469, 470, 472
Doliolaria larva, 146
Doliolida, 154
Domestic animals, 470, 498
Domestication, 430, 456, 460, 469, 470
Dormancy, 144, 173—174
Dormice, 471
Dorsal vessel, 410
Dorsiventral symmetry, 196
Drinking, 435
Drosophila, 172
Ducts, 74, 297
Dugesia gonocephala, 33, 65
Dulosis, 456, 471
Dung beetles, 472, 475
Duodenum, 283, 362
Dust cells, 405
Dytiscus, 68

E

Ears, 348
Earthworm, 198, 282, 289
   cephalization, 201
   circulation, 298
   circumenteric nerve rings, 360
   food storage, 434—435
   luminescence, 449
   segmentation, 204
   storage organs, 420
   turgor, 412
Ecdysial gland, 363
Ecdysis, 167, 169
Echinochrome, 323
Echinococcus, 152, 491
Echinodermata, 516
   asexual processes, 21
   blastopore fate, 130
   blood pigments, 324
   body openings, 256
   body wall muscle layers, 242—243
   cilia, 220
   circulatory systems, 302
   excretory devices, 338

flagella, 220
hard part constituents, 381
integument features, 375
luminescence, 449
message systems, 367
morphological features, 196—197
muscle phosphagens, 409
muscle striation, 408
pumping organs, 411
regeneration, 176
reproduction, 28, 91, 97
respiration, 313—314, 325
setae, 376
spermatozoa ducts, 254, 255
Echinoid, 285
Echinoidea, 391
Echinopluteus larva, 146
Echinospira larva, 146
Echiuroidea, 513
asexual processes, 20
blood pigments, 324
body openings, 256
body wall muscle layers, 242
chitin, 189
cilia, 220
circulatory systems, 302—303
colonies, 492
excretory devices, 337
flagella, 220
hard part constituents, 381
integument features, 375
message systems, 367
morphological features, 196—197
muscle phosphagens, 409
muscle striation, 408
reproduction, 28, 91, 97
respiration, 313, 325
setae, 376
spermatozoa ducts, 254, 255
tissue products, 246
Echoes, 431
Echolocation, 431
Eclosion, 140
Ectocommensal, 478
Ectoderm, 134, 237
Ectohormones, 361
Ectolecithal, 289
Ectomesenchyme, 240
Ectomesoderm, 133, 237
Ectoparasites, 457, 467
Ectoparasitism, 271—272, 461, 466—467
Ectotrachea, 388
Eels, 147, 154
Effectors, 365
Egestion, 286
Egg, see also Ova, 68—72, 79, 121—122, 136
yolk, 289—290
parasites, 463
Egg-mother cell, 63
Egg rafts, 79
Ejectisomes, 261

Elasmobranchiata, 392, 393, 415
Elastin, 190
Elaterids, 449
Electra pilosa, 152
Electron-transfer system, 214
Electroreceptors, 351
Eleocytes, 231, 243, 405
Elephants, 419, 461, 469, 471, 472
Elimination, 328
Embioptera, 492
Emboly, 127, 129, 133
Embryo, 71, 94, 112, 113, 135—141
defined, 122
development into adult, 143—158
Embryogenesis, 122, 126—135
Embryogeny, 113, 134
Embryology, see also specific topics, 111—142
apozygotes, 118—122
cleavage, 122—126
developmental stages, 112—113
embryo, 135—141
embryogenesis, 122, 126—135
Mesozoa, 116
orientation, 112—122
sponge, 116—118
zygotes, 118—122
Embryonic cavities, 399—400
Embryonic membranes, 135
Embryonic tissues, 237
Embryophores, 76, 79
Emergence, 140—141
Emplectonema kandai, 448
Enamel, 394
Enclosure of body, 257, 263
Encystment, 173
End of existence, 498—499
Endochorion, 71, 120
Endocommensal, 478
Endocrine glands, 362—363
Endocrine system, 341—368
Endocrinology, 362—365
Endocytosis, 225
Endoderm, 127, 128, 133, 134, 237
Endogamy, 49, 54, 106
Endolymph, 392
Endomesoderm, 133, 237
Endomixis, 31, 106, 499
Endoparasites, 467, 468
Endoparasitic Hymenoptera, 155
Endoparasitism, 271, 456, 461, 466—468
Endophoresis, 472
Endoprocta, 504
End organ, 345
Endoskeleton, 392—393, 411, 414—415
Endostyle, 282
Endotrachea, 388
Endozoic, 478
Energid, 7
Energy, storage, 422
Enslavement, see Slavery
Enterocoel, 137, 400, 402

Enterocoelous, 138
Enterocoely, 133, 137
Enterocrinin, 362
Enterogastrone, 362
Enteron, 266
Enteropneusta, 516
    asexual processes, 20
    blastopore fate, 130
    blood pigments, 324
    body openings, 256
    body wall muscle layers, 243
    cilia, 220
    circulatory systems, 302
    excretory devices, 338
    flagella, 220
    hard part constituents, 381
    integument features, 375
    luminescence, 449
    message systems, 367
    morphological features, 196—197
    muscle phosphagens, 409
    muscle striation, 408
    reproduction, 28, 92, 97
    respiration, 314, 325
    spermatozoa ducts, 254, 255
    tissue products, 246
Enteroxenus, 269, 274
Entolecithal, 289
Entomitosis, 227
Entomophagy, 272
Environmental control, 440
Enzymes, proteolytic, 285
Eosinophil, 405
Ephelota, 36
Ephemeroptera, 275, 286, 449, 475
Ephippium, 70
Ephyrae, 41, 146
Epiactis orikufera, 151
Epiboly, 127, 133
Epicauta, 153
Epicrine glands, 419
Epidermis, 64, 116, 373, 375
Epididymis, 75
Epigamy, 43
Epimorphic development, 156
Epimorphosis, 177
Epinephrine, 362
Epiparasitism, 466
Epiphytism, 469
Episodes, 85, 86, 94
Epistylis anastatica, 218
Epitheloid membrane, 373
Epitheliomuscular cells, 406
Epithelium, 239, 334, 421
Epitoke, 42, 77, 113, 155, 160, 250—252
Epitoky, 20, 37, 39, 42—43, 77, 155, 165
Epizoic, 478
Epizoism, 469
Equilibration, 343
Equilibrium, 348
Erichthus larva, 146

Ersea, 493
Erythrocytes, 224, 226, 231
Estivation, 173
Ethology, 429
Eudoxids, 113, 252, 493
Eudoxome, 493
Eudoxy, 40
Euglena gracilis, 269
Euglenoid movement, 436
Eumetazoa, 509
Eumitosis, 227
Ephausiid, 146, 449
Euplotes, 218
Eutely, 170—173
Evagination, 135
Evasion, 439
Evisceration, 444
Evolution, 22, 195, 224, 504
Exconjugants, 105
Excretion, 371
    adults, 327—340
    brown body, 332, 334
    brown funnels, 334
    chloragogen tissue, 334—335
    ciliated funnels, 333
    ciliated urns, 333, 336—337
    coxal glands, 331, 335
    diversity, 329, 337—338
    elimination distinguished, 328
    excretory pores, 337
    flame-cell system, 329—331, 335
    glomerular kidneys, 332
    glomerulus, 333—335
    lateral canal system, 332, 335
    liver, 332, 335
    Malpighian tubules, 331—332, 335
    mechanisms, 338—340
    mycetocytes, 333, 336
    nephridial kidney, 331, 336
    nephridium, 331, 336
    nephrocytes, 333, 336
    nephron kidneys, 332
    organs, see also specific types, 329—337
    pathways, 340
    protonephridia, 329, 336
    renettes, 332—333, 336
    solenocytes, 330—331, 336
    stomach epithelium, 334
    substances, 340
    urns, 333, 336—337
Excretophores, 335
Excretory organs, see Excretion
Excretory pores, 337
Exochorion, 71, 120
Exocrine glands, 455
Exogamy, 49, 106
Exolecithal, 289
Exoskeleton, 373, 392, 411, 414
Exovation, 140
Exploitation, 457—458, 460—477
    body parts, use of, 472

camouflage, 471
care of nonfeeding individuals, 473
care of offspring, 473—477
food, see also Food, 460—468
labor, use of, 469—471
man's purposes, 473
products, use of, 472
purpose, 460
shelter, 469
transplanted organelles, use of, 472—473
transport, 471—472
Exploited captives, 470—471
Expulsion, 257, 261—262
External gills, 310
External tube, 411
Extinct groups, 4, 508
Eyes, 346
Eye-spots, 346

F

Falcons, 461
Fanworms, 313, 316, 321
Fat, storage, 421
Fat body, 421
Feathers, 253, 378, 383, 392, 472
Fecampiidae, 278
Fecundation, 54
Feeding, see Food
Females, 96, 98—99, 160
Ferrets, 471
Fertilization, 32, 46—47, 52—59, 82, 84, 113
clonal, 47—48, 54—55, 88, 90—92
external, 56
fraternal, 54—55, 90—92
insemination, 56—57
internal, 56
ova, 68
polar body, 54—55, 59, 83
site of, 56
somatic, 32, 103, 106
spermatozoon migration, 57—58
spermatozoon transfer, 56—57
Fertilization membrane, 58, 71, 120
Fibrinogen, 284
Fibroin, 190, 383
Filarial worms, 474
Filter chambers, 285, 287
Filter-feeding, 272—273, 460
Final host, 478
Fin-rays, 393
Fireflies, 447—449, 454—455
Fish, see also specific types, 284
control of, 465
ectoparasitism, 466
electroreceptors, 351
entrapment of food, 434
feeding, 273
flotation, 445
flying, 437, 439

gills, 321
lateral line system, 390, 392
lungs, 318
lymph system, 300
mormyomasts, 231
nephron kidneys, 332
noxious secretions, 418
orientation, 431
parasitism, 464
poison organs, 418
sex determination, 103
stimuli, reception of, 344
teeth, 281
viviparity, 475, 476
yolk sac, 477
Fish-stealing birds, 468
Fission, 11, 28, 34, 38—39, 104, 498
Fissiparity, 40
Flagella, 217—221
Flagellar movement, 406
Flagellated chambers, 386
Flame bulb, 330—331
Flame cell, 231, 329—330, 335
Flatworms, 19, 249, 329, 406, 472
Flies, see also specific types, 156, 268, 466, 472, 475, 480
Floating, 228
Flotation, 444—445
Flukes, 465, 480
Flustra, 491
Flying, 436—437
Foetus, 112, 136
Follicular gestation, 475
Food, see also specific topics, 267—273
capture, 432—433
cleptobiosis, 468
competition for, 459
cultivation, 461—462
drinking, 435
ectoparasitism, 466—468
entrapment, 432, 434
exploitation for, see also other subtopics hereunder, 460—468
feeding, 267, 269—273, 282, 430
gleaning, 468
ingestion, 267
micropredation, 463
movement, 286
nutrition types, 269—273
parasitism, 464—466
plant-feeding, 463—464
predation, 462—463
provision of, 433—434
stealing, 468
storage, 422, 434—435
tools, 434
types, 267—269
utilization of, 266—267
Foraging, 464
Foraminifera, 205, 210, 211, 222, 223
Foregut, 279

Fossils, 507
Fossorial phyla, 441
Fowls, 471
Foxes, 471
Fragmentation, 11, 18, 22—23, 34, 38, 113, 443—444, 498
Fragments, 29—30, 113
Fraternal fertilization, see Fertilization
Free-living nematode, 309
Free martin, 207
Frog-hoppers, 288
Frogs, 286, 475
Frondose colony, 493
Frustulation, 20, 39—40, 113, 162
Frustules, 113, 252
Fucilia larva, 146
Function vs. structure, 183—192
Fungi, 461
Fungia, 491
Funnel, 253, 333, 334
Fur, 472
Fusion, 18, 58, 103—104, 498—499
Fusion nucleus, 59

G

Gall formation, 469
Gall makers, 464
Gall midges, 440
Gall wasps, 24, 440
Galvanotaxis, 430
Galvanotropism, 430
Gametes, 22, 27, 29—30, 38, 46—47, 49—50, 52—53, 61—72, 232, 251
    haploid, 47
    sponges, 116
    tissue source, 65
    types, 64
Gametocyte, 104
Gametogamy, 55
Gametogenesis, 46—47, 49, 51, 107, 113, 224
Gametogony, 35
Gametophores, 61, 76—79, 250, 252
Gametophyte, 164
Gamogenesis, 48
Gamogony, 35, 49—50, 55, 104
Gamones, 361
Gamont, 52, 55, 104, 160
Gamontogamy, 55
Ganglia, 356—357
Gastric caeca, 283
Gastric glands, 283—284
Gastric mill, 282
Gastrin, 362
Gastroblasts, 490
Gastrocoel, 399
Gastrodermis, 63, 277—278
Gastrodes, 151
Gastropoda, 77
Gastrotricha, 511—512

asexual processes, 20
blood pigments, 324
body openings, 256
body wall muscle layers, 242
cilia, 219—220
circulatory systems, 302
excretory devices, 337
flagella, 220
integument features, 375
message systems, 366
morphological features, 197
muscle striation, 408
reproduction, 28, 90, 97
respiration, 312, 325
setae, 375
spermatozoa ducts, 254, 255
tissue products, 246
Gastrovascular cavity (GVC), 266, 275, 277—278, 400
Gastrozooids, 207, 277, 494
Gastrula, 112, 126—134, 136
Gastrulation, 113, 117—118, 127—128
Gaur, 471
Gemmation, 41
Gemmiparity, 37
Gemmulation, 20—21, 23, 28, 35, 113, 173
Gemmules, 11, 20, 29—30, 34—35, 43—44, 113, 162, 173, 251
    detached, 252
    sponges, 116
Genetics, 22
Genetic sex determination, 103
Genome, 105, 224, 498—499
Genotypes, identical, 32
Genotypic sex determination, 103
Geographical polymorphism, 206
Geophilus carpophagus, 449
Geotaxis, 430
Geotropism, 430
Germarium, 62
Germ balls, 44, 94, 135, 139, 157, 238
Germ band, 136
Germ cell line, 107—108
Germ cells, 49, 108
Germ layers, 118, 127—128, 135
Germovitellarium, 75
Germplasm, 107, 139, 237, 239
Gerontology, 177
Gestation, 475—476
Giant fibers, 355
Giant grasses, 470
Gills, see also specific types, 276, 282, 287, 310, 315—317, 320—322
Giraffes, 419
Gizzard, 282
Glands, 378, 419—420
    antennal, 334
    associated, 76
    blood circulation, 301
    Cowper's, 76
    coxal, 331, 335

digestive, 283—284
endocrine, 362—363
exocrine, 455
green, 334
labial, 284
mandibular, 284
Mehlis', 76
moniliform, 387
nidamental, 71, 120
oesophageal, 284
oviducal, 71
pharyngeal, 284
proboscis, 336
prostate, 76
rectal, 287
repugnatorial, 455
salivary, 284
shell, 76
thymus, 304
yolk, 75
Glass-fish, 154
Gleaning, 461, 468
Glia, 240, 353
Glochidium larva, 146
Glomerular kidneys, 332
Glomerulus, 332—335
Glossina, 284
Glossobalanus minutus, 449
Glow worms, 449
Glucagon, 362
Glycogen, 421
Glycolysis, 191, 214
Gnathostomuloidea, 511
    asexual processes, 20
    blastopore fate, 130
    cilia, 220
    circulatory systems, 302
    flagella, 220
    respiratory mechanisms, 325
    sexual reproduction and sexuality, 97
Goats, 469, 470
Golfingia, 153
Gonactinia, 205
Gonadotrophins, 362
Gonads, 46—47, 61—64, 74, 77, 102
Gonangia, 114, 207, 473
Gonium, 490
Gonochorism, 28, 54, 96, 98—101
Gonocoel, 400
Gonoducts, 56, 73—74
Gonomery, 47, 49, 55, 83
Gonophores, 41, 61—62, 76—77, 155, 202, 476
    detached, 252
    multiple, 42
    polymorphism, 207
Gonopore, 73—74
Gonozooid, 207, 494
Gonyaulax, 448
Gordioidea, 512
    asexual processes, 20
    blood pigments, 324

body openings, 256
body wall muscle layers, 242
cilia, 220
circulatory systems, 302
excretory devices, 337
flagella, 220
integument features, 375
message systems, 366
molting, 167—168
morphological features, 196—197
muscle striation, 408
reproduction, 28, 90, 97
respiration, 312, 325
setae, 376
spermatozoa ducts, 254, 255
tissue products, 246
Gorgonia, 491
Gorgonin, 190
Gotte's larva, 146
Grantia, 117, 448
Granular clubs, 231, 278
Granulocyte, 405
Graptolitoidea, 490
Graptozoa, 189, 380, 509—510
Grasping, 435—436
Grasshoppers, 287, 465
Gravireceptors, 349
Gravity, 349, 431
Grazing, 464
Green gland, 335
Gregaloid colony, 493
Gregaloidy, 487
Gregarine protozoans, 218
Gregarinida, 205, 487
Growth, 112, 169—171
Grub larva, 146
Guanine, 222, 340
Guests, 457, 460, 469
Guinea pigs, 471
Gullet, 277, 282
Gustatory organs, 347
Gut, 266
Gymnospores, 34
Gymnostomata, 262
Gynandromorph, 11, 100, 222
Gynandromorphism, 101—102
Gynandromorphy, 96
Gynoecism, 100
Gynoecy, 100
Gynogenesis, 83, 103
Gyrocotyle, 152, 375
Gyrodactylus, 491

H

Habitats, 430, 440—443
Haemal system, 297
Haemerythrin, 323—324
Haemocoel, 64, 137, 296, 399—400, 403
Haemocyanin, 323—324

Haemocytoblast, 405
Haemoglobin, 323—324
Haemolymph, 296, 299, 304, 322
Haemoparasitism, 466
Haemovanadin, 323
Hagfish, 446
Hair, 253, 378, 383, 392, 472
Hair plates, 350
Hair sensillum, 348, 350
Haliclystus, 37
Halistauri, 448
Halteres, 349
Hamsters, 471
Hancock's organ, 347, 349
Haplodiploidy, 103
Haploid ova, 29
Haplomitosis, 227
Haplosis, 51
Haplozoon, 490
Haptocysts, 261
Harboring symbionts, 273
Hard parts, 279—384
Harmothoe, 211
    adventor, 468
Hatching, 140
Hearing, 343
Heart, 303—304, 410—411
Heat, 343
Hectocotyl, 251, 252
Hectocotylized arm, 57
Hectocotylus, 77
Hectocotyly, 77
Helicoplacoidea, 516
Heliocidaris, 154
Heliotropism, 430
Heliozoa, 211, 223, 261
Hemicellulose, 190
Hemichordata, 516
Hemimetabolous, 150
Hemimixis, 31, 106, 499
Hemiptera, 410
Hemiteles biannulatus, 466
Hemixis, 31
Hepatic caeca, 283
Hepatopancreas, 284
Herbivorous, 271
Herding, 469
Hermaphrodite, 11, 98—99, 160
Hermaphroditic, 101
Hermaphroditic gland, 61—62
Hermaphroditic organs, 61
Hermaphroditism, 28, 96, 99, 101—102
Hermit crabs, 465, 468, 471
Herpyllobiidae, 207
Heterandra formosa, 76
Heterochely, 177
Heterodontus, 211
Heterogamy, 49, 95, 106, 209
Heterogenesis, 95
Heterogenomic specimens, 104
Heterogony, 95

Heterokinesis, 103
Heteromorphic, 209
Heteromorphosis, 177
Heterophil, 405
Heteropolar polarity, 200
Heterozooid, 493
Heterozygote, 121
Hexacanth larva, 146
Hexacontium, 211
Hibernacula, 20, 30, 35, 173, 252
Hibernation, 173
Hindgut, 279
Hirudinea, 78
Histiocyte, 405
Histioteuthis bonelleii, 449
Histogenesis, 134
Histozoic, 466
Histriodrilus, 268
Holocrine glands, 419
Hologamete, 49, 52, 58, 62, 64, 72
Hologamy, 19, 49—50, 55, 59, 72, 104—106
Holometabola, 153
Holometabolous, 150
Holometabolous Insecta, 132
Holophytic, 271
Holothurioidea, 333, 391, 411
Holozoic, 271
Homalozoa, 515
Homing, 431
Homo sapiens, 4—5
    adults, 160
    artificial insemination, 57
    asexual processes, 25
    camouflage, 440
    cannibalism, 499
    competition for shelter, 459
    cooperation, 458
    cultivation of food, 461
    death, 498
    detached organs, 251
    domestication of animals, 470
    exploitation, 471—473
    flotation in air, 444
    food types, 268
    foster parents, 469
    germ cell sources, 108
    gerontology, 177
    locomotion, 437
    multiple-segment sequences, 93
    oxygen-carrying pigments, 323
    predator, 462
    sex determination, 103
    slavery, 471
    stimuli, reception of, 345
    storage of food, 434
    storage organs, 420
    varying span of individuals between reproductive
        occurrence, 87
Homoeosis, 150, 177
Homoeostasis, 422
Homolecithal, 289

Homopolar polarity, 200
Homoptera, 285, 333, 339, 475
Homozygote, 121
Honey, 272, 461
Honeybee, 65, 103, 217, 284
Honey guides, 268
Hookworms, 467
Hooves, 378, 383, 392
Hormones, 61, 76, 295, 360—365
Horns, 378, 392, 419
Horseflies, 433
Horsehair worms, 465, 467
Horses, 461, 469, 470, 472
Horseshoe crabs, 433
Host, see also specific types, 465, 467, 477—479
Host modification, 440
Houseflies, 466
Human orientation, 5—6
Humans, see *Homo sapiens*
Hyalosporina cambolopsisae, 58
Hybocodon, 490
Hybridization, 54
Hydatid cysts, 37
Hydra, 9—10, 19, 36—37
    cnidocils, 217
    development, 163
    digestive tract, 274
    exploitation, 472
    gullet, 277
    multiple-segment sequences, 89
    nematocysts, 417
    neurosecretions, 365
    storage organs, 421
    symmetry, 195
Hydranths, 65, 114, 207
Hydrocaulus, 493
Hydroids, 471
Hydropore, 129, 132
Hydrostatic movement, 405—406
Hydrostatic pressure, 412
Hydrozoa, 189
Hymenoptera, 39, 147, 275, 492
Hyolithelminthes, 512
Hypergamesis, 267, 290
Hypermastigina, 205
Hypermetamorphic Insecta, 147
Hypermetamorphosis, 115, 145, 148, 151, 155, 161
Hyperparasite, 466, 480
Hyperparasitism, 480
Hyperpredators, 480
Hypertrophy, compensatory, 177
Hypnozygote, 121
Hypochord, 416
Hypodermic impregnation, 68
Hypodermis, 373
Hypogenesis, 33, 95
Hypopharyngeal compound sense organ, 347
Hypophysis, 362

Hypostome, 276

I

Ichneumon fly, 466
Ichthyophthirius, 34
Identical twins, 39
Identification, 447
Ileum, 283
Illumination, 447
Imaginal discs, 132, 161, 238
Imagines, 155
Imago, 155, 160
Imbrication, 211
Implantation, organs, 456
Impregnation, 54, 68
Impulses and their transmission, 355
Inanition, 173
Inarticulata, 402
Inbreeding, 47—48, 54
Incubation, 476
Individuality, 9—11
Individuals, see also specific topics, 31, 250
    activities of, 427—451
    adults, 181—423
    asexual reproduction, 32—44
    attachment, 445—446
    autotomy, 443—444
    bioluminescence, 446—450
    bisexual reproduction, 45—80
    chains of, 41
    defined, 9
    development, 109—179
    end of existence, 498—499
    flotation, 444—445
    food, 432—435
    grasping, 435—436
    habitats, 440—443
    locomotion, 436—439
    origin of, see also other subtopics hereunder,
        13—108
    parthenogenesis, 81—85
    prehension, 435—436
    protection, 439—440
    reproduction, 15—32
    response, 429—432
    sequences of reproductive cycles, 85—96
    sexuality, 96—104
    structure, 188
    thermogenesis, 450
    treatment as, 11
Infra-buccal chamber, 280
Infusorigen larva, 146
Ingestion, 286, 371
Ingression, 128, 133
Ink sacs, 417—418
Inner ear, 392
Inquilinism, 469
Insecta, 71, 78, 120, 410
Insectivorous, 271
Insemination, 47, 53—54, 56—57, 82
Instar, 154, 169
Insulin, 362
Integuments
    adults, 369—384

bristles, 374—376
containment, 370—371
defined, 373
diversity, 372—373
functions, 370—372
hard parts, 379—384
histology, 374—378
invertebrates, 372—378
protection, 371
protozoa, coverings of, 372
setae, 374—378
skin of vertebrates, 378
spines, 374—376
support, 371
Interactions of animals, see also specific topics, 4,
        453—481
    communication, 454—455
    forms, 458
    reproductive behavior, 480
    symbiosis, 456—480
Intercalary host, 478
Intercellular spaces, 295—296
Interface, 309, 320
Intermediate host, 478
Intermedin, 362
Intermolt, 169
Interneurons, 356
Intersexes, 11, 100
Intersexuality, 96, 101—102
Intertentacular organ, 74
Intestinal gland, 335
Intestinal tract, see also Digestive tract, 266, 275,
        278—288
Intestine, 266, 278, 280, 283, 288—289
Intima, 388
Intussusception, 266
Invagination, 127, 129
Inversion, 117—118, 135, 157
Invertase, 284
Invertebrates, 5
Investion, 267
Involution, 128, 133
Inwandering, 133
Iodopsin, 346
Iridocytes, 222
Isaria, 288
Islets of Langerhans, 362
Isogametes, 49, 51, 58, 62, 64—66
Isogamety, 96
Isogamonty, 55, 105
Isogamy, 49
Isolecithal, 289
Isopod, 268, 431
Isopoda, 153, 310—311, 315, 321, 480
Isopolar polarity, 200
Isoptera, 492
Isotropy, 69
Ivory, 472
Ixodes, 275

J

Jackal, 459, 468, 477
Janthina, 445
Jaws, 281, 435
Jejunum, 283
Jellyfish, 5, 472
Jet-propulsion, 436, 438, 492
Johnston's organs, 348, 349
Jointed appendages, 435
Jumping, 436—437
Juvenile, 112, 144, 155

K

Kalymmocytes, 290
Karyogamy, see also Fertilization, 9, 28—29, 48,
        50, 52—55, 59, 82, 84
Keber's organ, 335
Kenozooids, 65, 207, 494
Kentrogen larva, 146
Keratin, 190, 383
Kerkring, valves of, 289
Kidney, 335
Kinaesthesis, 348
Kinetocysts, 261
Kinetopause, 173
Kinorhyncha, 512
    asexual processes, 20
    blood pigments, 324
    body openings, 256
    body wall muscle layers, 242
    cilia, 220
    circulatory systems, 302
    excretory devices, 337
    flagella, 220
    integument features, 375
    message systems, 366
    molting, 167
    morphological features, 196—197
    muscle striation, 408
    reproduction, 28, 90, 97
    respiration, 312, 325
    setae, 375
    spermatozoa ducts, 254, 255
    tissue products, 246
Klinotaxis, 431
Knight-Darwin Law, 55
Krebs citric acid cycle, 191, 214
Kupffer cells, 225, 405

L

Labial glands, 284, 335
Labor, use of, 469—471
Labyrinths, 348—349
Lacinularia, 491
Lacteals, 300
Lafoea, 490

Lamprey larva, 146
Lamp shell, 198
Lampyridae, 449
Lancelets, cephalization, 201
Lantern fish, 450
Larva, see also specific types, 39, 71, 94, 112
    definition, 144—145, 154
    development to adult, 143—158
    diporpa, 104
    direct development, 144
    dispersal, 148
    fate, 148
    function, 147—148
    fusion, 106
    indirect development, 144
    metamorphosis, see also Metamorphosis, 144,
        148—157
    neoteny, 157
    paedogenesis, 157
    penetration, 148
    reproduction of, 157
    tissues, 237—238
    types, 145—147
Larvacea, 168
Larviparity, 141, 473, 475—476
Larynx, 318, 320
Lasso cells, 211
Lateral canal system, 332, 335
Lateral line system, 390, 392
Latia neritoides, 449
Leaf-cutting ants, 461, 469
Leaf-miners, 464
Leather, 472
Lecathylus, 492
Lecudina tuzetae, 218
Leeches, 156, 176, 284
Lepidocystioidea, 516
Lepidoptera, 492
    cellulose, 189
    detection of airborne chemicals, 347
    larva, 146
    light production, 449
    poison organs, 418
    setae, functions of, 378
    viviparity, 475
Leptocephalus larva, 146
Leptodora, 156
Lernaeopodidae, 269
Leucons, 386
Leucosolenia, 117
Leukocytes, 225, 335, 405
Life cycles, 94, 113—114, 149, 159—179
    adult stage, 160—161
    change of form, 163
    composite, 165—166
    dormancy, 173—174
    eutely, 170—173
    growth, 169—171
    life history, 161—164
    metagenesis, 164—165
    molting, 166—169

    normal features, 161
    parasite, 479—480
    regeneration, 175—177
    senescence, 177—178
    uncontaminated, 48
Life history, 114, 161—164
Ligaments, 393
Light, 345—346, 351, 446—447
Light emissions, 455
Limivorous, 271
Limpet, 449
Linckia, 40, 161, 176
Lineus, 24, 25, 152
    sanguineus, 48
Lingula, 152, 189
Lions, 459
Lipoid membrane, 71
Lithocysts, 349
Lithostyles, 349
Live birth, 140
Liver, 284, 332, 335, 421
Lizards, 318, 418, 419, 443, 475, 477
Llamas, 471
Lobster, spiny, 212
Lobster eggs, 268
Locomotion, see also Movement, 228, 430, 436—
    439
Loligo, 417
Looping, 436
Lophomonas blattarum, 174
Lophophorata, 512
Lorica, 168, 223, 373, 413
Loxosoma, 152
Lumbricidae, 156
Lumbriculus, 33, 48
Luminescence, see Bioluminescence
Luminodermus sequoiae, 449
Lunar orientation, 431
Lungs, 311, 314, 317—318, 320
Lycaenid butterflies, 461
Lycophore larva, 146
Lymphatic system, 299—301, 304
Lymphoblasts, 301
Lymphocytes, 301, 335, 405
Lyriform organs, 350

M

Machopolyp, 494
Macrocilia, 218
Macrogametes, 64
Macrophage, 335, 405
Macrotrichia, 378
Macula, 350
Madreporite, 390—391
Maggot larva, 146
Male, 57, 96, 98, 160, 207
Mallophaga, 467
Malpighian tubules, 287, 331—332, 335
Mammals, storage organs, 420

Man, see *Homo sapiens*
Mandibular glands, 284
Man-made animals, 470
Mantispidae, 155
Mantle, 320, 374
Mantle lungs, 317
Manubrium, 276
Marsupials, 475
Marsupium, 75, 474, 476
Masking crabs, 462
Mastax, 281
Mates, competition for, 459
Mathevioidea, 513
Mating types, 56, 98—99
Matricin, 190, 383
Maturation, 113
Maxillary gland, 335
Mechanoreception, 348—351
Medialecithal, 289
Medusa bell, 410
Medusae, 39, 114, 160, 207
Medusoid, 493
Megalecithal, 289
Megalops larva, 147
Megalosphere, 165
Meganyctiphanes norvegica, 449
Meiosis, 29, 32—33, 38, 46—47, 50—52, 69, 105
Meiotic parthenogenesis, 28
Meissner's corpuscle, 349
Melampus, 152
Meliphagy, 272
Meloidae, 147, 155
Meloidogyne, 51, 119
Membrane, see specific type
Membranelle, 218—219, 438
Membranous labyrinth, 392
Menotaxis, 430
Meristem, 43
Mermis, 469
Mermithization, 440, 469
Merocrine glands, 419
Merogony, 34, 38, 106
Merozoites, 34, 38, 147
Mesenchyme, 63, 64, 239
Mesencoel, 401
Mesoblast, 237
Mesocestoides, 152
Mesoderm, 132—134, 237
Mesogloea, 117, 239
Mesolecithal, 289
Mesomitosis, 227
Mesonephros, 332, 335
Mesothelium, 137
Mesozoa, 509
  asexual processes, 20
  blastopore fate, 130
  blood pigments, 324
  body wall muscle layers, 242
  cilia, 220
  circulatory systems, 302
  embryology, 116

  excretory devices, 337
  flagella, 220
  integument features, 375
  message systems, 366
  morphological features, 196—197
  reproduction, 28, 90, 97
  respiration, 312, 325
  tissue products, 246
Metabolism, 191—192, 266
Metabolous, 150
Metacercaria larva, 147
Metagenesis, 95, 164—165, 209
Metamere, 204
Metamerism, 201—205
Metamitosis, 227
Metamorphosis, see also specific topics, 42, 135, 139, 144, 148—157, 164
Metanauplius larva, 147
Metanephridium, 331, 336
Metanephros, 332, 336
Metatrochophore, 153
Metazoa, 19, 147, 274—275, 509
Metecdysis, 169
Miastor, 172
Mica flakes, 372
Mice, 471
Micrococcus, 288
Microfilariae, 152
Microgametes, 64
Microhabitat, 440
Microlecithal, 289
Microorganisms, 469
Microphagous, 271
Micropredation, 271, 460, 463
Micropredators, 458, 462—463
Micropyles, 71, 119—120, 200
Microsphere, 165
Microsporidia, 480
Microtrichia, 378
Microtubules, 353
Microvili, 51
Midgut, 279
Migration, 438—439
  cell, 296—297
Milk, 461, 476
Millepora, 490
Mimicry, 440
Minks, 471
Miolecithal, 289
Miracidium larva, 147
Mites, 467, 472
Mithan, 471
Mitosis, 38, 46, 51, 224, 226—228
Mitraria larva, 147
Mixis, 31, 33, 48
Mixocoel, 403
Mnemiopsis leidyi, 448
Molecules, 4, 188
Moles, 434
Mollusca, 6, 513
  asexual processes, 20

blastopore fate, 130
blood pigments, 324
body openings, 256
body wall muscle layers, 242
chitin, 189
cilia, 220
circulatory systems, 302—303
colonies, 491—492
excretory devices, 337
flagella, 220
hard part constituents, 381
integument features, 375
luminescence, 449
message systems, 367
morphological features, 196—197
muscle phosphagens, 409
muscle striation, 408
pumping organs, 410
regeneration, 175
reproduction, 28, 91, 97
respiration, 313, 325
spermatozoa ducts, 254, 255
tissue products, 246
Molt, 169
Molting, 156, 166—169
Monastrea, 10
Moniliform glands, 387
Monkey, 285
Monoblastozoa, 509
asexual processes, 20
body wall muscle layers, 242
cilia, 220
flagella, 220
reproductive sequences, 90
tissue products, 246
Monocyte, 405
Monoecism, 61, 100
Monogenea, 466
Monogenesis, 33
Monogenetic, 95
Monogony, 33
Monopodial colony, 493
Monospermy, 56
Monosymmetry, 198
Monotomy, 38
Monotremes, 475
Monsters, 112
Moribund, 178
Mormyomasts, 231, 351
Morphallaxis, 177
Morphogenesis, 134—135
Morphogenetic cell movements, 118
Morphogenetic movements, 134
Morphology, 188
adults, 193—212
body arrangement, see also Body arrangement,
200—210
symmetry, see also Symmetry, 194—200
Morula, 122, 136
Mosquitoes, 433
Moth, 461

Motility, cells, 228—229
Mouflon, 470
Mouth, 117, 253, 275—276, 280
Mouthparts, 433
Movement, see also Locomotion, 228, 229, 250—
251, 286, 295—297, 348, 403—410, 436,
437
Mucocysts, 262
Mucopolysaccharides, 190
Mueller's larva, 147
Muggiaea, 490, 492
Mules, 461, 470
Muller's organ, 348
Multicellular individual, 11
Multicellularity, 8—9, 30
Multiple fission, 38—39
Musca, 403
Muscles, 240, 242—243, 350, 375, 406—410, 421
Muskrats, 471
Mussel, 472
Mutations, 32
Mutualism, 457, 478
Mycetocytes, 333, 336
Mycetophilid fly, 449
Mycetozoa, 104, 214, 216, 488
Myctophum, 450
Myelin sheath, 353
Myiasis, 466
Myochordotonal organs, 350
Myoglobin, 323
Myohaemerythrin, 323
Myonemes, 406
Myrmecophagous, 271
Myrmecophily, 478
Mysis, 147, 310, 315
Myxamoebae, 104, 216
Myxine, 154
Myxomycetes, 488, 490
Myzostomida, 514
asexual processes, 20
blood pigments, 324
body openings, 256
body wall muscle layers, 242
cilia, 220
circulatory systems, 302
excretory devices, 338
flagella, 220
hard part constituents, 381
integument features, 375
message systems, 367
morphological features, 196—197
muscle striation, 408
reproduction, 28, 91, 97
respiration, 313, 325
setae, 376
spermatophores, 77
spermatozoa ducts, 254, 255
tissue products, 246

N

Naiad, 154
Nails, 378, 383, 392
Nannozooecium, 494
Nannozooids, 65, 207, 494
Naphthoquinone, 323
Nares, 253, 276, 318, 320
Narwhal, 419
Nauplius, 147, 351
Nautilus, 445
Necrophagy, 271, 272
Nectochaeta, 147, 153
Nectonema, 376
Nectophores, 207, 410, 494
Nectosome, 493
Needham's sac, 77, 421
Nematocysts, 51, 71, 79, 223, 230, 417, 435, 472
Nematocyte, 417
Nematoda, 469, 512
    asexual processes, 20
    blastopore fate, 130
    blood pigments, 324
    body openings, 256
    body wall muscle layers, 242
    chitin, 189
    cilia, 220
    circulatory systems, 302
    climbing, 439
    egg coverings, 71
    excretory devices, 337
    flagella, 220
    host modification, 440
    integument features, 375
    message systems, 366
    molting, 167
    morphological features, 196—197
    muscle striation, 408
    reproduction, 28, 90, 97
    respiration, 312, 325
    setae, 376
    spermatozoa ducts, 254, 255
    tissue products, 246
    zygote covering, 120
Nematodinium, 223
Nematomenia banyulensis, 152
Nematophore, 494
Nematozooid, 494
Nemerteans, 19, 360
Neocoel, 399
Neoteny, 107, 148, 157
Nephridial kidney, 331, 336
Nephridiopore, 331
Nephridium, 331, 336
Nephrocytes, 226, 231, 333, 336
Nephromixium, 331
Nephron, 336
Nephron kidneys, 332
Nephrophagocytes, 225
Nephrostome, 331

Nereis, 468
Nerves, 351, 353—356, 358—359
Nervous system
    adults, 341—368
    brain, 356—358
    centralized, 352
    circum-enteric rings, 359
    conducting devices, 351
    ganglia, 356—357
    nerve cords, 358—359
    nerve nets, 351
    neurons, 352—354
Nestlings, 154
Neural plate, 135
Neural tube, 132
Neurite, 353
Neuroglia, 240, 353
Neurohormones, 361, 365
Neurohumors, 361, 365
Neurohypophysis, 362
Neuromasts, 390, 392
Neuronemertea aurantiaca, 356
Neurons, 352—354
Neuropile, 354
Neuroptera, 275, 288
Neurosecretions, 365—366
Neurosecretory granules, 353
Neurosensory cells, 345
Neurotoxin, 284
Neurotubules, 353
Neurula, 135—136
Neuters, 96, 99—101, 160
Neutrophil, 405
Nidamental gland, 120
Nissl substance, 353
Nitrogenous wastes, circulation, 295
Nociceptors, 348
Noctiluca, 448
    miliaris, 37
Noctuid moth, 288
Node of Ranvier, 354
Nonagria, 288
Noncellular, 8
Noradrenalin, 362
Norepinephrine, 362
Nostrils, 318, 320
Notila proteus, 106
Notochord, 135, 393, 411, 415—416
Notophthalmus, 154
Nourishment, protozoan, 273—274
Nuclear constancy, 172
Nuclear reorganization, 31, 96, 104—106
Nucleus, cells, 221
Nucula, 205
Nuda, 277
Nudibranchiata, 310
Nudibranchs, 316, 320, 449
Nurse cell, 52, 61, 69, 75, 103, 116, 119
Nutria, 471
Nutrients, circulation, 295
Nutriments for ovum and zygote, 289—290
Nutrition, 266—273

Nutritional organs, 75
Nymph, 154

O

Obelia, 23, 25, 36, 87, 95, 114, 165, 448
  gelatinosa, 194
Oceania, 448
Ocelli, 346
Octopus, 77, 252, 284
Odontostyle, 281—282
Oenocytes, 231
Oesophageal glands, 284
Oesophagus, 282
Offspring, exploitation for care of, 473—477
Oikopleura, 449
Olenus, 153
Olfactory organs, 347
Oligochaeta, 77—78
Oligomery, 203—204
Oligopod larva, 147
Omnivorous, 271
Oncomiracidium larva, 147
Oncosphere larva, 147
Oniscus, 317
Onuphin, 190
Onychophora, 514
  asexual processes, 20
  blastopore fate, 130
  blood pigments, 324
  body openings, 256
  body wall muscle layers, 242
  chitin, 189
  cilia, 220
  circulatory systems, 302—303
  excretory devices, 338
  flagella, 220
  hard part constituents, 381
  integument features, 375
  message systems, 367
  molting, 168
  morphological features, 196—197
  muscle striation, 408
  pumping organs, 410
  reproduction, 28, 91, 97
  respiration, 313, 325
  setae, 376
  spermatophores, 78
  spermatozoa ducts, 254, 255
  tissue products, 246
Oocyst, 121
Oocytes, 51, 53, 104
Ooecium, 474, 476
Oogenesis, 49, 51
Oogonia, 49, 62
Ookinete, 60, 121
Oophores, 79
Ootheca, 70, 476
Ootid, 51
Oozooids, 65, 494

Opalinid, 39
Opalinida, 505
Operculum, 71, 120
Ophiactis, 40
Ophiopluteus larva, 147
Ophiuroidea, 391
Ophrydium, 490
Ophryoscolecin, 190
Opiliones, 319
Opisthobranchiata, 199
Opisthorchis, 467
Optic gland, 363
Oral cavity, 280—281
Oral pore, 276
Oral stylets, 433
Organ of Bojanus, 336
Organelles, 188, 217, 416
Organismal concept, 428
Organismic viewpoint, 5
Organisms, 7—17
  cellularity, 7—9
  individuality, 9—12
  polymorphism, 12
  protozoa as animals, 7
Organogeny, 134
Organs, see also specific topics
  adults, 247—254
  asexual, 43—44
  auditory, 348
  blood circulation, 301—304
  body openings, see also specific types, 253
  body spaces, 399—403
  cavities, 399
  coelenteron, 277
  defense, 416—419
  definitions, 248
  detached, 251—253
  excretory, 329—337
  functions, 251
  gastrovascular cavity, 278
  gustatory, 347
  implantation, 456
  intestinal tract, 279—284
  locomotion, 436
  luminescent, 447—448
  lymph, 300—301
  miscellaneous, 397—423
  movement of, 250—251, 403—410
  olfactory, 347
  organ systems, compared, 249
  osmoregulation, 422—423
  pumping, 410—411
  reception, 343
  respiration, 309—311
  respiratory, 314—323
  secretory, 419—420
  sponges, 116—117
  storage, 420—422
  structure, 188
  supporting structures, 411—416
  tactile, 348—349

tissues compared, 248—249
transplants, 57, 253, 456
unicellular, 249—251
unique, 253
Organ systems, see also specific types, 250
  adults, 254—263
  alimentation, 257—258
  control, 257, 262—263
  definition, 254
  demanian system, 386—387
  enclosure, 257, 263
  expulsion, 257, 261—262
  functions, 257—263
  lateral line system, 390, 392
  organs compared, 249
  respiration, 257, 260—261
  skeletal system, 392—394
  spongiocoel, 386
  tracheal system, 387—389
  translocation, 257—260
  transport devices, 258—259
  tube systems, 259—260
  unique, 385—395
  water-vascular system, 389—391
Origin of individuals, see also Individuals, 13—108
Origin of cells, 216
Orthoptera, 475
Osculum, 74, 386
Osmoregulation, 422—423
Osphradium, 347
Ossicles, 383, 411
Ostia, 253, 386
Ostracodermi, 504
Ostrich, 119
Otocysts, 349
Outbreeding, 22, 54—55
Ova, see also Egg, 11, 19, 23, 30, 51—52, 62, 64,
       68—69
  amictic, 72
  diploid, 72
  diversity of, 69
  dormant, 72
  haploid, 29, 72
  isotropic, 72
  mictic, 72
  motility, 70
  nutriments for, 289—290
  penetration of, 58
  polymorphism of, 69—70
  terms, 72
  types, 72
  yolk, 70
Ovarian balls, 62, 421
Ovarian epithelium, 76
Ovarian gestation, 475
Ovary, 61—62, 116
Ovejector, 253
Ovicell, 474, 476, 493
Oviduct, 73—74
Oviparity, 140, 144, 476
Oviparous, 140, 476

Ovisac, 76
Ovotestis, 62, 99, 101
Ovoviviparity, 140—141, 144, 473, 474, 476
Ovoviviparous, 141, 476
Ovum, see Ova
Oxen, 461
Oxygen, 295, 308
Oxygen-carrying pigments, 323
Oyster, 471
Ozobranchus, 310

P

Pacinian corpuscles, 349
Paedogamy, 55, 106—107
Paedogenesis, 40, 107, 157
Pain, 343
Palintomy, 38
Palinurus, 212
Palpigradi, 310
Palpocils, 230
Palpon, 494
Palps or palpi, 349
Pangolin, 378
Panorpa, 487
Pantopoda, 156
Papulum, 321
Parabiosis, 469
Parabronchi, 321
Parachords, 416
Paraclone, 33
Paragastrula, 127
Paraglycogen, 190
Parahormones, 361
Paramecium, 24, 236, 417
  bursaria, 106
Paramitosis, 228
Paranephridial plexus, 336
Parapodium, 321, 410
Para-reproduction, 19
Para-reproductive processes, 104—106
Parasite, 438, 464—465, 479—480
Parasitic barnacle, 465
Parasitic control, 430, 465
Parasitic copepods, 145
Parasitic Crustacea, 274
Parasitic Hymenoptera, 24, 115, 139, 153
Parasitic insects, 115, 435
Parasitic males, 456
Parasitic nematodes, 474
Parasitic wasp, 434, 471
Parasitism, 464—466, 479
Parasitoid, 463
Parasitoidism, 461
Parasitology, 479—480
Paratenic host, 478
Parathormone, 362
Parathyroid gland, 362
Paratomy, 20—21, 29, 36—37, 39—40, 43
Parenchyma, 239

Parenchymula, 127, 147
Parental care, 430
Parthenogenesis, 18, 22, 28, 47—48, 81—85, 87—
    —93, 96
Parthenogenetic paedogenesis, 157
Parthenospore, 85
Partial constancy, 172
Parturition, 140
Pathogenicity, 464
Paurometabolous, 150
Pauropoda, 78
Pearl, 245, 472
Pecten, 367
Pectinatella, 491
Pectines, 253
Pedal disc, 44
Pedal laceration, 20, 39—40, 113
Pedicellariae, 253, 418
Pedicellina, 152, 491
Pelagia noctiluca, 448
Pelicans, 461
Pellicle, 223, 372
Pelomyxa palustris, 269
Penetration, 148
Pennatula, 491
Pentacrinoid larva, 147
Pentastomoidea, 514
    asexual processes, 20
    blood pigments, 324
    chitin, 189
    cilia, 220
    circulatory systems, 302
    excretory devices, 338
    flagella, 220
    hard part constituents, 381
    integument features, 375
    message systems, 367
    molting, 168
    morphological features, 196—197
    muscle striation, 408
    reproduction, 28, 91, 97
    respiration, 313, 325
    tissue products, 246
Pentidotea resecata, 431
Peranema trichophorum, 269
Periblast implantation, 75
Periblastula, 126, 133
Pericardial cavity, 401
Pericardial cells, 336
Periderm, 245, 373—374
Perikaryon, 354
Peripheral nerve systems, 352
Perisarc, 245, 373—374
Peristomial gills, 310, 321
Perithelium, 240
Peritoneal cavity, 401
Peritoneum, 137
Peritrich Ciliata, 217
Peritrophic membrane, 282

Periviseral cavity, 401
Perophora, 421
Petrobius, 73
Petromyzon, 154
Pexicysts, 262
Phaceloid colony, 493
Phagocata, 278
Phagocytes, 225, 301, 336, 405
Phagocytosis, 224—225, 272—274
Phagotrophy, 272
Phalangida, 387
Pharotaxis, 430
Pharyngeal gills, 310, 321
Pharyngeal glands, 284
Pharyngotremy, 282, 287, 316, 321
Pharynx, 277, 281—282, 321
Phengodidae, 449
Pheromones, 76, 361
Philine, 282
Phlebotomus, 410
Pholas, 447
    dactylus, 449
Phonoreceptors, 348
Phoresis, 472
Phoresy, 456, 472
Phoretic, 472
Phorocyte, 35, 123, 226, 230, 258—259
Phoronida, 512
    asexual processes, 20
    blastopore fate, 130
    blood pigments, 324
    body openings, 256
    body wall muscle layers, 242
    chitin, 189
    cilia, 220
    circulation, 297—298, 302—303
    colonies, 491
    excretory devices, 337
    flagella, 220
    hard part constituents, 380
    integument features, 375
    message systems, 367
    morphological features, 196—197
    muscle striation, 408
    regeneration, 175
    reproduction, 28, 90, 97
    respiration, 313, 325
    spermatozoa ducts, 254, 255
    tissue products, 246
Phorozooid, 494
Phosphagens, 409—410
Phosphoarginine, 409
Phosphocreatine, 409
Phosphoglycocyamine, 409
Phosphohypotaurocyamine, 409
Phospholombricine, 409
Phosphoopeline, 409
Phosphorescence, 447
Phosphorylation, 191
Phosphotaurocyamine, 409
Photoblepharon, 450

Photocytes, 447—448
Photogenesis, 446—447
Photogenic, 447—448
Photo-horotaxis, 430
Photophores, 447, 455
Photoreception, 345—346
Photosynthesis, 271, 273
Photosynthetic algae, 269
Phototaxis, 430
Phototropism, 430
Phyllirhoe bucephala, 449
Phyllopoda, 173
Phyllosoma, 147
Phyllozooids, 207
Phylogeny, 195, 409
Physalia, 10, 488, 490
Physogastry, 460
Phytoflagellate, 217
Phytohormones, 361
Phytomastigina, 223, 269
Phytomonadina, 115, 164
Phytophagous, 271, 464
Pigs, 470
Pilidium larva, 147
Pilot fish, 468, 477
Pinacocytes, 230
Pinnaglobin, 323
Pinnipedia, 272
Pinnules, 222, 231
Pinocytosis, 225, 272—274
Piroplasmea, 505
Piscicolidae, 316
Piscivorous, 271
Placentae, 75, 290, 473—476
Placentation, 141, 461, 473, 476
Placodea, 347
Placozoa, 509
Pladinium larva, 147
Planctosphaeroidea, 516
Plankton-feeding, 460
Plankton-filtering, 272
Plant-feeding, 272, 461, 463—464
Plant-parasitic nematodes, 440
Planula, 37, 39, 147
Plasmalemma, 372
Plasma membrane, 71, 372
Plasmodium, 7, 10—11, 104, 106, 121, 488
  vivax, 25
Plasmogamy, 83
Plasmogony, 22, 49, 83
Plasmotomy, 39
Plastogamy, 106
Plastron, 312, 321, 383
Plate organs, 217
Platyhelminthes, 511
  asexual processes, 20
  blastopore fate, 130
  blood pigments, 324
  body openings, 256
  body wall muscle layer, 242
  cilia, 220

circulatory systems, 302
colonies, 491
egg coverings, 71
excretory devices, 337
flagella, 220
hard part constituents, 380
message systems, 366
morphological features, 196—197
muscle phosphagens, 409
muscle striation, 408
reproduction, 28, 90, 97
respiration, 312, 325
setae, 375
spermatozoa ducts, 254, 255
tissue products, 246
Plecoptera, 195
Pleopod, 321
Plerocercoid larva, 147
Pleural cavity, 401
Pleurobranchia, 212
Plumatella, 10, 152
  fungosa, 37
Pluteus larva, 147
Pneumatophore, 207, 494
Pneumostome, 317, 321
Podia, 253, 389, 391, 435
Podochela hemphilli, 462
Podocysts, 20, 30, 35, 173, 252
Poecilogeny, 208—210
Pogonophora, 515
  asexual processes, 21
  blastopore fate, 130
  blood pigments, 324
  body openings, 256
  body wall muscle layers, 242
  chitin, 189
  cilia, 220
  circulation, 298, 302—303
  excretory devices, 338
  flagella, 220
  hard part constituents, 381
  integument features, 375
  message systems, 367
  morphological features, 196—197
  muscle striation, 408
  pumping organs, 410
  reproduction, 28, 91, 97
  respiratory mechanisms, 325
  setae, 376
  spermatozoa ducts, 254, 255
  tissue products, 246
Poison organs, 418
Polar bodies, 51, 54—55, 59, 83, 103
Polarity, 119, 200
Polian vesicle, 390—391
Pollard, 207
Pollen-feeding, 272
Polychaeta, 42, 77, 377, 410
Polyembryony, 11, 20—22, 24, 37, 39—41, 43,
  47, 55, 60, 90—92, 94, 121, 162, 168—
  169, 498

successional, 24, 41, 107, 148, 152, 157
twinning, 25
Polyenergid masses, 7
Polyisomere, 204
Polykrikos, 223
Polymegaly, 68
Polymorphism, 12, 67—70, 206—210
Polynoe, 474
Polyp, 39, 41, 114, 160
Polypheism, 208
Polyphenism, 210
Polyp-medusa, 165
Polypod larva, 147
Polypodium hydriforme, 118
Polypoid, 493
Polyspermy, 56, 58
Polystomium, 275—276
Polytrocha, 153
Polytrochula larva, 147
Pore cells, 116
Pore plates, 347
Porifera, 509
asexual processes, 20
blastopore fate, 130
blood pigments, 324
body openings, 256
body wall muscle layers, 242
chitin, 189
cilia, 220
circulatory systems, 302
colonies, 490
epidermis, 116
excretory devices, 337
flagella, 220
hard part constituents, 380
integument features, 375
luminescence, 448
message systems, 366
morphological features, 196—197
muscle phosphagens, 409
muscle striation, 408
pumping organs, 410
regeneration, 175
reproduction, 28, 97
respiration, 312, 325
spermatozoa ducts, 254, 255
tissue products, 245
Porocytes, 230, 258, 386
Porphyropsin, 346
Porpita, 332, 339, 490, 511
Porpoises, 461
Portuguease man-o'-war, 195
Postembryonic stages, 154—155
Posterior pituitary, 362
Postlarvae, 104
Praying mantises, 68
Predation, 271, 456, 460, 462—463, 498—499
Prehension, 435—436
Pre-oral ciliary organ, 347
Prey, 271—272
Priapuloidea, 512

asexual processes, 20
blood pigments, 324
body openings, 256
body wall muscle layers, 242
chitin, 189
cilia, 220
circulatory systems, 302
excretory devices, 337
flagella, 220
integument features, 375
message systems, 366
molting, 168
morphological features, 196—197
muscle striation, 408
reproduction, 28, 90, 97
respiration, 312, 325
setae, 376
spermatozoa ducts, 254, 255
tissue products, 246
Proboscis, 277, 284—285, 435
Proboscis gland, 336
Procercoid larva, 147
Procerodes lobata, 205
Procotyla, 10
Proctodaeum, 135, 137, 290
Proctostome, 74, 275—277, 314
Proecdysis, 169
Progenesis, 83
Progesterone, 362
Proglottids, 11, 41—42, 79, 156, 204, 251, 252
Prolactin, 362
Promitosis, 228
Promorphology, 198
Pronephros, 332, 336
Pronghorns, 419
Pronucleus, 53, 59, 105
Proprioception, 348—350
Prosobranch, 269
Protamoeba primitiva, 39
Protandrous organs, 61
Protandry, 55, 98, 101—102
Protaspis larva, 147
Protease, 284
Protection, 371, 372, 439—440
Prothoracic glands, 363
Prothrombin, 284
Protochordata, 516
Protoconch larva, 147
Protodrilidae, 77
Protogenesis, 36
Protogynous organs, 61
Protogyny, 55, 99, 101—102
Protonephridia, 329, 336
Protonychophora, 514
Protoplasm, 214—215
Protopterus, 154
Protostomatous, 129, 137
Protostome, 129
Protozoa, 7, 508—509
asexual processes, 20
cell functions, 229

cellularity of, 8—9
chitin, 189
cilia, 220
classifications of, 506
colonies, 490
coverings of, 372
diversity, 7
excretory devices, 337
flagella, 220
hard part constituents, 380
luminescence, 448
message systems, 366
nourishment, features of, 273—274
organelles for, 44
pumping organs, 410
reproduction, 28, 90, 97
respiration, 312, 325
tissue products, 245
Protrochula larva, 147
Protura, 156, 205, 319, 387
Proventriculus, 282
Przewalski horses, 470
Psammon, 210
Pseudochitin, 190
Pseudocoel, 64, 137, 399—401
Pseudocoelocytes, 231, 405
Pseudocoelomata, 511
Pseudocolony, 492—493
Pseudo-eggs, 20, 34, 39—40
Pseudogamy, 22, 47, 49, 83—84
Pseudohermaphroditism, 102
Pseudometamerism, 201—202, 204
Pseudoparasitism, 466
Pseudophyllidea, 152
Pseudoplacenta, 475, 476
Pseudopodia, 123, 405, 435
Pseudotrachea, 317, 321
Pseudova, 30, 47, 52, 64, 68, 71—72, 84
Pseudozooea larva, 147
Pterobranchia, 516
    asexual processes, 21
    blastopore fate, 130
    blood pigments, 324
    body openings, 256
    body wall muscle layers, 243
    cilia, 220
    circulatory systems, 302
    colonies, 492
    excretory devices, 338
    flagella, 220
    hard part constituents, 381
    integument features, 375
    message systems, 367
    morphological features, 196—197
    muscle striation, 408
    regeneration, 176
    reproduction, 28, 92, 97
    respiration, 314, 325
    spermatozoa ducts, 254, 255
    tissue products, 246
Ptychoderidae, 449

Pulmonary sac, 317
Pulmonata, 152
Pumping organs, 410—411
Pupa, 112, 115, 154, 156, 161
Puparium, 156
Pupation, 155—156, 174
Pupiparity, 141, 475—476
Pygochord, 416
Pyloric caeca, 283
Pyramidellidae, 267
Pyrophorus, 449
Pyrosoma, 10, 154, 449, 492

Q

Quinqueradiate, 198

R

Rabbits, 268, 471
Racquet organs, 253
Radial canals, 276, 390
Radiata, 510
Radiolaria, 205, 211, 223, 379, 412, 487
Radioles, 310, 321
Radiophrya, 490
Radula, 281, 433
Railletiella, 205
Rats, 471
Rattles, 455
Recapitulation theory, 178
Receptaculitida, 509
Receptaculum seminis, 75
Rectal bladder, 283
Rectal diverticula, 283
Rectal gill, 321
Rectal glands, 287
Rectal respiratory tree, 287, 314
Rectum, 283
Redia, 147, 157
Reduction bodies, 11, 30, 35, 174
Regeneration, 118, 135, 161—162, 175—177, 443
Regionation, 196, 205—206
Regression, 175
Regurgitation, 287, 473
Reindeer, 461, 469, 471
Remora, 468
Renettes, 231, 332—333, 336
Renilla, 243, 491
Renin, 362
Repetition, 201—206
Replacement principle, 18
Replication of molecules, 18
Reproduction, see also specific topics, 162
    adults only, 23
    ameiotic parthenogenesis, 28
    amphimixis, 29, 31—32
    animal, 15—32
    apomixis, 31—32

asexual, see also Asexual reproduction, 27—28, 32—44
bisexual, 26—27
body forms, 23
colonies, 494—495
conjugation, 27
definitions, 18—19
development vs., 23—26
diversity in, 15, 22—23, 28—29, 47
fragments, all new individuals from, 29—30
gametes, 27
larva, 157
meiotic parthenogenesis, 28
misconceptions, 19, 22—27
parameters, 27—31
process, 30
sexual, 27
simplicity of, 22—23
universality, 19
Reproductive behavior, 480
Reproductive bodies, 22—23, 29, 30, 47
Reproductive cycle, 87—89, 93—96
Reproductive openings, 253
Reproductive organs, see also specific organs, 60
    primary, 61—72
    secondary, 72—76
Reptiles, 318, 332, 378, 437, 477
Repugnatorial glands, 455
Reservoir host, 479
Resilin, 190
Resorption, 112, 135, 171
Respiration, see also specific topics, 257, 260—261, 371
    adults, 307—326
    aerobic, 308, 320
    air-breathing, 311—312
    anaerobic, 308, 320
    anoxybiotic, 320
    associated functions, 323—324
    carbon dioxide, 308
    cutaneous, 309, 320
    diversity of organs, 314—315
    energy release, 308
    exchange devices, 312—314
    fermentative, 308
    gills, 315—317, 320—322
    integumentary, 309, 320
    lungs, 317—318
    mechanisms, 309—314
    organs, 309—311, 314—323
    oxidative, 308
    oxybiotic, 320
    oxygen, 308
    oxygen-carrying pigments, 323
    pneustic, 321
    respiratory fluids, 322—323
    tracheae, 318—319
Respiratory horns, 312
Respiratory openings, 253
Respiratory trees, 311, 319, 321
Resting buds, 30, 35

Resting stage, 115
Reticulin, 190
Retinal, 346
Retrogression, 156—157
Retrogressive reproduction, 144
Rhabditis, 98
Rhabdopleura, 154, 211, 492
Rhagoletis cerasi, 414
Rhaphidiophrys, 490
Rheoreceptors, 350—351
Rheotaxis, 430
Rheotropism, 430
Rhinoceros, 419
Rhinophores, 347
Rhodopsin, 346
Rhopalia, 349
Rhorocyte, 75
Rhynchocoela, 132, 400, 511
    asexual processes, 20
    blastopore fate, 130
    blood pigments, 324
    body openings, 256
    body wall muscle layers, 242
    cilia, 220
    circulation, 297, 302—303
    egg coverings, 71
    excretory devices, 337
    flagella, 220
    hard part constituents, 380
    integument features, 375
    luminescence, 448
    message systems, 366
    morphological features, 196—197
    muscle phosphagens, 409
    muscle striation, 408
    pumping organs, 410
    regeneration, 175
    reproduction, 28, 90, 97
    respiration, 312, 325
    spermatozoa ducts, 254, 255
    tissue products, 246
    zygote covering, 120
Ricinulei, 319, 387
Rind, 357
Ring canal, 276, 390—391
Roaches, 475
Rosettes, 336, 386
Rostral canals, 392
Rotifera, 511
    asexual processes, 20
    blastopore fate, 130
    blood pigments, 324
    body openings, 256
    body wall muscle layers, 242
    cilia, 219—220
    circulatory systems, 302
    colonies, 491
    egg coverings, 71
    excretory devices, 337
    flagella, 220
    germ cell line, 107

integument features, 375
larva, 152
message systems, 366
morphological features, 196—197
muscle striation, 408
regeneration, 175
reproduction, 28, 90, 97
respiration, 312, 325
setae, 375
sex determination, 103
spermatophores, 77
spermatozoa ducts, 254, 255
tissue products, 246
zygote covering, 120
Royal jelly, 284
Ruminants, 419
Running, 436—437

S

Sabre-tooths, 419
Sacciform colony, 493
Sacoglossa, 268, 316
Saccoglossus horsti, 154
Sagartia, 104
Salamanders, 78, 107, 475
Salinella salve, 244, 509
Salivary glands, 284, 363
Salivary pump, 284, 410
Salt, storage, 421
Saprophagy, 271, 272
Saprotrophy, 272
Saprozoic, 271
Sapsucking, 272
Scale insects, 275, 433, 475
Scales, 378, 392—393
Scallops, 407
Scavenging, 272
Schizocoel, 132, 137, 138, 401—403
Schizogamy, 43
Schizogenesis, 36, 38
Schizogony, 34, 38, 40
Schizometamery, 40, 43, 175—176
Schizont, 34, 38, 51
Schizopod larva, 147
Schwann cell, 354
Scissiparity, 36, 40
Sclerasterias, 40
Sclerites, 414
Scleroblasts, 225, 230
Sclerotin, 190, 414
Scolex, 42
Scoli, 378
Scolioplanes crassipes, 449
Scolopale organs, 217
Scolophire, 348
Scolopophorous organ, 348
Scorpionida, 253, 355
Scutigera, 317
Scyphistoma, 39, 41, 147, 486

Scyphozoa, 189
Sea anemones, 273, 469, 471
Sea cucumbers, 176
Sea otters, 434
Seasonal polymorphism, 206, 208
Secondary reproductive organs, see also specific organs, 72—76
Secretin, 362
Secretory organs, see also Glands, 419—420
Seed feeders, 464
Segmentation, 85, 196, 201—205
Selachian, 450
Self-fertilization, 22, 47—48, 53—55, 59, 88, 90—92, 102
Sematophore, 57
Semicircular canals, 349, 392
Seminal vesicle, 75
Semiplacenta, 476
Senescence, 112, 177—178, 498
Senility, 178
Sense clubs, 349
Sense receptors, see also specific types, 344—351, 430
Senses, see also specific types, 342—344
Sensilla basiconica, 347, 351
Sensilla chaetica, 347
Sensillum, 345
Sensory cells, 345
Sensory cones, 350
Sensory hairs, 349
Sensory nerve cells, 345
Sensory nerve endings, 345
Sensory pits, 347
Sepia, 417
Sergestidae, 156
Sericin, 190
Serrule, 378
Sessile animals, 145
Setae, 222, 246, 374—378
Sex, 96, 99, 100, 102
Sex characters, 62
Sex chromosomes, 96, 102—103
Sex determination, 102—103
Sex differences, 98
Sex distribution and change, 100—102
Sex reversal, 96, 101—102
Sexuality, 19, 22, 96—104
Sexual polymorphism, 206—207
Sexual reproductive processes, see also Reproduction; specific terms, 18, 27, 49—60, 494
Shark, 477, 499
Shedding, 169
Sheep, 469, 470
Shells, see also specific types, 223, 374, 383, 411, 413, 472
Shelter, 459, 469
Shrews, 434
Shrikes, 434
Shrimps, 438
Siamese twins, 488
Siblings, 54

Siculozooid, 494
Siebold's organ, 348
Signalling, 430, 447
Silk, 245, 284
Silkworm, 222
Sinuses, 303
Siphonaptera, 467
Siphonophores, 252, 490, 492—494
Siphonosome, 493
Siphonozooids, 65, 494
Siphons, 253, 286—287, 321
Siphon tube, 287
Siphonula, 494
Sipunculoid, 285
Sipunculoidea, 513
    asexual processes, 20
    blastopore fate, 130
    blood pigments, 324
    body openings, 256
    body wall muscle layers, 242
    cilia, 220
    circulatory systems, 302
    excretory devices, 337
    flagella, 220
    hard part constituents, 381
    integument features, 375
    message systems, 367
    morphological features, 196—197
    muscle phosphagens, 409
    muscle striation, 408
    reproduction, 28, 91, 97
    respiration, 313, 325
    setae, 376
    spermatozoa ducts, 254, 255
    tissue products, 246
Skeletal system, 392—394, 411—415
Skin, 378
Skunks, 418
Slavery, 430, 456, 469, 471
Sleep, 174
Slime molds, 214
Slit sensillum, 348, 350
Slugs, 268
Smell, 343
Snails, 199, 445, 462, 471
Snakes, 418, 475, 477
Social behavior, 430
Social insects, 206, 492
Social parasitism, 471
Social polymorphism, 206—208
Societies, 430, 459
Soil-filtering, 272
Solenia, 276, 493
Solenocyte, 218, 231, 330—331, 336
Solpugida, 253, 319, 357, 387
Somatic skeleton, 393
Somatoplasm, 107, 237
Somatotrophin, 362
Somersaulting, 436—437
Somites, 135, 204
Sorites, 20, 30, 35, 113, 173, 252

Sound, detection of, 348
Sperm, 67, 68
Spermary, 62
Spermatheca, 75
Spermatocyte, 53
Spermatogenesis, 49
Spermatophores, 11, 57—58, 61, 67, 73, 77—78
Spermatozoa, 11, 30, 52—53, 61, 62, 64, 66—68
    migration, 57—58
    transfer, 56—57
Sperm ducts, 56, 73
Sperm-entry point, 119, 200
Spermiducal vesicle, 75
Sperm sacs, 75
Sphaeridia, 349
Sphaeriidae, 152
Spheroid colony, 493
Spicules, 71, 222, 224—225, 246, 379, 411—412
Spiculin, 190
Spiders, 211, 434—435, 437, 444
Spinal cord, 359
Spinax niger, 450
Spines, 246, 374—376, 378, 435
Spirachles, 314
Spiracles, 319, 321, 388
Spiracular gills, 310, 321
Spiralling, 289
Spiral valve, 279, 283, 289
Spitting organs, 418
Splanchnocoel, 399
Spleen, 304, 421
Sponge canals, 386
Sponges, 11, 19, 35, 258—259, 440
    cephalization, 201
    chambers, 386
    coloniality, 490
    division, 495
    embryology, 116—118
    inversion, 117—118
    number of basic tissue layers, 244
    organs, 116—117
    phagocytosis, 272
    reconstitution, 238
    regeneration, 175
    spicules, 225, 372
    tissues, 116—117
Spongin, 190, 383
Spongiocoel, 386, 400—401
Spore-feeding, 272
Spores, 22, 29—30, 34—35, 37, 38, 64
Sporocyst, 147, 157
Sporogony, 34—35
Sporont, 121
Sporophyte, 164
Sporosacs, 77, 250, 252
Sporozoites, 34, 38, 147
Spurs, 378
Squids, 252, 449
Squirrels, 433, 434, 437, 459
Starfish, 9, 176, 195, 280, 421
Star orientation, 431

Static organs, 349
Statoblasts, 11, 20, 30, 35, 43—44, 113, 173, 251, 252
Statocysts, 349
Statoreceptors, 349
Staurocoryne, 205
Steatocyte, 405
Steer, 462
Stenostomum, 491
Stereoblastula, 126, 133
Stereogastrula, 122, 127
Stiff cilia, 350
Stigmata, 319, 321
Stimuli, detection of, 342—351
    response to, 429—430
    sense receptors, 344—351
    senses, 342—344
Stolonization, 20—21, 37
Stolons, 41—42, 61, 94, 492, 493
Stomach, 282—283, 286, 334
Stomach pouches, 283
Stomata, 300—301
Stomatopoda, 146—147, 310
Stomias, 450
Stomoblastula, 126
Stomochord, 415—416
Stomodaeum, 135, 137, 290
Storage, food, 434—435
Storage organs, 75—76, 420—422
Stratum subcutaneum, 378
Strepsiptera, 63, 147, 153, 155, 272
Stridulating, 455
Strobilae, 41, 65, 493
Strobilation, 11, 20—21, 23, 37, 41—43, 113, 156, 201—202, 204, 486
Strobilus, 41
Stromatoporoidea, 510
Structure vs. function, 183—192
Sturgeon, 118
Style sac, 283
Stylets, 246, 281—282
Stylopid, 153
Subgenual organ, 348
Substellar organs, 350
Successional polyembryony, see Polyembryony
Suckling, 473
Suctoria, 505
Suicide, 498
Sun-compass, 431
Supporting structures, 411—416
Suspended animation, 174
Suspension-feeding, 272
Swarmers, 34, 36, 145, 151
Swim-bladder, 317, 321
Swimming, 436, 438
Swimming bell, 494
Swine, 469
Sycon, 117, 386
Syllis ramosa, 492
Symbiosis, see also specific topics, 430, 456—480
    commensalism, 477—478

    competition, 459
    cooperation, 459
    definitions, 456—458
    exploitation, 460—477
    host, see also specific types, 478—479
    mutualism, 478
    parasitology, 479—480
Symbranchus marmoratus, 310, 317
Symmetry, 194—200
Symparasitism, 466
Symphiles, 469
Symphyla, 78
Sympodial colony, 493
Synapses, 49, 353, 355—357
Synchronogamy, 101—102
Syncytial tissue, 7
Syncytium, 7
Synechthrans, 469
Synergids, 58, 224
Syngamy, 53, 58—59, 82
Syngony, 101
Synkaryon, 58—59, 105—106
Synoeketes, 469, 478
Syntomy, 39
Syringopora, 491
Syzygy, 41, 104, 106, 201—202, 486—488, 494

T

Tachyblaston ephelotensis, 36, 39
Tactile organs, 348—349
Tadpoles, 147, 154
Taenia, 467, 491
Taenidium, 319
Taenioidea, 152
Tagmata, 205
Tagmosis, 205
Tails, 436
Taming, 469
Tangoreceptors, 348—349
Tapeworms, 9, 36, 41, 79, 201—202, 204—205, 245, 433, 480
Tardigrada, 514
    asexual processes, 20
    blood pigments, 324
    body openings, 256
    body wall muscle layers, 242
    cilia, 220
    circulatory systems, 302
    excretory devices, 338
    flagella, 220
    hard part constituents, 381
    integument features, 375
    message systems, 367
    molting, 168
    morphological features, 196—197
    muscle striation, 408
    reproduction, 28, 91, 97
    respiration, 313, 325
    setae, 376

spermatozoa ducts, 254, 255
tissue products, 246
Taste, 343
Taste buds, 347
Taxis, 430
Tecnophagy, 272
Tectin, 190
Teeth, 281, 383, 393—394, 433
Tegmentum, 383
Tegument, 374
Teleosts, 392, 450
Teloblasts, 132—133, 139
Telolecithal, 290
Telotaxis, 431
Temnocephaloidea, 375
Temperature control, 295, 371—372
Tentacles, 435
Tentaculata, 276
Tentaculocysts, 349
Tentaculozooid, 494
Tentilla, 494
Tenuis larva, 147
Terebratulina, 152
Teredo, 268
Termites, 99, 107, 208, 433—435, 440, 443, 461,
    462, 469
Terrarium reptiles, 471
Terricolous phyla, 441
Territory, competition for, 459
Tertiary embryo, 10
Testacea, 223
Testacida, 190
Testis, 57, 62, 73, 252
Tetrad, 51
Tetrapods, 393
Tetrathyridium larva, 147
Thanatosis, 174
Theca, 136, 223, 374, 379, 411, 413
Thelytoky, 83
Thermogenesis, 450
Thermotaxis, 430
Thermotropism, 430
Thesocytes, 230
Thigmocytes, 231
Thigmotaxis, 430
Thigmotropism, 430
Thoracic ducts, 301
Thrips, 475
Thrixion, 466
Thymosin, 362
Thymus gland, 304, 362
Thyroid gland, 362
Thyrotrophin, 362
Thyroxine, 362
Tiedemann's bodies, 390—391
Tiger, 499
Tintinnida, 223
Tissues, see also specific types, 188, 236—250,
    406—407
Titusvillia, 490
Toads, 475

Tokophrya lemnarum, 474
Tomiparity, 38
Tongue, 281, 436
Tooth, see Teeth
Topogenesis, 134
Tornaria larva, 147
Torpidity, 174
Torpor, 174
Torsion, 135, 155, 199
Touch, 343, 348, 349
Toxicysts, 262
Trachea, 259, 314, 318—319, 322, 387—389
Tracheal gills, 310, 315, 322, 388
Tracheal lung, 317
Tracheoles, 222, 314, 318—319, 322, 388—389
Translocation, see also Circulatory system, 257—
    260, 404
Transparency, 212
Transplanted organelles, 472—473
Transplantation, 102, 456
Transport, see also Circulation; Movement, 258—
    259, 439, 471—472, 479
Trap for food, 432, 434
Trematoda, 375
Trematobdellidae, 276
Trephocyte, 405
Trichinella, 474
Trichocysts, 223, 262, 416—417, 435
Trichonympha, 218, 268
Trichoptera larva, 146
Trichosomoides, 57
Trilobites, 156
Triploblastic, 117
Triungulin larva, 147
Trochophore, 145, 147
Trophallaxis, 461, 473
Trophamnion, 476
Trophic membrane, 476
Trophobiosis, 462, 478
Trophoblast, 136, 237, 474, 476
Trophonemata, 475—476
Trophotaeniae, 475, 477
Trophozoite, 51, 55
Tropism, 430
Tropotaxis, 431
Trunks, 285
Trypanosoma, 33, 51, 439
Tube-feet, 389, 391
Tubes, 413—414
Tube systems, 259—260
Tubificids, 77
Tuft sensilla, 350
Tunic, 374, 411, 413
Tunicata, 517
    asexual processes, 21
    blastopore fate, 131
    blood pigments, 324
    body openings, 256
    body wall muscle layers, 243
    cilia, 220
    circulatory systems, 302—303

colonies, 492
excretory devices, 338
flagella, 220
hard part constituents, 381
integument features, 375
luminescence, 449
message systems, 368
morphological features, 196—197
muscle phosphagens, 409
muscle striation, 408
regeneration, 176
reproduction, 28, 92, 97
respiration, 314, 325
spermatozoa ducts, 254, 255
tissue products, 246
Tunicin, 190, 383
Turbellaria, 77, 175, 189, 375, 472
Turgor, 295, 411—412
Turkeys, 471
Turtles, 68, 318, 418
Tusks, 419
Twinning, 10—11, 25, 41, 121
Tympana, 455
Tympanal organs, 348
Typhlosole, 243, 283, 289, 420

U

Ultraviolet light, 345
Ultraviolet receptors, 346
Uncinni, 378
Undulating membrane, 218—219, 438
Ungulates, 469
Unicellular, 8—9
Unionidae, 152
Uniparous, 51
Unisexual, 100
Urea, 340
Urechis, 289
Ureotelic animals, 340
Ureter, 332
Uric acid, 340
Uricotelic animals, 340
Urnatella, 491
Urns, 250, 252, 333, 336—337
Urogastrone, 362
Uterine bell, 74
Uterine gestation, 475
Uterine milk, 475, 477
Uterus, 73—74

V

Vagina, 73—74
Valves, 301
Vas deferens, 56, 73
Vas efferens, 73
Vater's corpuscle, 348
Veins, 303

Velella, 10, 332, 339, 490, 510
Veliger larva, 147
Velums, 218
Vertebrata, 5, 517
asexual processes, 21
blastopore fate, 131
blood pigments, 324
body openings, 256
body wall muscle layers, 243
cilia, 220
circulation, 298, 302—303
egg coverings, 71
excretory devices, 338
flagella, 220
hard part constituents, 381
integument features, 375
luminescence, 450
message systems, 368
molting, 168
morphological features, 196—197
muscle phosphagens, 409
muscle striation, 408
pumping organs, 411
regeneration, 176
reproduction, 28, 60—61, 92, 97
respiration, 314, 325
skeletal system, 392—394
spermatozoa ducts, 254, 255
tissue products, 246
zygote covering, 120
Vexillifer larva, 147
Vibracula, 65, 207, 473, 494
Villi, 289
Visceral skeleton, 393
Vision, 343
Visual pigments, 346
Vitellarium, 75
Vitelline cells, 75
Vitelline membrane, 71
Viviparity, 118, 140—141, 144, 473, 475, 477
Vocal cords, 455
Vocalization, 455
Volvox, 10, 118, 487—488, 490, 492, 494—495
globator, 269
Vorticella, 472
Vorticellidae, 211

W

Walking, 436—437
Warble flies, 466
Warning coloration, 440
Wasps, 47, 208, 268, 468, 471, 475
Water, storage, 422
Water-borne chemicals, 347
Water buffalo, 471
Water channels, 136, 259
Waterfowl, 471
Water-vascular system, 389—391
Wax, 287

Whalebone, 280, 383
Whales, 280
Wild boar, 470
Wing, 253
Winter rigidity, 174
Wolves, 470, 499
Wood-borers, 464
Woodpeckers, 434
Worms, see specific types

X

Xenoparasitism, 466
Xylophilous, 464

Y

Yak, 471
Yolk, 70, 119, 289—290, 473, 477
Yolk cells, 71, 75, 121
Yolk glands, 75
Yolk sac, 71, 477
Y-organ, 363

Z

Zebu, 470

Zeppelina, 24, 33
   monostyla, 48
Zoarium, 493
Zona pellucida, 70
Zona radiata, 71
Zonite, 204
Zoochlorellae, 222
Zooea larva, 147
Zooecium, 373—374, 411, 413, 493
Zoogamy, 46
Zooids, 42, 65, 160, 493
Zoophagous, 271
Zoospores, 37
Zoosuccivorous, 271
Zoothamnion, 490
Zooxanthellae, 222
Zygogenesis, 48
Zygote, 11, 19, 23, 34, 39, 46, 51—52, 55, 59—
      60, 62, 68, 71—72, 104, 112, 118—123,
      232
   composite, 106
   nucleus, 58
   nutriments for, 289—290
   yolk food, 69
Zygotophores, 76, 79